Susanne A. Quallich, PhD, ANP-BC, NP-C, CUNP, FAANP, holds both an academic and a clinical appointment at the University of Michigan. Dr. Quallich is Clinical Adjunct Faculty at the University of Michigan School of Nursing, where she teaches primarily men's health and urology to BSN and MSN/DNP students. Her clinical appointment is within the Division of Andrology and Urologic Health, Department of Urology at Michigan Medicine, the Hospital of University of Michigan, where her patient case load includes independent evaluation and management of male patients with sexual and reproductive function concerns and independent evaluation, management, and teaching of chronic male genital pain patients. Dr. Quallich has been PI or co-PI on numerous research projects and has published more than 30 peer-reviewed journal articles in journals such as ***The Journal for NPs, Urologic Nursing, Journal of Advanced Nursing, American Journal of Men's Health, and Urologic Clinics of North America.*** She has published more than 30 books and chapters including Goolsby/Grubbs, *Advanced Assessment* (Davis) on the genitourinary system, multiple chapters in Black/Hawks, *Medical-Surgical Nursing* (Saunders/Elsevier, 2008), and several chapters in Stanley/Veith/Wakefield (eds), *Current Therapy in Vascular and Endovascular Surgery* related to postsurgical neurogenic impotence and drug therapy for erectile dysfunction (Elsevier, 2014). She recently coedited *The Nurse Practitioner in Urology* (Springer). She has been instrumental in defining the role of the nurse practitioner (NP) in urology and in developing a framework of competencies by which NPs can progress toward an expert urology NP role. Dr. Quallich has won numerous awards, including the ***Sigma Theta Tau, Rho Chapter*** Award for *Excellence in Nursing Practice* for 2018. She was inducted as a Fellow in the American Association of Nurse Practitioners based on her work in advancing men's health knowledge among NPs and advancing the specialty urology NP role.

Michelle Lajiness, MSN, FNP-BC, is a Urology Nurse Practitioner at The University of Toledo Medical College in Toledo, Ohio. She has been Master's prepared for over 28 years and has over 18 years of experience as an NP in urology. She co-edited *The Nurse Practitioner in Urology*, the only urology book published for nurse practitioners. She has published several articles and book chapters on urology topics and is a frequent invited speaker at the local, national, and international levels.

Kenneth A. Mitchell, MPAS, PA-C, is a certified physician assistant with over 22 years of clinical experience overall and over 20 years of experience in male erectile and sexual dysfunction. He actively promotes men's health and has participated in community outreach programs to educate men about sexual health. He has lectured both nationally and internationally on the subject of men's health and sexual dysfunction. Kenneth received his master's in physician assistant studies from the University of Nebraska Physician Assistant Program. He is a Fellow of the American Academy of Physician Assistants (AAPA), the Urological Association of Physician Assistants (UAPA), member of the Sexual Medicine Society of North America, Chair of the AUA APN/PA Membership Committee, Past President of UAPA, Past Chair of the Sexual Medicine Society of North America APN/PA Affairs Committee, and board member at-large of the American Society of Men's Health (ASMH).

Manual of Men's Health
A Practice Guide for APRNs and PAs

Editor

Susanne A. Quallich, PhD, ANP-BC, NP-C, CUNP, FAANP

Section Editors

Michelle Lajiness, MSN, FNP-BC

Kenneth A. Mitchell, MPAS, PA-C

SPRINGER PUBLISHING COMPANY

Springer Publishing Company, LLC
11 West 42nd Street
New York, NY 10036
www.springerpub.com

Acquisitions Editor: Margaret Zuccarini
Managing Editor: Cindy Yoo
Compositor: S4Carlisle Publishing Services

ISBN: 978-0-8261-9113-7
e-book ISBN: 978-0-8261-9114-4

18 19 20 21 22 / 5 4 3 2 1

Library of Congress Cataloging-in-Publication Data

Names: Quallich, Susanne, editor. | Lajiness, Michelle, editor. | Mitchell, Kenneth (Kenneth A.), editor.
Title: Manual of men's health : a practice guide for APRNs and PAs / editor, Susanne A. Quallich ; section editors, Shelley Lajiness, Kenneth Mitchell.
Description: New York : Springer Publishing Company, [2018] | Includes bibliographical references and index.
Identifiers: LCCN 2018028860| ISBN 9780826191137 | ISBN 9780826191144
Subjects: | MESH: Men's Health | Physician Assistants | Advanced Practice Nursing
Classification: LCC R697.P45 | NLM WA 306 | DDC 610.73/72069--dc23 LC record available at https://lccn.loc.gov/2018028860

Printed in the United States of America.

To my husband Len, and to my children, Danielle, Brianna, and Luke, for demanding that I live with them in moments.

And to my dogs, Titan and Rogue, for just demanding.

We are what we repeatedly do. Excellence, then, is not an act but a habit.

Aristotle

Contents

SECTION II OVERVIEW OF SPECIAL ISSUES IN MEN'S HEALTH

SECTION III UROLOGY AND PREVENTATIVE CARDIOLOGY

---

*Chapter 10 was reprinted with permission from Fenstermaker, M., Paknikar, S., Rambhatla, A., Ohl, D. A., Skolarus, T. A., Dupree, J. M. (2017). The State of Men's Health Services in the Veterans Health Administration. *Current Urology Reports 18*(11). doi:10.1007/s11934-017-0733-4

Contributors

Michelle Angie, MSN, CNP, NP-C Glickman Urological and Kidney Institute, Beachwood Family Health Center, Cleveland Clinic Foundation, Cleveland, Ohio

Jose Bauermeister, PhD, MPH Presidential Associate Professor of Nursing, Director, HIV Disparities Scientific Working Group, Center for AIDS Research, School of Nursing, University of Pennsylvania, Philadelphia, Pennsylvania

Yolanda Bone, DNP, APRN, FNP-BC Oncology Nurse Practitioner, Survivorship Coordinator, Christus St. Michael, West Temple Webber Cancer Center, Texarkana, Texas

Nancy Brownlee, MSN, APRN, FNP-BC Baylor College of Medicine, St. Luke's Medical Group, Houston, and Lake Jackson, Texas, Clinical Instructor, Adjunct Faculty, University of Texas Health Science Center, FNP Program, Houston, Texas

Jade Burns, PhD, RN, CPNP-PC Postdoctoral Fellow, National Clinician Scholars Program, University of Michigan School of Nursing, Center for Sexuality and Health Disparities, Ann Arbor, Michigan

Anne E. Calvaresi, MSN, CRNP, RNFA Urology Nurse Practitioner, Kimmel Cancer Center, Thomas Jefferson University, Philadelphia, Pennsylvania

Mashrin Lira Chowdhury, DO Department of Urology, Detroit Medical Center, Detroit, Michigan

Sara M. Drummer MSN, ARNP, FNP-BC, CUNP Florida Urology Associates, Orlando, Florida

James M. Dupree IV, MD, MPH* Assistant Professor, Division of Andrology and Urologic Health, Department of Urology, Michigan Medicine, Ann Arbor, Michigan

Hillary B. Durstein, MSN, APRN, NP-C Urology Nurse Practitioner, Robert J. Dole VA Medical Center, Wichita, Kansas

Kathleen Fasing, MS, ACNP Cardiology Nurse Practitioner, Department of Cardiology, Michigan Medicine, Ann Arbor, Michigan

Michael Fenstermaker, MD* Department of Urology, Michigan Medicine, Ann Arbor, Michigan

Sallyanne M. Fisher, APRN, FNP-BC, CUNP Urology Nurse Practitioner, Carl T. Hayden VA Medical Center, Phoenix, Arizona

Dalmacio Dennis Flores, PhD, ACRN Ruth L. Kirschstein NRSA Postdoctoral Research Fellow, Program for Sexuality, Technology, and Action Research, Department of Family and Community Health, School of Nursing, University of Pennsylvania, Philadelphia, Pennsylvania

Mikkel Fode, MD, PhD, FECSM Clinical Researcher, Department of Urology, Herlev and Gentofte Hospital, University of Copenhagen, Herlev, Denmark

Zane Giffen, MD Resident, Department of Urology, University of Toledo College of Medicine and Life Sciences, Toledo, Ohio

James Hotaling, MD, MS, FECSM Assistant Professor of Surgery (Urology), Andrology/Urology Center for Reconstructive Urology and Men's Health, University of Utah, Salt Lake City, Utah

Christian Fuglesang S. Jensen, MD PhD student, Department of Urology, Herlev and Gentofte Hospital, University of Copenhagen, Herlev, Denmark

Min Suk Jun, DO Department of Urology, Detroit Medical Center, Detroit, Michigan

Michelle Lajiness, MSN, FNP-BC Clinical Director, Pelvic Floor Dysfunction Rehabilitation Program, Department of Urology, University of Toledo College of Medicine and Life Sciences, Toledo, Ohio

Amy Leatherwood, MSN, FNP-BC Department of Radiation Medicine, Oregon Health and Sciences University, Portland, Oregon

MiChelle L. McGarry, MSN, RN, CPNP, CUNP, FAANP, FNAPNAP Certified Pediatric and Urology Nurse Practitioner, President and Director, Pediatric Effective Elimination Program Clinic & Consulting, PC, Highlands Ranch, Colorado

Adriana R. Messina, MSN, CRNP Urology Surgery, Department of Veteran Affairs, Wilmington, Delaware

Kenneth A. Mitchell, MPAS, PA-C Founding Program Director, Meharry Medical College, School of Graduate Studies and Research, Physician Assistant Sciences, Nashville, Tennessee

Mark A. Moyad, MD, MPH Jenkins/Pokempner Director of Preventive and Complementary Medicine, Michigan Medicine, Department of Urology, Ann Arbor, Michigan

Stanley Mukundi, MMS, PA-C Division of Andrology and Urologic Health, Department of Urology, Michigan Medicine, Ann Arbor, Michigan

Karen M. Myrick, DNP, APRN, FNP-BC, ANP-BC Associate Professor of Nursing, Joint Appointment Frank Netter School of Medicine, Quinnipiac University School of Nursing, Hamden, Connecticut

Jo Ann L. Nicoteri, PhD, CRNP, FNP-BC Assistant Professor, Family Nurse Practitioner, Department of Nursing/Student Health Services, University of Scranton, Scranton, Pennsylvania

Ruby Nzoma, DNP, RN-C Research Assistant, Wayne State University, Hutzel Women's Hospital, Detroit, Michigan

Dana A. Ohl, MD Professor, Division of Andrology and Urologic Health, Department of Urology, Michigan Medicine, Ann Arbor, Michigan

Sujay Paknikar, MD* University of Michigan School of Medicine, Ann Arbor, Michigan

Mari Parker, MSN, FNP-C, CUNP The Urology Group

George Byron Peraza-Smith, DNP, APRN, GNP-BC, AGPCNP-C, CNE Associate Dean for Academic Affairs, College of Nursing, Program Director, MSN Programs, United States University, San Diego, California

John Phoenix, APRN, FNP-C Nurse Practitioner, Huntridge Family Clinic, Las Vegas, Nevada

Rachel Prosser, PhD, APRN, CNP, AAHIVS, FAANP Research Manager of the HIV/AIDS Research, Hennepin County Medical Center, Medical Director for Rural AIDS Action Network (RAAN) of Minnesota, HIV Specialist for the MN Department of Corrections and Minnesota State Hospitals (MSOP), Owner of Positive Healthcare LLC, Minneapolis, Minnesota

Susanne A. Quallich, PhD, ANP-BC, NP-C, CUNP, FAANP Andrology Nurse Practitioner, Division of Andrology and Urologic Health, Department of Urology, Michigan Medicine, Ann Arbor, Michigan

Ashwin Raghavan, MD Resident, Department of Urology, University of Toledo College of Medicine and Life Sciences, Toledo, Ohio

Amarnath Rambhatla, MD* Wayne State University School of Medicine, John D. Dingell VA Medical Center, Detroit, Michigan

Michael Sanchez, DNP, CRNP, NP-C, FNP-BC, AAHIVS Assistant Professor, Johns Hopkins University, School of Nursing, Baltimore, Maryland

Mette L. K. Schmidt, PhD Department of Urology, Herlev and Gentofte Hospital, University of Copenhagen, Herlev, Denmark

Tariq Shah, PhD, HCLD, MPA Assistant Professor, Department of Urology, Department of Medical Education, College of Medicine and Life Sciences, University of Toledo, Toledo, Ohio

Michael Sheehan, RNFA, MSN, NP-C, CUNP Carson Urologists, Carson City, Nevada

Hilary Shreves, MSN, ACNP-BC Instructor/Nurse Practitioner, Department of Urology, Oregon Health & Science University, Portland, Oregon

Puneet Sindhwani, MD, MS Chairman, Department of Urology & Renal Transplantation, Kenneth A. Kropp Endowed Professor of Urology, University of Toledo College of Medicine and Life Sciences, Toledo, Ohio

Ted A. Skolarus, MD* Department of Urology, University of Michigan and Ann Arbor VA Healthcare System, Ann Arbor, Michigan

Jens Sønksen, MD, PhD, DSc Professor, Department of Urology, Herlev and Gentofte Hospital, University of Copenhagen, Herlev, Denmark

Kelley Taylor, RN, MSN, AG ACNP-BC Center for Reconstructive Urology and Men's Health, University of Utah, Salt Lake City, Utah

Joanne Thanavaro, DNP, AGPCNP-BC, AGACNP-BC, DCC, FAANP Associate Dean of Graduate Nursing Education, Associate Professor and Director of Advanced Practice Nursing, St. Louis, Missouri

Alice Ukaegbu, DNP, MSN, FNP-BC, RN Nurse Manager, Howard University Clinical Research Unit, College of Medicine, Washington, District of Columbia

Aaron Wallace, BS CHEK Practitioner, Level 3, Owner and CEO of Balance Your Fitness, Troy, Michigan

*These individuals did not contribute to this work. Their chapter originally appeared in *Current Urology Reports*.

Foreword

There has been a resurgence in attention to men's health in the last 10 years. However, the push to champion men's health has not been as robust as the goal of promoting initiatives in women's health.

Major studies looking at estrogen replacement therapy have redefined the way practitioners look at postmenopause support for women. Conversely, well-done studies on testosterone replacement therapy are uncommon, but are increasing in numbers recently.

Prostate cancer studies and prostate health promotion is going well, but has significantly lacked when compared to the well-funded and well-organized push for breast health over the last 20 to 30 years.

Attention needs to be given to men's health issues. This book, edited by Susanne Quallich, PhD, gives such attention to this group of problems. Dr. Quallich is uniquely suited to generate a book on this topic, having worked exclusively in the clinical treatment of men's health issues for almost 20 years. She is a well-recognized expert in clinical andrology and has a special expertise in the treatment of male genital pain; her PhD work centered on idiopathic testis pain in men.

Dr. Quallich has separated the book into three sections: general men's health issues; special issues; and finally, conditions seen in urological and cardiology practices.

Section I gives the reader tools that will allow a general approach to health challenges facing men. Men have a propensity to avoid medical system contact and intervention and generally try to avoid seeking medical treatment. These roadblocks to treatment need to be addressed either directly or with the help of family members and/or significant others. Direct outreach to the patients is another method that may be helpful. The authors also address special situations, such as the adolescent male, who may be even more prone to avoid medical contact for male issues.

In Section II, the writers explore more specific situations in men's health. Different venues for men's health delivery are explored, including the Veterans Health Administration system and free-standing men's health clinics. Mark Moyad, an international expert in alternative medicine, has a contribution on nutritional and dietary supplements for men. Finally, the concept of urology as a portal to men's general health is discussed. This leads to the last section of the book, discussing specific urological conditions.

Section III homes in on specific issues, including types of male sexual dysfunction, infertility, prostate problems, and male-specific cancers. Controversies in PSA screening for prostate cancer are addressed, as well as issues facing the urological cancer survivor. The last three chapters are devoted to an incredibly important topic: the relationship between men's health issues and cardiovascular disease. This link is inextricable and provides the rationale as to why practitioners of men's health maladies are really the portal to men's general health.

The editor and authors of this book should be congratulated on their undertaking. This information is important and impactful, and will hopefully serve as an impetus for practitioners to seriously address men's health issues. This push will improve quality of life for men suffering from these conditions, but will also lead to greater scrutiny of general health issues and lead to general health improvement in the male population.

Dana A. Ohl, MD, FECSM
Professor of Urology, University of Michigan
Head, Division of Andrology and Urologic Health

Jens Sønksen, MD, PhD, DMSci
Chair Professor of Urology, University of Copenhagen
Adjunct Secretary General, European Association of Urology

Preface

My first jobs after graduation as a nurse practitioner in 1996 involved the care of men almost exclusively at the John D. Dingell Veterans Administration Medical Center (VAMC) in Detroit, Michigan, which was followed a few years later by a transfer to the Ann Arbor VAMC. Veterans are a unique population of men, and it was a difficult decision to leave that environment, because these men were special. I had never really intended to stay long at either of those jobs, and certainly never intended to make a career out of taking care of men and striving to improve the care of men. But I was recruited to the University of Michigan Health System, now Michigan Medicine, and my role within urology eventually focused on the care of men within a specialized area of urology: andrology, or sexual and reproductive health complaints. I think of andrology as a specialty that offers some of the greatest quality-of-life interventions that can be offered to men. Andrology offers opportunities to help men regain sexual function and intimacy, or the potential to have biologic children. My practice continues to change and has grown to include the quality-of-life interventions that can be offered with a thorough approach to the evaluation and management of chronic genital pain and chronic pelvic pain in men.

This book, then, offers a unique perspective to any healthcare provider wishing to focus more on the care of men, a perspective that has been refined over my 22 years of caring for adult men in the clinical setting. It concentrates on topics that are unique to men; for this reason, a large section of the book is dedicated to those urologic topics pertinent to men. After all, in many specialties there is little to no difference in clinical management between men and women for most conditions.

This is not a textbook, nor is it an exhaustive review of the literature regarding men and illness, nor is it meant to present meticulous evidence-based guidelines for urologic care—these perspectives can be found elsewhere in the literature and online. This book is meant to guide the reader toward topics that may not have previously been considered "men's health" such as the needs of teens and young adult men. The clinically based chapters offer clinical pearls and websites that may be of use to providers and patients alike. Furthermore, this book presents unique perspectives on selected men's health issues, discussions that are not present to date in other men's health books.

As luck would have it, I have never left the men's health arena, and for those who may feel that healthcare has been short-sighted regarding *women's* health, I offer the gentle reminder that there has never been a "men's health NP" nor is there dedicated training for any profession as a "men's health specialist"—no parallel to the gynecologist. Those who are interested in this field are self-taught, and pick up skills on the job, specific to the particular environments in which we work. This is one of the greatest strengths of this emerging field of men's health—the variety of multidisciplinary providers who bring their unique perspective and skills to these topics and to the clinical care of our husbands, fathers, brothers, and sons, as you will note as you review the contributors.

I have been honored to work with many established authors as we moved this book forward, as well as having the pleasure of coaching and coauthoring many newer or first-time authors. It is my hope that this book will act as a signpost, one that can introduce you to the world of men's health, or encourage you to learn more in directions that perhaps you had not considered.

Susanne A. Quallich

SECTION I

General Men's Health

CHAPTER 1

Introduction to the Complexity in Defining Men's Health

Kenneth A. Mitchell

INTRODUCTION

The definition of men's health has undergone a significant change over the last several decades. Several factors ranging from marketing to social determinants have diluted a once clearly expressed definition. The World Health Organization (WHO) in the 1940s defined men's health as a state of complete physical, mental, and social well-being, as experienced by men, and not merely the absence of disease or infirmity. These aspects of health often relate to structure such as male genitalia or to conditions caused by hormones specific to, or most notable in, males (World Health Organization [WHO], 1948). Health experts at the time acknowledged the definition and attempted to educate men and boys about the importance of incorporating healthy lifestyle habits to establish and maintain good health throughout the life span.

However, efforts by healthcare professionals since that time have been ineffective at reducing the morbidity and mortality rates of men versus those of women. Numerous studies have confirmed that over the past several decades, men have continued to have a significantly shorter life span than women. The Global Burden of Disease study led by the Institute for Health Metrics and Evaluation (2013) showed that throughout the period from 1970 to 2010, women had a longer life expectancy than men. Furthermore, it was observed that over that 40-year period, female life expectancy at birth increased from 61.2 to 73.3 years, whereas male life expectancy rose from 56.4 to 67.5 years. The data indicate that the gap in life expectancy at birth widened between the sexes to men's disadvantage over that span of 40 years (Wang et al., 2012).

The past several decades have seen an increased interest in men's health by healthcare providers largely related to advertising and the availability for both Food and Drug Administration (FDA)-approved and over-the-counter supplements designed to improve a man's health by enhancing sexual performance or restoring a youthful physical appearance. The public interest in men's health has been further accentuated by a constant barrage of conventional media advertising combined with relentless online advertising redefining the public's perceived definition of men's health to only be related to a condition of failure to maintain sexual function, sexual prowess, vitality, and manhood. Critics, including medical experts, have challenged this redefined perception of men's health as unethical and propagating an unwarranted antiaging movement leading to medical treatments that yield no clinical benefit and/or may be harmful (The Guardian, 2008). This new definition of the healthy male feeds into the societal perception that good health in a man at any age is measured by the ability to achieve unrealistic, if not mythical, sexual prowess and physical appearance, while simultaneously ignoring the health issues that impact men's morbidity and mortality worldwide. Consequently, the promise of "turning back the clock" and increasing masculinity has perpetuated, if not worsened, the lack of engagement by men with the healthcare system.

HEALTH DISPARITY

The disparity in men's health is believed to be attributed to several factors including economic, social, and ethnic considerations; accessibility to healthcare; and men's perceived attitudes toward healthcare. The *Los Angeles Times* reported in 2000 that three times as many men as women had not seen a doctor in the previous year when surveyed. Furthermore, one in three men had no regular doctor, and nearly one-quarter said they would wait "as long as possible" before seeking medical advice for any health-related condition (Los Angeles Times, 2000). Globally, the evidence supports that men tend to be in worse health than women. The UCL Institute of Health Equity conducted a retrospective study of the WHO European Region that indicated by 2010 women were outliving men by an average of almost 6 years. In the region with the lowest life expectancy at birth, central sub-Saharan Africa, men were living 5.3 years less than women on average. The biggest difference in life expectancy between men and women was seen in Eastern Europe, which showed women in the Russian Federation were outliving men by an average of 11.6 years. According to the Global Health 2035 report, countries classified as "least developed" and "less developed" by the United Nations showed adult mortality rate fell faster among women than among men between 1992 and 2012 (Jamison et al., 2013; UCL Institute of Health Equity, 2013). The Centers for Disease Control and Prevention (CDC) National Vital Statistics Report 2016 showed similar findings in the United States, indicating that the overall life expectancy for females is 81.2 years, while for males, it is 76.4 years. Racial differences further showed that for non-Hispanic white males, life expectancy did not change (76.5 years), while for non-Hispanic white females, life expectancy decreased by 0.1 year to 81.1 years. Life expectancy for the non-Hispanic black population was 75.2 years in 2014, an increase of 0.1 year compared with 2013. For non-Hispanic black males, life expectancy increased by 0.2 year to 72.0, while life expectancy for non-Hispanic black females remained unchanged since 2012 (78.1 years; National Vital Statistics Report, 2016).

Social Determinants

Studies in the United States have pointed toward social determinants as being a major contributing factor for men's health disparities. Bruce et al. reviewed several key articles that support the concept that social factors can have implications for disease, disability, and premature death. The authors indicate that it has been long established that poverty, education, geography, family, race, and ethnicity are important social determinants of health and healthcare (Bruce, Roscigno, & McCall, 1998; Marmot, 2014; Marmot & Allen, 2014). These authors go on to suggest that identification of men's health disparities is not simply examining racial and ethnic disparities among men, but includes efforts to consider how sex and gender interact with other social determinants to create population-specific patterns of health among men (Griffith, Metzl, & Gunter, 2011).

THE IMPACT OF GENDER ON MEN'S HEALTH

It is widely known that in many societies, men have shorter lives than women despite men having social and economic advantages relative to women. Experts have identified several factors that contribute to the gender disparity, noting the profound impact that masculinity has on health behaviors; the male ideal of masculinity greatly contributes to the lack of engagement with the healthcare system. Male socialization, social connectedness, and work-life balance have also been shown to significantly impact overall health. The perception of masculinity begins early in boyhood and is perpetuated throughout the psychological and physical developmental stages, and has been identified as a key factor leading both men and boys to risk-taking and self-harming behavior. Societal expectation of male emotional responses further contributes to self-denial of access to the healing effects of emotional release, and valuing physical, emotional, and mental health. Healthcare providers must consider and understand the variability of masculine identity and behavior over the course of a man's life as well as the cultural and ethnic background, sexual identity, socioeconomic status, and geographical locations as factors.

Behavioral scientists attempting to explain behaviors of men relating to health and wellness considered evolution and adaptation as part of the explanation. However, the belief that remnants of primitive behaviors, and the impulses behind the behaviors, contribute to the consistent belief that men are invincible or refractory to illness and thus put off seeking medical attention is highly unlikely. Researchers in the United States and Europe have conducted research that suggests masculine norms of self-control, self-reliance, taking risks, competitiveness, and seeking dominance may explain why boys begin and grow to maturity behaving recklessly, are hesitant or reluctant to seek medical advice, because of conforming to societal masculine ideology.

In 2007, the University of Nevada researchers reported results of a study that ranked 172 men based on their score on the Bem Sex Role Inventory (BSRI) questionnaire. The BSRI was developed in 1971 by Dr. Sandra Lipsitz Bem, and it characterizes the subject's personality as masculine, feminine, androgynous, or undifferentiated. The BSRI is based on gender stereotypes and measures how well individuals fit into their perceived or traditional sex role (Bem, 1977). The resulting score can reveal much about how cultural expectations have changed over the last 45 years, as well as provide some insight into personality traits of the person being tested. Researchers from the University of Nevada reported those with high masculinity scores were more responsive to a skin cancer message that appealed to controlling fears (e.g., wearing sunscreen regularly will relieve worry about getting skin cancer) rather than a message about mitigating the danger (wearing sunscreen regularly will reduce your exposure to ultraviolet light) (Harvard Health Letter, 2008). Several experts have suggested that simply being a "man" and upholding masculine ideals is a possible risk factor for poor health (Courtenay, 2000).

In 1995, several researchers introduced the concept of hegemonic masculinity. This ideal refers to the perception of what it means to be a "real" man. These traits include stoicism, the appearance of being strong and brave, and risk-taking behaviors (Gough, 2006). These studies have led researchers to believe that deep-rooted culturally held social norms influence men's behavior, specifically avoiding accessing healthcare as a demonstration of masculinity. Moreover, men being proactive with healthcare-seeking behavior are viewed as possessing more feminine traits, thus further threatening masculine identity (Courtenay, 2000). Furthermore, health-seeking behavior may be construed as "deviant" within the masculine arena. Societal acceptance of the typical male model of masculinity leads to the assumption that men have no interest in their health and men are viewed as a stereotype belonging to a homogeneous group with similar behaviors in all manners. This portrayal is the example by which young boys and adolescent males pattern their behavior, and is the target of advertising to men seeking men's health solutions. Gough (Gough, 2006) suggests that the mere use of the term "men's health" alludes to the view that all men are the same, perpetuating the belief that all men are seeking similar healthcare outcomes.

HEALTHCARE PROVIDERS' ATTITUDES TOWARD MEN'S HEALTH

The anticipation for an oral on-demand treatment for erectile dysfunction marked the beginning of a cultural revolution regarding male sexual dysfunction. On March 27, 1998, Viagra (sildenafil) represented one of the most successful launches of an FDA-approved medication in the history of the pharmaceutical industry (IMS Health, 1998). Similarly, in 2002, topical testosterone gels were approved by the FDA with sales following a similar trajectory to sildenafil. In that first year, there was an 87% increase in sales and a continued increase that ranged from 8% to 32% from year to year from 2002 to 2008 (IMS Health, 2002). Consequently, healthcare providers faced increasing demands for evaluation and management of erectile dysfunction and hypogonadism (e.g., ED and low T). The increased demand on general practitioners (GPs) to provide management of these two diagnoses, combined with increasing demands from all other provided services, increased administrative workload, a shrinking physician workforce, media pressure, and resulting patient demand, all greatly contributed to a negative clinical bias toward men's health by many healthcare providers.

In a qualitative UK study, 10 male GPs aged 35 to 53 years were interviewed to gain insight into their experience regarding the health-seeking behaviors of their male patients (Hale, Grogan, & Willott, 2010). The study specifically examined male GP perceptions of their patients' health needs and their views on how and why men arrive at a decision to seek help. The study further explored the GPs' own beliefs about health and health behaviors to investigate whether those beliefs influenced or biased their consultations with their male patients. Interestingly, the findings suggested that the GPs' attitude toward working men who had little contact with healthcare services was positive. The GPs ascribed this behavior as their patients demonstrating hegemonic masculinity through nonattendance at healthcare clinics. One physician stated, "the working guys come in with stuff that stops them from working" (Hale et al., 2010, p. 706). In contrast, nonworking men who consulted with their GP more frequently were criticized, alluding to the fact that they presented with health problems that were not "real." This view was further evidenced by one GP comparing nonworking men to housewives and trivializing their attendance in the clinic. He specifically described "non-working men who've got the attendance profile that you associate with non-working women" (Hale et al., 2010, p. 706). In contrast, men who presented within a masculine framework, maintaining a stoic identity, coerced into an office visit by a spouse or significant other, or communicating that the visit was delayed until the problem became "real" were viewed as more legitimate. Perhaps a more alarming finding in the study suggested that the GPs' negative attitude toward nonworking male patients might be nonverbally communicated (Hale, Grogan, & Willott, 2007). The study further indicated that some males felt male GPs held negative attitudes related to their use of healthcare services. Further evidence revealed that the GPs' own health-seeking behaviors were not dissimilar to those of their male patients in that the GPs also adhered to stoicism, a characteristic they viewed positively within their working male patients. Although this was a small study, the findings suggest that healthcare providers must carefully consider the possibility that male patients may feel that they are viewed negatively by their GP for their healthcare-seeking practices. The adverse effect on both the consultation and the frequency of visits by male patients can further contribute to the patterns of healthcare-seeking behavior among male patients.

HEALTHCARE-SEEKING BEHAVIOR DIFFERENCES BETWEEN MEN AND WOMEN

The American Academy of Pediatrics (AAP) publishes and regularly updates Recommendations for Preventive Pediatric Health Care (American Academy of Pediatrics, 2017) with recommendations for both boys and girls outlined from birth until the age of 21. Despite the recommendations, and as boys and girls age into adulthood, the level and reasons for engagement with the healthcare system between the two groups take two very different and distinct paths. In the United States, men and women typically begin their engagement with healthcare at birth. As children, both boys' and girls' continuance with the healthcare system is largely in part due to parental direction. School physical requirements or sports physical examinations through high school and/or college ensures that young men continue some level of engagement with the healthcare system until they complete their education or sports careers. However, once young men are no longer required to undergo physical exams and/or seek healthcare for sports injuries, they typically disengage from the healthcare system. This pattern of engagement with the healthcare system perpetuates the male notion to only seek medical care when an injury or illness occurs. In contrast, the pattern of engagement with the healthcare system for girls typically continues well into adulthood for reproductive reasons beginning with reaching the age of menarche, progressing to pregnancy and childbirth, and ultimately perimenopause and menopause. From an early age, men are directed to seek medical care only when something is wrong rather than make efforts to prevent illness or injury.

THE MEDIA AND MEN'S HEALTH

The media has been long been implicated in reproducing and reinforcing male stereotypes and often characterizes men as all being the same (Gough, 2006). This portrayal further perpetuates the stereotypical attractive, physically fit, highly masculine, and affluent male as being the symbol of health and wellness. Health promotion initiatives are typically designed and underpinned by these symbols of hegemonic masculinity with the intent of luring the male to seek products or services that will help him become like the symbolic portrayal of male health and wellness (Robertson & Williamson, 2005). However, other factors portrayed in the media, such as ethnicity, socioeconomic status, and sexuality may have a similar or greater impact on healthcare-seeking behavior (Coles et al., 2010; Galdas, Cheater, & Marshall, 2004).

The findings of a study carried out by Cole et al. (Coles et al., 2010) observed 82 men aged 40 years and over in two deprived boroughs in North West England. This qualitative study aimed to explore men's understandings of their health within a social context. Their results partially supported the idea that men should be targeted using an understanding of hegemonic masculinity, but the participants' comments also revealed a challenge to notions that men should be targeted exclusively in this manner. Many of the participants did not welcome being stereotyped by advertising, and thus rated existing health promotion material poorly. Furthermore, participants equally expressed their dislike of the stereotypical portrayals of the masculine body as young and athletic as they did images depicting men as excessive beer drinkers. The findings support that it is not necessarily the norm for men to frequent "typical male spaces" for purposes of drinking, attending sporting events, and the like. One participant stated, "A lot of men don't go to pubs, a lot of men don't go to clubs, a lot of men don't go to sports fixtures and stuff like that. More men go around supermarkets" (Coles et al., 2010, p. 933). The authors concluded that a range of health promotion strategies should be used and in diverse locations. It can be further concluded that some media campaigns for men's health products may further drive men away from the healthcare system for fear of not attaining the promised results.

THE INTERNET AND MEN'S HEALTH-SEEKING BEHAVIOR

The use of the Internet for men's health has grown exponentially over the past 25 to 30 years. In 2013, 43% of adults had used the Internet to find health-related information via websites such as NHS Direct, compared to approximately 18% in 2007 (Office for National Statistics, 2013). Internet users gather health information for various purposes, including for the preparation before or following a medical consultation, to gain information regarding prescribed medication, for self-diagnosis purposes, or for help with managing a long-term condition. Despite the potential benefits of Internet use in this area, researchers have raised several concerns related to the adverse effect it could have. These fears include social isolation, website credibility (Hardy, 1999), a pathway to unconventional and unproven healthcare, misleading health information, and arriving at an incorrect self-diagnosis (Larner, 2006).

Male patients seek information from the Internet typically to avoid the embarrassment of seeking medical care related to sexual dysfunction and/or general healthcare concerns. Concerns have been raised regarding the threat of challenging healthcare providers by patients wanting to discuss the information they obtained on the Internet (Nwosu & Cox, 2000). Researchers refer to this as "deprofessionalization," defined as a shift in the control from the healthcare provider as the gatekeeper of health information to the patient having access to this privileged information. The Internet is often the first place that men will visit to seek out health information (Pollard, 2007). A wide range of information can be accessed including email, chat rooms, online support groups, websites, and instant messaging. Benefits of using the Internet for health have been described, which may be attractive to some men as it supports the traditional male behavioral norms of invincibility, resilience, self-reliance, and stoicism. However, as mentioned previously, men are not a homogeneous group; thus, the effectiveness of this approach for all men cannot be assumed.

The use of the Internet to influence the health-seeking behavior of men includes the fact that it provides access to a voluminous supply of information that can be updated readily; is easily accessed, fast, and low-cost; and offers confidentiality and anonymity, and it enables men to maintain a sense of autonomy. Despite the potential benefits of using the Internet for men's health issues, several concerns have been identified including quality of the information, outdated information, Internet "addiction," disparities in Internet access, user health literacy requirements, and searching skills (Pollard, 2007).

MEN'S HEALTH REPORTS

In 2016, researchers conducted the Men's Health: Perceptions from Around the Globe survey (www.gamh.org). The survey was commissioned by Sanofi Consumer Health Care in cooperation with Global Action on Men's Health (GAMH), the Men's Health Network (MHN), Men's Health Forum (MHF) UK, Australian Men's Health Forum (AMHF), and Men's Health Education Council (MHEC). The survey was conducted among 2,000 demographically representative adults in eight countries (Australia, France, Germany, Italy, Poland, Sweden, the United Kingdom, and the United States) examining attitudes toward men's health. The survey was carried out from August 31 to September 10, 2016 by Opinium Research (Europe and Australia) and Harris (USA). This initiative marked one of the most comprehensive global surveys ever conducted investigating men's perceptions of their health.

The findings from the study revealed that the majority of men wanted to take greater control of their health and wellness. Furthermore, participants reported they were as confident as women that they could do so. The survey results challenged several well-established norms of healthcare-seeking behavior of men. Specifically, the survey showed that 87% of men wanted to take charge of their health, while 83% of the men were confident in managing their own health, and felt like they knew what to do when they had a health problem. Interestingly, 55% of men agreed there is plentiful information online to help them choose the right medication, while almost half of all men cited visiting a doctor as their first response when faced with a health problem and 80% of men believed that pharmacists can deal with nonserious and nonchronic health conditions. The conclusions identified significant changes in men's attitudes and approaches to their healthcare. The findings further indicated significant opportunities for policy makers around the world who are looking for ways to improve men's health and well-being as part of more efficient and effective healthcare services.

In the state of Tennessee (TN), data on Men's Health have been reported in 2010, 2012, 2014, and 2017; the 2017 Tennessee Men's Health Report Card is the latest edition that monitors the health and well-being of men in TN. The goal is to use the data to develop strategies to improve the health and well-being of men in the state. Remarkably, the TN Men's Health Report Card continues to distinguish Tennessee as the only state in the United States that has regularly published a report card to guide the planning, implementation, and evaluation of programs and policies to improve men's health (Griffith, 2017). The data collected come from the Tennessee Department of Health and the U.S. Census Bureau, and indicate that men comprise slightly less than half of the state's population in TN. Significant findings from the report are as follows:

- Men had a 5-year shorter life expectancy at birth than TN women (73.8 years vs. 78.8 years).
- The life expectancy at birth for both men and women in the state is more than 2 years shorter than the national averages of 76.3 years for men and 81.2 years for women.
- Caucasian men have a 5-year shorter life expectancy at birth than Caucasian women (74.5 years vs. 79.2 years).
- African American men have a 7-year shorter life expectancy than African American women (70.8 years vs. 77.9 years).
- Heart disease and cancer were the leading causes of death for African American men, Caucasian men, men in each grand division of the state, and men 35 years old and older.

Comparisons of men in east TN, middle TN, and west TN indicated a larger gap in life expectancy between men and women in west TN than is found in east and middle TN, and men in west TN have a shorter life expectancy than men in east and middle TN. Nearly half of the deaths of men in TN were attributed to heart disease and cancer, which is reflective of the CDC reports on the 10 leading causes of death among men nationally. For men 18 to 34 years old, the leading cause of death was unintentional injuries (including accidental drug overdoses) not including motor vehicle accidents, while the second leading cause of death for young adult men was suicide.

Data reports and surveys on the state of men's health, such as this exemplar from the state of TN, are useful and will continue to play an integral role in the development of effective initiatives and policies to equip healthcare providers and community leaders with the resources necessary to improve the health of men.

CHANGING ATTITUDES AND PERCEPTIONS OF MEN'S HEALTH

Healthcare providers and the public are becoming increasingly aware of the health disparity that exists between men and women. Academic and private practice groups are offering more men's health services than ever before. In a survey conducted by Cleveland Clinic, they reported younger generations of fathers are significantly more likely to have a father/father figure who talks to them about their health (millennials: 84% vs. baby boomers: 48%) (Cleveland Clinic, 2016). However, 32% of fathers currently don't talk to their family about their health issues and concerns because they don't want to worry people. Eighty-five percent of fathers who talk to their son(s) about health started the conversation when their son(s) were under 16 years old. Racial differences in responses indicated that 50% of African American fathers whose family didn't openly talk about health issues and concerns wanted to break the pattern of silence with their own families.

Two-thirds (62%) of Hispanic fathers who participated in this Cleveland Clinic (Cleveland Clinic, 2017) study said that their family hid family health issues from them as a kid but talked to them more about health as an adult. Meanwhile, 31% of Hispanic fathers reported they wanted to talk to their sons about health topics but struggled to find the right words. The survey also indicated that of the more than 500 U.S. males over the age of 18, who are currently fathers or father figures to a boy, and who had a father and/or father figure growing up, approximately 62% responded wishing that their own father/father figure had talked to them more about health topics. In fact, 47% said that they didn't know about their family health history until they started to go to the doctor as an adult (Cleveland Clinic, 2017). These responses demonstrate that men are beginning to understand the importance of maintaining their health and communicating to their sons at a younger age to do the same. Healthcare providers are responding to the increased awareness by offering more men's health services in their practices.

THE SCOPE AND FUTURE OF MEN'S HEALTH

Men's healthcare continues to be a controversial area of medicine. The emphasis on sexual health has clouded the original definition of men's health and has contributed to the increasing disparity in this area of medicine. Relentless marketing of sexual dysfunction and hypogonadism have skewed both the public and healthcare provider's perception of the true threats to the health and wellness of men. Controversial information surrounding the effects of treatment for erectile dysfunction and hypogonadism has further compounded the public misconception of men's health. The desire by men to treat sexual dysfunction has created an industry of men's health centers appearing in cities throughout the United States offering treatments for erectile dysfunction and "low T" and guaranteeing results. Men are lured into these centers with the promise of alleviating the embarrassment and worry of erectile and sexual dysfunction equating improved sexual prowess with wellness and vitality. Often, these centers are staffed with healthcare providers not adequately trained to evaluate and treat men suffering from these ailments. Typically, the style of patient engagement feeds the masculine traits of stoicism and anonymity and further perpetuates men's lack of engagement with the healthcare system. Healthcare providers have felt the increasing demand for treatments with expectations of restoring youthful appearances and sexual prowess without addressing the underlying causes that threaten the health and well-being of men.

The CDC reports that the top three leading causes of death in men have remained consistent (heart disease, cancer, and accidents). Despite the efforts by healthcare providers to address men's health issues, minimal progress has occurred toward reducing the morbidity and mortality of men versus women. The emergence of advanced practice providers (APPs) in the discipline of men's health has already made a significant impact in the delivery of men's healthcare. True Men's Health clinics staffed with well-trained APPs are increasing in number throughout the United States providing quality evidence-based care to men.

Healthcare providers in the 21st century have many more considerations regarding the care of men including working directly with lesbian, gay, bisexual, and transgender (LGBT) patients and their partners to address the needs of men in these communities. Addressing barriers unique to caring for gay and bisexual men requires additional considerations and training (Chapters 11 and 16). Standard men's health questionnaires are biased toward a heterosexual, heteronormative male patient population, and often don't adequately assess the symptoms associated with certain conditions like erectile dysfunction, side effects from urological surgeries such as a radical prostatectomy, or placement of a penile prosthesis that can affect gay men differently.

The challenge of men's health will require that the medical community be actively involved with creating public awareness of men's health issues. Seizing opportunities to inform men and their significant others about the true threats to men's health and wellness will be critical to improving engagement of men with the healthcare system. Additionally, focused education in men's health should become standard in the curriculum where *any* healthcare provider undergoes training. Population health studies that continue to investigate and identify the specific variables that impact the disparity of men's health will be paramount to developing healthcare policy that ensures access to men's health services. Lastly, the combination of increased public awareness and improved training of healthcare professionals will lead to a culture change in which young men remain engaged with the healthcare system throughout the life span with the hope of closing the life expectancy gap between men and women.

REFERENCES

American Academy of Pediatrics. (2017). Recommendations for preventive pediatric health care bright futures. Retrieved from https://www.aap.org/en-us/Documents/periodicity_schedule.pdf

Bem, S. L. (1977). On the utility of alternative procedures for assessing psychological androgyny. *Journal of Consulting and Clinical Psychology, 45*(2), 196–205. doi:10.1037/0022-006X.45.2.196

Bruce, M. A., Roscigno, V. J., & McCall, P. L. (1998). Structure, context, and agency in the reproduction of black on-black violence. *Theoretical Criminology, 2*(1), 29–55. doi:10.1177/1362480698002001002

Cleveland Clinic. (2016). 2017 MENtion It Survey. Retrieved from https://newsroom.clevelandclinic.org/wp-content/uploads/sites/4/2017/08/CC-MENtion-It-Survey-Media-Deck_FINAL.pdf

Cleveland Clinic. (2017). MENtion It. Retrieved from https://health.clevelandclinic.org/2017/09/american-dads-sons-keep-health-themselves-infographic

Coles, R., Watkins, F., Swami, V., Jones, S., Woplf, S., & Stainstreet, D. (2010). What men really want: A qualitative investigation of men's health needs from the Halton and St Helens Primary Care Trust men's health promotion project. *British Journal of Health Psychology, 15*, 921–939. doi:10.1348/135910710X494583

Courtenay, W. H. (2000). Constructions of masculinity and their influence on men's well-being: A theory of gender and health. *Social Science and Medicine, 50*, 1385–1401. doi:10.1016/S0277-9536(99)00390-1

Galdas, P. M., Cheater, F., & Marshall, P. (2004). Men ad health help-seeking behavior: Literature review. *Journal of Advanced Nursing, 49*(6), 616–623. doi:10.1111/j.1365-2648.2004.03331.x

Gough, B. (2006). Try to be healthy, but don't forgo our masculinity: Deconstructing men's health discourse in the media. *Social Science and Medicine, 63*, 2476–2488. doi:10.1016/j.socscimed.2006.06.004

Griffith, D. (2017). Tennessee men's health report card. Retrieved from https://www.vanderbilt.edu/crmh/2017TNMensHealthReportCard.pdf

Griffith, D. M., Metzl, J. M., & Gunter, K. (2011). Considering intersections of race and gender in interventions that address U.S. men's health disparities. *Public Health, 125*(7), 417–423. doi:10.1016/j.puhe.2011.04.014

Hale, S., Grogan, S., & Willot, S. (2007). Patterns of self-referral in men with symptoms of prostate cancer. *British Journal of Health Psychology, 12*, 403–419. doi:10.1348/135910706X118413

Hale, S., Grogan, S., & Willott, S. (2010). Male GPs' views on men seeking medical help: A qualitative study. *British Journal of Health Psychology, 15*, 697–713. doi:10.1348/135910709X479113

Hardy, M. (1999). Doctor in the house: The Internet as a source of lay health knowledge and the challenge to expertise. *Sociology of Health and Illness, 21*(6), 820–835. doi:10.1111/1467-9566.00185

Harvard Health Letter. (2008, June). Masculinity and men's health. Retrieved from https://www.health.harvard.edu/newsletter_article/Masculinity_and_mens_health

IMS Health. (1998). Retail and Provider Perspective, and National Prescription Audit.

IMS Health. (2002). Retail and Provider Perspective, and National Prescription Audit.

Institute for Health Metrics and Evaluation. (2013). *The global burden of disease: Generating evidence, guiding policy*. Seattle, WA: Author.

Jamison, D. T., Summers, L. H., Alleyne, G., Arrow, K. J., Berkley, S., Binagwaho, A., … Yamey, G. (2013). Global Health 2035: A world converging within a generation. *Lancet, 382*, 1898–1955. doi:10.1016/S0140-6736(13)62105-4

Larner, A. J. (2006). Searching for medical information: Frequency over time and by age and gender in an outpatient information population in the UK. *Journal of Telemedicine and Telecare, 12*, 186–188. doi:10.1258/135763306777488816

Los Angeles Times. (2000). Men tend to avoid health care, Study says. Retrieved from http://articles.latimes.com/2000/mar/14/news/mn-8681

Marmot, M. (2009). Action on health disparities in the United States: Commission on Social Determinants of Health. *JAMA, 301*(11), 1169–1171.

Marmot, M., & Allen, J. J. (2014). Social determinants of health equity. *American Journal of Public Health, 104*(S4), S517–S519.

National Vital Statistics Reports. (2016). Deaths: Final data for 2014. Retrieved from https://www.cdc.gov/nchs/data/nvsr/nvsr65/nvsr65_04.pdf

Nwosu, C. R., & Cox, B. M. (2000). The impact of the Internet on the doctor patient relationship. *Health Informatics Journal, 6*, 156–161. doi:10.1177/146045820000600308

Office for National Statistics. (2013). Internet Access—Households and Individuals. Statistical Bulletin. Retrieved from http://www.ons.gov.uk/ons/dcp171778_322713.pdf

Pollard, J. (2007). Working with men via the Internet. In A. White & M. Pettifer (Eds.), *Hazardous waist tackling male weight problems* (pp. 186–197). Oxford, NY: Radcliffe.

Robertson, S., & Williamson, P. (2005). Men and health promotion in the UK: Ten years further on? *Health Educational Journal, 64*, 293–301. doi:10.1177/001789690506400402

The Guardian. (2008). Ten years on: It's time to count the cost of the Viagra revolution. Retrieved from https://www.theguardian.com/theobserver/2008/feb/24/controversiesinscience

UCL Institute of Health Equity (2013). *Review of social determinants and the health divide in the WHO European Region: Final report*. Copenhagen, Denmark: World Health Organization, Regional Office for Europe. Retrieved from http://www.euro.who.int/__data/assets/pdf_file/0004/251878/Review-of-social-determinants-and-the-health-divide-in-the-WHO-European-Region-FINAL-REPORT.pdf

Wang, H., Dwyer-Lindgren, L., Lofgren, K. T., Rajaratnam, J. K., Marcus, J. R., Levin-Rector, A., … Murray, C. J. L. (2012). Age-specific and sex-specific mortality in 187 countries, 1970–2010: A systematic analysis for the Global Burden of Disease Study 2010. *Lancet, 380*, 2071–2094. doi:10.1016/S0140-6736(12)61719-X

WHO Definition of Health. (1948). Preamble to the Constitution of the World Health Organization as adopted by the International Health Conference, New York, 19–22 June 1946; signed on 22 July 1946 by the representatives of 61 States (Official Records of the World Health Organization, no. 2, p. 100) and entered into force on 7 April 1948. Retrieved from http://apps.who.int/gb/bd/PDF/bd47/EN/Constitution-en.pdf

CHAPTER 2

A Brief Discussion of Issues in Men's Health Seeking

Mari Parker

INTRODUCTION: DISPARITIES IN MEN'S HEALTH

The discipline of men's health remains relatively new when one compares it with the history of women's health as a specialty. This is further influenced by the fact that no individual specialty exists to claim ownership for "men's health" and men's health specialists can come from fields as diverse as psychology, urology, cardiology, and family practice. When it comes to healthcare, there are clearly different patterns between women's and men's health (Chapter 1) (Addis & Mahalik, 2003; Courtenay, 2000a; 2000b; Hooper & Quallich, 2016). There is abundant literature that supports the concept that women are more open to the idea of preventive healthcare, in part due to the recognition of prenatal and pregnancy care, as well as their role as caregiver for children. Women are simply more likely to pursue routine healthcare, as the socialization to the need for routine healthcare begins with the acknowledgment that once they become sexually active they should be having routine pelvic examinations and Pap smears. There is no reciprocal socialization for men to receive routine preventive healthcare, historically until age 50, when men are informed that they should have a screening rectal examination and prostate-specific antigen (PSA) test for prostate cancer as well as a routine screening colonoscopy. This created some clear differences in how men and women conceptualize healthcare and, in particular, preventive healthcare.

Why are there differences between men and women's healthcare behaviors? What increased hazards do men face because they do not seek healthcare? What are the health conditions that men are at increased risk for developing? Why is it that men don't take care of themselves as well as women do? Are there opportunities to change the status quo, and to find ways to encourage men to take measures to improve their health? These are the sort of questions that an expansive view of men's health seeks to investigate.

There are legitimate physiologic, social, and cultural differences between men and women. Values of masculinity and femininity are passed down from birth through toys children play with, family and social traditions (Bruce, Griffith, & Thorpe, 2015), and various media, everything from fairy tales, to song lyrics, and television shows—a discussion that is well beyond the scope of this chapter. For example, John Gray, in his 1992 work *Men Are From Mars, Women Are From Venus*, suggests that members of the opposite sex are different based on their needs, desires, behavior, and means of communication. The title itself promotes the idea that men and women are very different and there are an abundance of books on this stated difference between genders: *Men, Women, and the Mystery of Love; Cold Hard Truth on Men, Women, and Money; Man, Woman, and Child;* and even *Men, Women, and Chain Saws: Gender in the Modern Horror Film.*

The American Psychological Association (APA) equates these gender differences more with societal expectations than with biology. A meta-analysis by Hyde (Hyde, 2005) reviewed 46 studies conducted during the last two decades of the 20th century with the results that men and women are more similar than different in terms of psychological variables, leadership, cognitive ability, motor behaviors, moral reasoning, and personality. Hyde concluded that any differences may be more the result of the measurement context than a true gender-based difference, and that in most of the studies reviewed, gender-based differences were non-existent. The media tends to exaggerate the stereotypical differences and the consequences of that affect both adults and children at home, schools, and in the workplace (American Psychological Association [APA], 2014). Most people have heard the assumptions that boys are told they are better at math and sciences than girls, for example; this may be only a function of the fact that there continue to be more men than women in math and science careers. The types of beliefs create consequences for children as well. Hyde (Hyde, 2005) reports girls' performance in school may begin to suffer toward the end of high school based on societal expectations alone rather than on any factor that has to do with gender. These assumptions extend into adulthood, with assumptions such that men are rewarded for aggressive behavior, while women are not expected to show the same aggressive personality traits.

These differences can carry over into attitudes about health and illness as well, both as patients and providers. Health disparities between men and women have increased in the last 40 years, and presently women outlive men on average by 5 years; in 2017, the life expectancy for men was 76.1 years, while the life expectancy for women was 81.1 years (National Center for Health Statistics, 2017). The gender gap is due, in part, to men's greater exposure to occupational hazards, increased risk-taking behaviors, and health behaviors related to masculinity (Baker et al., 2014). Men tend not to visit a doctor annually for screenings and only go when ill; they are also less likely to report symptoms while at the doctor's office or clinic (Baker, 2015). Some differences between men and women are based in biology, but others are formed as the result of gender roles formed through societal and cultural pressures and how an individual or his culture and social influences create a definition of health or illness.

It is also significant to note that the national Office of Women's Health was established in 1991. There has been no parallel "Office of Men's Health" yet established that would serve the same function nationally in coordinating research strategies, public policy coordination, public and private partnerships, and other activities that would encourage healthy lifestyle and disease knowledge among men. This contributes to the disparity in health seeking among men as there is no national office coordinating research and education activities for U.S. men. This office was initially suggested with the Men's Health Act of 2001 (originally HR 632; Senate Bill 1028 in 2003), but little progress has been made on its passage in several years. This proposal for a national office eventually stalled and died in congressional subcommittee. One could conclude that men's health issues have been marginalized on the national level, and have not seen any improvements or protections of male gender–specific healthcare services with the initiation of the Patient Protection and Affordable Care Act (PPACA) (111th United States Congress, 2014).

This disparity in coordination of services extends to the state level; many states have an office of women's health but only six states have a formal process for recognition of issues of men's health. Only New Hampshire has a specific Office of Men's Health, while many other states have a combined office of men's and women's health.

Prevention Issues

A hard look at the statistics reveals areas of concern and needed improvement in men's health. According to the Centers for Disease Control and Prevention (CDC, 2017a), the leading causes of death in men of all ages in the United States in 2014 were heart disease,

TABLE 2.1 Leading Causes of Death in Males in the United States, 2014

1	Heart disease	6	Diabetes
2	Cancer	7	Suicide
3	Unintentional injuries	8	Alzheimer's disease
4	Chronic lower respiratory diseases	9	Influenza and pneumonia
5	Stroke	10	Chronic liver disease

Source: Centers for Disease Control and Prevention. (2017a).

cancer, and accidental injuries (CDC, 2017; Table 2.1), while lung, prostate, and colorectal cancers were the leading causes of cancer deaths. Despite the fact that overall cancer death rates from 2010 to 2014 have decreased by 1.8% per year for men, the death rates due to liver, pancreas, and brain cancers have increased (Jemal et al., 2017). Risk reduction strategies (for lung cancer) and improved screening efforts (prostate and colorectal cancer) may help lessen the impact of these diseases over time. Deaths from each of these diseases can be lessened with appropriate education and prevention strategies, and the majority of these causes of death are preventable. Annual health screening for heart disease, hypertension, diabetes, and cancer would identify men at risk and lead to prevention or treatment. Delays in treatment often equate to worse prognosis and more time and money spent on treatments.

Many factors contribute to men's poor prevention and health seeking. These issues can be as basic as access, especially for minority men, but socioeconomic factors play a considerable role in risk as well, as many men may simply not know the screening schedules for annual PSA tests and colonoscopy (Gilbert, Elder, & Thorpe, 2016) while having difficulty navigating the process of making appointments and establishing trust with their provider. For some minority groups, this difficulty establishing trust has its roots in gender socialization that dictates that illness or asking for help is a sign of weakness and a decline in masculinity. Furthermore, these disparities are influenced by conscious and unconscious stereotyping, particularly for minority men, and this is heavily influenced by both historical and societal inequities, a discussion that is beyond the scope of this chapter. Several authors have explored racism, bias in care provision and bias in public health information as it pertains to both men and women of minority status (Ford & Airhihenbuwa, 2010; Jones et al., 2008; Smedley, Stith, & Nelson, 2002).

Self-Care Practices

Men's lack of health-seeking behaviors ultimately equates to poorer health outcomes and a heavier burden on the healthcare system (Baker et al., 2014). Separate from looking at causes of death, it is also striking that many men simply do not follow good health habits, and take care of themselves poorly. The National Center for Health Statistics data from 2015 looked at men 18 years and over: 12.4% were in fair or poor health, 29.9% had five or more drinks in 1 day in the past year, only 52.4% met the 2008 federal physical activity guidelines for aerobic exercise through leisure-time activity, and 16.7% currently smoked cigarettes (CDC, 2017a; 2017b). More alarming, a third of men ages 20 and over were obese or suffered from hypertension: 34.5% were obese, 32.6% measured high blood pressure or were taking an antihypertensive medication (CDC, 2017b).

Further statistics from the CDC compare the health of male veterans and nonveterans aged 25 to 64 in the United States between the years 2007 and 2010. Veterans were more likely to have two or more chronic conditions, report serious psychological distress more often, and have more work limitations than nonveterans. Self-reporting of being in fair or poor health and having two or more chronic conditions increased with age among both veterans and nonveterans (CDC, 2017c).

Interestingly, many of the early health studies focused solely on men; the earliest medical and drug trials were done exclusively with men as participants. It wasn't until the Framingham Study in 1948 on cardiovascular disease that more than half the participants were women. This was a stark contrast to most epidemiological studies at that time (Mahmood, Levy, Vasan, & Wang, 2014). That has changed in the current healthcare and health awareness environments; breast cancer research clearly elevated the visibility of a disfiguring illness and by doing so created a grassroots awareness of the importance of research studies and clinical trials for women's health issues. While women have embraced research and disease awareness, men have been less likely and slower to do the same. Only recently has prostate cancer awareness grown with its own ribbon (light blue) and month (September). Also, June is Men's Health month, although it is not uncommon to find providers who are unaware that the National Institutes of Health (NIH) and societies such as the American Society of Men's Health promote men's health awareness during each June because the second Sunday in June is Father's Day.

Authors from various disciplines have begun to identify social and cultural factors that inhibit men from health seeking and engaging in preventive healthcare practices. For example, gender roles and masculinity often conflict with health-seeking behaviors. Masculinity is viewed as emotional control, independence, and dominant or aggressive behaviors, all of which are negatively impacted by seeking healthcare or getting treatment for illnesses (McCreary, 1994; Vogel, Heimerdinger-Edwards, & Hubbard, 2011). The need for emotional control or fear of vulnerability, as well as psychological issues of embarrassment, anxiety, and fear related to using healthcare services, often deters men from getting needed care. Corporate expectations for men to work long days are rewarded monetarily and are valued by society, not giving men much time or access to healthcare or healthy behaviors. Health risks are often underestimated or symptoms minimized by men again owing to ideals of masculinity. When men do have health issues, they often view symptoms as not significant enough to warrant getting help. They focus on physical ailments rather than on psychological problems and they spend less time in doctor's appointments and receive less advice during those appointments than women. This poor communication with health professionals and obstacles of access to the system (difficulty making appointments, lack of knowledge of how to acquire care, and costs) are barriers to men (Hooper & Quallich, 2016, Krader, 2017; Yousaf, Grunfeld, & Hunter, 2015).

Men must overcome the barrier of not seeking care, but when they do seek care, there may be additional roadblocks that prevent them from getting the help they need. According to Hyde et al. (2016), men with prostate cancer have very specific needs that are not always met. More than half the participants in a study of men with localized prostate cancer identified areas of concern regarding sexuality and cancer-specific needs that were not addressed while undergoing care. Sexuality concerns that were identified included changes in sexual feelings and relationships. Prostate cancer–specific needs of greatest concern were losing their sense of masculinity and urinary incontinence. Men who were older, had less education, and had depression were less likely to seek help when needed. However, those who had better outcomes on sexual, urinary, and bowel domains and were older had fewer unmet needs (Hyde et al., 2016). Another factor that influenced help-seeking behaviors was erectile function. "[H]elp-seeking was associated with better sexual function and this may reflect that men who sought help had better outcomes. Alternatively, it may suggest that men were more likely to seek support for sexuality needs if they had better sexual function. This latter interpretation is consistent with prior research suggesting severity of erectile dysfunction deters help-seeking" (Hyde et al., 2016).

The recognition that men do not do as well as women in seeking healthcare, and the identification of some of the underlying reasons, allows the provider an opportunity to select strategies that may be available to influence and change individual men's, or group of men's, behavior to lead to more positive outcomes. The areas to manage include novel techniques to deliver healthcare information to men with community dialogues, media advertising, family support structures, national public health initiatives, and improved access to health insurance.

Men look for answers to health questions in nontraditional settings. A recent study on African American male preferences for where and from whom they receive health information revealed interesting results. From a self-survey of 512 African American men from Indiana (Indiana's Black Men's Health Study—BMHS), it was determined that factors such as age, income, and education determined if information from formal versus informal places and persons was preferred (Parker, Hunte, & Ohmit, 2017). Individuals with lower incomes preferred informal sources, such as a minister, barber, or family member, for their health information. Those who preferred to get their health information from a formal source (such as a doctor or nurse) were older men, were college graduates, had health insurance, and earned an income of more than $35,000/year. One of the most notable findings from this study was *where* these men preferred to get their health information. College-educated men preferred informal places such as the barbershop, church, or place of work. Older men, possibly due to the onset of more chronic health conditions, preferred formal places—doctor's office, hospital, or health fair. Social support, such as being married and feelings of discrimination, were not factors that affected health information in this study (Parker, 2017; Parker et al., 2017). This unique study concluded that a community effort to make available resources in a variety of areas outside the health fields improved healthcare literacy, and its authors suggested education for community leaders to facilitate getting men into the health arena for screenings and preventive care. Information about screenings and disease prevention obtained at the barber shop or churches may be more effective than holding health fairs at the hospital or clinic. These locations may be more effective than the shopping malls or grocery stores, which traditionally may attract more women. Rather than trying to change the societal notions of masculinity, identifying factors and working with them may increase the number of men who get care, which is the ultimate goal.

OTHER DIRECTIONS

Traditional media and social media are both robust outlets for dissemination of health information to men, especially teen and young adult men (Chapter 6). The rise of testosterone replacement therapies prescribed in recent years was driven by direct-to-consumer advertising (Morgentaler et al., 2014) that led more men to inquire about testosterone (Chapter 29), and then seek provider visits. It was found that "[e]ach exposure to a testosterone advertisement was associated with a monthly relative increase of 0.6% in new testosterone testing, 0.7% in treatment initiation, and 0.8% in initiation without recent testosterone serum measurement" (Krader, 2017). Although it is encouraging that men may have increased visits to their healthcare providers and discussed symptoms with them, it is suspected that many men may have been given testosterone replacement therapy without measurement in serum testosterone by providers who may not be familiar with diagnosis and management guidelines.

Social and societal attitudes affect many aspects of men's healthcare, and social support from family and friends plays a notable role in how men receive health information. Men receive more social support from female partners than male friends and tend to use avoidance coping mechanisms to deal with stress and illness (Hooper & Quallich, 2016; Keogh, 2015). Incorporating men into their spouse's healthcare may be an avenue to pursue.

Warner and Frey (Warner & Frey, 2013) looked at the "Well-Man Visit"—a preconception evaluation to optimize reproduction. They found this provided an excellent opportunity to promote healthy behaviors related to general health, including maintaining a healthy weight and regular exercise, disease prevention and screenings, stress reduction, and avoidance of risky behaviors (Warner & Frey, 2013).

Development and implementation of national and global initiatives are crucial in making a noted change. Few countries in the world have produced policies on men's health. Brazil, in 2009, and Australia, in 2010, were followed by Ireland's National's Men's Health Policy 2008–2013. A review of these policies confirms that dedicated national policies with attention to men's health are necessary to improve men's poorer survival rates. These policies mention risk factors—previously mentioned in this chapter—that contribute to men's poorer survival: greater levels of occupational exposures to physical and chemical hazards, behaviors associated with male norms of risk-taking and adventure and masculinity, and the fact that men are less likely to visit a doctor when ill and less likely to report symptoms when visiting a doctor (Baker, 2015).

The United States' national initiative on health, Healthy People 2020, promotes healthy behaviors in many areas, including physical activity, tobacco use, mental health, responsible sexual behavior, immunization, and access to healthcare services (CDC, 2014). Among initiatives aimed at males, several goals have been met: increasing the proportion of men who discussed PSA testing with their healthcare provider, increased aspirin use in males aged 45 to 79 with a history of cardiovascular disease, reduction in new hepatitis B infections among high-risk males, and a reduction in the prostate cancer death rate.

But other male-specific initiatives have not yet been met: a reduction in the number of new AIDS cases among adolescent and adult men who have sex with men (MSM), an increase in the proportion of sexually experienced males aged 15 to 44 years who received reproductive health services, and multiple initiatives on abstinence, condom use, formal instruction on sexually transmitted disease (STD) and AIDS prevention as well as increasing discussions between parents and adolescent males about these issues (Chapters 5 and 6).

There is room for additional improvements. Education in schools at all grade levels can promote a new concept of masculinity that is framed to include health-seeking behaviors. In the workplace, health information can be disseminated and health screenings can be promoted. Marginalized men—minorities, the prison population, and MSM—should be an increasing focus of health promotion as they have a higher burden of disease and early death (Baker et al., 2014) (see also Chapters 11, 12, 16, and 17).

Financial concerns and lack of healthcare insurance may pose formidable barriers to men if they want to seek healthcare. The Healthy People 2020 initiative goal of improving access to healthcare for all Americans finds the roadblocks to accessing healthcare are the high cost of care, inadequate or no insurance coverage, lack of availability of services, and lack of culturally competent care. Not surprisingly, disparities that affect access to healthcare include sex, sexual orientation, and gender identity, as well as race (Cheatham, Barksdale, & Rodgers, 2008), ethnicity, socioeconomic status, and age. Increasing access to a primary care provider improves access to preventive care and promotes healthy behaviors. The PPACA has taken several important steps to make it easier and more affordable for men, including minority men and single men to obtain healthcare coverage, although recent data regarding the success of these particular perspectives of the PPACA are sparse.

CONCLUSION

Understanding men's health behaviors is paramount in changing the statistics of men's disease and death. This is a fundamental investigation as there are racial and ethnic factors that directly influence a man's perceptions about self-care and health seeking. Actions to change men's health behaviors must recognize these societal roles of men and masculinity and focus on encouraging healthy behaviors and making more opportunities for preventive care. Working with societal norms in place now may require some ingenuity and creative measures to get health information to men in nontraditional settings. Global initiatives are also important to guiding healthcare to address concerns with men's preventive health and mortality; it highlights the value of culturally specific information about health issues and health screening needs. Health seeking for men is a complex process of education, self-confidence, and access. Education of the general population, as well as healthcare providers, is critical to making changes and improving men's health; as this education becomes increasingly successful, men will gain knowledge and skills by which to optimize their health and manage their own chronic conditions.

REFERENCES

111th United States Congress. (2010). Compilation of patient protection and affordable care act. Retrieved from http://housedocs.house.gov/energycommerce/ppacacon.pdf

Addis, M. E., & Mahalik, J. R. (2003). Men, masculinity, and the contexts of help seeking. American Psychologist, *58*(1), 5. doi:10.1037/0003-066X.58.1.5

American Psychological Association. (2014, August). Think again: Men and women share cognitive skills. Retrieved from http://www.apa.org/research/action/share.aspx

Baker, P. (2015). National men's health policies: Can they help? Trends in Urology & Men's Health, *6*, 24–26. doi:10.1002/tre.493

Baker, P., Dworkin, S. L., Tong, S., Banks, I., Shand, T., & Yarney, G. (2014). The men's health gap: Men must be included in the global health equity agenda. *Bulletin of the World Health Organization, 92*, 618–620. doi:10.2471/BLT.13.132795

Bruce, M. A., Griffith, D. M., & Thorpe, R. J., Jr. (2015). Social determinants of men's health disparities. *Family & Community Health, 38*(4), 281–283. doi:10.1097/FCH.0000000000000083

Centers for Disease Control and Prevention. (2014, May 20). Healthy people 2020. [Online documents]. Retrieved from http://www.cdc.gov/nchs/healthy_people/hp2020.htm

Centers for Disease Control and Prevention, U. S. Department of Health and Human Services. (2017a, May 28). Leading Causes of Death (LCOD) in Males United States, 2014 (current listing). Retrieved from https://www.cdc.gov/healthequity/lcod/index.htm

Centers for Disease Control and Prevention. (2017b, July 2). *Men's Health*. Retrieved from https://www.cdc.gov/nchs/fastats/mens-health.htm

Centers for Disease Control and Prevention. (2017c, July 2). The Health of Male Veterans and Nonveterans Aged 25-64: United States, 2007–2010. Retrieved from https://www.cdc.gov/nchs/products/databriefs/db101.htm

Cheatham, C. T., Barksdale, D. J., & Rodgers, S. G. (2008). Barriers to health care and health-seeking behaviors faced by black men. *Journal of the American Academy of Nurse Practitioners, 20*(11), 555–562. doi:10.1111/j.1745-7599.2008.00359.x

Courtenay, W. H. (2000a). Constructions of masculinity and their influences on men's well-being: A theory of gender and health. Social Science and Medicine, *50*, 1385–1401. doi:10.1016/S0277-9536(99)00390-1

Courtenay, W. H. (2000b). Behavioral factors associated with disease, injury, and death among men: Evidence and implications for prevention. The Journal of Men's Studies, 9, 81–142. doi:10.3149/jms.0901.81

Ford, C. L., & Airhihenbuwa, C. O. (2010). The public health critical race methodology: Praxis for antiracism research. *Social Science and Medicine, 71*, 1390–1398. doi:10.1016/j.socscimed.2010.07.030

Gilbert, K. L., Elder, K., & Thorpe, R. J. (2016). Health-seeking behavior and meeting the needs of the most vulnerable men. In J. J. Heidelbaugh (Ed.), *Men's health in primary care* (pp. 33–44). Cham, Switzerland: Humana Press.

Hooper, G. L., & Quallich, S. A. (2016). Health seeking in men: A concept analysis. *Urologic Nursing, 36*(4), 163–172. doi:10.7257/1053-816X.2016.36.4.163

Hyde, J. S. (2005). The gender similarities hypothesis. *American Psychologist, 60*(6), 581–592. doi:10.1037/0003-066X.60.6.581

Hyde, M. K., Newton, R. U., Galvao, D. A., Gardiner, R. A., Occhipinti, S., Lowe, A., ... Chambers, S. K. (2016). Men's help-seeking in the first year after diagnosis of localised prostate cancer. *European Journal of Cancer Care, 26*, 1–12. doi:10.1111/ecc.12497

Jemal, A., Ward, E. M., Johnson, C. J., Cronin, K. A., Ma, J., Ryerson, B., ... Weir, H. K. (2017). Annual Report to the Nation on the Status of Cancer, 1975-2014, Featuring Survival. *Journal of the National Cancer Institute, 109*, 9. doi:10.1093/jnci/djx030

Jones, C. P., Truman, B. I., Elam-Evans, L. D., Jones, C. A., Jones, C. Y., Jiles, R., ... Perry, G. S. (2008). Using "socially assigned race" to probe white advantages in health status. *Ethnicity and Disease, 18*, 496–504.

Keogh, E. (2015). Men, masculinity and pain. *Pain, 156*(12), 2408–2412. doi:10.1097/j.pain.0000000000000328

Krader, C. G. (2017, May 4). Study: Consumer ads prompt men to seek TRT. *Urology Times*, 11–15. Retrieved from www.urologytimes.modernmedicine.com/urology-times/news/study-consumer-ads-prompt-men-seek-trt

Mahmood, S. S., Levy, D., Vasan, R. S., & Wang, T. J. (2014). The framingham heart study and the epidemiology of cardiovascular diseases: A historical perspective. *Lancet, 383*(9921), 999–1008. doi:10.1016/S0140-6736(13)61752-3

McCreary, D. R. (1994). The male role and avoiding femininity. *Sex Roles, 31*(5), 517–531. doi:10.1007/BF01544277

Morgentaler, A., Khera, M., Maggi, M., & Zitzmann, M. (2014). Commentary: Who is a candidate for testosterone therapy? A synthesis of international expert opinions. *The Journal of Sexual Medicine, 11*(7), 1636–1645. doi:10.1111/jsm.12546

National Center for Health Statistics. (2017). Mortality in the United States, 2016. Retrieved from https://www.cdc.gov/nchs/data/databriefs/db293.pdf

Parker, L. J. (2017). Factors associated with black men's preferences for health information. *Health Promotion Practice, 18*(1), 119–126. doi:10.1177/1524839916664488

Parker, L. J., Hunte, H., & Ohmit, A. (2017). Discrimination in health care: Correlates of health care discrimination among black males. *American Journal of Men's Health, 11*(4), 999–1007. doi:10.1177/1557988315585164

Smedley, B. D., Stith, A. Y., & Nelson, A. R. (2002). *Unequal treatment: Confronting racial and ethnic disparities in healthcare*. Washington, DC: National Academies Press.

Vogel, D. L., Heimerdinger-Edwards, J. H., & Hubbard, A. (2011). "Boys Don't Cry." Examination of the links between endorsement of masculine norms, self-stigma, and help-seeking attitudes for men from diverse backgrounds. *Journal of Counseling Psychology, 58*(3), 368–382. doi:10.1037/a0023688

Warner, J. N., & Frey, K. A. (2013). The well-man visit: Addressing a man's health to optimize pregnancy outcomes. *The Journal of the American Board of Family Medicine, 26*(2), 196–202. doi:10.3122/jabfm.2013.02.120143

Yousaf, O., Grunfeld, E. A., & Hunter, M. S. (2015). A systematic review of the factors associated with delays in medical and psychological help-seeking among men. *Health Psychology Review, 9*(2), 264–276. doi:10.1080/17437199.2103.840954

CHAPTER 3

Basics of Sports Injury Assessment

Karen M. Myrick

■ INTRODUCTION

Each sport has its own "brand" of injuries, based on the specific movements that are endemic to that sport. But there are certain similarities among all sports that determine the risk for injury: anatomy, gender, age, training variables, engagement with stretching and warm-up prior to activity, individual history of prior injuries, and appropriate gear for the activity. Other factors influence the incidence of injury as well, including an individual's gait, strength, and overall biomechanics. These risk factors include medication and supplement use as well as nutrition, medical comorbid conditions, and prior surgeries.

This chapter discusses the basics of common sports injuries in men and provides the framework for the mechanism and evaluation of these injuries. A full discussion of the orthopedic examination relative to each condition is beyond the scope of this chapter, but a fundamental understanding of the anatomy and the basic maneuvers for evaluation will help in identifying the next steps for assessment of these potential complaints.

■ ACHILLES TENDON RUPTURE

Identification

The Achilles tendon is the largest tendon in the body and injuries to this tendon can affect both competitive and recreational athletes; over 80% of ruptures are due to recreational activities and occur in individuals with preexisting Achilles tendon issues (Leppilahti & Orava, 1998). These injuries tend to occur with activities such as running, jumping, sudden acceleration, and sudden deceleration. Certain conditions such as vascular diseases and neuropathy can contribute to rupture as well. Fluoroquinolone antibiotics are rarely associated with Achilles tendon rupture (Sode, Obel, Hallas, & Lassen, 2007), and oral glucocorticoids may increase the risk of tendinopathy (Jones, 1985). The identification of Achilles tendon ruptures occurs in the context of a comprehensive history and physical examination, and the use of diagnostic imaging. A stepoff at the Achilles tendon is typically found with complete tendon ruptures; the tendon should be palpated with the patient dorsiflexing and plantar-flexing the foot. Some patients with the complete tendon rupture are able to continue to ambulate on that leg. The findings on physical examination include a positive Thompson's test, which is performed by squeezing the calf, testing the integrity of the tendon, and is an accurate means for diagnosing a complete Achilles tendon rupture. The test is positive when there is no passive plantar flexion of the foot when the calf of the affected side is squeezed.

Suspected Achilles tendon injuries can be confirmed by a variety of imaging techniques, but it is primarily a clinical diagnosis. An ultrasound scan by a skilled musculoskeletal ultrasound technologist will be capable of evaluating the tendon for tears and determining the level of the tendon injury. The ultrasound test also helps distinguish between a true rupture and other potential pathology. The best imaging modality is MRI for evaluating the integrity of the Achilles tendon (Kruse, Stafilidis, & Tilp, 2017) and providing greater anatomic detail and accuracy.

Management

Rates of nonoperative management are on the rise with advances in nonoperative treatment, whereas in the past, operative management was most common (Park, Jeong, Choi, & Kim, 2017; Zellers, Cortes, & Silbernagel, 2016). The initial treatment consists of the patient being placed in a posterior splint in a slightly equinus position (plantar flexion) to keep the tendon approximated, and provided with crutches to avoid weight bearing on the injured side. This nonoperative treatment should be continued for 12 weeks, while patients who undergo surgery may need 2 to 3 months off from any work that requires walking.

Referral

Men with suspected or known Achilles tendon tears should be seen in consultation with an orthopedic surgeon. Treatment in either a nonoperative or operative fashion should begin urgently; therefore, follow-up within 3 to 7 days is prudent. The risks and benefits of operative versus nonoperative management should be discussed at length with the orthopedic surgeon.

■ GROIN STRAIN OR SPORTS HERNIA

Groin strains are common in sports in which athletes are involved in frequent changes in direction, and sports in which activity comes in bursts, instead of constant motion, and when no hernia is found. Groin strains can be classified as adductor, iliopsoas, inguinal, or pubic-related groin pain (Mosler et al., 2017). Other terms for this condition include hockey groin, sportsman hernia, or athletic pubalgia. All of these terms describe a condition causing persistent unilateral pain in the groin and represent a clinical diagnosis. This condition results from chronic, repetitive trauma or stress to the musculotendinous portions of the groin, and overuse of the lower abdominal muscles and contributes to the development of the groin strain.

Identification

Men may present with complaints of lower abdominal or groin pain that is nonspecific. With symptoms that are nonspecific and insidious in onset, a delay in diagnosis from the time of initial presentation may occur. A thorough history is important in diagnosing a sports hernia, as the mechanism of injury is considered to be overuse. The symptoms are often worse with activity and improve with rest (Cohn, Lerebours, & Strauss, 2015).

Physical examination includes a digital palpation of the inguinal ring through invagination of the scrotal pouch in men (Santilli et al., 2016). Palpation in a positive inguinal hernia case yields a protrusion of a mass in the inguinal ring. Obtaining plain radiographs is useful in illuminating differential diagnoses. With normal radiographic findings, a dynamic high-resolution ultrasound scan is indicated.

The typical presentation for a patient with groin strain is pain in the groin area, with a history of acute injury; groin strain is most commonly identified in men involved in high-intensity sports such as hockey or soccer. A common mechanism of injury is kicking or an abrupt change in direction. Pain during adduction is the hallmark sign of a groin strain (Chaudhari, Jamison, McNally, Pan, & Schmitt, 2014). Coughing or sneezing may aggravate the pain but may also enable the individual to localize his pain to the groin. Examination of the individual in the frog-leg position while he adducts against resistance from the provider suggests a sports hernia, in the absence of finding an inguinal hernia.

Imaging may be unnecessary in patients who present with groin strain. The only indications for imaging techniques would be for those patients who are not improving within a 4- to 6-week period. As is typical with most soft tissue injuries, physiology allows for soft tissue healing within a 6-week period.

Management

Athletes in sports in which changing directions frequently is common have tried to prevent and treat groin strains by wearing compression shorts (Chaudhari et al., 2014). As a muscle strain, these injuries heal well with relative rest, ice, compression, and elevation. Gentle stretching is usually started once the pain has decreased, and cross friction massage has been used as a modality to assist in recovery as well.

Patients who are diagnosed with a sports hernia should be evaluated for the impact this disorder has on their activities of daily living and the effect the condition has on their ability to participate in sports at a level that they desire. Any patient unable to return to his desired level of performance and play should be referred for physical therapy and further evaluation.

Men who have been diagnosed with an inguinal hernia should be referred to a general surgeon for a discussion of surgical repair.

Referral

These soft tissue injuries are typically managed by the primary care provider, but refractory cases may be referred to a sports medicine or orthopedic specialist, who may choose to proceed with imaging studies such as MRI or an ultrasound examination. Refractory cases may be considered as lasting a period of longer than 6 to 8 weeks, and may require exploratory surgery. A referral for physical therapy will assist the athlete in returning to play and in identifying any underlying muscle imbalances.

TRANSIENT QUADRIPARESIS

Transient quadriparesis is also known as a "stinger" or "burner" and describes temporary neuropraxis that results from a stretch or compression of the upper roots of the brachial plexus (Tosti, Rossy, Sanchez, & Lee, 2016), a direct blow to the supraclavicular fossa, or a combination of neck hyperextension and ipsilateral lateral flexion. The condition is most common in athletes who participate in contact sports, such as rugby, wrestling, or football, and signifies peripheral nerve dysfunction and injury. This condition is typically transient but can lead to prolonged weakness and time lost from participation in athletics; furthermore, this injury tends to recur and create additional disability and pain.

Identification

After a history of a stretch or compression injury, patients typically present with symptoms of a radiating pain that is fleeting in the upper extremities to weakness and numbness that may last a few weeks (Tosti, Rossy, Sanchez, & Lee, 2016). Immediately after contact, the individual may report burning pain in the supraclavicular area that can radiate down the affected arm; generally, he will describe a circumferential, nondermatomal pattern to the pain. It is imperative that the provider rule out other causes of the symptoms, prior to diagnosing the condition as transient quadriparesis, and investigate a history of previous similar injuries. These conditions include disc herniation, and fracture of the cervical or thoracic vertebrae. Physical examination may yield evidence of muscle atrophy (if this is a recurrent injury) or tenderness and spasm along with maladaptive use of the affected shoulder and arm. Strength, sensation, and reflexes should be examined on the affected side.

There is no role for imaging, if the symptoms are transient, except in the case of suspected cervical spine involvement. In this instance CT or MRI may be appropriate, based on clinical presentation. If the condition does not resolve, there may be a role for electrodiagnostic studies to aid in the identification and localization of the affected nerve roots.

Management

The management of a transient quadriparesis consists of supportive care, and rehabilitation that focuses on strengthening and correcting any strength deficits, sport-specific therapy, and range of motion acquisition. Repetitive evaluation may occur at the following week and weekly thereafter until the condition normalizes. Any potential predisposing factors such as postural abnormalities must also be identified. Return to play is generally granted after patients have full resolution of their symptoms, are pain free and neurologically intact, and have regained full strength and full range of motion (Huang, Anissipour, McGee, & Lemak, 2015). Athletes are advised to always use protective equipment to protect the injured area, and cannot be fully cleared for activity until symptoms are not provoked during practice or warm-up for the designated activity.

Referral

Referral to a qualified physical therapist is recommended. Patients who present with symptoms that are not improving, or that continue beyond a few weeks, should be referred to neurosurgery for further evaluation. Typically, prior to referral to neurosurgery, an MRI scan should be completed.

ACROMIOCLAVICULAR JOINT INJURIES

The acromioclavicular (AC) joint is diarthrodial with an intra-articular disc surrounded by a dense capsule and ligamentous support (Roberson & Tokish, 2016). The coracoclavicular (CC) ligaments provide the primary restraint to superior displacement of the clavicle (Roberson & Tokish, 2016). The AC joint injury is a common condition, and more common in the contact athlete (Roberson & Tokish, 2016), occurring from direct trauma to the superior or lateral aspect of the shoulder when the arm is adducted, such as occurs with a fall onto the shoulder. The degree of injury is directly related to the force applied, and direct trauma can displace the shoulder and scapula in relation to the clavicle.

Identification

In most cases, the injury is identified without imaging studies being absolutely necessary, based on a history of the suspected injury and examination of the joint itself. Men should first be asked about the precise mechanism of injury. The injury can also occur with a fall onto an outstretched hand. Physical examination will help identify the extent of the injury and examination findings can range from tenderness over the AC joint to potential visible deformity of the shoulder. All of the shoulder components should be palpated for tenderness, which will suggest the extent of the involved structures. Abduction of the arm across the body can also be performed; if this produces pain, it helps confirm the diagnosis of an AC joint injury.

All patients who present with potential AC separation should have bilateral AC views taken with plain radiography. The Rockwood classification for AC joint injuries identifies type I as no displacement in the CC ligament distance between the injured side and the noninjured side (Rockwood, 1984). Type II is defined as minimal displacement, type III is defined as <100% increase in the distance, type IV is posterior displacement through the trapezius, type V is >100% increase in the CC distance, and type VI is subacromial or subcoracoid displacement (Rockwood, 1984). In some instances, ultrasound evaluation of the shoulder may be an important adjunct to plain x-ray films.

Management

Conservative management is effective for treating patients with grade 1–3 injuries. Conservative treatment consists of physical therapy, return to normal range of motion, decreasing inflammation and pain, return of full function and strength, and sport-specific training. A key to full recovery is to gradually increase resistance and avoid activities that cause pain to the affected shoulder.

Referral

Referral is recommended for a course of 4 to 8 weeks with a physical therapist. Referral to an orthopedic surgeon is recommended for grade 3 and above injuries.

SCAPHOID FRACTURE

Scaphoid fractures commonly occur after a fall onto an outstretched hand and may not be immediately apparent on x-ray studies taken after the injury. If the mechanism of injury involves a fall onto an outstretched hand, the provider should assume a scaphoid fracture until proved otherwise; this injury accounts for up to 10% of all hand fractures (Geissler, 2001). Fractures occur as a result of direct axial compression of the scaphoid bone or hyperextension of the wrist.

Identification

The mechanism of injury for scaphoid fractures is a fall onto an outstretched hand, often referred to as FOOSH, but this is a radiographic diagnosis. Early identification and treatment are of utmost importance in improving outcomes of scaphoid fractures (Rambau & Rhee, 2015). Pain will localize to the radial side of the wrist proximal to the thumb, but swelling may be present on the opposite side. Focal tenderness may be noted at one of three locations, indicating a fracture: the volar prominence (Kohyama, Kanamori, Tanaka, Hara, & Yamazaki, 2016); the anatomic snuffbox; or distal to the distal radius located just to the ulnar side of the extensor carpi radialis tendon (Lister's tubercle).

Delays of even 4 weeks for treatment can lead to significantly higher rates of delayed union and nonunion (Rambau & Rhee, 2015). Imaging studies should include standard posteroanterior (PA) and lateral views of the wrist, as well as slightly supinated with ulnar deviation while clenching the hand into a fist. This maneuver extends the scaphoid and permits thorough evaluation of its entire length (Rambau & Rhee, 2015). Plain radiographs should be evaluated for ligament disruption as a clue to scaphoid fracture. CT or MRI within 72 hours of the injury may provide a more rapid diagnosis.

Management

Nonoperative treatment consists of immobilization in a thumb spica cast for 2 to 6 months. Immobilization is important, especially in the absence of clear diagnosis. Return to sport is possible with a cast that is suitable for the sport that the athlete is playing. Identification of this injury is key as there is a very high percentage of nonunion of this fracture, highlighting the need for follow-up x-rays to confirm the fracture is healing.

Referral

Up to 45% of athletes with late presentation to hand surgery were initially diagnosed with a sprain. It is important to refer and treat any patient who presents with pain in the wrist or hand who has sustained an injury from a fall onto an outstretched hand, or with an open fracture. Referral to a hand surgeon is the optimal procedure for further evaluation and treatment, especially knowing the close monitoring required during healing of fracture.

BOXER'S FRACTURE: FIFTH METACARPAL NECK FRACTURE

A boxer's fracture is aptly named for the common mechanism of injury during which it occurs—a punch or striking an object with a closed fist—but may also result from a fall onto the outstretched hand, although this is an uncommon mechanism for this particular injury (Joyce et al., 2013). Blunt force trauma to the back of the hand can also result in a boxer's fracture. The boxer's fracture is a fracture of the fifth metacarpal neck and is common in young men (Dunn, Kusnezov, Orr, Pallis, & Mitchell, 2016). The boxer's fracture is the most common fracture of the hand accounting for 20% of all fractures (Dunn et al., 2016).

Identification

Patients will present with the chief complaint of hand pain, after punching an object with a closed fist, and may have noticed a visible deformity as well. Men are likely to present with a swollen and focal tenderness over the fractured metacarpal; if there is tenderness and ecchymosis on the palmer surface of the hand, this is likely to confirm the diagnosis of fracture. A neurologic examination of the hand must be done to confirm that there is no neurologic or vascular compromise as a result of the injury. The hand should be carefully examined for any open wounds; if the injury occurred as the result of a fight, the open wound may have been sustained while striking a tooth, raising concerns for contamination of the wound.

This is a radiographic diagnosis. Radiographs of the hand should include anteroposterior, lateral, and oblique views. The findings of a fifth metacarpal fracture and angulation at the neck of the bone indicate a boxer's fracture.

Management

The boxer's fracture is typically treated in a nonoperative fashion with immobilization in a splint or cast for 6 weeks. Ideally, repeat radiographs after 3 weeks are taken to assure that there is no change in the alignment of the fracture. An ulnar gutter splint will successfully immobilize fractures of the fifth metacarpal neck. Men with this injury will benefit from appropriate analgesic medication and ice to improve overall comfort level in the 2 to 3 days after the injury. In healthy men, this injury should heal in 4 to 6 weeks. Patients can be cleared to return to their sport and everyday activity when they are pain free and have regained their complete range of motion.

There may be a treatment delay after sustaining this injury. Providers may notice decreased hand function, an increased level of pain, and alterations to the degree of bony healing on radiographs. This scenario would necessitate referral to a hand surgeon, especially in the presence of increased pain and deformity of the hand.

Referral

Referral is indicated for patients who have a rotational deformity or greater than 30 degrees of angulation in the fracture or open metacarpal neck fractures, especially if associated with any neurovascular impairment (Joyce et al., 2013). Rotational deformity and angulation greater than 30 degrees has been associated with long-term discomfort and functional deficits (16). It is best to refer the patient with findings of angulation or rotation to a hand surgeon for evaluation and treatment, and for exploring the option for surgical intervention.

ANKLE SPRAIN

Ankle sprains are one of the most common musculoskeletal injuries that primary care providers will see in practice. The ligaments of the ankle provide a variety of functions including mechanical stability and proprioceptive and location information, and direct the motion of the joint. Half of ankle sprains occur during athletic activity, and they are more common in males than in females in the 15- to 24-year old range (Myrick, 2014). The mechanism of injury will determine the location of the sprain:

- *Lateral sprain* results with inversion of the plantar-flexed foot, causing damage to the entire lateral ligament complex of the ankle. This injury is less common but can be more debilitating and results in significant instability of the ankle.
- *Medial sprain* is far less frequently seen, owing to the strength of the ligament. The mechanism of injury is more likely to cause a fracture of the medial malleolus of the ankle, rather than a medial ankle sprain.
- *Syndesmotic sprain* (high ankle sprain) results after dorsiflexion or eversion of the ankle, and contributes to chronic instability of the ankle itself. This injury is most commonly seen in contact sports.

Identification

Men presenting with an ankle strain must be queried about the mechanism of injury, whether they could walk after the injury, and whether there was a history of previous ankle injury. Men will present with ankle pain that began with a traumatic injury; the majority of ankle sprains occur with excessive inversion of the joint (Myrick, 2014) and involve injury to the soft tissue and ligaments of the ankle. Key points of the physical examination include inspection for gross abnormalities, swelling, and ecchymosis; and palpation for point tenderness; and a neurovascular assessment. Tenderness over the ligaments as a nonspecific finding that could indicate injury. Special tests include the anterior drawer test, talar tilt test, and squeeze test (Myrick, 2014) (Table 3.1); the ankle should be examined for pain with gentle inversion and eversion of the joint.

If a patient exhibits positive bony tenderness on physical examination, radiographs should be obtained and consist of anteroposterior, lateral, and oblique/mortise views.

Management

Treatment without any significant residual laxity includes the principles of RICE, or rest, ice, compression, and elevation (Myrick, 2014). Activity should be encouraged during the recovery phase and may consist of non-weight-bearing activity including swimming. When tolerated, pedaling a stationary bicycle starting with low resistance is also a good recommendation.

Referral

If excessive laxity is found on physical examination, or felt by the patient once he returns to activity, referral to an orthopedic surgeon is recommended. If radiographs are obtained, and they show any widening of the ankle mortise, referral to an orthopedic surgeon is indicated (Myrick, 2016).

TABLE 3.1 Special Tests for Evaluation of Ankle Sprain

Maneuver	Description
Squeeze test	Compression of the fibula against the tibia at the mid-calf level. Will elicit pain in the region of the anterior tibiofibular ligament (anterior to the lateral malleolus and proximal to the ankle joint) indicating a syndesmotic sprain.
External rotation stress test	Stabilize leg proximal to the ankle joint while grasping the plantar aspect of the foot and rotating the foot externally relative to the tibia. Test is positive if pain in the region of the anterior tibiofibular ligament (anterior to the lateral malleolus and proximal to the ankle joint).
Anterior drawer test	Detects excessive anterior displacement of the talus on the tibia. Patient's foot in the neutral position (slightly plantar-flexed and inverted); lower leg is stabilized by the examiner with one hand; with the opposite hand, the examiner grasps the heel while the patient's foot rests on the anterior aspect of the examiner's arm. Test is positive if steady anterior force applied to the heel reveals laxity. Has limited usefulness in the acute setting.
Talar tilt test	Detects excessive ankle inversion; limited usefulness in the acute setting. With the ankle in neutral position, gentle inversion force is applied to affected ankle; degree of inversion is compared with the uninjured side.

ANTERIOR CRUCIATE LIGAMENT TEAR

The anterior cruciate ligament (ACL) stabilizes the knee, and a tear in this ligament is one of the most common traumatic knee injuries. It is estimated that more than 120,000 ACL injuries occur in the United States each year (Myrick, 2016), but the actual instance may be higher as there is no mechanism for tracking the incidence of ACL in the general population. It has been suggested that the rates of ACL injury are increasing (Weinberg, Williamson, Gebhart, Knapik, & Voss, 2017), and this injury is more common in football, tennis, soccer, and basketball, and is generally noted in athletes (low-energy injury) and trauma victims (high-energy injury). However, it is worth noting that the majority of ACL tears occur in noncontact athletic scenarios.

The precise mechanism of injury hasn't been definitely established for this injury, but weakness and disparity in the hamstrings and poor biomechanics could be contributing factors. Increased friction and traction of the playing surface may be a factor, especially when coupled with a particular shoe type (e.g., basketball court). The typical injury occurs with a running or jumping athlete who decelerates rapidly, pivots, and changes direction, creating a lateral stress on the knee. If the injury occurs as a result of contact, the mechanism usually involves a direct blow that causes hyperextension; this mechanism is more common in football.

Identification

Patients typically present after either a contact or noncontact injury with a mechanism that includes either a valgus force or hyperextension of the knee joint. Patients may or may not have felt or heard a "pop" at the time of the injury, and typically a large joint effusion is present shortly after the time of injury (Myrick, 2016; Chapter 6). ACL injuries are typically due to sudden deceleration, from hyperextension of the knee or pivoting in place.

TABLE 3.2 Special Tests for Evaluation of ACL Tear

Maneuver	Description
Lachman test	Injured knee is placed in 30° of flexion and stabilized at the femur with one hand, as the other hand pulls the proximal tibia interiorly. Increased movement suggests ACL injury.
Pivot shift test	Begin with knee in extension; hold lower leg with one hand and internally rotate the tibia while placing stress on the knee with the other hand. This will cause subluxation if the ACL is torn, resulting in a "clunk" in the knee as the tibia is reduced. Has limited usefulness in the acute setting owing to patient guarding.
Anterior drawer test	Patient is supine and knee is flexed at 90°. Proximal tibia is gripped with both hands and pulled anteriorly; test is positive if there is anterior movement. Has limited usefulness in the acute setting.

ACL, anterior cruciate ligament.

The physical examination includes inspection; palpation; testing of mobility, strength, and stability; and performance of special tests of ACL integrity (Table 3.2) that are most sensitive and specific for ACL injury. These tests can be limited in their specificity by the degree of guarding and patient pain.

While plain x-rays may be completed in the setting of trauma, radiographs cannot diagnose ACL tears. MRI is the best imaging choice to confirm this diagnosis; alternatively, this diagnosis can be confirmed via knee arthroscopy (which is considerably more invasive than MRI).

Management

Once an ACL injury is suspected, the patient should wear a knee immobilizer and be given crutches to maintain a non-weight-bearing status. Acute management consists of the RICE protocol (rest, ice, compression, and elevation of the affected extremity). Over-the-counter medication is typically sufficient to control pain. Physical therapy referral to enhance balance, strengthen adjacent structures, and improve core strength can help prevent subsequent reinjury.

Referral

Referral to an orthopedic surgeon is warranted for discussion of treatment options, which include surgical intervention. ACL injuries can be managed either operatively or conservatively depending on the degree of injury, damage to adjacent structures, and the desire to preserve athletic performance. Men who experience knee instability may also be appropriate candidates for surgical repair.

■ EPICONDYLITIS

Epicondylitis can be medial or lateral, and is the inflammation of the tendons of the forearm and the muscle and tendon area around the outside of the elbow. This is also known as tennis elbow or golfer's elbow, but there are multiple recreational and occupational activities that can lead to epicondylitis. Typically, epicondylitis results from an overuse injury or repetitive strain/gripping associated with wrist extension or flexion (Buchanan & Hughes, 2017), such as with poor form for tennis backhand. A degenerative overuse has been suggested as the mechanism of injury, and tennis and golf are not the only activities that induce the problem (Buchanan & Hughes, 2017). Smoking, obesity, repetitive movement for 2 hours a day, and managing physical loads over 50 pounds appear to be contributing risk factors for the development of epicondylitis, as does an age between 45 and 54 (Shiri, Viikari-Juntura, Varonen, & Heliövaara, 2006). Complaints are divided into lateral pain and medial pain.

Identification

Patient presentation includes a patient who is complaining of chronic elbow pain, and can typically point to either the lateral or medial side of the joint. A history of overuse or new activity is typically reported, and there will be reports of varying degrees of impact on recreational and work activity. Physical examination would rule in or out other causes of the discomfort, such as a radiculopathy (Myrick, 2016). Lateral epicondylitis is identified by pain with palpation of the lateral epicondyle and proximal wrist extensor muscles, pain with wrist extension and elbow in full extension, and pain with wrist flexion and elbow in full extension. Medial epicondylitis is identified by pain with palpation of the medial epicondyle and proximal wrist extensor muscles, pain with resisted wrist extension and elbow in full extension, and pain with terminal wrist flexion and elbow in full extension. Imaging studies are helpful if the presentation is not straightforward, but are usually unnecessary as part of the initial evaluation of this complaint.

Management

Conservative treatment is the mainstay of epicondylitis. This consists of stretching, limiting activities, epicondylitis straps, and icing. Management can also include splints or a counterpoint brace, avoiding activities that exacerbate the pain, and physical therapy to modify the actions that contribute to the injury. Oral nonsteroidal anti-inflammatory drugs (NSAIDs) are helpful in the short term, and topical NSAIDs may improve comfort level with acute injury.

Referral

If conservative treatment fails, referral to an orthopedic surgeon for steroid injections or surgical intervention is suggested (Buchanan & Hughes, 2017) if there is limited improvement after 6 months of conservative management.

CONCUSSION

A concussion is an injury to the brain that results in temporary loss of normal brain function (Myrick, 2015). The American Academy of Neurology defines concussion as a trauma-induced alteration in mental status that may or may not involve loss of consciousness (American Academy of Neurology, 1997). In the United States, contact sports (football, soccer, and rugby) are significant contributors to the incidence of concussion, but nonsport causes are prevalent as well (motor vehicle accidents, falls, and recreational accidents). Mild concussion or traumatic brain injuries are also common among soldiers.

Injury results from cortical contusions due to coup and contrecoup injuries, and the resulting axonal injury. There is no role for imaging, as there are no findings on MRI or CT scan. Many cases of concussion do not have external signs of head trauma.

Identification

Concussions can be identified by the history of a fall with head trauma, or a blow to the head, as part of the patient's history of the present illness. Early symptoms include memory loss, or an inability to recall events immediately before and after the injury. The individual may repeatedly ask the same question(s). Symptoms may progress over minutes to hours to headache, vertigo, nausea/vomiting, and a lack of awareness of surroundings; symptoms may continue to progress to light sensitivity, sleep disturbance, and mood or cognitive issues.

The examination includes a thorough history along with a thorough neurologic assessment and mental status examination, and attention to vision. The most prevalent signs of concussion commonly include incoordination, postural instability, disorientation or an inability to focus attention, slurred speech, confusion, amnesia, and nausea or vomiting (American Academy of Neurology, 1997). Several standardized tools have been suggested for the evaluation of suspected concussion, including the Post-Concussion Symptom Scale and Graded Symptom Checklist, the Immediate Post-Concussion Assessment and Cognitive Testing (ImPACT), the Westmead Post-Traumatic Amnesia Scale (WPTAS), the Galveston Orientation and Amnesia Test (GOAT), and the Military Acute Concussion Evaluation (MACE).

A CT scan without contrast is recommended for those patients with concerning or rapidly progressive neurologic deficits during the initial assessment. These indications include skull fracture, seizures, two or more episodes of vomiting, any sign of basilar skull fracture, use of anticoagulants, and age 65 or older (Stiell et al., 2017). MRI is not usually indicated in the acute setting. Any patient with suspected complications should be admitted to the hospital for observation, especially in the case of older patients who may not have an adequate support system that can monitor them at home.

Management

Recognizing the typical recovery for signs and symptoms of concussion is paramount for identifying problems with recovery and rehabilitation from the injury. Three vital considerations in the management of concussion include identifying neurologic emergencies after injury, management of neurologic sequelae, and prevention of chronic/cumulative brain injury. Recovery is defined as the absence of symptoms at rest and no provocation or return of symptoms with exertion (Colvin et al., 2009). Management will be based on the symptoms and needs will be based on the residual symptoms. In the case of uncomplicated concussions, adults will benefit from rest for at least 24 hours and a gradual return to activity and exercise or athletics.

The number of concussions before retiring from play is a subject of considerable debate. Some believe that any more than three concussions puts an athlete at greater risk of permanent neurocognitive impairment; the decision to continue in the sport remains personal with medical guidance. There are available guidelines (Box 3.1) to guide the provider in determining when athletes should return to activity.

BOX 3.1 GUIDELINES ON RETURN TO PLAY AFTER CONCUSSION

2012 Consensus Statement on Concussion in Sport

McCrory, P., Meeuwisse, W. H., Aubry, M., Cantu, B., Dvřák, J., Echemendia, R. J., ... Turner, M. (2013). Consensus statement on concussion in sport: the 4th International Conference on Concussion in Sport held in Zurich, November 2012. *British Journal of Sports Medicine, 47*(5), 250–258. doi:10.1136/bjsports-2013-092313

(continued)

BOX 3.1 GUIDELINES ON RETURN TO PLAY AFTER CONCUSSION (*continued*)

2013 American Academy of Neurology Systematic Review and Evidence-Based Guideline

Giza, C. C., Kutcher, J. S., Ashwal, S., Barth, J., Getchius, T. S. D., Gioia, G. A., ... Zafonte, R. (2013). Summary of evidence-based guideline update: Evaluation and management of concussion in sports: Report of the Guideline Development Subcommittee of the American Academy of Neurology. *Neurology, 80*(24), 2250–2257. doi:10.1212/wnl.0b013e31828d57dd

2013 American Medical Society for Sports Medicine Position Statement

Harmon, K. G., Drezner, J. A., Gammons, M., Guskiewicz, K. M., Halstead, M., Herring, S. A., ... Roberts, W. O. (2012). American Medical Society for Sports Medicine position statement: Concussion in sport. *British Journal of Sports Medicine, 47*(1), 15–26. doi:10.1136/bjsports-2012-091941

Referral

When a patient presents with symptoms lasting longer than 7 to 10 days, or has symptoms that are not improving or are concerning, referral to a neuropsychologist or sports medicine provider is warranted to rule out postconcussion syndrome.

CONCLUSION

Certain sports-related injuries are more likely to happen in the male population. This chapter has provided an overview of assessment and physical examination points that will be useful when evaluating men presenting with sports-related injuries. When these injuries occur in men who are older, it may prompt a functional assessment examination as well.

CLINICAL PEARLS

- Acute Achilles tendon rupture is most likely to occur in men when sudden shear stress is applied to an already weakened tendon.
- "Burners" are commonly brief and self-limited, but full recovery can take weeks or even months, and frequent reexamination is mandatory.
- Severe shoulder injuries should be referred urgently to an orthopedic specialist for operative management to avoid permanent neurologic or vascular deficits.
- The scaphoid bone in the wrist has a tenuous blood supply that runs from distal to proximal leading to the high percentage of nonhealing fractures.
- Fifth metacarpal neck fractures result in dorsal angulation of the apex of the fracture, causing loss of the usual knuckle contour and aiding in identification of fracture.
- Initial treatment of an uncomplicated ankle sprain consists of rest, ice, compression, elevation (RICE), early mobilization, and support orthosis with early weight bearing to promote early return to activity.
- Men who sustain an athletic-related ACL injury will report feeling a "pop" in the knee, acute swelling thereafter, and a feeling that the knee is unstable; almost all patients with an acute ACL injury manifest a knee effusion.

(*continued*)

■ **CLINICAL PEARLS (*continued*)**

- Evidence supporting specific treatments for epicondylitis is sparse; symptomatic management is recommended with consideration for physical therapy for strengthening.
- All men with mild concussion should be medically evaluated, and then observed for at least 24 hours owing to the risk of potential complications.

RESOURCES FOR THE CLINICIAN

The American Academy Orthopedic Surgeons: www.orthoinfo.org
The American College of Sports Medicine: www.acsm.org

RESOURCES FOR THE PATIENT

The American College of Sports Medicine public site: www.acsm.org/public-information
Centers for Disease Control and Prevention: www.cdc.gov/traumaticbraininjury/symptoms.html
The Concussion Legacy Foundation: concussionfoundation.org/concussion-resources?gclid=EAIaIQobChMItvDwxIvf1wIVgrrACh398Ad9EAAYASAAEgKYm_D_BwE

REFERENCES

American Academy of Neurology. (1997). Practice parameter: The management of concussion in sports (summary statement). Report of the Quality Standards Subcommittee. *Neurology, 48*, 581–585. doi:10.1212/WNL.48.3.581

Buchanan, B., & Hughes, J. (2017). *Tennis Elbow (Lateral Epicondylitis)*. Island, FL: StatPearls Publishing LLC.

Chaudhari, A., Jamison, S., McNally, M., Pan, X., & Schmitt, L. (2014). Hip adductor activations during run-to-cut maneuvers. *Journal of Sport Sciences, 32*(14), 1333–1340. doi:10.1080/02640414.2014.889849

Cohn, R., Lerebours, F., & Strauss, E. (2015). Sports hernia and extra-articular causes of groin pain in the Athlete. *Bulletin of the Hospital for Joint Diseases, 73*(2), 90–99.

Colvin, A., Mullen, J., Lovel, M., West, R. V., Collins, M. W., & Groh, M. (2009). The role of concussion history and gender in recovery from soccer-related concussion. *American Journal of Sports Medicine, 37*(9), 1699–1704. doi:10.1177/0363546509332497

Dunn, J., Kusnezov, N., Orr, J., Pallis, M., & Mitchell, J. (2016, May/June). The boxer's fracture: Splint immobilization is not necessary. *Orthopedics, 39*(3), 188–192. doi:10.3928/01477447-20160315-05

Geissler, W. B. (2001). Carpal fractures in athletes. *Clinics in Sports Medicine, 20*(1), 167–188. doi:10.1016/S0278-5919(05)70254-4

Huang, P., Anissipour, A., McGee, W., & Lemak, L. (2015). Return-to-play recommendations after cervical, thoracic, and lumbar spine injuries: A comprehensive review. *Orthopedic Surgery, 8*(1), 19–26. doi:10.1177/1941738115610753

Jones, J. G. (1985). Achilles tendon rupture following steroid injection. *JBJS, 67*(1), 170. doi:10.2106/00004623-198567010-00025

Joyce, C., Kelly, J., Chan, J., Colgan, G., O'Brian, D., McCabe, J., & Curtin, W. (2013). Second to fourth digit ratio confirms aggressive tendencies in patients with boxers fractures. *Injury, 44*, 1636–1639. doi:10.1016/j.injury.2013.07.018

Kohyama, S., Kanamori, A., Tanaka, T., Hara, Y., & Yamazaki, M. (2016). Stress fracture of the scaphoid in an elite junior tennis player: A case report and review of the literature. *Journal of Medical Case Reports, 10*, 8. doi:10.1186/s13256-015-0785-3

Kruse, A., Stafilidis, S., & Tilp, M. (2017). Ultrasound and magnetic resonance imaging are not interchangeable to assess the Achilles tendon cross-sectional-area. *European Journal of Applied Physiology, 117*(1), 73–82. doi:10.1007/s00421-016-3500-1

Leppilahti, J., & Orava, S. (1998). Total Achilles tendon rupture. A review. *Sports Medicine, 25*(2), 79. doi:10.2165/00007256-199825020-00002

Mosler, A., Weir, A., Eiral, C., Farooq, A., Thorborg, K., Whiteley, R., ... Crossley, K. (2018). Epidemiology of time loss groin injuries in a men's professional football league: a 2-year prospective study of 17 clubs and 606 players. *British Journal of Sports Medicine, 52*(5), 292–297. doi:10.1136/bjsports-2016-097277

Myrick, K. (2014). Clinical assessment of ankle sprains. *Journal of Orthopaedic Nursing, 33*(5), 244–248. doi:10.1097/NOR.0000000000000083

Myrick, K. (2015). Head injuries in soccer. *Rehabilitation Nursing, 41*(4), 197–201. doi:10.1002/rnj.249

Myrick, K. (2016). *Orthopedic and sports medicine case studies for nurse practitioners*. New York, NY: Springer Publishing Company.

Park, Y., Jeong, S., Choi, G., & Kim, H. (2017). How early must an acute Achilles tendon rupture be repaired? *Injury*, 48, 776–780. doi:10.1016/j.injury.2017.01.020

Rambau, G., & Rhee, P. (2016). Evaluation and management of nondisplaced scaphoid waist fractures in the Athlete. *Operative Techniques in Sports Medicine, 24*, 87–93. doi:10.1053/j.otsm.2016.01.005

Roberson, T., & Tokish, J. (2016). Acromioclavicular joint injuries in the contact Athlete. *Operative Techniques in Sports Medicine, 15*, 254–262. doi:10.1053/j.otsm.2016.09.004

Rockwood, C. (1984). Injuries to the acromioclavicular joint. In C. A. Rockwood Jr. & D. P. Green (Eds.), *Fractures in the adult* (2nd ed., pp. 860–910). Philadelphia, PA: JB Lippincott.

Santilli, O., Nardelli, N., Santilli, H., Tripoloni, D., Santilli, O. L., Santilli, H. A., & Tripoloni, D. E. (2016). Sports hernias: Experience in a sports medicine center. *Hernia, 20*(1), 77–84. doi:10.1007/s10029-015-1367-4

Shiri, R., Viikari-Juntura, E., Varonen, H., & Heliövaara, M. (2006). Prevalence and determinants of lateral and medial epicondylitis: A population study. *American Journal of Epidemiology, 164*(11), 1065–1074. doi:10.1093/aje/kwj325

Sode, J., Obel, N., Hallas, J., & Lassen, A. (2007). Use of fluroquinolone and risk of Achilles tendon rupture: A population-based cohort study. *European Journal of Clinical Pharmacology, 63*(5), 499–503. doi:10.1007/s00228-007-0265-9

Stiell, I. G., Wells, G. A., Vandemheen, K., Clement, C., Lesiuk, H., Laupacis, A., ... Eisenhauer, M. A. (2001). The Canadian CT Head Rule for patients with minor head injury. *Lancet, 357*(9266), 1391–1396. doi:10.1016/S0140-6736(00)04561-X

Tosti, R., Rossy, W., Sanchez, A., & Lee, S. (2016). Burners, stingers, and other brachial plexus injuries in the contact athlete. *Operative Techniques in Sports Medicine, 24*, 273–278.

Weinberg, D., Williamson, D., Gebhart, J., Knapik, D., & Voss, J. (2017). Differences in medial and lateral posterior tibial slope: An osteological review of 1090 Tibia comparing age, sex, and race. *American Journal of Sports Medicine, 45*(1), 106–112. doi:10.1177/0363546516662449

Zellers, J., Cortes, D., & Silbernagel, K. (2016). From acute Achilles tendon rupture to return to play—A case report evaluating recovery of tendon structure mechanical properties, clinical and functional outcomes. *International Journal of Sports Physical Therapy, 11*(7), 1150–1159.

CHAPTER 4

Genitourinary History and Physical Examination for the Adult Male Patient

Nancy Brownlee

INTRODUCTION

When the male patient presents with urologic concerns, it is helpful to have resources to facilitate obtaining a thorough history. The American Urological Association (AUA) has practice guidelines for urologic patient care (American Urological Associations Guidelines, 2015). This is quite helpful in providing direction for the assessment, depending on the specific symptoms or concerns of the patient. Men will present with issues related to changes with urination, pain or discomfort, new lesion/appearance on genitalia, urine odor or color changes, and alterations in sexual performance. The urologic evaluation includes kidney, bladder, prostate and genitalia (Lajiness, 2017).

Concerns in the urologic system include, but are not limited to, stone disease, cancer, benign prostate hyperplasia, urination difficulties/concerns, hematuria, pain of any kind within the urinary system and genitalia, and erectile dysfunction (ED). There can also be hormone deficiencies, or concerns with fertility and/or sexually transmitted diseases (STDs). Questioning of symptoms, onset, duration, progression, and any treatment and current medications is based on the presenting complaint. A review of systems is always necessary, and should include concerns such as fatigue, obesity, unexplained fevers, neurologic history, diabetes, heart disease, smoking history, depression, rectal bleeding, and autoimmune disease.

A medication history is vital (as it is for all patients), and men of all ages should be asked specifically about virility supplements, over-the-counter products to increase testosterone or fertility, and over-the-counter products to improve erectile function, because many patients do not view these as "medications."

Many men will exhaust the Internet trying to find an explanation to their symptoms, and may present with a list of diagnoses that they feel are most pertinent. Ultimately, a thorough knowledge of the male genitourinary (GU) anatomy and a focused history will enable evaluation of the presenting complaint.

HISTORY

Many of the pertinent points of the history can be gathered in advance of the provider's first contact with the patient, through use of paper or electronic intake forms. Men should be asked about the presence of similar complaints in the past, regardless of the presenting complaint. Establish the start of puberty, and roughly when they started shaving as a way to confirm normal physiologic and endocrine development; asking about previous paternity also helps confirm that their endocrine status was normal in the past. Ask about any activity that may put the groin at risk (contact sports) and any potential exposure to environmental toxins.

Generally, any presentation with GU complaints will involve a brief sexual history, including number and gender of partners and the history of using protection for sexual activity. Any history of unprotected sex should be disclosed as are new partners and onset of signs and symptoms of pain and/or discharge and new lesions or skin abnormalities. Testing, evaluation, treatment, and reporting will proceed according to current Centers for Disease Control and Prevention (CDC) guidelines (CDC, 2015).

Family history can be important as well. Ask about testicular or other GU malignancies specifically, a general history of any cancers or prostate or bladder problems in other family members (including female relatives with bladder conditions), and other members of family with complaints similar to the patient's presenting complaint.

MALE SURGICAL HISTORY

Even in young men, the history should include investigation of any procedures they may have had as an infant or small child, including orchidopexy (bringing testis down into the scrotum), hernia repair and age (include presence/absence of mesh if known), hypospadias or epispadias repair and age at time of repair, previous prostate procedures, or any surgery that may have compromised the structure or function of their reproductive or GU system. These procedures may change the physical examination findings. Always specifically ask about a history of vasectomy, as many men do not consider this surgery, but it can help sort out any findings in the scrotum, such as an indurated epididymis.

INVESTIGATING SPECIFIC SYMPTOMS

Urinary symptoms are a common presentation in multiple settings, including retail clinics. Ask the patient if he has ever seen blood in his urine or been told there was microscopic blood, and if any treatment or follow-up took place. If, during the stream, he has noticed blood (initially, midstream, terminal), this can help narrow the differential diagnosis. Nocturia is also an important indicator of an enlarged prostate or incomplete bladder emptying. Assess for a history of urologic cancer (self or family), urinary tract infection, stones, sleep apnea, or diabetes. After an infection is ruled out, a helpful tool to use to assess urinary function is the International Prostate Symptom Score (IPSS), also referred to as the AUA symptom score (AUASS; Barry, 1992). This information can provide objective assessment of urination patterns.

Symptoms of urgency, frequency, and/or nocturia may be a result of the patient having overflow incontinence, may occur because he never completely empties his bladder, or may be due to an enlarged prostate or neurologic concern (Chapters 25 and 32). Ask the patient if he leaks urine at any time and under what circumstances; incontinence will drive men to seek evaluation with primary care or urology. It is imperative that if a patient complains of frequent urination, leakage, or incomplete bladder emptying, a postvoid residual (PVR) is imperative. If a bladder scanner is not available in the office, a more invasive approach is to catheterize the patient. This is not ideal, but if there is no urology office in the vicinity for referral, it can be helpful with a diagnosis. This avoids the common pitfall of placing a male patient on overactive bladder medication for urgency/frequency without confirming that he was emptying his bladder, and avoids any risk for urinary retention. Male patients may be given medication presumptively to relax or shrink their prostate as well as an overactive bladder medication simultaneously, and have not ruled out the cause of their symptoms.

When a patient requests a prostate examination and a prostate-specific antigen (PSA) blood test for cancer screening, a discussion will need to take place about recommended guidelines. The AUA guidelines do not recommend screening in patients ages 40 to 54 unless they have urination symptoms or family history of prostate cancer (American Urological

Associations Guidelines, 2015) (Chapter 26). There is a higher incidence of prostate cancer in African American males and men with first-degree relatives diagnosed with prostate cancer, and PSA can be checked at an earlier age (United States Preventative Services Task Force, 2017). Men with this history can also be referred for additional counseling and testing to a urologist who specializes in prostate cancer management.

Microscopic hematuria can also result from a urinary tract infection or stones. Flank pain and pain radiating to the groin can be a sign of impending stone passage. A stone workup may be warranted if there is a history of stones and the pain follows the course of stone passage. Pyelonephritis may be present if they have a history of urinary tract infections and present with hematuria and flank pain. Hematuria can also occur with previous urologic trauma, penile injury, or urogenital trauma. Ask about straddle injuries that may also cause hematuria, such as cycling, sports injury, horseback riding, or any activity that involves pressure or kick/hit to the genitalia. Inquire if the patient has noticed a split urinary stream or spray during urination; this is an indication of possible urethral stricture that may have resulted from a previous injury.

Bladder cancer is also a concern in patients with hematuria, especially those who have a history of smoking due to the direct association with smoking (cigarettes or cigars) or people who have worked around chemicals (Gilbert & Porter, 2015). Hematuria or microhematuria and/or urinary symptoms can be a first symptom of bladder cancer and warrant a hematuria workup. This patient would be referred to urology, especially if there is a history of gross or painful hematuria. Additionally, bladder pain along with suprapubic distention needs to be assessed. You will need to check the PVR along with the presentation of hematuria because of the possibility of clot retention, even though the patient may not complain of urination difficulty at the visit. Bladder pain may also cause urgency and frequency of urination. Ask the patient if there is relief after urination and then pain again as the bladder begins to refill; this could be a symptom of interstitial cystitis or bladder inflammation and would need to be further evaluated by urology.

Blood in the semen may also occur after an injury and will resolve after a few weeks. If hematospermia is the only symptom, and no hematuria is present, it is usually benign and resolves spontaneously, although it is quite distressing to men. A referral to urology for further evaluation is recommended and is not considered an emergency (Gerber & Brendler, 2012).

A patient may also present with concerns about his fertility status. If he has never had children and is not sure if he is fertile, a semen analysis is recommended. Referral to urology, or preferably an andrologist or male fertility specialist, is appropriate if there is an abnormal semen report for further evaluation. If the patient has had children and is now concerned about his fertility, a semen analysis and fertility testing for the partner may be reasonable recommendations.

Another concern is ED in the male patient without evidence of hypogonadism, hyperprolactinemia, or depression. Ask the patient if he has nocturnal erections; absence of these can indicate an organic (physiologic) nature to this complaint when they have previously had normal erectile function (Lue, 2012). Comorbid conditions will need to be assessed as are issues such as loss of libido, fatigue, current medications, cardiovascular disease, smoking, diabetes, previous pelvic radiation, and any neurologic disease. He may need to be referred for medical management of his other disease processes prior to the treatment of any ED.

Additional questions would concern any genital pain, difficulty with ejaculation and orgasm, and any deformities or curves observed in his penis during erections that cause him or his partner pain. This can be a sign of Peyronie's disease, which is plaque or scar tissue in his penis causing a curve during erection (Levine, Rybak, Corder, & Farrel, 2013). A history of Dupuytren's hand contracture is associated with Peyronie's disease and may help confirm the diagnosis.

A low testosterone level can cause a decrease in libido. There is also a questionnaire available from the AUA called sexual health inventory for men (SHIM). Ask about fatigue and sleep apnea, which also affects the testosterone level if untreated. It is important to have the testosterone level checked in the morning on two separate mornings to test for true low testosterone, although this is one of the most controversial areas in men's health (Morgentaler et al., 2015).

Scrotal pain or orchialgia will need to be evaluated, and a scrotal ultrasound scan is the single best test to rapidly screen for urgent issues (Marchese, 2016) (Chapter 23). For example, a patient may report scrotal pain and further examination may show that he has a heaviness in his scrotum that is new and actually painless; a scrotal ultrasound scan can rule out a testicular tumor.

Conditions such as paraphimosis, priapism, and testicular torsion are considered urologic emergencies and must be referred immediately to the nearest emergency department for treatment and resolution. Urologic emergencies are typically seen in an emergency department and referred for follow-up to urology or primary care, depending on the nature of the emergency.

PHYSICAL EXAMINATION

After a thorough history has been obtained, how to further target the physical examination may become clear. The GU physical examination includes kidney, bladder, prostate, and external genitalia. Any areas of concern or tenderness can be examined at the completion of the examination so as not to make the patient initially uncomfortable. If providing a full physical examination, examining the genitals last can help reduce embarrassment and allows time for the patient to become comfortable with the interaction. If he is accompanied by his partner, always ask him directly if he would like him/her present during the genital examination. Always assess for secondary sexual characteristics as a metric for endocrine status; establish that his apparent development is consistent with his chronologic age (Table 4.1). Privacy is always a priority and will be maintained throughout the examination; if his partner is present, give the patient the option to have the partner remain in the room or wait outside during the examination.

Depending on any complaints the patient may have, he may be asked to lay flat on the examination table for examination of the lower abdomen. It will be inspected for any abnormalities and examined for tenderness or distention (fullness) in the suprapubic area where the bladder is located. Depending on the complaint of the patient and the history, a noninvasive scan of the bladder may be done in the office to check if there is any remaining urine in the bladder after urination, PVR. While the patient is supine, the provider may pinch or brush the inner thigh with a finger to evaluate the cremasteric reflex. This checks for testicular torsion or twisting of the testicle that can be quite painful and is considered a urologic emergency. If the patient has relief from pain when the testicle is elevated, this is called Prehn's sign; this points to inflammation of the epididymis, but is not a reliable finding.

Place the patient in the sitting position and assess the kidneys. Check for costovertebral tenderness by making a fist and lightly press or tap on each side to elicit any pain or

TABLE 4.1 Tanner Stages in the Male

Stage 1	No hair, or fine pigmented; testes 2.5 cm; penis length <6 cm
Stage 2	Scant hair to base of symphysis pubis; testicular enlargement (2–3 cm diameter), enlarged scrotum; little change to penis
Stage 3	Increased pigmented hair that spreads across symphysis pubis; testes 3.5 cm diameter, scrotal skin thins, darkens, wrinkles; penis lengthens
Stage 4	Hair fills in pubic triangle; scrotum darkens, testes 4–4.5 cm diameter; penis to 11–17 cm length flaccid, glans increases in size
Stage 5	Hair extends to medial thighs and toward umbilicus; testes 4.5 cm or greater; genitalia fully grown

Source: Adapted from Tanner, J. M. (1962). *Growth at adolescence* (2nd ed.). Oxford, England: Blackwell Scientific Publications.

tenderness. If the patient has a smaller frame, a bimanual examination of the kidneys may be done to check for enlargement of the kidney.

Ask the patient to lower his trousers and undergarments in the standing position to expose his genitalia. Supine or lying flat is an option if the patient is unable to be in the standing position. If the patient is in the standing position, a visual inspection can be made of the proper anatomical location of the scrotum and penis. The penis will be inspected for any lesions or skin abnormalities, glans penis size should be proportional to the penis, and the skin should be smooth. Next, it will be palpated for lumps, indurations, or lesions upon closer inspection. If uncircumcised, the foreskin will be retracted to view the urethral opening or meatus, which should be positioned centrally at the tip of the glans penis and appear as a pink slit or round opening. It will be compressed to inspect the inside and assess for lesions and discharge or excretions. Replace the foreskin over the meatus following the examination. The penile shaft itself should be smooth or slightly wrinkled and largely hairless; the color of the skin varies, and may suggest the site of circumcision. The dorsal vein may be prominent.

Each testicle will be palpated separately, noting whether both testicles are descended. Examine for appropriate size and location of the testicle. Ideally the examination room should be warm, to avoid activation of the cremaster muscle (Table 4.2) and subsequent retraction of the testes. The epididymis will be identified on top of each testicle, and will be palpated for any tenderness, a common site for inflammation and scrotal pain. The vas deferens that carries the sperm will also be identified in the scrotal sac along with the spermatic cord.

If scrotal enlargement is reported over a period of time and is painless, a hydrocele may be present and may be identified by transillumination with a penlight or examination light in a darkened room. If the history is consistent with a hernia, a stethoscope can be used to

TABLE 4.2 Specific Maneuvers for the Male Genital Examination

Cremasteric Reflex
One or both testicles elevate due to the action of the cremaster muscle in response to downward touching of the scrotum. Reflex is prompted by a cool room/cold temperatures—reflex may be engaged prior to any contact.
Digital Rectal Examination (DRE)
Gloved, lubricated finger is inserted into the anus and swept across the surface of the prostate; also involves estimation of anal sphincter tone. Normal examination yields symmetrical, nontender, walnut-sized gland that is free of nodules, with a smooth rubbery consistency; seminal vesicles cannot be palpated.
Neurologic Examination
Perianal sensation: reflexive contraction of external anal sphincter ("anal wink") if neurologically intact, as a result of brushing the anus with a cotton swab Bulbocavernosus reflex: contraction of anal sphincter and bulbocavernosus muscles as a result of insertion of the gloved finger into the anus and squeezing glans penis *(These tests are most helpful when evaluating sensory complaints or erectile dysfunction in apparently neurologically intact males.)*
Valsalva Maneuver to Evaluate for Varicocele
Ideally the patient is standing in a warm room (to avoid activating the cremaster reflex). Asking him to perform the Valsalva maneuver will reverse flow into the pampiniform plexus of the scrotum, and result in distention of the vessels ("bag of worms" if varicocele of sufficient size) that can be noted on examination.

Source: Adapted from Quallich, S. A. (2018). Male reproductive system. In M. J. Goolsby & L. Grubbs, L, eds. *Advanced assessment: Interpreting findings and formulating differential diagnoses*. Philadelphia, PA: F. A. Davis.

listen for bowel sounds in the enlarged scrotum. A dilated or tortuous vein that is obvious as the patient performs the Valsalva maneuver is indicative of a varicocele, known as the "bag of worms." Third, examine for inguinal hernias on each side. Ask the patient to turn his head and cough; this is to protect the provider, as well as induce the Valsalva maneuver to cause any "loose" material to move into the inguinal canal.

Next, in order to examine the prostate, ask the patient to turn around and lean over the examination table, resting his weight in his forearms (this position relaxes the pelvic floor). This examination may also be done in the side-lying position, if he is unable to bend over. The prostate is a walnut-sized organ located at the base of the bladder. It is best palpated by placing the gloved index finger and using sufficient lubricant in the rectum and pressing downward, then sweeping from one side to the other. The gland is assessed for estimated size, any nodules, firmness, and/or tenderness. The anus and rectum will be examined for any internal or external hemorrhoids, abscesses, excoriations, tenderness, or fissures.

CONCLUSION

There are maneuvers and vital points to the male history that will aid in the assessment of male GU complaints. Many of these insights will be picked up "on the job" as needed. Table 4.3 provides direction for the normal presentation and possible abnormal findings that may need additional evaluation. Older men may benefit from a more specific examination that assesses their functional status (Table 4.4), which can be especially relevant when deciding between medications and nonpharmacologic treatments.

TABLE 4.3 Adult Male Physical Examination Guide

Structure	Normal Findings	Abnormalities (Possible Cause)
Penis	Foreskin is easily retracted and replaced Urethral meatus midline Smooth penile shaft Average measurements of adult men age > 25: 12.4 ± 1.6 cm when flaccid	Phimosis—tightened foreskin (balanitis) Fibrotic plaque (Peyronie's disease) Urethral meatus not centrally located: ventral (hypospadias); dorsal or along the penile shaft (epispadias) Vesicles/lesions (herpes, ulcers, warts)
Testis(es)	Bilateral, oval, rubbery consistency, smooth Average measurements of adult men age > 25: 5.2 ± 0.6 cm, 15–18 mL each	Firm or hard area (tumor) Absent (undescended testes, Klinefelter's syndrome—less than 2 cm) Atrophied (hypogonadism/testosterone replacement, aging, anabolic steroid use)
Epididymis	Palpable as ridge of tissue posterior to or above each testis	Tender on palpation, pain, swelling (epididymitis) Mass (spermatocele, cyst) Indurated (postvasectomy, epididymal cyst)
Scrotal skin	Hair and sweat glands Loose skin	Small pustules (hair follicle infection) Sebaceous cysts Stretched or enlarged unilaterally (hydrocele, spermatocele, or mass)

(continued)

TABLE 4.3 Male Physical Examination Guide (*continued*)

Prostate	Size of walnut	Asymmetry, hard nodule (tumor)
	Flattened, heart-shaped configuration with a midline furrow	Boggy (softer than normal) and exquisitely tender (prostatitis)
	Consistency of contracted thenar eminence of thumb	Enlarged (benign prostatic hyperplasia)
	Average measurements of adult men age >25: 20 g, may be larger with age	
Inguinal canal (hernia)	No bulges with Valsalva maneuver	Distinct bulge that descends against the tip of the finger in the external ring (hernia)

TABLE 4.4 Specifics for Assessing Older Males

Older males can benefit from light and moderate physical activity. However, low muscle strength, mobility disability, poor balance, and frailty can limit participation in activities of daily living as well as engagement in beneficial levels of physical activity. Few studies have examined gender differences regarding variables impacting physical activity engagement in older adults. The factors may be multidimensional and involve biological, social, and psychological influences. Prior to engaging an older male in a new regimen of physical activity, a comprehensive assessment is required. The following is a list of variables to consider prior to prescribing the type, frequency, and intensity of physical activity in the older male.

Dimension	Assessment	Available Tools	Reference
Biological	Grip strength	Hand dynamometer	Crimmins et al. (2008)
	Mobility and balance	Short Physical Performance Battery (SPPB)	Gurlanik (2011)
	Frailty	Fried Frailty Phenotype	Fried et al. (2001)
Social	Social support	Social Support for Physical Activity	Sallis et al. (1987)
Psychological	Depression	Geriatric Depression Scale	Yesavage et al. (1982)

CASE STUDY

CH is a 46-year-old male who has been plagued by left-sided scrotal and testicular pain for almost a year that sometimes limits his physical activities. He has been able to continue his exercise habits, which consist of mountain biking and kayaking with his teenage children, but may have a few days of significant scrotal and testicular pain afterward that sometimes radiates into the left inguinal region and sometimes even in his left lower quadrant. The pain is "achy, dull, bothersome" and "occasionally nauseating." Athletic underwear has helped somewhat when he is engaging in these activates, but he will still have a dull ache afterward. He works as an IT specialist for a local automotive parts supplier. He denies any issues with erection or libido, and denies any risk for sexually transmitted diseases (STDs). His pain increases somewhat after ejaculation.

Past medical history is largely unremarkable. He takes over-the-counter medication for gastric reflux disease, and acetaminophen or ibuprofen as needed. He reports no surgeries as an infant or child, no personal or family history of cancer. He thinks

(*continued*)

CASE STUDY (*continued*)

that he may have a tumor, although he has not noticed any change to the size of his left testicle.

He has seen many providers in his primary care practice and been treated with anti-inflammatory drugs, antibiotics, and a short course of narcotic pain medication for "chronic epididymitis" with minimal improvement to his pain complaint. Two previous ultrasound scans have been negative for testicular malignancy.

He is eventually referred to a urology provider. A generalized physical examination is normal. He has a circumcised phallus without plaques or lesions, and a centrally placed meatal opening. Testes are both present in the scrotum and are normal size and consistent; they are nontender. Subtle sperm granulomas are present in the vas deferens bilaterally. He has bilateral epididymal induration and enlargement, left much more pronounced than the right; palpation of the left epididymis reproduces his complaints of pain. He has no evidence of hernias on examination. His pain is localized with a careful physical examination to his left epididymis; the urology provider confirms that he had a vasectomy 8 years ago and diagnoses postvasectomy pain syndrome. He is treated with a 30-day course of an anti-inflammatory agent, and given a return visit in 6 weeks for routine follow-up.

CLINICAL PEARLS

- Male genital examination is best done in a warm room to avoid activation of the cremaster reflex.
- Always ask if there is a history of a vasectomy.
- DRE is best performed at the end of the physical examination.
- Palpation is the most important part of the male genital examination.
- Auscultation and percussion are rarely indicated in evaluation of male GU complaints, except with suspected herniation of bowel into the scrotum or as part of complete physical examination.

REFERENCES

American Urological Associations Guidelines. (2015). Retrieved from http://www.auanet.org/guidelines

Barry, M. J., Fowler, F. J. Jr, O'Leary, M. P., Bruskewitz, R. C., Holtgrewe, H. L., Mebust, W. K., & Cockett, A. T. (1992). The American Urological Association symptom index for benign prostatic hyperplasia. *The Journal of Urology, 148*, 1549–1557. doi:10.1016/S0022-5347(17)36966-5

Centers for Disease Control and Prevention. (2015). 2015 Sexually transmitted diseases treatment guidelines. Retrieved from https://www.cdc.gov/std/tg2015/default.htm

Crimmins, E., Guyer, H., Langa, K., Ofstedal, M. B., & Wallace, R. (2008). *Documentation of physical measures, anthropometrics and blood pressure in the health and retirement study*. Ann Arbor, MI: Survey Research Center, University of Michigan

Fried, L. P., Tangen, C. M., Walston, J., Newman, A. B., Hirsch, C., Gottdiener, J., … McBurnie, M. A. (2001). Frailty in Older Adults: Evidence for a Phenotype. *The Journals of Gerontology Series A: Biological Sciences and Medical Sciences, 56*(3), M146–M157. doi:10.1093/gerona/56.3.m146

Gerber, G. S., & Brendler, C. B. (2012). Evaluation of the urologic patient: History, physical examination, and urinalysis. In A. J. Wein, L. R. Kavoussi, A. C. Novick, A. W. Partin, & C. A. Peters (Eds.), *Campbell-Walsh urology* (10th ed., pp. 73–84). Philadelphia, PA: Saunders Elsevier.

Gilbert, S. M., & Porter, M. (2015). Patient navigation and cancer navigation programs. In S. P. Lerner, M. P. Schoenberg, & C. N. Sternberg (Eds.), *Bladder cancer: Diagnosis and clinical management* (pp. 368–370). Hoboken, NJ: Wiley Blackwell.

Gurlanik, J. (2011). Assessing physical performance in the older patient. Retrieved from https://www.nia.nih.gov/research/labs/leps/short-physical-performance-battery-sppb

Lajiness, M. J. (2017). Assessment of men. In D. K. Newman, J. F. Wyman, & V. W. Welch (Eds.), *Core curriculum for urologic nursing* (1st ed., pp. 247–255). Pittman, NJ: SUNA.

Levine, L., Rybak, J., Corder, C., & Farrel, M. R. (2013). Peyronie's disease plaque calcification—Prevalence, time to identification, and development of a new grading classification. *Journal of Sexual Medicine, 10*(12), 3121–3128. doi:10.1111/jsm.12334

Lue, T. F. (2012). Physiology of penile erection and pathophysiology of erectile dysfunction. In A. J. Wein, L. R. Kavoussi, A. C. Novick, A. W. Partin, & C. A. Peters (Eds.), *Campbell-Walsh urology* (10th ed., pp. 688–720). Philadelphia, PA: Saunders Elsevier.

Marchese, K. (2016). Evaluation and management of common scrotal conditions. In M. Lajiness & S. Quallich (Eds.), *The nurse practitioner in urology* (1st ed., pp. 39–50). Basel, Switzerland: Springer International Publishing.

Morgentaler, A., Miner, M. M., Caliber, M., Guay, A. T., Khera, M., & Traish, A. M. (2015). Testosterone therapy and cardiovascular risk: Advances and controversies. *Mayo Clinic Proceedings, 90*, 224–251. doi:10.1016/j.mayocp.2014.10.011

Sallis, J. F., Grossman, R. M., Pinski, R. B., Patterson, T. L., & Nader, P. R. (1987). The development of scales to measure social support for diet and exercise behaviors. *Preventive Medicine, 16*(6), 825–836. doi:10.1016/0091-7435(87)90022-3

United States Preventative Services Task Force. (2017). Providing clinicians and patients with important information to help guide decisions about prostate cancer screening. Retrieved from https://screeningforprostatecancer.org

Yesavage, J. A., Brink, T. L., Rose, T. L., Lum, O., Huang, V., Adey, M., & Leirer, V. O. (1982). Development and validation of a geriatric depression screening scale: A preliminary report. *Journal of Psychiatric Research, 17*(1), 37–49. doi:10.1016/0022-3956(82)90033-4

CHAPTER 5

Male Adolescent Health: Addressing a Critical Need

MiChelle L. McGarry

INTRODUCTION

The male adolescent is a patient rarely seen in primary care, and there are many possible reasons for this. In some cases their parents may see them as healthy and not needing to see a healthcare provider; for others the idea of masculinity may mean that many males do not go to the doctor until they absolutely have to or are forced to. Despite the possible reasons for this group of young men not seeking healthcare, particularly preventive, male adolescents have many healthcare needs. For this reason, it is important for the healthcare provider to have a good grasp on the needs of this male population in order to weave anticipatory guidance into any healthcare visit opportunity. Some of the varied areas that are important to address are mental health, substance abuse, sexuality, family planning, immunizations, transition from the family home, unintentional injury and violence, and relationships, to name a few. This chapter will provide a broad overview of issues pertinent to adolescent male health, providing a framework for providers wishing to focus on the care of this unique population.

DEFINITION OF ADOLESCENCE

The most common reasons for an adolescent male to seek healthcare is for the obligatory sports physical examination or for an injury. There are certainly needs here, but there are many more needs that often go unaddressed. One of the challenges in providing adolescent male healthcare is considering who their care provider should be. Adolescence is defined by the American Academy of Pediatrics (AAP) by age, development, and social roles. The AAP defines adolescence as up to 21 years of age. Supporting the incorporation of the young adult population, the National Initiative to Improve Adolescent Health identifies 10 to 24 years of age as their target population (Bell, Breland, & Ott, 2013). Given this, pediatricians are often seeing the adolescent male patient, but male adolescents may well be seeing internal medicine or family practice healthcare providers too, possibly more often than adolescent females because of the predominance of female pediatricians and possible preferences for a male provider. And even this poses a dilemma: does the provider acquiesce to this request, which has the potential to sexualize the patient–provider role, and is a matter-of-fact approach that this is business and healthcare better serve the male adolescent? These are decisions that healthcare providers need to make and then determine how they will communicate the decision to the patient. Adolescent males, in fact, have both pediatric and adult concerns much of the time, meaning that any provider evaluating this population group must be aware of, and comfortable with, discussing the entirety of these healthcare needs.

DEVELOPMENTAL COMPONENTS OF ADOLESCENCE

Adolescence is a period during which many developmental goals that will promote the transition into healthy adulthood may be achieved. These goals may at times be in direct opposition to the risk-taking behaviors that are also associated with adolescence, especially male adolescence. According to Muyle et al. (2009), when compared with females, adolescent males have a higher mortality rate, less engagement in primary care, and higher levels of unmet healthcare needs such as nutrition, immunizations, and risk prevention. The Centers for Disease Control and Prevention's (CDC) Healthy 2020 objectives offer a relevant overview of potential adolescent healthcare needs for both adolescents and young adults in the clinical setting. These objectives address chronic illness, mortality, unintentional injury, violence, mental health and substance abuse, and sexual and reproductive health (U.S. Department of Health and Human Services, 2013).

DEVELOPMENTAL TASKS AND THEIR EFFECTS WHEN INTERVIEWING AND EXAMINING AN ADOLESCENT MALE IN THE HEALTHCARE SETTING

It is important to remember that physical and emotional maturation do not always correlate and the interview needs to occur at the cognitive level of the male adolescent, regardless of age and/or size. In fact, in larger children, there can often be unrealistic expectations in school and this should be discussed proactively. If there has been a relationship with the patient and the provider in childhood, the cognitive level is much easier to ascertain. If the patient is new, it is important to have a casual conversation initially discussing school, grades, hobbies, and extracurricular activities, during which a skilled provider will be able to get a good assessment of where to begin the conversation around health topics and anticipatory guidance. Using open-ended questions and being very careful to use neutral words and tones are essential as the process of puberty can cause a patient to feel self-conscious.

Furthermore, it is common for adolescents to easily misperceive adult statements and feel judged when that was not the intent of the healthcare provider at all. Some of the verbiage that can be very useful is:

- "Tell me more about that."
- "Can you explain that to me?"
- "What did you think about that?"
- "What did you think was good about that choice or decision?"
- "What do you think the possible consequences of that choice or decision might be?"

It is also helpful to avoid asking how they "feel" about something as they are often not self-aware of feelings and this can shut a conversation down.

According to Erikson (1963), the developmental stage of adolescence is identity versus role confusion; this is the fifth of eight stages that occur during a child's development and occurs from about 12 to 18 years of age. During this stage, adolescents search for a sense of self and personal identity, through an intense exploration of personal values, beliefs, and goals (McLeod, 2013). This is a time for teens to explore their own identity while inventing and reinventing themselves, hopefully in an environment of respect and appreciation between parents and teens. Some of the tasks that adolescents may acquire during this time are obtaining a job outside the home, being independent in homework completion, and maintaining their own schedule. During this time adolescents also examine their family's beliefs in comparison to their peers in order to develop their own personal philosophies. This allows for closer friendships and a transition of the parents from an authority role to a more equal relationship. Dating and driving with their inherent risks are also things more adolescents do. Experimentation with drugs, alcohol, and smoking may also occur, often due to peer pressure and the desire to show their independence by "disobeying" parental rules. Finally, with the increased freedom, meals can become sporadic and not occur with the family, fast food consumption increases, and snacking can become a habit.

This development stage offers insight into why adolescents may struggle to accurately hear and implement what their healthcare provider is saying to them. This is also the reason that many adolescents have conflicts with their parents in this stage of life. They are transitioning, at greatly varying rates, from being children to being adults, and this transition is complex for both children and parents, involving biologic/hormonal, social, psychosocial, and emotional turmoil. This is also a stage in life when the preference is to be with peers over parents and adults. A healthcare provider needs to acknowledge this and find his/her own comfortable way to communicate and relate to the male adolescent patient.

A useful interviewing technique is to incorporate the anticipatory guidance into the physical examination. This could mean talking about bicycle helmet, seat belt use and car safety while doing the head examination; discussing smoking concerns and education while examining the lungs; and the importance of exercise and physical activity while doing the musculoskeletal examination.

Another common piece to being an adolescent is being resistant to parents, teachers, and others they view as authority figures as the adolescent is attempting to establish autonomy and independence. This is often softened by empathy and acknowledging that the patient does not want to be there, but that it will be as useful as you can make it. Adolescents can also be known for answering questions as they perceive the healthcare provider wants them to; this is the time when open-ended questions and "tell me more" statements can be very helpful.

Another potential issue for providers when evaluating this age group is whether parents are in the room for the interview and/or examination. This issue also raises ethical and legal questions; it is imperative for the healthcare provider caring for the adolescent male to be very aware of the current state laws and regulatory items pertaining to this in regard to reproductive and mental health and confidentiality. This is especially relevant for nurse practitioners (NPs); their primary license must include the care of adolescents.

Deciding how to address the issue of the parent being present for the examination can be a difficult process, as the parents are also learning how to let their children grow up. Despite laws that protect adolescents, it is often best practice to encourage them to have their parents involved in their decisions. Healthcare providers can be pivotal in assisting in good communication between adolescents and their parents. But when this cannot be done, the teen male needs to have private access to discussions with his healthcare provider. When the teen has been a patient of the provider throughout childhood, it is helpful if the provider can start to initiate discussions about potentially controversial subjects (such as peer pressure, sexual activity, substance use) with the child and the parent both in the room as the child begins to near adolescence. This makes it routine for the visit to discuss these types of issues and also offers the provider an opportunity to counsel the parent about their responses to their child. It is beneficial to encourage them to have an open mind and not to react quickly should an issue or concern arise. Some examples of this are "making a deal" with the tween and the parent that honesty is best:

- If the child does become sexually active, wouldn't the parent rather know and be sure that there is protection against pregnancy and sexually transmitted infections (STIs)?
- Wouldn't the parent rather be called to come and get the child if he ends up in a compromising situation, instead of the child staying in the unsafe situation because he is not sure how the parent will react if he calls and asks to be picked up.
- If the child has questions about alcohol, is it not best that this experimentation be done in the safe environment with his own parents and not friends?

This honesty perspective can be very helpful in supporting the relationship between the teen and his parents.

The examination of the genitalia presents another potential source of controversy for the provider. It is essential that this be done, yet teens are often embarrassed about this. They should be given a choice on whether their parents are there or not. That said, it is recommended that there be a chaperone or that the parent stands outside the door to the examination room with it cracked slightly open or behind a closed curtain so that they can hear all that is going on to protect both the teen and the provider.

OTHER IMPORTANT DISCUSSIONS TO HAVE WHENEVER POSSIBLE

Physical Activity

Fifty-seven percent of adolescent males report being physically active for the recommended 60 minutes per day, 5 days a week (CDC, 2014). Encouraging regular and enjoyable physical activity promotes optimal health and weight and is likely to extend into adult habits. The time that adolescents spend inside, with the availability of technology, has greatly decreased outside time, which usually equates to exercise (CDC, 2014). There is no question that starting exercise habits earlier in life has more potential to see those habits maintained throughout the life span. While young boys should not begin activities such as weight training until puberty, many teens may gravitate toward activities that offer opportunities for cross-training or team sports in high school. These activities may also be dictated by geography and specific rural, suburban, and urban settings.

Concussion

There is much more awareness about concussions recently and this information has been in the mainstream news frequently over the last few years. It is important to remember that the apparent severity of the head injury does not necessarily correlate with the possibility or severity of a possible concussion. According to the Colorado Children's Hospital Concussion Program, even a "mild" concussion must be taken seriously as it is an injury to the brain. Most people recover completely from one concussion. This can take a few days to a few weeks. Severe sequelae can also happen, so it is good practice to include a healthcare professional in concussion care. Many states have instituted standardized training protocols for both recreational and scholastic coaches, trainers, and athletic staff. Supportive care after a concussion includes safety and restricting the situation in which another concussion can occur such as sports and other athletic and recreational activities. Extra sleep after a concussion is also important to supportive care as well as good nutrition and fluid intake. Adolescents who are recovering from concussions may also need educational accommodations such as modification in the amount and due dates of makeup work for days missed owing to the initial injury, educational breaks during the day, flexibility of due dates for assignments given after the adolescent returns to school, and possibly modifying test schedules until the adolescent has recovered. The Sports Medicine Center at Colorado Children's Hospital has a good Return to Play Protocol. This protocol includes six steps to be moved through in 6 days beginning after the student has resolution of all concussion-related symptoms. These steps are relative rest to include a walk outside, then light aerobic exercise, such as brisk walking or riding a stationary bike. The next two steps are noncontact sport–specific activity for 30 to 45 minutes; examples are skating for a hockey player or dribbling a soccer ball for a soccer player. From here, an adolescent can move to noncontact sport–specific drills for 1 to 2 hours such as resistance training or use of blocking pads in football. Finally, if the adolescent patient tolerates this progression well, then they need a medical clearance to return to full-contact practices in their sport followed by return to competitive play. There are commonly concussion programs at children's hospitals and with the expertise they possess, they should be utilized early in concussion care.

Obesity

Twenty percent of males 12 to 19 years old were obese in 2011 to 2012; this is one in five, and is defined as a body mass index (BMI) at or above the 95th percentile (Ogden, Carroll, Kit, & Flegal, 2014). Obesity can lead to many problems in both adolescence and adulthood, including cardiovascular disease, type 2 diabetes, and musculoskeletal problems. One significant problem contributing to obesity in this population is "convenient" food, which is highly processed with decreased nutrition. Many adolescent males truly don't know how to make a meal if the food is not already prepared. This is a significant health issue that is best addressed as early as possible. Some tricks that may help include having adolescents learn to read nutrition labels and giving them ranges for their sodium, fat, and calorie intake. Providers can suggest avoiding foods that have chemicals in them—foods with ingredients that they can't read or pronounce. Portion control is also important in this age group as is encouraging them to eat at least three meals a day. Breakfast is important and many adolescents do not eat it (Ogden et al., 2014). If an adolescent has weight gain that is not on a consistent growth curve and does not match his height trajectory, referral to a nutritionist for the adolescent and family/household members who are responsible for meal preparation is indicated. It is important to include the adolescent in all of these meetings so that they can be empowered with education as they express independence and are not eating at home as consistently. According to the CDC, a male with a BMI in the 85th to 95th percentile is considered obese and should be encouraged to get input from a nutritional resource. Another option, depending on income, is providing information about food delivery services. These can actually be cost-effective as well as providing balanced nutrition and portion control.

Chronic Conditions

There are not much data separating the incidence in adolescent females versus males, but 18% of 12- to 17-year olds have one chronic condition and 13% have more than two chronic conditions (The Child and Adolescent Health Measurement Initiative, 2017). It is critical for a healthcare provider to engage the adolescent male in the management of his chronic disease as soon as he is developmentally ready. This can be very hard for parents, who may have spent the child's entire life advocating for them and managing their chronic health condition.

The most common chronic healthcare condition is asthma, affecting 21% of all students in 2013 (CDC, 2013). Supporting and suggesting a timeline for this transition and intentionally getting information directly from the patient can be ways to encourage empowerment and autonomy in the adolescent male's healthcare of his chronic condition.

Mental Health

In 2013, 21% of surveyed adolescent males in the United States reported having symptoms of depression in the last 12 months (CDC, 2013). Of students, both male and female, who were diagnosed with a major depressive episode, more than 6 in 10 did not get treatment (Substance Abuse & Mental Health Services Administration, 2014). There are a variety of tools available to have adolescents complete in order to assess their mental health, and it is important to really read these and go over them with the patient. To express a concern on the tool and not have it addressed by the adolescent male's healthcare provider can make a poor situation worse, as they feel invalidated and misunderstood. Healthcare providers of male adolescents must develop and feel comfortable with both verbiage and body language to use when asking about mental health issues, and especially if the teen has thought of harming himself. The ease with which the provider can do this will go far to encourage the male adolescent to feel safe and give honest answers. Any time there is risk of self or other harm, immediate referral to a mental health specialist is indicated. Whenever possible, a professional specifically trained in child and/or adolescent mental health is preferable.

SUICIDE RISK

According to the CDC, in 2013, suicide was the third leading cause of death in adolescents between the ages of 10 and 24 years. The CDC estimates that 4,600 youths in this age group in the United States die from suicide each year. The CDC also reports that males in the age group of 10 to 24 years are much more likely to commit suicide than females at a rate of 81% to 19%. This disparity continues throughout the life span. Firearms are the most commonly used method of suicide for all males with a rate of 56.9%. These statistics underscore the need to discuss these issues with our male adolescent patients at each opportunity we have because of their often infrequent visits to primary care. Doing so not only lets them know that their primary care provider is available for these types of discussions, if they should ever need to talk, but also may happen just at the time that the adolescent male patient needs to have support and a safe place to talk about his plans and the difficulties that have caused him to have a suicidal plan. The provider needs to be able to have the conversation confidently and empathetically and then take the steps to ensure that the adolescent male patient is transported directly to an appropriate mental health provider for immediate support and care. This also means that the provider needs to be aware of the services available in the area as well as how to transport patients to them and the intake process to ensure that a patient in this situation does not fall through the cracks.

ATTENTION DEFICIT HYPERACTIVITY DISORDER

Adolescent males are more than twice as likely to be diagnosed with attention deficit hyperactivity disorder (ADHD) as adolescent females at a rate of 16% in 2013 (Bloom, Jones, & Freeman, 2013); untreated ADHD can affect academic and relationship successes. The intake portion of any well-visit should include questions about attention and how the male adolescent does with focus at school. Before any intervention is undertaken, it is important to get evaluations from teachers and both parents, all independently. There are many published tools with scoring available to assist the primary care healthcare provider of the male adolescent in determining if, ADHD, or another diagnosis is affecting the patient. If interventions are not helpful or symptoms continue to worsen after interventions are begun or there is not a clear ADHD diagnosis, referral to a child/adolescent mental healthcare provider is indicated.

Sexual Activity and Sexual Orientation

In 2013, in the United States, 48% of male students aged 15 to 19 had had sexual intercourse (Goesling, Colman, Trenholm, Terzian, & Moore, 2014). This carries the risk of STIs, unintended pregnancy, and emotional distress. A vast majority of males between the ages of 12 and 19 (82%) reported feeling pressured by friends to have sex (National Campaign to Prevent Teen and Unplanned Pregnancy, 2010). The Internet and the ease of video streaming have had influence in these high numbers of males feeling pressured to have sex by outside influences. Male adolescents have easy access to pornography, which may give them very unrealistic ideas and opinions about what sexual activity is, may give them unrealistic expectations of the experience, and may fail to emphasize that sex does not promote a relationship between or among participants.

Social media platforms play a significant role in the lives of male adolescents as well. These have the potential to greatly influence a male adolescent's view of reality when it comes to many topics, including sexual intercourse. Male adolescents do not always realize that anyone can be and say anything online and it is not an accurate portrayal.

Sexting is another issue that needs to be addressed with male adolescents by their healthcare providers and parents both. It is important that the healthcare provider for adolescent patients be well aware of the laws in the state in which they practice, in regard to sexting and the transmission of nude pictures, as these activities have the potential to have an adolescent male labeled a sex offender. Reviewing these facts can often help the male adolescent patient to consider the potential consequences of what he may perceive as harmless actions.

Another important topic to cover is that of statutory rape. Again, the laws vary from state to state, but many adolescents, both males and females, are not aware that even if the intercourse is consensual, there could still be rape charges brought and a conviction. These things could greatly affect a male adolescent's life, including finishing school, going to college, and his future career.

It is also important for the healthcare provider to ask adolescent males about what they have learned in the school setting about sexuality and sexual activity. Schools in America have taken a progressively more and more involved presence in messages and teaching about these issues that may conflict with adolescents and/or their families' views. Schools also may potentially give the message that there is "safe" sex in their efforts to try to protect young men from STIs and unintended pregnancies, but there is no "safe sex," only safer sex. This is important to discuss with the adolescent male at every opportunity, especially because these young men also have the responsibility even if they are not the one who gets pregnant or catches the infection. It may be helpful to give a pointed visual for a young man in the primary care setting explaining that every time he has intercourse or sexual contact of any kind with any partner, regardless of gender, he is essentially having the activity with every individual whom has ever had any sexual relationship with that partner.

Another area that the healthcare provider needs to be comfortable discussing with male adolescent patients is that of gender identity and homosexuality. The primary care provider must be able to have frank and nonjudgmental conversations, in both verbal and body language, about these issues with every patient so that there is a safe place for the adolescent male patient to be honest in order to get accurate and needed health information. These issues are discussed in greater detail in other chapters in this book.

Substance Abuse

The majority of adolescents, both male and female, reported being substance free in 2013 (Child Trends, 2016). But this number decreased with age and progression through adolescence, with 86% of eighth graders not using substances to 52% of 12th graders not using substances (Child Trends, 2016). Half of all adolescent patients are using some drugs or alcohol, making it imperative that this topic be addressed at any contact with teens. This can be done during sports physicals and injury or illness visits, which are the times that providers are more likely to have access to adolescent male patients.

TOBACCO AND MARIJUANA

Most smoking begins in adolescence according to Johnston, O'Malley, Miech, Bachman, and Schulenberg (2015). In 2014, 7% of high school seniors, males and females, reported being a daily smoker and more teenagers smoked electronic cigarettes than tobacco cigarettes (Miech, Johnston, O'Malley, Bachman, & Schulenberg, 2014). This is a topic that still necessitates discussion with male adolescent patients, explaining to them what happens to the lungs when they smoke. There are ideas in the adolescent age group that "natural things" such as marijuana are safe to smoke, making it imperative that the healthcare provider address these issues even if the patient does not tell you that it is his belief. It is also important to address marijuana use in particular, as it is becoming legalized in more and more states in the United States. Male adolescents need to know what the local laws are. Teens need to have discussions with their healthcare provider about the safety of marijuana use during this time of growth and ongoing cognitive development, including consequences seen with frequent use: impaired judgment and short-term memory; altered motor skills; possible paranoia; bronchitis; and impaired brain development and lower IQ with frequent use during adolescence (Volkow, Baler, Compton, & Weiss, 2014).

ALCOHOL

In 2013, 34% of male adolescents reported drinking alcohol in the last month (CDC, 2014), and most adolescents (male and female) reported that they engaged in binge drinking (CDC, 2012). Healthcare providers can often be surprised at the candor their male adolescent patient will have, if they ask the questions about alcohol use. It is vital to discuss both the laws and the safety concerns not only with drinking themselves, but also being in the company of peers who are drinking and especially driving.

Educational Attainment

Healthy students are better students than their less healthy peers (National Center for Chronic Disease Prevention and Health Promotion, 2014). The relationship between health and education may be due to the increased earning and employment potential education can provide for adults (Telfair & Shelton, 2012), often termed the anticipated "return on investment." It is not unusual to have an adolescent, especially a male, tell his healthcare provider that he doesn't need school. Arguing this will not change his opinion, but having him do a quick budget while in clinic might. In order to do this, providers need to know the going rental rate, gas rate, minimum wage, and transportation costs for the area. Often this is an open-ended discussion: "well, let's look at how that might work out for you." This discussion may help the male adolescent see reality and decide that staying in school and even possibly attending a trade school or college after high school is, in fact, worth the effort.

Math Proficiency

In 2013, only 36% of male eighth graders were proficient in math and that number dropped to 28% in the 12th grade (U.S. Department of Education Institute of Education Sciences National Center for Education Statistics, 2014). Ask patients about their grades, as parents may not be aware of what they are until the end of a semester; this is rapidly changing as school districts take advantage of technology platforms that notify parents/guardians of grades weekly, and more frequently when grades are poor. Male adolescents may be embarrassed or overwhelmed and not aware of resources to help them with their schoolwork. Healthcare providers caring for adolescents can provide a resource, helping teens to have awareness of these resources in their community.

Writing Proficiency

Male students in the eighth grade had a writing proficiency of 17% and in the 12th grade 21% in 2011 (U.S. Department of Education Institute of Education Sciences National Center for Education Statistics, 2011). Again, assess how your male adolescent patients are doing in school in the humanities and be aware of resources and some reasons that writing is important in their adult future.

Healthy Relationships

DATING VIOLENCE

In 2013, 7% of male high school students in the United States reported that they had been intentionally physically hurt by their partner (CDC, 2014). This number is likely underreported. In general, in adult medicine, healthcare providers have improved tremendously in asking questions about personal and relationship safety in the home. Adolescent male patients should be asked the questions in relation to romantic relationship as well as familial relationships as are planned for female patients of all ages. It seems prudent here to also address sexual preferences and gender identity, as these are issues that are being seen in greater numbers in the adolescent population. Ask the questions in a matter-of-fact and neutral fashion, so that the adolescent male patient could both relate his preferences, while providing an attitude that prevents him from reacting in a discriminatory way to the question. Healthcare providers need to model nondiscriminatory behaviors and words.

BULLYING

Sixteen percent of male high school students reported in 2013 that they had been bullied at school in the last 12 months (CDC, 2014). Cyberbullying is also increasing; male adolescent patients should be reminded that cyberbullying is real and needs to be addressed just as in-person bullying does. Support reasonable parental access to teenagers' phones in order to support and assist them, not only when dealing with cyberbullying, but in identifying it. This also is useful in helping the adolescent to use his phone appropriately in all communications. Encourage your male adolescent not to send a text or a picture that they would not want to sit down and show their parents; these discussions give them boundaries in which to function safely.

PREVENTABLE ACCIDENTS

Traffic accidents were the leading cause of adolescent death in 2015. Drowning took the lives of 57,000 adolescents in the United States in 2015, and two-thirds of these deaths were males (World Health Organization, 2017). Seat belt safety and following state's laws regarding who and how many can be in the car with a new driver and then what time frame before that changes can be very useful to go over with your male adolescent patient. It provides them with a layer of accountability in addition to parents. It is also important to ask your patients if they know how to swim, and to talk to them about how even if they know how to swim, water and alcohol can often affect that ability in a negative way.

Helmet use is another very important health safety topic for adolescent males who often think that helmet use is only for little kids. Explaining to them how even a fall on grass that hits the wrong way can damage the brain and some potential consequences can sometimes help to increase helmet usage.

MALE ADOLESCENT IMMUNIZATIONS

Healthcare providers must stay current on the recommended immunizations for adolescents, especially as lack of immunizations can create conflict with school systems. In general, adolescents should be immunized for the following (Immunize, 2017):

- Hepatitis B, which may have happened in infancy, but can happen at any age
- Tdap, given at 11 to 12 years of age
- Td, given every 5 to 10 years after the Tdap, depending on the circumstances and recommendations
- Varivax, which may have been given in childhood
- MMR, which may have been administered in childhood
- Hepatitis A
- Influenza
- Meningococcal, given at 11 to 12 and again at 16 to 18 years of age
- Meningococcal B, given at 16 to 18 years of age by choice
- Human papillomavirus (HPV), given as two doses before 15 years of age and three doses after 15 years of age

A special note about HPV vaccine in male adolescents, as it is often viewed as the immunization to prevent cervical cancer and so there may be a general belief that males will not benefit from it. HPV vaccination is recommended for both boys and girls at ages 11 to 12 (CDC, 2016). Every year in the United States around 11,000 men get cancers caused by HPV infections. HPV infections can cause cancers of the anus and rectum, mouth/throat (oropharynx), and penis in men, and cases of anal cancer and cancers of the mouth/throat are on the rise (CDC, 2016). Unlike cervical cancer, there are no screening tests for these cancers, so they are often caught at a later stage when they are more difficult to treat. Many of the cancers caused by HPV infection in both men and women could have been prevented by HPV vaccination.

CONCLUSION

Know the core health issues that may be affecting your male adolescent patient. Encourage communication between parents and their adolescent male as well as with you. Guide male adolescents to build a variety of healthy responsible relationships. Realize that some male adolescents may be dealing with issues of sexuality, substance abuse, physical and/or emotional abuse, isolation, and the work of their adolescent developmental stage. Regardless of the reason for the visit and/or the clinical setting, provide thorough care to your male adolescent patient. Use the hooks such as the sports physical or injury visit to keep young men engaged with you and communicating about their lives, including their health.

REFERENCES

Bell, D. L., Breland, D. J., & Ott, M. A. (2013). Adolescent and young adult male health: A review. *Pediatrics, 132*(3), 545–546. doi:10.1542/peds.2012-3414

Bloom, B., Jones, L., & Freeman, G. (2013). *Summary health statistics for U.S. children: National Health Interview Survey, 2012*. Washington, DC: National Center for Health Statistics. Retrieved from https://www.cdc.gov/nchs/data/series/sr_10/sr10_258.pdf

Centers for Disease Control and Prevention. (2012). Fact sheets: Underage drinking. Retrieved from http://www.cdc.gov/alcohol/fact-sheets/underagedrinking.htm

Centers for Disease Control and Prevention. (2013). Asthma and schools. Retrieved from https://www.cdc.gov/healthyyouth/asthma/index.htm

Centers for Disease Control and Prevention. (2014). Youth risk behavior surveillance-United States, 2013. *Morbidity and Mortality Weekly Report, 63*(4). Retrieved from http://www.cdc.gov/mmwr/pdf/ss/ss6304.pdf

Centers for Disease Control and Prevention. (2016). HPV Vaccine is Cancer Prevention for Boys, too! Retrieved from https://www.cdc.gov/features/hpvvaccineboys/index.html

The Child and Adolescent Health Measurement Initiative. (2014). National Survey of Children's Health 2011/12. Retrieved from http://childhealthdata.org/browse/survey?q=2456&r=1

Child Trends Databank. (2016). Illicit drug use. Retrieved from https://www.childtrends.org/?indicators=illicit-drug-use

Erikson, E. H. (Ed.). (1963). *Youth: Change and challenge*. New York, NY: Basic books.

Goesling, B., Colman, S., Trenholm, D., Terzian, M., & Moore, K. A. (2014). Programs to reduce teen pregnancy, sexually transmitted infections, and associated sexual risk behaviors: A systematic review. *Journal of Adolescent Health, 54*(5), 499–507. doi:10.1016/j.jadohealth.2013.12.004

Immunize.org. (2017). Retrieved from http://www.immunize.org/catg.d/p2022.pdf

Johnston, L. D., O'Malley, P. M., Miech, R. A., Bachman, J. G., & Schulenberg, J. E. (2015). *Monitoring the Future national results on drug use: 1975-2014: Overview, key findings on adolescent drug use*. Ann Arbor, MI: Institute for Social Research, The University of Michigan. Retrieved from http://www.monitoringthefuture.org//pubs/monographs/mtf-overview2014.pdf

McLeod, S. A. (2013). Erik Erikson. Retrieved from https://www.simplypsychology.org/Erik-Erikson.html

Miech, R. A., Johnston, L. D., O'Malley, P. M., Bachman, J. G., & Schulenberg, J. E. (2014). *E-cigarettes surpass tobacco cigarettes among teens*. Ann Arbor, MI: University of Michigan. Retrieved from http://www.monitoringthefuture.org/pressreleases/14drugpr_complete.pdf

Muyle, T. P., Park, M. J., Nelson, C. D., Adams, S. H., Irwin C. D. Jr., & Brindis, C. D. (2009). Trends in adolescent and young adult health in the United States. *Journal of Adolescent Health, 45*(1), 8–24. doi:10.1016/j.jadohealth.2009.03.013

National Campaign to Prevent Teen and Unplanned Pregnancy. (2010). Science Says No. 6. The sexual attitudes and behavior of male teens. Retrieved from www.teenpregnancy.org

National Center for Chronic Disease Prevention and Health Promotion. (2014). *Health and academic achievement*. Atlanta, GA: Centers for Disease Control and Prevention. Retrieved from http://www.cdc.gov/healthyyouth/health_and_academics/pdf/health-academic-achievement.pdf

Ogden, C. L., Carroll, M. D., Kit, B. K., & Flegal, K. M. (2014). Prevalence of childhood and adult obesity in the United States, 2011-2012. *JAMA, 311*(8), 806–814. doi:10.1001/jama.2014.732

Substance Abuse & Mental Health Services Administration. (2014). *Results from the 2013 National Survey on Drug Use and Health: Mental health detailed tables*. Table 2.6B. Retrieved from http://www.samhas.gov/data/sites/default/files/2013MHDetTabs/NSDUH-M_HDetTabs2013.htm#tab2.6B

Telfair, J., & Shelton, T. L. (2012). Educational attainment as a social determinant of health. *North Carolina Medical Journal, 73*(5), 358–365.

U.S. Department of Education Institute of Education Sciences National Center for Education Statistics. (2011). National Assessment of Educational Progress (NAEP), 2011 Writing Assessments. Retrieved from http://nces.ed.gov/nationsreportcard/naepdata/dataset.aspx

U.S. Department of Education Institute of Education Sciences National Center for Education Statistics. (2014). National Assessment of Educational Progress Mathematics assessments (NAEP), 2013, 2011, 2009, 2007, 2005, and 2003 Mathematics assessments. Retrieved from htttp://nces.ed.gov/nationsreportcard/naepdata

U.S. Department of Health and Human Services. (2013). Adolescent health. Retrieved from https://www.healthypeople.gov/2020/topicsobjectives2020/overview.aspx?topicid=2

Volkow, N. D., Baler, R. D., Compton, W. M., & Weiss, S. R. (2014). Adverse health effects of marijuana use. *New England Journal of Medicine, 370*(23), 2219–2227. doi:10.1056/NEJMra1402309

World Health Organization. (2017). Adolescents: Health risks and solutions. Fact Sheet. Retrieved from www.who.int/mediacenter/factssheets/fs345/en

CHAPTER 6

Adolescent Males and the Media

Jade Burns

■ INTRODUCTION

Poor sexual health outcomes (such as sexually transmitted infections [STIs] and early sexual initiation) among youth remain a concern within the United States (Bull, Levine, Black, Schmiege, & Santelli, 2012). Adolescents and in particular subgroups such as young African American males are at the greatest risk of acquiring STIs and engaging in risky sexual behavior in comparison to their adolescent counterparts (Cornelius & Lawrence, 2009). In some circumstances, these youth do not have access to regular healthcare or health education (Bull et al., 2012). Barriers may include transportation and less access to convenient clinic locations (Bull et al., 2012). Adolescent males and young adults require access to appropriate information to make informed decisions regarding their personal and sexual health (Saewyc, 2012).

One way to support the sexual health information needs of adolescent males and young adults is to consider how they obtain information about sex. Social media as a platform for information dissemination may be one approach as an estimated 73% of teens currently use social media to access a variety of information, including material related to sexual health (Bull et al., 2012). Social media is defined as a mode of content sharing in virtual communities, with photos, videos, and live updates using electronic devices such as phones, mobile apps, computers, and tablets that are Internet based (Boyd & Ellison, 2010; Kim, & Ko, 2012). Social media is believed to be an effective way to provide the information that adolescent males and young adults need to make the appropriate sexual health decisions. Moreover, it may help delay behaviors such as early sexual debut, multiple partners, and unprotected sex.

To date, in clinical practice, providers have done relatively less to examine the benefits of social media and its relationship to safer sex behaviors. Given that adolescents and young adults often feel uncomfortable discussing sensitive topics, using social media may provide an avenue to facilitate and empower this population to discuss these sexual matters and other risk behaviors to potentially promote behavior change (Sznitman et al., 2011). Moreover, with the high expectations for youth to maintain contact with one another online, social media may be an optimal mechanism for evidence-based information sharing about risk behaviors including condom use (Dunne, McIntosh, & Mallory, 2014). This chapter provides a brief overview of social media and the Internet. It also specifically discusses evidence that social media and other forms of technology can be used to improve the sexual health of adolescent and young adult males with an emphasis on African American male youth.

AN OVERVIEW OF SOCIAL MEDIA AND RISK BEHAVIORS

Facts and Statistics

As adolescent risk behaviors persist, concerning sexual health, there have been widespread rates of STIs and HIV among all adolescents, and reducing adolescent sexual risk behavior is a persistent issue (Kann et al., 2016; Hutchinson, & Montgomery, 2007). Overall, adolescents and young adults ages 15 to 24 years comprise nearly half of the estimated 19 million new cases of STIs within the United States (Kann et al., 2016). While rates of HIV have been relatively reduced in the United States, males make up 80% of those diagnosed with HIV infection between ages 13 and 19 (Kann et al., 2016). Subgroups, such as African Americans, are being most heavily impacted by STIs such as gonorrhea and chlamydia infection (Guttmacher Institute, 2013; Kann et al., 2016). According to the Youth Risk Behavior Surveillance (Kann et al., 2016), the overall prevalence of ever having sexual intercourse, and having had sex before the age of 13 years, was highest among males. Minority groups such as African American males received the least amount of information in school regarding HIV and AIDS, as compared with other males (Eaton et al., 2012). It is clear that increasing rates of HIV and STIs, inadequate health education, and risky sexual behavior pose threats to the health and well-being of adolescent male and young adult communities.

Regarding sexual health, social media is believed to be an effective way to provide the information that adolescent males and young adults need to make in relation to sexual health decisions and may help delay behaviors such as early sexual debut, multiple partners, and unprotected sex. Currently, an estimated 73% of teens use social media to access a variety of information, including material related to sexual health (Bull et al., 2012). Little is known about the intersection of social media and its effect on youth regarding knowledge and decision-making behavior around condom use. Clinicians should know that using this type of technology may be useful in improving engagement and quality care in this unique population (Wong, Merchant, & Moreno, 2014).

SOCIAL MEDIA: BACKGROUND, CHARACTERISTICS, AND TYPES

Use of the Internet has grown exponentially since the first email in 1975, and some reports estimate that more than 500 social media sites exist today. Facebook, YouTube, Twitter, Google, Instagram, and Snapchat are the most common Internet-based sites (Craig, 2013; Curtis, 2013). Social media uses a personal profile created by the owner of the account. The owner can share updates on his or her personal status, or exchange messages either publicly or privately (Jones, Baldwin, & Lewis, 2012). Unlike traditional media (e.g., television, magazines), social media allows for the rapid transfer of information; messages are not solely created by marketing groups with a specific intent, but rather by individuals of any age, ethnic background, or socioeconomic status and can be about any topic (Jones et al., 2012, Moreno et al., 2009).

Regardless of the validity of the message, the ideas expressed allow individuals to state an opinion, and in turn, may go viral through multiple online channels by way of sharing links or posting messages (Thackeray, Neiger, Hanson, & McKenzie, 2008; Vance, Howe, & Dellavalle, 2009). As seen in Table 6.1, social media can be classified into five different categories that include collaborative websites, blogs, content communities, social networking sites, and virtual game social worlds (Albarran, 2013; Kaplan & Haenlein, 2010).

TABLE 6.1 Classification of Social Media

Collaborative Websites	Blogging (and Microblogging)	Content Communities	Social Networking Sites	Virtual Social/Game/ World	Communication/ Messengers
Wikipedia/ Wikia	***Twitter**	YouTube	***Facebook**	Second Life	***WhatsApp**
***AskFM**	***Tumblr**	Ted	Yelp	Smeet	***Kik**
answer.com	WordPress	Vimeo	the new MySpace	In Worldz	Facebook Messenger
about.com	Blogger (Google)	***Snapchat**	***LinkedIn**	IMVu	Skype
Encarta	Quora	***Vine**	Academia.edu		Line
Whisper	Facebook notes	Pheed	***Instagram**		Viber
Sarahah	Square Space	Flickr	***Pinterest**		GroupMe
Yik Yak	***LinkedIn**	Slideshare	***Kik**		WeChat
		Trendspottr	Meet up		Houseparty
		YouNow	Musical.ly		
		Reddit	Twitch		
		Periscope	***Google+**		
			Tinder		

*Not inclusive of all social media sites that exist today.

Note: Bold—preferred adolescent sites as of November 2017.

Source: Curtis, A. (2013). The brief history of social media. Retrieved from http://www2.uncp.edu/home/acurtis/NewMedia/SocialMedia/SocialMediaHistory.html; Duggan, M. (2015). *The demographics of social media users*. Washington, DC: Pew Research Center; Lenhart, A. (2015). Teens, social media and technology overview 2015: Smartphones facilitate shifts in communication landscape for teens. Washington, DC: Pew Research Center. Retrieved from http://assets.pewresearch.org/wp-content/uploads/sites/14/2015/04/PI_TeensandTech_Update2015_0409151.pdf

POPULAR SOCIAL MEDIA SITES

Facebook

Facebook has more than 2 billion users worldwide (Facebook.com). Its mission is to "give people the power to build community and bring the world closer together" (Facebook.com). It is the most widely used social media site among American youth ages 13 to 17 and is used by 71% of all adolescents (Lenhart, 2015). The site allows individuals to post comments, pictures, or videos (pre-taped or live); ask for recommendations for places to eat, travel, or shop; and create online blogs, business pages, or advertisements. The site has a mobile messenger to send text messages online or to your phone. People can also send money to one another. Additionally, individuals can "Like" each other's statuses. The site is used mainly on a desktop, mobile, or a tablet. This site is open to those ages 13 years and older (Facebook, 2017).

Instagram

Launched in 2010, Instagram is a site that is used mainly through a mobile app on a tablet or smartphone. As of 2012, it is owned by Facebook and has more than 300 million users (instagram-press.com/our-story). Instagram is a photo sharing site that has an eye-catching filter and other branded apps. Instagram brands include "Boomerang" (looping of videos and pictures on the Instagram), "Hyperlapse" (videos that can be recorded on one's phone and posted at an accelerated speed), and "Layout" (creates collages of photos; instagram-press.com/brand-assets). This app has a private message feature, and individuals can "like" photos, create live videos, and advertise on the app. This site is open to those ages 13 years and older (Instagram Privacy Policy, n.d.).

Snapchat

Founded in 2011, Snapchat is also referred to as Snap Is, a social media site and app that uses cameras to communicate with people. Snapchat users film moments from the camera phone and post them online. Picture or videos taken form a collection of moments that create a story. The app also allows the person to add geo-filters, an image-adjusting feature, that displays overlays such as colors, text caption to videos, and more (Snapchat, 2017a). Persons must be 13 years or older to create an account or use services from Snapchat (2017b).

Twitter

Launched in 2006, Twitter is a social media site that provides breaking news and entertainment in sports, personal opinions, politics, and everyday interests in 140 characters or less. Individuals can retweet other people's post or news announcements. Twitter's mission is "Give everyone the power to create and share ideas and information instantly, without barriers" (https://about.twitter.com/en_us/company.html; Twitter, 2017). Twitter is infamous for its hashtags; to follow a story or event, look up the hashtag of interest on the site.

SOCIAL MEDIA, ADOLESCENTS' ACCESS, AND TIME SPENT USING SOCIAL MEDIA

Adolescents are among the top users of social media (Jones et al., 2012). For the vast majority of teens, social media "is accessible anytime, anywhere, and on any digital device" (p. 208), including cell phones, laptops, and tablets (Allison et al., 2012). According to O'Keeffe and Clarke-Pearson's study (O'Keeffe, & Clarke-Pearson, & Council on Communications and Media, 2011), adolescents spend around 22% of their time logging onto their favorite social media sites and may visit those sites as many as 10 times per day. Additionally, social media has been identified as one of the most common extracurricular activities of children and adolescents (Jones et al., 2012; O'Keeffe et al., 2011).

Overall, Facebook, which is still the most popular, remains dominant as 71% of teens who are 13 to 17 years old use the site; the toughest competitors of Facebook include Instagram, Snapchat, and Twitter (Lenhart, 2015). Personal preference is an important variable in the popularity of any given social media platform, with use tied to income and gender (Kaplan & Haenlein, 2010). For example, boys admit to using Facebook more, while girls use Instagram and Tumblr social media sites (Lenhart, 2015). As social media grows, a teen using one form of social media at a time is less common, and teens enjoy combining these multiple platforms to express their thoughts, ideas, and identities (Boyd, 2014; Lenhart, 2015).

Benefits and Risks

Social media may be instrumental in adolescent development. For example, it allows peer group involvement because everyone is welcome; provides identity exploration; fosters independence; and allows youth to develop all of these tasks simultaneously (Allen, 2014). Studies have shown that social media and networking sites play an integral role in the development of a healthy sense of cultural identity as well as a positive sense of self-identity (Byrne, 2007). The results from an earlier Internet study using Black Planet found that the most popular forums for African Americans using social media included building relationships, heritage and identity, religiosity, and spirituality (Byrne, 2007).

Social media can also be used for anonymous communication because it creates a safe space that may help reduce stigma by bringing confidentiality to the forefront, which is critical to an adolescent's self-expression (Allen, 2014). Despite its benefits, the risks for adolescents must be considered. These risks include privacy concerns, minimal parental supervision, little accountability, as well as adolescents becoming entrapped in a "time sink," which refers to losing track of time spent on networking sites (Allen, 2014). Another important risk is inappropriate online contact, illustrating the need for better methods to balance anonymity and safety (Yager & O'Keefe, 2012).

AFRICAN AMERICAN ADOLESCENTS AND YOUNG ADULTS AND SOCIAL MEDIA

In one study, nearly all of African Americans ages 18 to 29 used a social media site (96%) (Smith, 2014). Among African American late adolescents (ages 18–24), Instagram and Twitter were especially appealing and were more widely used than any other social media sites (Duggan & Brenner, 2013). Younger African Americans (ages 18–29) "have shown high levels of 'tweeting' and comprise 22% of Twitter users as compared to 16% of whites" (Smith, 2014). Studies have also shown that African American adolescents have had a presence on Pinterest (Albarran, 2013). Topics that were "pinned" included hair care, hairstyles, and black fashion (Albarran, 2013).

Regarding privacy, Madden et al (Madden et al., 2013) found that African American adolescents were less likely to reveal their true identity on their profiles on social media. Privacy is important to consider because adolescents are looking for ways to establish their identity among their peers. Therefore, how much they reveal regarding their image online is important to consider when modeling certain behaviors (Moreno et al., 2009). Understanding how youth may want to be viewed online is complex. Self-presentation may be portrayed online in multiple identities (i.e., expressing explicit behaviors) not only to protect their privacy but also to establish an alter ego (Boyd & Ellison, 2010).

Cyberbullying

Cyberbullying is commonly defined as "an aggressive, intentional act or behavior that is carried out by a group or an individual, using electronic forms of contact, repeatedly and over time against a victim who cannot easily defend him or herself" (Chassiakos et al., 2016). According to the YRBS, cyberbullying has increased since 2012 with 14.8% of adolescents being electronically bullied, and more than 19.8% of students having ever been bullied on school grounds (Kann et al., 2014). It is recognized as a global phenomenon affecting various cultures groups and has severe consequences such as school refusal, depression, and even suicide (Twitter, 2017). The increasing number of adolescents online predisposes them to engage in dangerous online and aggressive communications (Ang, 2015).

Cyberbullying may, in fact, have greater gain than traditional bullying as the perpetrator has a larger audience to target, can hide his/her identity, can post visible messages, can stay posted and remain in the "cloud," and can have constant accessibility (Kim, Colwell, Kata, Boyle, & Georgiades, 2017). In turn, cyberbullying has been associated with key behavioral problems such as physical violence, and alcohol and tobacco use (Kin et al., 2017). Providers should pay close attention to their review of systems (psychiatric assessment) and history of present illness (HPI) of recurring emotional and behavioral problems that may be more apparent in this population (see Box 6.1).

BOX 6.1 HPI QUESTIONS TO ASK ADOLESCENT MALES AND YOUNG ADULTS

Reason for visit, screening for risk behaviors

- What brings you in today?
- Questions and concerns?
- General health questions?
- Annual/sports physical?
- Employment verification?
- Follow-up visit?
- Partner has symptoms?
- Treatment for positive test results?

General

- Fatigue, fever, chills, or weight gain/loss
- Appetite
- Activity

Head, Ears, Eyes, Nose, Throat (HEENT)

- Headache
- Sore throat
- Swollen glands

Skin

- Unusual growth on genitalia
- Pruritus
- Growth/lesion
- Rash

Genitourinary (GU)

- GU symptoms
- Hematuria
- Dysuria
- Polyuria
- Male GU
  - Penile (pain, lump, swelling, lesion, reddening, discharge)
  - Testicular (pain, swelling, lump)
  - Scrotum (pain, lesion, swelling, lump)
  - Blood in semen or fishy odor to semen

Neurological

- Dizziness
- Lightheadedness
- Headaches

Psychological

- Loss of interest in activities
- Sadness

(continued)

BOX 6.1 HPI QUESTIONS TO ASK ADOLESCENT MALES AND YOUNG ADULTS (*continued*)

- Feeling like you are going to harm yourself or others
- Do you feel safe or stressed
- Difficulty sleeping
- Mood swings

HPI, history of present illness.

Other Risk Behaviors and Social Media

A risk behavior is defined as an action that could potentially jeopardize an individual's physical, psychological, and/or emotional health, and is a distinct feature of adolescent development (Burns, Dunn, Brady, Starr, & Blosser, 2016). The need to gain independence, maturity, or even friends may propel this behavior. Some factors that contribute to risk taking include poor academic performance, lack of appropriate role model or association with those displaying deviant behavior, lack of social support, low self-esteem, depression, illiteracy, poverty, and lack of sleep (Burns et al., 2016). Likewise, adolescents and young adults are resilient. Therefore, there are protective factors that enable these individuals to make healthier lifestyle choices; some factors include high self-esteem and sense of worth, having goals, academic success, parental engagement, supportive family environment, civic and community involvement, and access to recreation and sports (Burns et al., 2016).

In addition to sexual risk behaviors, social media has been studied with other adolescent and young adult risk behaviors such as alcohol and other drug use and tobacco use. Studies have found that similar to traditional television media, adolescents who have been exposed to risky behaviors like sexual and substance abuse behaviors are associated with these behaviors (Chassiakos et al., 2016). Moreover, newer evidence has shown that adolescent-displayed behaviors online have showcased illegal alcohol use or overuse, risky sexual behavior, and those behaviors that cause self-harm, for example, self-injury (Chassiakos et al., 2016). Other clinically relevant topics of social media and risk behaviors include predicting college drinking, exposure to marijuana and substance-related content on social media sites, and how to promote HIV and STI testing in youth (Cabrera-Nguyen, Cavazos-Rehg, Krauss, Bierut, & Moreno, 2016; Dowshen, Lee, Lehman, Castillo, & Mollen, 2015; Yaeger & Moreno, 2017).

Clinical Concepts of Adolescent Male and Young Adult Health: Adolescent Development

Historically, adolescence has been defined as a unique period of development when one experiences hormonal and pubertal changes, develops new friendships, and experiences identity development. For some theorists, it includes a time of storm and stress in which adolescents yearn for exploration and activity that may involve conflict with parents, risky behavior, and mood changes (Arnett, 1999). It may be defined from multiple perspectives that include biological (defined by puberty), sociological (defined by roles), psychological (defined by stages), and historical perspectives (Arnett, 1999; Muuss, 1996). These aspects should be studied from such formats that consider personal experiences of general well-being, the capacity to perform expected roles, and the health potential of the adolescent (Millstein, Nightengale, Petersen, Mortimer, & Hamburg, 1993).

Moreover, adolescent development is also dependent on context, which influences the way in which an adolescent reaches maturity, socializes, or creates his identity. These settings include family, peers, neighborhood, school, and the American society (Caldwell, 2012; Muuss, 1996). As these circumstances change throughout an adolescent's life, they provide opportunities to help shape the behavior of the youth in ways that can establish a healthy lifestyle as he emerges into adulthood (Millstein, et al., 1993).

There are four phases of adolescent development for male youth (Arnett, 2015; Burns et al., 2016; Lerner & Steinberg, 2009):

Early Adolescence (Ages 11–14)

- Physical—Tanner stages for sexual maturity reach up to stage 3 or 4.
- Cognitive—Daydreaming, reasoning, and problem-solving skills develop.
- Social and Emotional—Mood swings. Renegotiate relationship with the parent and other significant mentors or family members. Intimate relationships start to form with peers. The adolescent will prefer to spend more time with friends at this stage. Desire greater privacy. Devote more time to electronic devices (texting, social media). Appearance may matter more at this stage.
- Sexual Development and Behavior—Initiation of puberty, wet dreams, masturbation occurs.

Middle Adolescence (Ages 15–17)

- Physical—Development near completion. Interested in body attractiveness.
- Cognitive—Abstract thinking is in its primitive stage; creativity and intellectual curiosity develops. Poor judgment.
- Social and Emotional—Egocentric individuals. Peer group involvement is most important and intense. In this stage, adolescents spend double the time with their peers than family members. Peer pressure to experiment in sexual activity occurs. May engage in more risk-taking behaviors such as smoking and drinking.
- Sexual Development and Behavior—Sexual energy is at its highest here. Dating and casual relationships. Sexual behavior is now in its exploratory phase.

Late Adolescence (Ages 18–21)

- Physical—Puberty is complete.
- Cognitive—Adult learning and reasoning and judgment skills develop. Understand risks, benefits, and consequences of a given situation.
- Social and Emotional—Relationships with parents and family members are renegotiated and gain importance. Value system defined. Enter workforce, college, or technical training programs.
- Sexual Development and Behavior—Sexual behavior becomes more expressive. Intimate relationships form.

Emerging Adult Population (Ages 21–25)

Can start as early as 18 years of age and may end as late as 29 years of age

- Physical—Development complete.
- Cognitive—Still learning to take responsibility for one's actions, making independent decisions, and securing financial independence.

- Social and Emotional—Transitioning from finishing education (high school, undergraduate, or graduate), and entering the workforce with the intent to find job stability. Finding relationships that are self-fulfilling including marriage and parenthood at a later stage in life. Period of independent exploration.
- Sexual Development—May have a series of sexual and intimate relationships before commitment takes place.

HUMAN SEXUALITY

Human sexuality is a process that begins at birth and ends at death (DeLamter & Freidrich, 2002). During adolescence, sexual orientation, identity, and gender attitudes are formed. Adolescent sexuality can be examined from either a biological or social perspective. Sigmund Freud describes sexual behavior as a result of socially shaped and learned patterns. (Miller, Norton, Fan, & Christopherson, 1998). Family characteristics, culture, parental values, early and steady dating, and peer influence can affect the expression of behavior and arousal between females and males (Miller et al., 1998).

ASSESSMENT OF RISK BEHAVIORS

Clinicians should assess all adolescents at their visit for risk-taking behavior. When interviewing the patient, clinicians should keep in mind to be open, nonjudgmental, and transparent, and to establish rapport when communicating with the adolescent (Burns et al., 2016). It is also essential to ensure and maintain privacy during the visit. Listed below are tools that can assess for risk-taking behavior:

- ***Home, Education/employment, Eating, Activities, Drugs, Sexuality, Suicide/ Depression, and Safety*** (HEEADSSS) screening tool (available at www.contemporarypediatrics.com/modern-medicine-feature-articles/heeadsss-30-psychosocial-interview-adolescents-updated-new-century-fueled-media). Examples of red flags include risky sexual activity, poor academic performance, drinking and driving, involvement in gangs, mood disorders, and physical inactivity (Burns et al., 2016). The result of not screening for these behaviors may include an increase in STIs, decreased school attendance, school failure, and incarceration (Burns et al., 2016).
- ***Rapid Assessment for Adolescent Preventive Services*** (RAAPS) risk assessment screening tool. Addressing risk-taking behavior is essential in reducing the morbidity and mortality outcome that adolescents may face (Darling-Fisher, Salerno, Dahlem, & Martyn, 2014). The RAAPS assessment is a validated screening tool that helps provide screening for key adolescent risk behaviors in a time-efficient manner (Darling-Fisher et al.; 2014). The strengths of the tool is that it is user friendly and composed of a 21-item questionnaire that can be filled out by the patient in approximately 5 to 7 minutes, and the provider can assess risk in a short period of time (Darling-Fisher et al.; 2014). The tool is culturally sensitive with health messages that are evidence based and tailored by age (38). RAAPS is frequently used in school-based and community health settings as well as in juvenile detention and youth serving organizations (Possibilities for Change, 2017). Providers can request a copy or view a webinar about RAAPS at www.possibilitiesforchange.com
- ***CRAFFT screening tool*** **(**Table 6.2**)**. Endorsed by the American Academy of Pediatrics (AAP), this tool is recommended to screen for alcohol and substance abuse and use in adolescent youth (Center for Adolescent Substance Abuse Research, 2009; Roberts, Gabrielli, & Van Hook, 2009). The screening

tool comprises six questions that are used to screen for these disorders that are highly associated with health problems such as "school failure, respiratory diseases and high-risk sexual behaviors" (Roberts et al., 2009).

Anticipatory Guidance

Anticipatory guidance for adolescent males and young adults should come from an open and honest discussion and be age appropriate. Items to discuss with this population include skills that can assist with decision making to reduce risky behaviors and understanding that self-care, physical activity, and good nutrition are essential in facilitating a healthy lifestyle. Clinicians should focus on not only knowledge but also incorporating skill building that can help to sustain positive behavior.

Discussions of responsibility and life choices should take place. Encourage these youth to build relationships with parents, friends, and positive male mentors (Burna et al., 2016). Discuss health promotion and risk reduction information with adolescents. Provide resources that extend outside the clinic (e.g., where to get condoms, emergency plan, mental health resources, school health programs; Burns et al., 2016). Respect their peers and themselves. Encourage parent–adolescent communication or discussion with a supportive adult (preferably male) regarding risk behaviors and accurate information about sex. Provide information about how to handle emotions and peer pressure. Help them learn how to manage time and activities. Encourage these youths to learn new skills and set goals as they transition to their next developmental phase (Hagan, Shaw, & Duncan, 2017).

TABLE 6.2 CRAFFT Screening Tool

To be administered orally by the clinician. Begin: "I'm going to ask you a few questions that I ask all my patients. Please be honest. I will keep your answers confidential."	
During the PAST 12 MONTHS, on how many days did you:	
1.	Drink more than a few sips of beer, wine, or any drink containing alcohol? Say "0" if none.
2.	Use any marijuana (pot, weed, hash, or in foods) or "synthetic marijuana" (like "K2" or "Spice")? Say "0" if none.
3.	Use anything else to get high (like other illegal drugs, prescription or over-the-counter medications, and things that you sniff or "huff")? Say "0" if none.
CRAFFT is a mnemonic acronym of the first letters of keywords in the six screening questions. The questions should be asked exactly as written.	
C	Have you ever ridden in a CAR driven by someone (including yourself) who was "high" or had been using alcohol or drugs?
R	Do you ever use alcohol or drugs to RELAX, feel better about yourself, or fit in?
A	Do you ever use alcohol/drugs while you are by yourself, ALONE?
F	Do you ever FORGET things you did while using alcohol or drugs?
F	Do your family or FRIENDS ever tell you that you should cut down on your drinking or drug use?
T	Have you gotten into TROUBLE while you were using alcohol or drugs?
Notice to Clinic Staff and Medical Records: The information on this page is protected by special federal confidentiality rules (42 CFR Part 2), which prohibit disclosure of this information unless authorized by specific written consent. A general authorization for release of medical information is NOT sufficient.	

Source: © John R. Knight, MD, Boston Children's Hospital. (2018). All rights reserved. Reproduced with permission. For more information, contact ceasar@childrens.harvard.edu

HEALTH PROMOTION FOR ADOLESCENT MALES AND YOUNG ADULTS

The behavior of the adolescent male and young adult is key to their growth and development. Focusing on responsible sexual behavior, building healthy relationships with partners, learning about intimacy, interpersonal skills, and engaging this population may help to increase health-promoting behaviors (Office of Adolescent Health, U.S. Department of Health and Human Services, 2013). Additionally, understanding their perspective on teen pregnancy, fatherhood, family planning, and childbearing can assist with strategies to reduce teen pregnancy (Office of Adolescent Health, U.S. Department of Health and Human Services, 2013). One study revealed that getting famous people to post messages or using certain social media sites are just a few innovative ways to capture the attention of young African American males (Burns, 2016). Moreover, this population can learn best from each other and desire to be in groups to discuss sensitive topics such as sexual health (Burns, 2016). Finding creative ways to initiate communication with this population such as the use of social media may be helpful and valuable to improve treatment rates, and to provide an opportunity to disseminate accurate information. Using these sites may also reinforce some skills related to sexual health knowledge, like condom use (Burns, 2016). Lastly, in a qualitative study it was found that the following sites (listed in order of preference) are easy to use for health information by young African American males and young adults: #1 YouTube, #2 Facebook, #3 Twitter, and #4 Instagram (Office of Adolescent Health, U.S. Department of Health and Human Services, 2013). Messages must be educational, accessible, brief, clear, and engaging (Burns, 2016).

CLINICAL RECOMMENDATIONS FOR PROVIDERS

Healthcare providers are all valuable resources in disseminating and using this type of information for the adolescent male and young adult population. Social media may be useful in promoting healthy behaviors and facilitating healthy lifestyle changes among this population. More attention needs to be given to our males and their health needs. Recruitment into clinics and health service research need to improve. Understanding that their needs and preference may change based on environment and circumstance also needs to be considered. Finding creative ways to initiate communication with this population such as the use of social media may be helpful and valuable to improve treatment rates, and to provide an opportunity to disseminate accurate information. Using these sites may also reinforce some skills related to sexual health knowledge, like condom use. Finally, understanding what sites this population is using, how they use them, and what factors can motivate them to use this platform for preventive health information may remove barriers and provide an opportunity for them to make safe decisions involving their personal health.

In conclusion, persistence needs to be stressed when providing clinical care and anticipatory guidance for youth. Healthcare providers need to reach out to this population in any possible safe format. Despite the challenges that remain in understanding how using this mode of communication can be used for health promotion efforts (e.g., STI prevention), clinicians need to strategically find a way to incorporate these methods into clinical practice. As adolescents and more specifically male subgroup populations (racial and ethnic minorities, sexual and gender minorities) navigate through these sites, they are challenged daily by what they experience in their social and media contexts. They need to be prepared to handle risky situations both in person and online. Understanding how they navigate these systems will not only give clinicians a view into what they may struggle with, but it can also help supportive influences like nurses, healthcare providers, the community, and researchers to better understand the role of social media. This insight will ultimately help healthcare providers be available and present when needed to help them navigate through these channels productively.

CASE STUDY

A 19-year-old African American male presents to a local Teen Clinic requesting a complete physical examination. The resident of a community organization program patient is requesting the completion of a health appraisal form and a copy of his immunization record.

The patient denied any health complaints or concerns at this visit. Medications include Latuda 40 mg once daily. He is allergic to grass, pollen, and coconut and has suffered from hay fever. Past medical history is significant for depression. The patient denied any recent visit to urgent care or emergency room. He also denied recent illnesses, injuries, or hospitalizations. A review of systems reveals no significant health concerns or history.

Social history includes homelessness for about one year, daily use of tobacco products, and social use of alcohol and marijuana. The patient denied use of any illicit drugs. He is sexually active with same-sex partners.

Physical examination was essentially benign with the exception of obvious hyperpigmented macules noted in bilateral palms which patient denied were itchy or painful. He reports that they were noted about 1 month ago and that his feet had the same "spots." The patient denied recent illness or fevers; he also denied weight loss or fatigue.

Differential diagnosis included general viral exanthems, HIV infection, and syphilis. The patient was asked about the presence of any ulcer or sores that healed, partners with known or suspected HIV infections, and partners with penile sores or lesions. Sexual history was obtained that revealed one current partner but a history of commercial sex worker that was sometimes unprotected.

Based on the current physical findings an anal examination was performed that revealed no obvious ulcers or lesions.

Laboratory investigations included urinalysis; testing for gonorrhea, chlamydia, and HIV; rapid plasma reagin (RPR) test for syphilis; complete blood count (CBC); and comprehensive metabolic profile (CMP) (Tables 6.3 and 6.4).

Education was provided regarding the increased risk of HIV infection, syphilis, and human papillomavirus (HPV) infection with MSM (men who have sex with men) activity. The treatment for syphilis was initiated, and education and rationale were provided. Specific to this visit was the anal examination, which without this patient's specific history would not have been done.

Anticipatory guidance was provided related to tobacco use, alcohol use, marijuana, and high-risk sexual behavior. Cessation was encouraged, condoms were provided, and the patient was provided a Next Steps Partner Notification card for partner to receive services in the local Teen Clinic.

Social media could have been used in this visit to provide the patient with education specific to syphilis as well as the risk associated with receptive partners in MSM sexual activity. Technology could be used to provide education on the appropriate way to apply condoms and to provide examples/scenarios on how to discuss the use of condoms and HIV status with partners.

(continued)

■ CASE STUDY (*continued*)

TABLE 6.3 Helpful Billing and Procedural Codes: *ICD-10*

Z68	BMI
Z68.52	BMI, 5th percentile to 85th percentile
Z68.54	BMI, greater than 95th percentile
Z68.53	BMI, 85th percentile to less than 95th percentile
A56, A56.8	Chlamydial infection (other sexually transmitted diseases)
A74.9	Chlamydial infection unspecified
A56.4	Chlamydial infection of pharynx
Z11.8	Chlamydial disease, Screening for
Z70	Counseling related to sexual attitude, behavior, and orientation
Z30	Counseling for surveillance of contraceptives, unspecified
Z13.89	Depression, Screening for
Z71.3	Dietary counseling and surveillance
A54.9	Gonorrhea
Z11.3	Gonorrhea, Screening for
A60.0	Herpes
A60.01, A60.02	Herpes of penis and other male genital organs
Z72.5	High-risk sexual behavior
B20	HIV
Z11.4	HIV, Screening for
Z71.7	HIV, Counseling for
Z20.6	HIV, Exposure to
A63.0	HPV/Genital Warts
Z23	Immunizations
Z00.129	Routine Child Health Examination (12–17)
Z00.121	Routine Child Health Examination (12–17), abnormal findings
Z00.0	Routine Health Examination >18 years of age
Z00.01	Routine Health Examination >18 years of age, abnormal findings
Z11.3	STIs, Screening for
Z20.2	STIs, Exposure to
A51, A5.2	Syphilis
Z11.3	Syphilis, Screening for
A59.9	Trichomoniasis

BMI, body mass index; ICD-10, *International Classification of Diseases*, 10th ed; STIs, sexually transmitted infections.

Source: SuccessEHS. (2017). Billing and coding. Retrieved from https://www.greenwayhealth.com

(*continued*)

CASE STUDY (*continued*)

TABLE 6.4 Helpful Billing and Current Procedural Terminology (CPT) Codes

2000F	Blood pressure measured
85025	CBC (includes DIFF/Platelets)
87591	Chlamydia. Gonorrhea RNA, TMA
87491	Chlamydia. Gonorrhea RNA, TMA – Throat
82465	Cholesterol, Total
80053	Comprehensive Metabolic Panel
82565	Creatinine W/EGFR
87255	Culture, Herpes Simplex, Rapid
10060	Drainage of Skin Abscess
J3490	Drug Unclassified Injection
86003	Food Allergy Profile
87070	Genital Culture, Routine
82947	Glucose, Plasma
85014	Hematocrit
85018	Hemoglobin
83036	Hemoglobin A1C
87389	HIV 1/2 Antigen/Antibody, Fourth generation
87536	HIV 1 DNA Quant
87529	HSV 1/2 PCR
87255	Herpes Simplex Rapid Culture
86695	Herpes Simplex Virus Type 1-Specific AB, IgG
86696	Herpes Simplex Type 2-Specific AB, IgG
83540	Iron, Serum
83550	Iron, TIBC, & Ferritin Panel
80061	Lipid Panel
J0558	Penicillin G Benzathine Injection
86580	PPD Test
86480	Quantiferon TB GOLD
86003	Respiratory Allergy Profile
86592	RPR
88175	Trichomonas Test for Males
84434	TSH
81001	UA/Culture
84520	Urea Nitrogen, BUN
81000	Urinalysis
82306	Vitamin D, 25-Hydroxy
99173	Visual Acuity
87070	Culture, Aerobic Bacteria
87081	Streptococcus, Group B Culture

BUN, blood urea nitrogen; CBC, complete blood count; DIFF, differential; DNA, deoxyribonucleic acid; EGFR, epidermal growth factor receptor; HSV, herpes simplex virus; IgG, Immunoglobulin G; PCR, polymerase chain reaction; PPD, purified protein derivative; RNA, ribonucleic acid; RPR, rapid plasma reagin; TIBC, total iron-binding capacity; TMA, Transcription-Mediated Amplification; TSH, thyroid-stimulating hormone; UA, urinalysis.

SOCIAL MEDIA AND INTERNET RESOURCES FOR PROVIDERS

- AAP Media Use Plan: www.healthychildren.org/English/media/Pages/default.aspx
- Advocates for Youth: www.advocatesforyouth.org/publications/1142-icuidate; www.advocatesforyouth.org/publications/publications-a-z/2302-the-reproductive-and-sexual-health-of-young-men-of-color
- Association for Reproductive Health Professionals: www.arhp.org/MethodMatch
- Bright Futures: brightfutures.aap.org/materials-and-tools/tool-and-resource-kit/Pages/adolescence-tools.aspx
- CDC HIV stats: www.cdc.gov/hiv/group/index.html
- CDC information Risk Behaviors (ages 12–19): www.cdc.gov/parents/teens/risk_behaviors.html
- Go Ask Alice: www.goaskalice.columbia.edu
- Kids Health: kidshealth.org/en/teens/nemours.html
- Mental Health Resources for Young Adults: www.adolescenthealth.org/Resources/Clinical-Care-Resources/Mental-Health/Mental-Health-Resources-For-Adolesc.aspx
- National Survey of Sexual Behavior: www.nationalsexstudy.indiana.edu
- Office of Adolescent Health: www.hhs.gov/ash/oah
- The Guttmacher Institute: www.guttmacher.org/state-policy/explore/overview-minors-consent-law
- Twitter/Facebook/Instagram sites
  - CDC STD: CDCSTD
  - Center for Sexuality and Health Disparities: SexualityLab
  - Healthy People 2020: GoHealthyPeople2020
  - Kinsey Institute: kinseyinstitute
  - SAMHSA: samhsa.gov
  - Stop Bullying: StopBullyingGov
  - Stop Teen Suicide: Help_sts
  - Teen Parent Connection: TeenParentNP
  - Teen Substance Abuse: ASKDrugAbuse
  - Visions Teen: VisionsTeen
  - What Works Youth HIV: whatworksythHIV
  - Youth HIV and AIDS Day: YouthAIDSDAY
- YB Men Project: www.ybmenproject.com/team

REFERENCES

Albarran, A. (Ed.). (2013). *The social media industries*. New York, NY: Routledge.

Allen, K. (2014). Social media use and social connectedness in adolescents: The positives and the potential pitfalls. *Educational and Developmental Psychologist, 31*, 18–31. doi:10.1017/edp.2014

Allison, S., Bauermeister, J. A., Bull, S., Lightfoot, M., Mustanski, B., Shegog, R., & Levine, D. (2012). The intersection of youth, technology, and new media with sexual health: Moving the research agenda forward. *Journal of Adolescent Health, 51*(3), 207–212. doi:10.1016/j.jadohealth.2012.06.012

Ang, R. P. (2015). Adolescent cyberbullying: A review of characteristics, prevention and intervention strategies. *Aggression and Violent Behavior, 25*, 35–42. doi:10.1016/j.avb.2015.07.011

Arnett, J. J. (1999). Adolescent storm and stress, reconsidered. *American Psychologist, 54*(5), 317. doi:10.1037/0003-066X.54.5.317

Arnett, J. J. (2015). *The Oxford handbook of emerging adulthood.* New York, NY: Oxford University Press.

Boyd, D. (2014). *It's complicated: The social lives of networked teens.* New Haven + London: Yale University Press.

Boyd, D. M., & Ellison, N. B. (2010). Social network sites: Definition, history, and scholarship. *IEEE Engineering Management Review, 38*(3), 16–31. doi:10.1109/EMR.2010.5559139

Bull, S. S., Levine, D. K., Black, S. R., Schmiege, S. J., & Santelli, J. (2012). Social media-delivered sexual health intervention: A cluster randomized controlled trial. *American Journal of Preventive Medicine, 43*(5), 467–474. doi:10.1016/j.amepre.2012.07.022

Burns, C. E., Dunn, A. M., Brady, M. A., Starr, N. B., & Blosser, C. G. (2016). *Pediatric primary care* (6th ed.). St. Louis, MO: Elsevier.

Burns, J. (2016). *In their public space: A qualitative analysis of young African American males' views of social media as a mode for condom use education* [Doctoral Dissertation]. University of Michigan. Retrieved from https://deepblue.lib.umich.edu/handle/2027.42/120861

Byrne, D. N. (2007). Public discourse, community concerns, and civic engagement: Exploring black social networking traditions on BlackPlanet.com. *Journal of Computer-Mediated Communication, 13*(1), 319–340. doi:10.1111/j.1083-6101.2007.00398.x

Cabrera-Nguyen, E. P., Cavazos-Rehg, P., Krauss, M., Bierut, L. J., & Moreno, M. A. (2016). Young adults' exposure to alcohol-and marijuana-related content on twitter. *Journal of Studies on Alcohol and Drugs, 77*(2), 349–353. doi:10.15288/jsad.2016.77.349

Caldwell, C. (2012). Theory research and practice [Power Point Slides]. Retrieved from https://ctools.umich.edu/portal/site/d0684939-46a5-4a9a-a9a5-3a4c0641f07b/page/fca50a44-0e6a-496e-a3da-ba777f6c0642

Center for Adolescent Substance Abuse Research. (2009). Children's Hospital Boston. Retrieved from www.ceasar.org

Chassiakos, Y. R., Radesky, J., Christakis, D., Moreno, M. A., Cross, C., Hill, D., ... Swanson, W. S. (2016). Children and adolescents and digital media. *Pediatrics, 138*(5), pii: e20162593. doi:10.1542/peds.2016-2593

Cornelius, J., & Lawrence, J. (2009). Receptivity of African American adolescents to an HIV-prevention curriculum enhanced by text messaging. *Journal for Specialists in Pediatric Nursing, 14*, 123–131. doi:10.1111/j.1744-6155.2009.00185.x

Craig, R. (2013). How many social media sites will survive? Retrieved from http://www.huffingtonpost.ca/randall-craig/social-mediasites_b_2925234.html?view=screen

Curtis, A. (2013). The brief history of social media. Retrieved from http://www2.uncp.edu/home/acurtis/NewMedia/SocialMedia/SocialMediaHistory.html

Darling-Fisher, C. S., Salerno, J., Dahlem, C. H. Y., & Martyn, K. K. (2014). The rapid assessment for adolescent preventive services (RAAPS): Providers' assessment of its usefulness in their clinical practice settings. *Journal of Pediatric Health Care, 28*(3), 217–226. doi:10.1016/j.pedhc.2013.03.003

DeLamater, J., & Friedrich, W. (2002). Human sexual development. *The Journal of Sex Research, 39*(1), 10–14. Retrieved from http://www.jstor.org/stable/3813417

Dowshen, N., Lee, S., Lehman, B. M., Castillo, M., & Mollen, C. (2015). IknowUshould2: Feasibility of a youth driven social media campaign to promote STI and HIV testing among adolescents in Philadelphia. *AIDS and Behavior, 19*(Suppl 2):106–111. doi:10.1007/s10461-014-0991-9

Duggan, M. (2015). *The demographics of social media users.* Washington, DC: Pew Research Center.

Duggan, M., & Brenner, J. (2013). *The Demographics of Social Media Users-2012.* Washington, DC: Pew Research Center's Internet & American Life Project.

Dunne, A., McIntosh, J., & Mallory, D. (2014). Adolescents, sexually transmitted infections, and education using social media: A review of the literature. *The Journal for Nurse Practitioners, 10*(6), 401–408.e2. doi:10.1016/j.nurpra.2014.03.020

Eaton, D. K., Kann, L., Kinchen, S., Shanklin, S., Flint, K. H., Hawkins, J., ... Centers for Disease Control and Prevention. (2012). Youth risk behavior surveillance—United States, 2011. *Morbidity and Mortality Weekly Report. Surveillance Summaries, 61*(4), 1–162. Retrieved from https://www.cdc.gov/mmwr/preview/mmwrhtml/ss6104a1.htm

Facebook. (2017). Minors and safety. Retrieved from https://www.facebook.com/about/privacy/minors

Guttmacher Institute. (2013). Facts on American Teens' Sexual and Reproductive Health (pp. 1–4). Retrieved from http://www.guttmacher.org/pubs/FB-ATSRH.pdf

Hagan, J. F., Shaw, J. S., & Duncan, P. M. (2017). *Bright Futures* (*Pocket Guide*; 4th ed.). Elk Grove Village, IL: American Academy of Pediatrics.

Hutchinson, M. K., & Montgomery, A. J. (2007). Parent communication and sexual risk among African Americans. *Western Journal of Nursing Research, 29*(6), 691–707. doi:10.1177/0193945906297374

Instagram Privacy Policy. (n.d.). Retrieved from https://help.instagram.com/155833707900388

Jones, K., Baldwin, K. A., & Lewis, P. R. (2012). the potential influence of a social media intervention on risky sexual behavior and Chlamydia incidence. *Journal of Community Health Nursing, 29*(2), 106–120. doi:10.1080/07370016.2012.670579

Kann, L., Kinchen, S., Shanklin, S. L., Flint, K. H., Hawkins, J., Harris, W. A., ... Zaza, S. (2014). Youth risk behavior surveillance-United States, 2013. *MMWR Surveillance Summaries, 63*(4), 1–168.

Kann, L., McManus, T., Harris, W. A., Shanklin, S. L., Flint, K. H., Hawkins, J., ... Zaza, S. (2016). Youth risk behavior surveillance—United States, 2015. *MMWR Surveillance Summaries, 65*(6), 1–174. doi:10.15585/mmwr.ss6506a1

Kaplan, A. M., & Haenlein, M. (2010). Users of the world, unite! The challenges and opportunities of Social Media. *Business Horizons, 53*(1), 59–68. doi:10.1016/j.bushor.2009.09.003

Kim, A. J., & Ko, E. (2012). Do social media marketing activities enhance customer equity? An empirical study of luxury fashion brand. *Journal of Business Research, 65*(10), 1480–1486. doi:10.1016/j.jbusres.2011.10.014

Kim, S., Colwell, S. R., Kata, A., Boyle, M. H., & Georgiades, K. (2017). Cyberbullying victimization and adolescent mental health: Evidence of differential effects by sex and mental health problem type. *Journal of Youth and Adolescence, 47*(3), 661–672. doi:10.1007/s10964-017-0678-4

Lenhart, A. (2015). *Teens, social media and technology overview 2015: Smartphones facilitate shifts in communication landscape for teens*. Washington, DC: Pew Research Center.

Lerner, R. M., & Steinberg, L. (2009). The scientific study of adolescent development: Historical and contemporary perspectives. In R. M. Lerner & L. Steinberg (Eds.), *Handbook of adolescent psychology: Vol. 1. Individual bases of adolescent development*. Hoboken, NJ: John Wiley & Sons, Inc. doi:10.1002/9780470479193

Madden, M., Lenhart, A., Cortesi, S., Urs, G., Smith, A., & Beaton, M. (2013). *Teens, social media, and privacy*. Washington, DC: Pew Research Center. Retrieved from http://www.pewinternet.org/Reports/2013/Teens-Social-Media-And-Privacy.aspx

Miller, B. C., Norton, M. C., Fan, X., & Christopherson, C. R. (1998). Pubertal development, parental communication, and sexual values in relation to adolescent sexual behaviors. *Journal of Early Adolescence, 18*, 27–52. doi:10.1177/0272431698018001002

Millstein, S. G., Nightingale, E. O., Petersen, A. C., Mortimer, A. M., & Hamburg, D. A. (1993). Promoting the healthy development of adolescents. *JAMA, 269*(11), 1413–1415.

Moreno, M. A., Vanderstoep, A., Parks, M. R., Zimmerman, F. J., Kurth, A., & Christakis, D. A. (2009). Reducing at-risk adolescents' display of risk behavior on a social networking web site: A randomized controlled pilot intervention trial. *Archives of Pediatrics & Adolescent Medicine, 163*(1), 35–41. doi:10.1016/S0084-3954(09)79302-9

Muuss, R. E. (Ed.). (1996). *Stanley Hall's biogenetic psychology of adolescents* (6th ed.). New York, NY: McGraw-Hill.

Office of Adolescent Health, US Department of Health and Human Services. (2013). *Adolescent health topics: Sexually transmitted diseases*. Rockville, MD: Office of Adolescent Health. Retrieved from http://www.hhs.gov/ash/oah/adolescent-health-topics/reproductive-health/stds.html

O'Keeffe, G. S., & Clarke-Pearson, K.; Council on Communications and Media. (2011). Clinical report-The impact of social media on children, adolescents, and families. *Pediatrics, 127*(4), 800–804. doi:10.1542/peds.2011-0054

Possibilities for Change. (2017). What is RAAPS? Retrieved from http://www.possibilitiesforchange.com/raaps

Roberts, T., Gabrielli, J., & Van Hook, S. (2009). *Performing preventative services: A bright futures handbook* (pp. 103–111.). Elk Grove Village, IL: American Academy of Pediatrics.

Saewyc, E. M. (2012). What about the boys? The importance of including boys and young men in sexual and reproductive health research. *The Journal of Adolescent Health, 51*(1), 1–2. doi:10.1016/j.jadohealth.2012.05.002

Smith, A. (2014). *African Americans and technology use*. Washington, DC: Pew Research Center.

Snapchat. (2017a). Geofilters. Retrieved from https://www.snapchat.com/geofilters

Snapchat. (2017b). Snap Inc. terms of service. Retrieved from https://www.snap.com/en-US/terms

SuccessEHS. (2017). Billing and coding. Retrieved from https://www.greenwayhealth.com

Sznitman, S., Vanable, P. A., Carey, M. P., Hennessy, M., Brown, L. K., Valois, R. F., ... Romer, D. (2011). Using culturally sensitive media messages to reduce HIV-associated sexual behavior in high-risk African American adolescents: Results from a randomized trial. *Journal of Adolescent Health, 49*(3), 244–251. doi:10.1016/j.jadohealth.2010.12.007

Thackeray, R., Neiger, B. L., Hanson, C. L., & McKenzie, J. F. (2008). Enhancing promotional strategies within social marketing programs: Use of Web 2.0 social media. *Health Promotion Practice, 9*(4), 338–343. doi:10.1177/1524839908325335

Twitter. (2017). Our mission. Retrieved from https://about.twitter.com/en_us/company.html

Vance, K., Howe, W., & Dellavalle, R. P. (2009). Social internet sites as a source of public health information. *Dermatologic Clinics, 27*(2), 133–136. doi:10.1016/j.det.2008.11.010

Wong, C. A., Merchant, R. M., & Moreno, M. A. (2014). Using social media to engage adolescents and young adults with their health. *Healthcare, 2*(4), 220–224. https://doi.org/10.1016/j.hjdsi.2014.10.005

Yaeger, J. P., & Moreno, M. A. (2017). The role of age and setting in adolescents' first drinking experience for predicting college problem drinking. *Journal of American College Health, 65*(7), 506–512. doi:10.1080/07448481.2017.1341767

Yager, A. M., & O'Keefe, C. (2012). Adolescent use of social networking to gain sexual health information. *The Journal for Nurse Practitioners, 8*(4), 294–298. doi:10.1016/j.nurpra.2012.01.016

CHAPTER 7

Musculoskeletal Manifestations of Stress in Men

Aaron Wallace

INTRODUCTION

Stress in any person manifests as a myriad of different physical symptoms in both men and women, including insulin resistance, weight gain, thyroid dysfunction, gastrointestinal issues, and increases in joint pain. However, actually measuring stress is difficult to do, as increases in cortisol can be caused by many different sources, including acute physical stressors such as car accidents, chronic overexercise, postural changes due to acute traumas, or chronic long-term occupational stressors. Behavioral stressors that can drive short- and long-term increases in stress can be disturbance of sleep patterns, emotional traumas, smoking, alcohol or drug abuse, and nutritional deficiencies. Each of these factors is individual in nature, and even though differences in joint pain are seen in men versus women, each patient has his or her own set of stressors that must be addressed to reduce the risk of chronic joint pain.

To help understand the individual needs of each patient, one must first understand the root causes of musculoskeletal pain. The CHEK (Corrective Holistic Exercise Kinesiology) Practitioner Survival Totem Pole Model will help demonstrate a distinct method for efficiently assessing the root cause of stress and musculoskeletal pain in men. This can also be adapted for use in women, as the assessment process will create individualized recommendations based on the results of the assessment process.

The CHEK Practitioner Survival Totem Pole Model (Figure 7.1) is designed to help integrate care for each patient and determine which stressors are driving the musculoskeletal pain in each patient. Each section of the totem pole represents an essential survival function that dysfunction in one or more areas can increase stress and alter posture, increasing the risk of musculoskeletal pain. The following sections explain the evaluation of stressors as they separate into the levels of the totem pole that represent basic physiologic processes, beginning at the top and traveling downward.

BREATHING

Breathing and Stress Hormone Release

Even though suboptimal breathing techniques are not clinically detrimental to health in the short term, any long-term deviations to breathing techniques can cause increases to stress and alter posture in several detrimental ways (Table 7.1). The suboptimal breathing pattern that many patients display when dealing with joint pain, for example, is upon inhalation the shoulders and chest will rise indicating use of the accessory respiratory muscles to pull the lungs upward, decreasing air pressure in the lungs, and drawing air into the lungs. Breathing this way increases the ventilation rate and increases cortisol release (Argyropoulos et al., 2002).

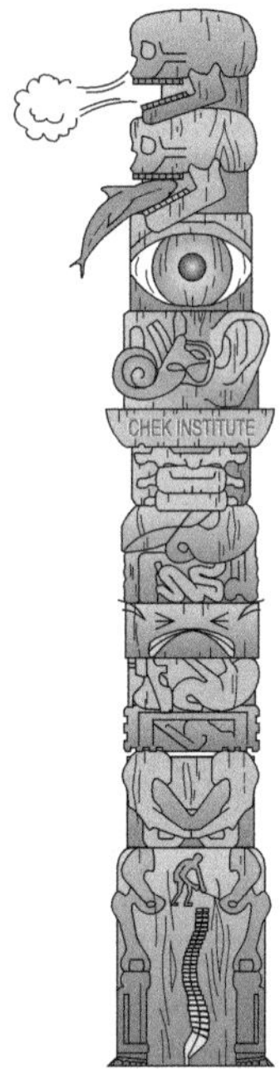

FIGURE 7.1 Corrective Holistic Exercise Kinesiology (CHEK) Practitioner Survival Totem Pole Model.

TABLE 7.1 Selected Causes Contributing to Compromised Breathing and Potential Consequences

Cause	Potential Consequences
Pain	Forward head posture
Muscular asymmetry	Breathing pattern
Spinal or core muscular asymmetry	Mouth breathing at night
Mastication/bite	Headaches
Poor sleep	TMJ disorders
Mental–emotional	Neck and low back pain
Ergonomics	Tendency for pronation injuries in ankles
Occupation	
Studying	
Nutrition/allergy	
Exercise technique	
Stress	

Diaphragmatic breathing is contraction of the diaphragm, which pulls the lungs downward allowing the abdominal cavity organs to push outward on the abdominal muscles forward for the initial two-thirds of the breath. The last third of the breath will allow for multidimensional movement of the rib cage by letting the rib cage rise upward, forward and backward, and laterally on both sides. This decreases the tone of the sympathetic nervous system and lowers cortisol release, lowering resting blood pressure and heart rate and decreasing muscle spasm symptoms (Ma et al., 2017). Without teaching proper resting breathing patterns to patients, decreasing overall stress in the body and joint pain can be more challenging.

Breathing and Postural Changes

Postural changes can happen with the chronic use of accessory respiratory muscles including the sternocleidomastoid, scalenes, upper trapezius, and others. When these muscles are chronically tightened owing to increased tension from reversed breathing patterns, the cranium moves forward due to the origin and insertion of these accessory respiratory muscles. This results in excess upper cervical extension, as the head moves forward to keep the eyes looking forward due to vestibuloocular reflexes. As described in the Lovett reactor system (Lawerence & Samson, 1988), movements in the upper cervical spine are mirrored in the lumbar spine; for example, C1 vertebra and L5 vertebra will both move in the same plane together whenever one of them moves. As C1 extends as the cranium moves forward, L5 will extend as well, resulting in more lumbar extension at rest. This will narrow the foraminal openings through which the nerves travel out of the spinal cord in the lower lumbar and sacral areas, putting the patient at higher risk for nerve compression and pain syndromes as a result.

Forward head posture (FHP) can also be caused by some form of blockage in the nasal passages or sinuses. Reasons for chronically blocked nasal passages can include traumatic physical injury and enlargement of adenoidal tissue, tonsils, and inferior turbinates. In a classic longitudinal study, Wenzel, Henriksen, and Melsen (1983) observed that with the decrease in nasal resistance after corticoid therapy there was a decrease in the craniovertical angle; that is, the reversal of upper airway obstruction minimized FHP. With the cranium positioned forward, breathing through the nasal cavities is maximized, and mouth breathing is also facilitated; as the cranium moves forward into this position, the previously described changes in posture will occur. Abnormal head positions include chin up, chin down, tilting of the head or face turned to the right or left, or a combination of any of these abnormal head positions—many of which are easily noted in people using handheld electronic devices.

TEMPOROMANDIBULAR JOINT DYSFUNCTION AND POSTURE

Temporomandibular joint (TMJ) dysfunction causes are complex and multifactorial. Often the exact cause is unknown; contributing factors include poor occlusion, micro- or macrotrauma to the TMJ, joint laxity, muscular trigger points altering TMJ range of motion, inflammation in the joint capsule, and psychosocial factors including chronic stress, depression, anxiety, or pain syndromes such as fibromyalgia. Because this disorder can be multifactorial in nature, an individual evaluation is necessary to determine if intervention is needed.

In humans and animals, changing occlusion causes immediate changes in postural muscle activity, head posture, and visual focusing. Poor occlusion is also correlated with scoliotic changes in the spine. Scoliotic changes in the spine can be highly variable depending on a variety of factors, but the excess rotation and side-bending on the spine can contribute to one-sided compression of various levels of the spinal column, contributing to lower lumbar and sacral compression.

VISION AND POSTURAL IMBALANCES

According to Tedorescu (2015), abnormal head position is adopted to improve visual acuity, avoid diplopia, or obtain a more comfortable binocular vision. The head can be turned or tilted toward the right or the left with the chin rotated upward or downward, or a combination of these positions. Tens of millions of Americans are estimated to suffer from undiagnosed eye conditions (Maino, 2010). There is commonly a reason for an abnormal or compensatory head position, and the patient often may adopt it unconsciously. The cause may be an ocular, muscular, skeletal, or neurologic disease; very rarely it may be a habit, without any reason to adopt it.

Kraft, O'Donoghue, and Roarty (1992) studied a 5-year sample of patients treated with strabismus surgery and noted the presence of compensatory head postures (CHPs). In this sample, 56.7% of the total population sample, 71.2% of the superior oblique palsy cases, and 100% of nystagmus of congenital motor nystagmus presented with CHP. CHPs contribute to postural changes in other sections of the body, increasing the risk of compression of the nerves of the spine.

INNER EAR FUNCTION AND POSTURE

The vestibular system regulates our ability to have both static and dynamic postural control. One of the most common symptoms of vestibular dysfunction is dizziness, but dizziness can also have other causes, including cervicogenic or vertebrobasilar insufficiency (VBI). The assessment to determine the exact cause of dizziness will be helpful to the patient; symptoms of dizziness will make it more difficult for the patient to adhere to a rehabilitation program for musculoskeletal causes of any undiagnosed chronic pain. General dizziness has a wide etiology and can arise from various body systems, including low blood pressure, endocrine and cardiac disease, hyperventilation, and drug interactions. Hyperventilation can be caused by mouth breathing due to FHP as described in Wenzel et al. (1983).

Cervicogenic dizziness is characterized by imbalance or disequilibrium, which is commonly associated with neck pain stiffness or headache. This type of dizziness is not well understood but may occur during whiplash-associated disorder (WAD) as a result of a flexion-extension injury, such as that seen with a car accident. Pain and headache are often immediate, but dizziness or disequilibrium manifest latently after whiplash injuries, and headaches and neck pain are also highly correlated with C1 misalignment. VBI dizziness symptoms may present as any of the four subtypes of dizziness, including vertigo, presyncope, disequilibrium, and nonspecific dizziness. VBI dizziness may occur following trauma but often has no known causative event. VBI may be the result of internal vascular compression such as that caused by atherosclerosis or may be the result of external factors such as mechanical compression from hypertonic musculature, osteophytes, cervical fracture, or dislocation and altered head postures.

Peripheral vestibular disorders such as benign paroxysmal positional vertigo (BPPV) account for a large proportion of dizziness cases (Rashad, 2010). Neuhauser et al. (2008) reported that vestibular disorders affect 25.2% of those who experience moderate to severe dizziness over a lifetime, and within this group 2.4% suffer from BPPV (Walther, 1988). The calcium carbonate crystals that are normally located in the inner ear can be displaced into the semicircular canals causing them to abnormally sense gravity. This can arise idiopathically or after trauma, inflammation, or degeneration of the inner ear. Although less common, viral or bacterial infections may also cause long-term damage to the vestibular nerve. If the dizziness symptoms persist for several months after a bacterial or viral infection, vestibular rehabilitation therapy is necessary to help the brain during the compensation phase (Oostendorp, van Eupen, van Erp, & Elvers, 1999).

Relief of long-term chronic musculoskeletal stress can be a useful tool for the provider in helping the patient with unexplained chronic pain. Dizziness and other vestibular dysfunction will alter a patient's righting reflexes, which in turn will alter one's posture negatively, creating a higher risk from musculoskeletal disorders and subsequent nerve compression. Proper diagnosis, referral, and treatment of the causes of dizziness, vestibular or otherwise, can help the patient progress through a rehabilitation program for the musculoskeletal system by reducing the risk of nerve compression.

C1 SUBLUXATION AND POSTURAL DYSFUNCTION

As discussed in previous sections, the relationships of the visual and occlusal planes have a direct effect on posture throughout the rest of the body. The alignment of the upper cervical spine also has a direct effect on the posture of the rest of the spine through the Lovett reactor system. Synergistic relationships occur at the segments of C1-L5, C2-L4, C3-L3, and C4-L2 while the remaining segments exert counter-rotational relationships (Walther, 1988).

Through its effect on the central nervous system, subluxation of C1 can create postural distortions that include pelvic girdle malalignment, a short or contracted leg, spinal imbalance, and displacement of the body's center of gravity (Seeman, 1978). The National Upper Cervical Chiropractic Association estimates over 10,000 different variations of C1-C2 misalignment grouped into four different categories (Fielding & Hawkins, 1977). The changes in the body as a result of C1 misalignment are believed to result primarily from three different effects: the influence of mechanoreceptors and nociceptors of the upper cervical spine; traction of the cord by the dentate ligaments; and shifts in the center of gravity of the head and pelvis. According to Paul Chek's chapter *in Chiropractic Approach to Head Pain* (Chek, 1994):

> Atlas adjustment has an effect on the entire nervous system, primarily through its effect on joint mechanoreceptors. They are located mainly in the superficial layers of the fibrous capsule and are more numerous on those aspects of the joint capsule that undergo the greater changes in stress during natural joint movement. Subluxation may similarly produce opposite results through the same mechanisms. . .Because of the mechanics of C0-C1 and C1-C2 joints, any subluxation of the atlas or axis will likely disturb head posture through coupled movement. Displaced laterally, C1 is positioned to be the interference that causes a loss of the inhibitory influences of the reticular formation in the brainstem at its caudal end on the extensor muscles. (p. 28)

Muscle tension will also affect the subluxation and the degree of the subluxation of the facets. Clinically, alterations to the muscle tone, most often hypertonicity, are palpable in association with both atlas subluxation complex (ASC) and FHP, and active trigger points can be expected. This again leads to several mechanisms for developing a pain spasm cycle with relative ischemia and high potential for pain referral into the craniofacial region.

The center of gravity of the head is slightly above the auditory meatus on a horizontal line at the midsagittal plane of the head. The center of gravity of the body lies in the midsagittal plane and somewhat anterior to the upper sacral spine. It is reported to be 4 cm in front of the first sacral vertebra in the standing anatomic position; abnormal neck posture contributes to activation of the nociceptive receptor system, resulting in reflexogenic effects on motor unit activity in neck and limb musculature. Clinically, this manifests in distortions of head and neck posture and gait that are associated with cervical pain, and suggest an origin for cervicogenic headaches. Examination may reveal bilateral or unilateral swelling and thickening of the muscles with atlas (C1) displacement, and exert pressure on one or both superior cervical ganglion. Alterations to head–neck posture will indicate the need for a thorough upper cervical evaluation. When one segment becomes misaligned, there will be compensatory malalignment of another segment to maintain a balanced position and posture.

There is a connection between low back and cervical spine, as indicated by the Lovett reactor system, that can commonly be overlooked by clinicians and patients alike. This connection may be responsible for low back and leg pain; the significance of low back and leg pain to craniofacial pain becomes evident in patients who develop craniofacial symptoms secondary to chronic low back complaints. These men, who demonstrate subclinical craniofacial symptoms, may have become clinical through summation of back and/or leg pain. But most patients experiencing both headache and low back pain can be treated, often by correction of upper cervical subluxation and posture. For example, the ASC can be hypothesized to contribute to unexplained penis pain by altering posture at the lumbar and sacral portions of the spine.

VISCERAL ORGAN ASSESSMENT

Digestive System Inflammation and Posture and Pain

Chronic inflammatory bowel disease (IBD) can have diverse and multidimensional causes. There are is a relationship between IBD and the hypothalamic–pituitary–adrenal (HPA) axis, and this can contribute to increased inflammation in the sacroiliac area, including sensory nerves located in the genitalia. This may be a potential contributor from IBD syndromes to unexplained pelvic/genital pain in men. Axial arthropathies, including sacroiliitis and ankylosing spondylitis, have been associated with IBD, but this is independent of disease activity (Evans & Pardi, 2007). Patients with more extensive IBD and colonic involvement in Crohn's disease have much higher risk of joint complications.

In brief, the central nervous system relays neural, endocrine, and circulatory messages to the gut via the brain-gut axis, reflecting changes in corticotropin-releasing hormone, mast cell activity, neurotransmission at the autonomic nerve system, and intestinal barrier function, all affecting the pathogenesis of animal colitis and human IBD. Stress triggers the hypothalamic–pituitary axis and the activation of the autonomic nervous system, causing an increase in cortisol levels and proinflammatory cytokines such as tumor necrosis factor-alpha, interleukin 8, interleukin 1 beta, and interleukin 6 (Brzozowski et al., 2016). Acute or chronic stress enhances the intestinal permeability, weakening the tight junctions and increasing bacterial translocation into the intestinal wall. An increased microbial load in the colonic tissue, excessive cytokine release, and a partially blunted immune reactivity in response to stress result in its negative impact on IBD (Brzozowski et al., 2016).

A connection with IBD severity as the result of nutrient deficiencies has been reported as well. Owing to this process of chronic inflammation, and chronic use of medications, patients with IBD are also at increased risk of nutritional factor deficiencies, including iron, calcium, vitamin D, vitamin B_{12}, folic acid, zinc, magnesium, and vitamin A. Zinc deficiency plays a role in inflammation, mainly elevating inflammatory response as well as damage to host tissue (Gammoh & Rink, 2017). Vitamin D deficiency may lead to lower functional capacity, and clinically, vitamin D levels should be checked in musculoskeletal pain patients at risk of vitamin D deficiency (Çalık & Aygün, 2017). Magnesium, vitamin B_{12}, and zinc deficiencies are associated with an increased risk of myofascial pain syndrome (Okumus et al., 2017). However, no single common diet is suitable for all IBD patients. Each patient is unique and dietary recommendations must be tailored for each patient, depending on the course of the disease, past surgical procedures, and type of pharmacotherapy (Owczarek, Rodacki, Domagała-Rodacka, Cibor, & Mach, 2016). As with other sections of the CHEK survival totem pole, this section is meant to show that each patient should be given individual evaluation for underlying chronic IBD and seek appropriate referral to help assist proper multidisciplinary treatment.

A comprehensive review of the musculoskeletal effects of visceral dysfunction is presented by Barral (Barral, 2005; 2007). These resources list several visceral dysfunctions with concomitant osseous restrictions, some of which are pertinent to thoracic, lumbar, and sacral pain symptoms.

ASSESSMENT OF MUSCULOSKELETAL STRESS SUMMARY

When compiling possible treatment options for undiagnosed genital pain in men, proper assessment protocols for each level of the survival totem pole can help with proper referral to correct the specialist for each patient (Table 7.2). Because one-on-one time is limited with each

TABLE 7.2 Corrective Holistic Exercise Kinesiology (CHEK) Assessments

Totem Level	Specific Test	Rationale	Method
Breathing Assessment	Forward Head Posture (FHP) Testing	Evaluation of possible nasal breathing restriction as contributor to FHP	Use a caliper with the patient in a standing position facing straight forward Can use a therapeutic grade peppermint oil to increase space in nasal cavities If the patient's head position moves into a more retracted position by more than 1 cm, this is evidence of FHP FHP may be causing narrowed nasal passages or contributing to lumbar and sacral nerve compression *Consider referral to an ENT physician, allergist, or craniosacral therapist*
	Diaphragmatic Breathing Assessment	Helps to determine if the patient's breathing pattern is contributing to FHP, increased risk of lumbar and sacrum nerve compression, and preventing multidimensional expansion of the rib cage	Asking patient, while he is standing, to take a deep breath, observing the muscular activation Observe where the movement of breathing begins Deep inhale continues multidirectional (anterior, posterior, lateral, and upward) movement from the rib cage, due to contraction of the intercostal muscles, and a small rise in the chest cavity should be observed Breathing with the chest and shoulders rising upon inhaling, suggests that the sternocleidomastoid, scalene, and upper trapezius muscles are being overactivated, increasing the risk of FHP May add to stress on the lumbar spine due to decreased range of motion in the thoracic spine *Referral to ENT physician, skilled manual therapist, physical therapist, or CHEK practitioner can help the patient improve his breathing pattern*

(*continued*)

TABLE 7.2 Corrective Holistic Exercise Kinesiology (CHEK) Assessments (*continued*)

Totem Level	Specific Test	Rationale	Method
Atlas Assessment	Supine Cranioventral Glide	Evaluates for atlas/axis misalignment	Have the patient lie supine on a table with legs extended. Gently grasp the cranium with both hands and passively glide the cranium ventrally and laterally one side at a time without cervical rotation, flexion, or extension After several repetitions in each direction, visually assess the range of right motion vs. left motion Significant range of motion difference is a red flag for an atlas-axis misalignment *Consider referral to an NUCCA chiropractor if range of motion is significantly different between sides*
	March Test	Evaluation for possible C1 misalignment	Begin by having the patient close his eyes and march in place, bringing him perpendicular to the floor, while also moving the arms in opposition (similar to a soldier marching) After 2–3 minutes of marching with his eyes closed, if he starts to move in a different direction (such as marching in a circle), this may indicate possible C1 misalignment C1 rotation to one side causes a one-sided tightening of the longissimus and iliocostalis muscles Induces a rotational torque on the torso slowly inducing the patient to rotate while marching *Consider referral to an NUCCA chiropractor, physical therapist, Blair chiropractor or Level 3 CHEK Practitioner*
Temporomandibular Joint (TMJ) Assessment	Deviation in Opening/Closing, Subjective Assessments	Changes in the occlusal plane will alter spinal postures, increasing risk for lumbar and sacral nerve compression	Visually assess position of the mandible: are the lower lips pulled to one side as compared with upper lips, are the muscles of one side of the mandible overdeveloped, etc. Have the patient show the teeth, and slowly open and close the mandible several times Note deviations upon opening or closing *Consider referral to TMJ specialist or skilled TMJ manual therapist to release possible trigger points in the musculature controlling the mandible*

Vision Assessment	Eye Chart: Right vs. Left Eye	Undiagnosed eye conditions can alter posture, potentially increasing the risk of nerve root compression	Perform a simple eye chart examination to test for acuity *Consider referral for additional visual testing or to a neuromuscular therapist for release of trigger points in the ocular muscles*
Vestibular Assessment	Past Pointing	Tests for vestibular nerve dysfunction	Place one finger on each hand straight up in the air at shoulder level of the patient; have patient raise his arms up above his head with index fingers pointed out, and bring his arms down to touch the fingers Repeat with the eyes closed *Consider referral to an ENT physician for more extensive vestibular evaluation if he cannot touch the outstretched fingers with eyes closed*
	Neck Torsion Test	Evaluates for possible cervicogenic dizziness vs. vestibular dizziness	While the patient's head is held stationary, the patient rotates the trunk and if the patient experiences symptoms, this is a possible sign of cervicogenic dizziness vs. vestibular dizziness *Consider referral to an ENT physician for more extensive vestibular evaluation*
	Sustained Neck Rotation Test	Tests for vertebrobasilar artery insufficiency	Place the patient in a supine position and perform passive extension followed by passive cervical rotation Rotation should be performed in both directions If the patient displays dizziness, nausea, syncope, dysarthria, dysphagia, disturbances of the hearing or vision, paresis, or paralysis with the symptoms getting worse as the time held in extension and rotation increases, this is a positive sign for VBI *Refer urgently to neurology for evaluation of possible positional arterial compression*
Visceral Organ Assessment	Inflammatory Bowel Disease (IBD) Assessment	Assessment of organ systems such as the thyroid, adrenals, and other hormonal systems	Can be useful in developing a multidisciplinary approach to stress management *Results may be helpful in determining the need for gastroenterology referral*

CHEK, Corrective Holistic Exercise Kinesiology; ENT, ear, nose, and throat; NUCCA, National Upper Cervical Chiropractic Association; VBI, vertebrobasilar insufficiency.

patient, these assessments can be used to determine if referral is needed for more in-depth assessment procedures by specialists in these areas.

Musculoskeletal stress can contribute to various joint pain syndromes throughout the body. The challenge for any provider is to understand that changes in posture that can increase the risk of undiagnosed genital pain are multifactorial and require a more holistic integrated approach to each patient's treatment. The CHEK survival totem pole can be a useful guide to assessing the possible underlying causes of musculoskeletal pain and postural distortion that can increase the risk of nerve compression in a patient with persistent or chronic pain.

REFERENCES

Argyropoulos, S. V., Bailey, J. E., Hood, S. D., Kendrick, A. H., Rich, A. S., Laszlo, G., … Nutt, D. J. (2002). Inhalation of 35% CO_2 results in activation of the HPA axis in healthy volunteers. *Psychoneuroendocrinology, 27*, 715–729. doi:10.1016/S0306-4530(01)00075-0

Barral, J. P. (2005). *Visceral manipulation (revised)*. Seattle, WA: Eastland Press.

Barral, J. P. (2007). *Visceral manipulation II (revised)*. Seattle, WA: Eastland Press.

Bhattacharyya, N., Baugh, R. F., Orvidas, L., Barrs, D., Bronston, L. J., Cass, S., … Haidari, J. (2008). Clinical Practice guideline: Benign paroxysmal positional vertigo. *Otolaryngology—Head and Neck Surgery, 139*, S47–S81. doi:10.1016/j.otohns.2008.08.022

Brzozowski, B., Mazur-Bialy, A., Pajdo, R., Kwiecien, S., Bilski, J., Zwolinska-Wcislo, M., … Brzozowski, T. (2016). Mechanisms by which stress affects the experimental and clinical Inflammatory Bowel Disease (IBD): Role of Brain-Gut Axis, *Current Neuropharmacology, 14*(8), 892–900. doi:10.2174/1570159X14666160404124127

Çalık, Y., & Aygün, Ü. (2017). Evaluation of vitamin D levels in patients with chronic low back-leg pain. *Acta orthopaedica et traumatologica turcica, 51*(3), 243–247. doi:10.1016/j.aott.2017.03.006

Chek, P. (1994). Posture and craniofacial pain. In D. D. Curl (Ed.), *Chiropractic approach to head pain* (pp. 121–162). Baltimore, MD: Williams & Wilkins.

Evans, P. E., & Pardi, D. S. (2007). Extraintestinal manifestations of inflammatory bowel disease: Focus on the musculoskeletal, dermatologic, and ocular manifestations. *Medscape General Medicine, 9*(1), 55.

Fielding, J. W., & Hawkins, R. J. (1977). Atlanto-axial rotatory fixation. (Fixed rotatory subluxation of the atlanto-axial joint). *The Journal of Bone and Joint Surgery, 59*(1), 37–44. doi:10.2106/00004623-197759010-00005

Gammoh, N., & Rink, L. (2017). Zinc in infection and inflammation. *Nutrients, 9*(6), pii: E624. doi:10.3390/nu9060624

Kraft, S. P., O'Donoghue, E. P., & Roarty, J. D. (1992). Improvement of compensatory head postures after strabismus surgery. *Ophthalmology, 99*(8):1301–1308. doi:10.1016/S0161-6420(92)31811-1

Lawerence, E. S., & Samson, G. S. (1988). Growth and development influences on the craniomandibular region. In S. L. Kraus (Ed.), *TMJ disorders management of the craniomandibular complex* (pp. 241–274). New York, NY: Churchill Livingstone.

Ma, X., Yue, Z. Q., Gong, Z. Q., Zhang, H., Duan, N. Y., Shi, Y. T., … Li, Y. F. (2017). The effect of diaphragmatic breathing on attention, negative affect and stress in healthy adults. *Frontiers in Psychology, 8*, 874. doi:10.3389/fpsyg.2017.00874

Maino, D. (2010). The binocular vision dysfunction pandemic. *Optometry & Vision Development, 41*(1), 6–13.

Neuhauser, H. K., Radtke, A., von Brevern, M., Lezius, F., Feldmann, M., & Lempert, T. (2008). Burden of dizziness and vertigo in the community. *Archives of Internal Medicine, 168*, 2118–2124. doi:10.1001/archinte.168.19.2118

Okumus, M., Ceceli, E., Tuncay, F., Kocaoglu, S., Palulu, N., & Yorgancioglu, Z. R. (2010). The relationship between serum trace elements, vitamin B12, folic acid and clinical parameters in patients with myofascial pain syndrome. *Journal of Back and Musculoskeletal Rehabilitation, 23*(4), 187–191. doi:10.3233/BMR-2010-0264

Oostendorp, R. A. B., van Eupen, A., van Erp, J. M. M., & Elvers, H. (1999). Dizziness following whiplash injury: A neuro-otological study in manual therapy practice and therapeutic implication. *Journal of Manual Manipulative Therapy, 7*, 123–130. doi:10.1179/106698199790811609

Owczarek, D., Rodacki, T., Domagała-Rodacka, R., Cibor, D., & Mach, T. (2016). Diet and nutritional factors in inflammatory bowel diseases. *World Journal of Gastroenterology, 22*(3), 895–905. doi:10.3748/wjg.v22.i3.895

Rashad, U. M. (2010). Patients with benign paroxysmal positional vertigo and cervical spine problems: Is Epley's maneuver contraindicated and is a purpose new maneuver effective and safer? *Journal of Laryngology and Otology, 124,* 1167–1171. doi:10.1017/S0022215110000927

Seeman, D. (1978). Biomechanics of the upper cervical spine. *The Upper Cervical Monograph, 2*(5), 6–10.

Tedorescu, L. (2015). Anomalous head postures in strabismus and nystagmus—Diagnostic and management. *Rom J Ophthalmol, 59*(3), 137–140.

Walther, D. S. (1988). *Applied kinesiology synopsis* (p. 70). Pueblo, CO: Systems D.C.

Wenzel, A., Henriksen, J., & Melsen, B. (1983). Nasal respiratory resistance and head posture: Effect of intranasal corticosteroid (Budes-onide) in children with asthma and perennial rhinitis. *American Journal of Orthodontics, 84*(5), 422–426. doi:10.1016/0002-9416(93)90005-R

CHAPTER 8

Health Screening and Immunization Issues for Adult Men

Alice Ukaegbu

INTRODUCTION

The U.S. Preventive Services Task Force (USPSTF) is composed of nationally recognized experts specializing in preventive health and evidence-based medicine. Detailed, up-to-date, preventive health screening guidelines or timelines are set by expert preventive health task forces such as USPSTF and the Agency for Healthcare Research and Quality (AHRQ). According to USPSTF, the main purpose of preventive health services is the preservation of health and quality of life.

According to an article written by the American Heart Association (2017) there are 10 reasons why some men decline routine health screening: the assumption that probably nothing is wrong with them, lack of insurance, not having a doctor, lack of money, lack of time, the thought that providers do not do anything for them, their preference to simply "tough it out," claim of phobia, nagging from their significant other to get a check up, and not wanting to hear what the providers have to say. Despite these and other reported reasons, it is unclear why men commonly refuse to undergo regular health screening; and therefore should be encouraged to do so (American Heart Association, 2017).

The way to detect health issues before they start is through regular health screening and assessments. Early identification of health problems improves chances for health treatment and cure. Age, health, family history, lifestyle choices (i.e., diet, activity level, smoking), and other significant factors influence what type and how often one needs healthcare. According to the AHRQ (Agency for Healthcare Research and Quality, 2012), men are 32% more likely than women to be hospitalized for long-term complications of diabetes and are more than twice as likely as women to have a leg or foot amputated due to complications related to diabetes. Men are 24% more likely than women to be hospitalized for pneumonia that could have been prevented by getting immunized (Agency for Healthcare Research and Quality, 2012). The purpose of this chapter is to identify essential health screening and immunization issues and guidelines for the adult male.

ABDOMINAL AORTIC ANEURYSMS

An abdominal aortic aneurysm (AAA) is an enlargement of the aorta at the level of the abdomen. The force of blood pumping can split the layers of the arterial wall, allowing blood to leak in between the layers or burst, resulting in severe immediate bleeding and death. Aortic aneurysms were the primary cause of 9,863 deaths in 2014 and in 2009, was identified as a contributing cause in more than 17,215 deaths in the United States. About two thirds of people who have an aortic dissection are male, and men who have a history of smoking are three to five times more likely to develop an AAA (Centers for Disease Control and Prevention [CDC], 2015). The USPSTF recommends men aged 65 to 75 years who have ever smoked, be screened one time with ultrasound screening for AAA even if they are asymptomatic (USPSTF, 2017).

ALCOHOL MISUSE: SCREENING AND BEHAVIORAL COUNSELING

One of the most common issues in the primary care population across the United States is alcohol misuse. Approximately 21% of adult males report engaging in risky or hazardous drinking, and the prevalence of current alcohol dependence is about 4% (U.S. Prevention Services Task Force, 2016a). Alcohol misuse plays a contributing role in a wide range of health conditions, such as hypertension, gastritis, liver disease and cirrhosis, pancreatitis, certain types of cancer (e.g., breast and esophageal), cognitive impairment, anxiety, and depression (U.S. Prevention Services Task Force, 2016a). Alcohol misuse has also been implicated as a major factor in injuries and death as a result of trauma, falls, drowning, fires, motor vehicle crashes, homicide, and suicide (Moyer, 2013a).

Screening for alcohol misuse in men begins at age 18 years; no specific frequency is recommended. Clinicians should use their discretion based on history and presentation. Instruments for screening for alcohol misuse include Alcohol Use Disorders Identification Test (AUDIT), the abbreviated AUDIT-Consumption (AUDIT-C), and single-question screening (e.g., the National Institute on Alcohol Abuse and Alcoholism [NIAAA] recommends asking, "How many times in the past year have you had 5 (for men) drinks in a day" (Moyer, 2013a).

BLOOD PRESSURE SCREENING

High blood pressure puts men at risk for the leading causes of death in United States, including heart disease and stroke. About 75 million American adults (32%) have high blood pressure, or 1 in every 3 adults; out of this number, only about half have their high blood pressure under control (Merai et al., 2016), making hypertension a major contributor to the national epidemic of cardiovascular disease and stroke. High blood pressure is called a "silent killer" because it has no warning signs or symptoms, and many men may not know they have it because of a lack of screening (CDC, 2017g).

Blood pressure screening is one of the screening tests recommended by USPSTF for adult men ages 18 and older (U.S. Prevention Services Task Force [USPSTF], 2016b). Individuals are to be screened every 2 years if their blood pressure remains less than 120/80 mmHg. If the systolic blood pressure reading is between 120 and 139 mmHg or diastolic blood pressure reading is between 80 and 89 mmHg, and in people at risk for high blood pressure (including obese individuals and African Americans), blood pressure screening should be performed annually. A blood pressure check is one of the most easily accessed tests in men, as many neighborhood pharmacies and workplaces have a screening booth. Furthermore, blood pressure screening is routinely offered during health fairs conducted by various health organizations (USPSTF, 2016b).

COLORECTAL CANCER SCREENING

Colorectal cancer is the second leading cancer killer in the United States. Colorectal screening is an important tool for changing this statistic because it helps in early detection of precancerous polyps and early identification of abnormal bleeding in the rectum with subsequent early treatment (CDC, 2017a). Colorectal screening is suggested for asymptomatic males 50 years or older, with average risk of colorectal cancer but no family history of known genetic disorders that predispose them to lifetime risk of colorectal cancer, a personal history of inflammatory bowel disease, previous adenomatous polyp, or previous colorectal cancer. Screening can be done using fecal occult blood testing, sigmoidoscopy, or colonoscopy; men can be screened earlier than 50 years of age depending on family history of colorectal cancer. Screening can continue until 75 years considering overall health and prior screening history. Several screening strategies are used in colorectal screening including the following:

Stool Tests

The guaiac-based fecal occult blood test (gFOBT) is done to determine the presence of blood in the stool and it uses the chemical guaiac. It is recommended once a year. The fecal immunochemical test (FIT) is also done to detect blood in the stool using antibodies. The FIT-DNA test (also referred to as the stool DNA test) combines the FIT with a test that detects altered DNA in the stool. For this test, an entire bowel movement is collected and sent to be checked for cancer cells. It is done once every 1 or 3 years.

Flexible Sigmoidoscopy

This test is done with the insertion of a short, thin, flexible lighted tube for the identification of polyps or cancer inside the rectum and lower third of the colon and it is done every 10 years with a FIT every year.

Colonoscopy

Colonoscopy remains the gold standard for colorectal cancer screening and it can also be used for early identification and intervention in removing identified polyps. This procedure is similar to flexible sigmoidoscopy; the screening is done using long, thin, flexible lighted tube to check for polyps or cancer inside the rectum and the entire colon. Colonoscopy also is used as a follow-up test for any abnormality found during one of the other screening tests and it is to be done every 10 years. According to Vashi (2014) many adults avoid colonoscopy due to fear of pain and only about 52% to 54% of adults within the ages of 50 to 75 years screen with this procedure (Vashi, 2014).

Computed Tomography (CT) Colonography

CT colonography, also known as virtual colonoscopy, uses x-rays and computers to produce images of the complete colon, which are shown on a computer screen for analysis, and it is to be done every 5 years. It does not allow for treatment of any identified lesions; men would need to undergo a traditional colonoscopy.

CHOLESTEROL SCREENING

Cholesterol is a waxy, fat-like substance needed by the body, but excess cholesterol can build up on the walls of the arteries and in the blood, leading to heart disease and stroke. High cholesterol is asymptomatic; lowering cholesterol can reduce the risk of heart attack, needing heart bypass surgery or angioplasty, and dying of heart disease. Some behavior modifications by men such as exercising, eating a healthy diet, and smoking cessation will help prevent high cholesterol and reduce levels.

Lipid disorder screening should be performed in men ages 20 to 35 years who are at increased risk for cardiovascular heart disease (CHD). Other people have the risk of elevated lipids owing to disease or certain conditions such as diabetes, history of previous CHD or atherosclerosis, family history of cardiovascular disease, tobacco use, hypertension, and obesity (body mass index ≥ 30 kg/m^2). Lipid screening is recommended every 4 to 6 years for those with normal lipid levels, but more often in those with elevated risk for heart disease, stroke, or high levels of low-density lipoprotein (LDL) cholesterol or low levels of high-density lipoprotein (HDL) cholesterol (National Center for Chronic Disease Prevention, 2017). The preferred screening tests for dyslipidemia are serum lipid profile (total cholesterol, HDL cholesterol, and LDL cholesterol) in nonfasting or fasting blood samples.

DEPRESSION

Depression is both a serious medical illness and a significant public health issue; it is one of the leading causes of disease or injury worldwide. Depression is the most common type of mental illness, affecting more than 26% of the U.S. adult population (CDC, 2016a). USPSTF (2014a) updated its recommendation on the screening of depression in adult male population ages 18 years and older: screening is to be performed in these men using efficient assessment tests including the Patient Health Questionnaire, the Hospital Anxiety and Depression Scales (HADS), and the Geriatric Depression Scale in older adults. The exact screening interval for depression is unknown, but clinical judgment should be used in considering at-risk patients. Men who have not been screened before and individuals with a history of depression, unexplained somatic symptoms, or comorbid psychological conditions should be screened (USPSTF, 2014a).

DIABETES MELLITUS

Diabetes mellitus (DM) is a disease characterized by a sustained increase of blood glucose levels above normal. The prevalence of type 2 diabetes mellitus is on the rise; approximately 9% of the adult U.S. population currently has been diagnosed with DM. Diabetes is a primary cause of blindness, renal disease, amputation, and a subsequent increase in mortality risk, primarily from cardiovascular events. A fasting plasma glucose level of 126 mg/dL or higher on two separate tests performed on two separate days establishes the diagnosis of diabetes (CDC, 2015b).

The USPSTF (2015a) final statement recommends test for high blood glucose as part of cardiovascular risk screening in adults aged 40 to 70 years who are overweight or obese. Men of some ethnic groups (African Americans, American Indians, Alaska Natives, Asian Americans, Hispanic or Latinos, Native Hawaiians, or Pacific Islanders) are considered high-risk and should be screened earlier for diabetes. Men with normal blood sugar levels should be screened every 3 years. USPSTF also recommends that men identified with high glucose levels should be referred to behavioral counseling interventions to promote a healthy diet and physical activity.

HEPATITIS SCREENING

Hepatitis B Screening

In the United States approximately 700,000 to 2.2 million persons are unaware they have chronic hepatitis B virus (HBV) infection (USPSTF, 2014b). In the United States, adult males who are considered at high risk for HBV infection include people from countries with a high prevalence of HBV infection, HIV-positive persons, injection drug users, household contacts of persons with HBV infection, and men who have sex with men (USPSTF, 2014b).

These guidelines relate to asymptomatic, adult males at high risk for HBV infection (including those at high risk who were vaccinated before being screened for HBV infection). Periodic screening may also be useful in patients with ongoing risk for HBV transmission, for example, active injection drug users, men who have sex with men, healthcare and public safety workers, people with HIV, people who are in close contact with someone infected with HBV, and patients receiving hemodialysis. According to USPSTF, there was inadequate evidence to determine screening frequency and interval; thus, this decision is left to the discretion of the clinician (USPSTF, 2014b). Identification of chronic HBV infection based on serologic markers is considered accurate. Immunoassays for detecting hepatitis B surface antigen (HBsAg) have a reported sensitivity and specificity of greater than 98% (USPSTF, 2014b).

Hepatitis C Screening

Hepatitis C virus (HCV) is the most common chronic blood-borne pathogen in the United States and a leading cause of complications from chronic liver disease. The prevalence of the anti-HCV antibody in the United States is approximately 1.6% in no institutionalized persons (Moyer, 2013b). The USPSTF (USPSTF, 2016c) recommends screening for HCV infection in persons at high risk for infection; it is also recommended that a one-time screening for HCV infection be done in adult males born between 1945 and 1965. HCV infection is most likely undiagnosed in asymptomatic adult males born between 1945 and 1965. In addition, men with high risk for HCV infection including past and present injection drug users, men having sex with men, men born to a mother with HCV infection, those who are intranasal drug users, those who have acquired an unregulated tattoo or who have other percutaneous exposures, and those receiving a blood transfusion before 1992 should be screened periodically (Moyer, 2013). Anti-HCV antibody testing followed by polymerase chain reaction testing for viremia is accurate for identifying patients with chronic HCV infection.

HIV SCREENING

HIV weakens the immune system by destroying important cells that fight disease and infection. No effective cure exists for HIV infection, but screening leads to early detection and early treatment, which reduces complications (CDC, 2017b). According to U.S. Department of Health and Human Services (USPSTF, 2017) an estimated 1.2 million persons in the United States are currently living with HIV infection, but less than half of those diagnosed have their viral load under control. Early identification and treatment of HIV in men will decrease the progression of AIDS, AIDS-related events, and deaths in men with immunologically advanced disease defined as a CD4 count less than 0.200×10^9 cells (CDC, 2016b).

The recommendation by USPSTF (2016d) is for healthcare providers to screen for HIV infection in adolescents and adults ages 15 to 65 years. Earlier assessment is preferred for younger adolescents and older adults who are at increased risk. The conventional serum test for diagnosing HIV infection is the repeatedly reactive immunoassay followed by confirmatory Western blot or immunofluorescent assay. The test is highly accurate (sensitivity and specificity, >99.5%), and results are available within 1 to 2 days from most commercial laboratories (USPSTF, 2016d).

SYPHILIS SCREENING

Syphilis is a systemic disease caused by *Treponema pallidum*. The disease has been divided into stages based on clinical findings, helping to guide treatment and follow-up. In 2014, the total number of syphilis cases reported for all stages (including 458 cases of congenital syphilis) and all ages in the United States was 63,450, which is a 12.3% increase from the previous year (USPSTF, 2016e).

The USPSTF recommends screening for syphilis infection in asymptomatic sexually active men who are at increased risk for infection. Current screening tests for syphilis rely on detection of antibodies rather than direct detection of the organism. Screening for syphilis infection is a two-step process involving an initial nontreponemal test (Venereal Disease Research Laboratory [VDRL] or rapid plasma reagin [RPR] test) followed by a confirmatory treponemal antibody detection test (fluorescent treponemal antibody absorption [FTA-ABS] or *Treponema pallidum* particle agglutination.

LUNG CANCER SCREENING

Lung cancer is a disease in which out-of-control cell growth starts in the lungs. Lung cancer is by far the leading cause of cancer death among both men and women; about 1 out of 4 cancer deaths are from lung cancer counterpart (American Cancer Society, 2017). Each year, more people die from lung cancer than from colon, breast, and prostate cancers combined. The American Cancer Society estimates that in the United States for 2017 there were about 116,990 new cases of lung cancer in men and about 84,590 deaths in men resulting from lung cancer counterpart (American Cancer Society, 2017). The most significant risk factor for lung cancer is smoking, and black men are about 20% more likely to develop lung cancer than their white counterparts (American Cancer Society, 2017). Men who smoke cigarettes are 15 to 30 times more likely to be diagnosed with or die from lung cancer than people who do not smoke. The risk of lung cancer increases with the number of cigarettes one smokes each day and rises with age, but decreases over time if one quits smoking (CDC, 2017c).

According to USPTF (2015c) screening for lung cancer targets men ages 55 to 80 years who have a history of 30 pack-years of smoking, who are presently smoking, or who have quit within the past 15 years. Lung cancer screening is recommended for adult men who have no symptoms but who are at high risk for developing the disease because of their smoking history. Assessment is done with low-dose computed tomography (LDCT). Screening may not be appropriate for patients with considerable comorbid conditions, especially those men who are in the upper end of the screening age range (USPSTF, 2015b). It is also recommended that screening be discontinued if the individual has not smoked for over 15 years.

LATENT TUBERCULOSIS INFECTION

Tuberculosis is one of the infectious respiratory diseases that causes extensive health burden worldwide. In the United States about 9,563 new cases of tuberculosis were recounted in 2015 and an estimated 1.5 million deaths related to tuberculosis infection occurred worldwide (USPSTF, 2016f). The USPSTF recommendation relates to asymptomatic males 18 years of age and older at increased risk for tuberculosis, including prevalence of active disease and increased risk of exposure. Other people at elevated risk include persons who were born in, or are former residents of, countries with intensified tuberculosis occurrence and persons who live in, or have lived in, high-risk congregate settings (e.g., homeless shelters and correctional facilities). The screening interval for latent tuberculosis infection (LTBI) depends on specific risk factors; screening frequency could range from one-time only screening among persons who are at low risk for future tuberculosis exposure to annual screening among those who are at continued risk of exposure, including healthcare workers and students of all levels.

Two types of screening tests for LTBI are currently available in the United States: the Mantoux tuberculin skin test (TST) and interferon gamma release assay (IGRA) blood test. IGRA screening is preferred for Individuals who have received bacille Calmette–Guérin vaccination or persons who may be unlikely to return for TST interpretation. The skin test is done with the intradermal placement of purified protein derivative and reading of response within 48 to 72 hours later. IGRA is done with a single venous blood sample and laboratory processing within 8 to 30 hours after collection (USPSTF, 2016f).

OBESITY

More than one third (36.5%) of U.S. adults are diagnosed as obese, the incidence of obesity in the United States is high, exceeding 30% in adult men (CDC, 2017d). Obesity is related to various health complication issues in men, including elevated risk for coronary heart disease, type 2 diabetes mellitus, and numerous types of cancer, gallstones, and disability. Research indicates the presence of two or more comorbid conditions results in high usage of healthcare services with consequent higher costs noted among obese men. Furthermore, obesity has been linked with an increased risk of death in adult men younger than 65 years; it contributes to ischemic heart disease, diabetes, respiratory diseases, and cancer in adult men (CDC, 2017d).

According to USPSTF, calculation of obesity is done by body mass index (BMI), which is a measure of weight to height, or by measuring waist circumference. Those with BMIs of 30 kg/m^2 or above are termed obese, and those ranging from 25 to 29.9 are overweight. A BMI of 18.5 to 25 kg/m^2 indicates a normal weight. Waist circumference size 40 inches and above for men is related with higher heart disease, stroke, high blood pressure, and diabetes risks (Agency for Healthcare Research and Quality, 2014). The recommendation by USPSTF (2016g) is for the screening of obesity in all adult men and patients with a BMI of 30 kg/m^2 or higher. As a part of this recommendation men identified with obesity should be included in the intensive weight loss and behavioral intervention program, which is found to improve their risk factors for development of comorbid conditions. No screening interval was identified (USPSTF, 2016g).

SKIN CANCER SCREENING

Skin cancer is one of the most common types of cancer among men in the United States. Research indicates men are two to three times more likely to acquire nonmelanoma basal cell and squamous cell skin cancers than women and the risk of the disease increases as lifetime exposure to sun accumulates. The majority of men diagnosed with melanoma are white men over age 55; overall, 1 in 33 men will develop melanoma in their lifetimes (Anderson, 2017). According to the American Academy of Dermatology (Torres, 2016) men should perform self-examination about every 3 months to check for new or changing skin lesions and should include head-to-toe skin assessment during routine annual physical preventive examination.

The American Academy of Dermatology (2017) encourages all men to frequently observe their skin for signs of skin cancer and follow up with a board-certified dermatologist if any unusual spots, itching, or bleeding are observed on their skin. Those with an increased risk of melanoma or a history of skin cancer should also check with a dermatologist to determine how often to follow up with a provider for formal checks.

IMMUNIZATIONS IN ADULT MEN

Herpes Zoster

In the United States almost 1 out of every 3 people will develop shingles, also known as zoster or herpes zoster, in their lifetime. Anyone who has had chickenpox is at risk of developing shingles later in life, with about half of all cases of shingles occurring in men age 60 years or older. Varicella zoster virus (VZV) is the organism that causes shingles (CDC, 2016c). The

Centers for Disease Control and Prevention (CDC) recommends that people age 60 years and older get one dose of herpes zoster vaccine (HZV) regardless of whether they had a prior episode of herpes zoster. This vaccine reduces the risk of developing shingles by 51% and postherpetic neuralgia (PHN) by 67%, and is given as a single dose (CDC, 2016c). Adult men with malignant conditions, including those that affect the bone marrow or lymphatic system, or who receive systemic immunosuppressive therapy and adult men with HIV infection and $CD4^{+}$ T-lymphocyte count <200 cells/μL should not receive HZV (American Association for Clinical Chemistry, 2017).

Influenza

According to the CDC (2016d), the estimated number of flu-related hospitalizations since 2010 ranged from 140,000 to 710,000, and flu-related deaths are estimated to have ranged from 12,000 to 56,000 during flu season. Influenza (flu) is a contagious respiratory illness caused by influenza viruses that infect the nose, throat, and lungs. Annually in the United States, millions of people are sickened, hundreds of thousands are hospitalized, and thousands or tens of thousands of people die from the flu (CDC, 2016d). This includes people age 65 years and older and people of any age with certain chronic medical conditions such as diabetes, asthma, and heart disease.

Pneumococcal Vaccination

Pneumococcal disease causes thousands of infections, such as meningitis, bloodstream infections, pneumonia, and ear infections in the United States annually. A pneumococcal vaccine decreases the rate of hospitalization by preventing severe disease from becoming worst. Two pneumococcal vaccines are recommended for adult men: 13-valent pneumococcal conjugate vaccine (PCV13, Prevnar13) and 23-valent pneumococcal polysaccharide vaccines (PPSV23, Pneumovax) (CDC, 2017e).

A single dose of the PCV13 is recommended for adult men 65 years or older who have not previously received PCV13. PCV13 is also given to men 19 years or older with certain medical conditions who have not previously received PCV13. A single dose of PPSV23 is recommended for adults 65 years or older, regardless of previous history of vaccination with pneumococcal vaccines, and no additional doses of PPSV23 should be administered. PPSV23 is given to men ages 19 through 64 years with certain medical conditions including lung diseases, cardiovascular disease, diabetes, liver disease, alcoholism, and cochlear implant and those who smoke cigarettes. It is also recommended for adults 19 years or older with conditions that weaken the immune system, including HIV infection, organ transplantation, leukemia, lymphoma, and severe kidney disease. A second dose may be indicated depending on the medical condition (CDC, 2015a).

Human Papillomavirus

Human papillomavirus (HPV) vaccine is for protection from most of the cancers caused by HPV, a common virus that can lead to cancer. Nearly 80 million people—about 1 in 4—are currently infected with HPV in the United States, and about 14 million people, including teens, become infected with HPV each year (Bradford, 2017). A 2017 study published in the *Journal of the American Medical Association Oncology* found that nearly half of American men under the age 60 have an HPV infection (Bradford, 2017).

The CDC recommends HPV vaccine for adult males ages 11 through 21 years who have not received any HPV vaccine. HPV vaccination is also recommended for men up to ages 22 to

26 years for men having sex with men and men with compromised immune systems including HIV. There is a new recommendation by the Food and Drug Administration (FDA) for use of a two-dose schedule for boys who initiate the vaccination series at ages 9 through 14 years. Three doses remain recommended for persons who initiate the vaccination series at ages 15 through 26 years and for immunocompromised persons (Meites, Kempe, & Markowitz, 2017).

Measles, Mumps, Rubella

The measles, mumps, rubella (MMR) vaccine protects against all three of those vastly contagious diseases. The number of measles cases in the United States is on the rise because more and more people aren't immunized. A single dose of MMR vaccine is recommended for U.S citizens born after 1957 or later without acceptable evidence of immunity to measles, mumps, or rubella unless there is medical contraindication including immunodeficiency, such as HIV infection and $CD4^+$ T-lymphocyte count below 200 cells/µL, malignancy, and immunosuppressive therapy. Men who have not received MMR vaccine and have never had measles and adult men with HIV infection and $CD4^+$ T-lymphocyte count at or above 200 cells/µL for at least 6 months who do not have evidence of measles, mumps, or rubella immunity should receive two doses of MMR vaccine at least 28 days apart. MMR vaccine is also recommended for teachers, healthcare workers, and anyone traveling outside the United States. Acceptable evidence of immunity to measles, mumps, or rubella in adults includes men born before 1957, documentation of receipt of MMR vaccine, and laboratory evidence of immunity or disease (CDC, 2017f).

Tetanus, Diphtheria, and Acellular Pertussis Vaccination

Respiratory diphtheria is an acute and communicable infectious illness caused by strains of *Corynebacterium diphtheriae, and* tetanus is a noncommunicable disease caused by *Clostridium tetani*. Administration of tetanus and diphtheria toxoid and acellular pertussis (Tdap) vaccine protects against tetanus, diphtheria, and pertussis. Adult men who have not been given the Tdap vaccine or those whose pertussis vaccination status is not known should receive one dose of Tdap vaccine followed by a tetanus toxoid (Td) booster every 10 years. Adult men are encouraged to receive Tdap vaccine irrespective of when a tetanus or diphtheria toxoid-containing vaccine was last received. Adult men with an unknown or incomplete history of a three-dose primary series with tetanus and diphtheria toxoid-containing vaccines should complete the primary series including one dose of Tdap. Adult males who have not been vaccinated should receive the first two doses at least 4 weeks apart and the third dose 6 to 12 months after the second dose.

CONCLUSION

As of February 2018, there is a new *Recommended Immunization Schedule for Adults Aged 19 Years or Older, United States* available from the CDC, and it can be found on their website (www.cdc.gov/vaccines/schedules/downloads/adult/adult-combined-schedule.pdf). It forms the basis for this summary chapter. One of the key points with adult vaccinations is that if an individual's vaccination status is not clear, the CDC recommends moving ahead with any suspected missing vaccines. Providers should also be aware that although intervals for multidose vaccines are recommended, a delay between doses will not affect the ultimate effectiveness of the vaccine. Any potential cases of vaccine-preventable diseases must be reported to the local or state health department, and any suspected postvaccination events should be reported to the Vaccine Adverse Event Reporting System online.

REFERENCES

Agency for Healthcare Research and Quality. (2012, December). Healthy Men. Retrieved from https://archive.ahrq.gov/patients-consumers/patient-involvement/healthy-men/index.html

Agency for Healthcare Research and Quality. (2014, June). Section 2. Recommendations for Adults (continued). Retrieved from http://www.ahrq.gov/professionals/clinicians-providers/guidelines-recommendations/guide/section2c.html

American Academy of Dermatology. (2017). Skin cancer. Retrieved from https://www.aad.org/media/stats/conditions/skin-cancer

American Association for Clinical Chemistry. (2017, July). Screening Tests for Adults (50 and Up). Retrieved from https://labtestsonline.org/understanding/wellness/e-over50-1/e-over50-14

American Cancer Society. (2017). Key statistics for lung cancer. Retrieved from https://www.cancer.org/cancer/non-small-cell-lung-cancer/about/key-statistics.html

American Heart Association. (2017). The top 10 reasons men put off doctor visits. Retrieved from https://www.heart.org/HEARTORG/Conditions/Heart-Disease---The-Top-10-Reasons-Men-Put-Off-Doctor-Visits_UCM_433365_Article.jsp

Anderson, L. (2017). 14 Essential Health Screenings That All Men Should Consider. Retrieved from https://www.drugs.com/slideshow/health-screenings-men-need-1128

Bradford, A. (2017). HPV (human papillomavirus): Symptoms and treatment. Retrieved from https://www.livescience.com/53799-what-is-hpv.html

Centers for Disease Control and Prevention. (2015a). Pneumococcal vaccine timing for adults make sure your patients are up to date with pneumococcal vaccination. Retrieved from https://www.cdc.gov/vaccines/vpd/pneumo/downloads/pneumo-vaccine-timing.pdf

Centers for Disease Control and Prevention, U.S. Department of Health and Human Services. (2015b). Basics about diabetes. Retrieved from http://www.cdc.gov/diabetes/basics/diabetes.html

Centers for Disease Control and Prevention. Program Performance and Evaluation Office. (2016a, March). Depression. Retrieved from https://www.cdc.gov/nchs/fastats/mental-health.htm

Centers for Disease Control and Prevention. (2016b). Today's HIV/AIDS epidemic. Retrieved from https://www.cdc.gov/nchhstp/newsroom/docs/factsheets/todaysepidemic-508

Centers for Disease Control and Prevention. (2016c, August). Shingles overview. Retrieved from https://www.cdc.gov/shingles/about/overview.html

Centers for Disease Control and Prevention, National Center for Immunization and Respiratory Diseases. (2016d). Influenza (Flu). Retrieved from https://www.cdc.gov/flu/protect/keyfacts.htm

Centers for Disease Control and Prevention, Division of Cancer Prevention and Control. (2017a). Colorectal (Colon) cancer. Retrieved from https://www.cdc.gov/cancer/colorectal

Centers for Disease Control and Prevention, Division of HIV/AIDS Prevention, National Center for HIV/AIDS. (2017b). HIV/AIDS. Retrieved from https://www.cdc.gov/hiv/basics

Centers for Disease Control and Prevention, Division of Cancer Prevention and Control. (2017c). Lung cancer. Retrieved from https://www.cdc.gov/cancer/lung/statistics/index.htm

Centers for Disease Control and Prevention, Division of Nutrition, Physical Activity, and Obesity, National Center for Chronic Disease Prevention and Health Promotion. (2017d). Overweight & Obesity. Retrieved from https://www.cdc.gov/obesity/index.html

Center for Disease Control and Prevention. (2017e). Pneumococcal vaccination. Retrieved from https://www.cdc.gov/pneumococcal/vaccination.html

Center for Disease Control and Prevention. (2017f). Adult immunization schedule by vaccine and age group-shell. Retrieved from https://www.cdc.gov/vaccines/schedules/hcp/imz/adult-shell.html

Centers for Disease Control and Prevention, Division for Heart Disease and Stroke Prevention, National Center for Chronic Disease Prevention and Health Promotion. (2017g). High Blood Pressure. Retrieved from https://www.cdc.gov/bloodpressure/

Meites, E., Kempe, A., & Markowitz, L. E. (2017). Use of a 2-dose schedule for human papillomavirus vaccination-updated recommendations of the Advisory Committee on Immunization Practices. *American Journal of Transplantation, 17*(3), 834–837. doi:10.1111/ajt.14206

Merai, R., Siegel, C., Rakotz, M., Basch, P., Wright, J., Wong, B., & Thorpe, P. (2016). CDC grand rounds: A public health approach to detect and control hypertension. *MMWR. Morbidity and Mortality Weekly Report, 65*(45), 1261–1264. doi:10.15585/mmwr.mm6545a3

Moyer, V. A. (2013a, August). Screening and behavioral counseling interventions in primary care to reduce alcohol misuse: USPSTF recommendation statement. Retrieved from http://annals.org/aim/article/1722524/screening-behavioral-counseling-interventions-primary-care-reduce-alcohol-misuse-u

Moyer, V. A. (2013b). Screening for hepatitis C virus infection in adults: USPSTF recommendation statement. *Annals of Internal Medicine, 159*(5), 349–357. doi:10.7326/0003-4819-159-5-201309030-00677

Torres, A. (2016, January). AADA provides input on skin cancer screening recommendation. Retrieved from https://www.aad.org/media/news-releases/aada-provides-input-on-skin-cancer-screening-recommendation#sthash.1hi8hbRc.dpuf

U.S. Prevention Services Task Force. (2014a). Final recommendation statement: Depression in adults: Screening. Retrieved from https://www.uspreventiveservicestaskforce.org/Page/Document/RecommendationStatementFinal/depression-in-adults-screening

U.S. Prevention Services Task Force. (2014b). Final recommendation statement: Hepatitis B virus infection: Screening. Retrieved from https://www.uspreventiveservicestaskforce.org/Page/Document/RecommendationStatementFinal/hepatitis-b-virus-infection-screening-2014

U.S. Prevention Services Task Force. (2015a). Blood pressure in adults (hypertension): Screening. Retrieved from http://www.uspreventiveservicestaskforce.org/uspstf07/hbp/hbprs.htm

U.S. Prevention Services Task Force. (2015b). Final diabetes screening guideline questions & answers. Retrieved from http://www.diabetesnc.com/downloads/1215/USPSTF_QA_120315.pdf

U.S. Prevention Services Task Force. (2015c). Final update summary: Lung cancer. Retrieved from https//www.uspreventiveservicestaskforce.org/PageSummaryFinal/Lung-cancer-screening

U.S. Prevention Services Task Force. (2016a). Alcohol misuse: Screening and behavioral counseling interventions in primary care. Retrieved from https://www.uspreventiveservicestaskforce.org/Page/Document/UpdateSummaryFinal/alcohol-misuse-screening-and-behavioral-counseling-interventions-in-primary-care

U.S. Prevention Services Task Force. (2016b). Final update summary: High blood pressure in adults: Screening. Retrieved from https://www.uspreventiveservicestaskforce.org/Page/Document/UpdateSummaryFinal/high-blood-pressure-in-adults-screening

U.S. Prevention Services Task Force. (2016c). Final recommendation statement: Hepatitis C: Screening. Retrieved from https://www.uspreventiveservicestaskforce.org/Page/Document/RecommendationStatementFinal/hepatitis-c-screening.

U.S. Prevention Services Task Force. (2016d). Final recommendation statement: Human Immunodeficiency Virus (HIV) infection: Screening. Retrieved from https://www.uspreventiveservicestaskforce.org/Page/Document/RecommendationStatementFinal/human-immunodeficiency-virus-hiv-infection-screening

U.S. Prevention Services Task Force. (2016e). Final recommendation statement: Syphilis. Retrieved from https://www.uspreventiveservicestaskforce.org/Page/Document/RecommendationStatementFinal/syphilis-infection-in-nonpregnant-adults-and-adolescents

U.S. Prevention Services Task Force. (2016f). Final recommendation statement: Latent Tuberculosis Infection: Screening. Retrieved from https://www.uspreventiveservicestaskforce.org/Page/Document/RecommendationStatementFinal/latent-tuberculosis-infection-screening

U.S. Prevention Services Task Force. (2016g). Final recommendation statement: Obesity in adults: Screening and management. Retrieved from https://www.uspreventiveservicestaskforce.org/Page/Document/RecommendationStatementFinal/obesity-in-adults-screening-and-management

U.S. Department of Health and Human Services. (2017, January). Leading causes of death in males United States. Retrieved from https://www.cdc.gov/men/lcod/index.htm

Vashi, P. G. (2014, March), Colonoscopy Still the 'gold standard' for colorectal cancer screening. Retrieved from www.cancercenter.com/discussions/blog/colonoscopy-gold-standard-for-colorectal-cancer-screening

CHAPTER 9

Controversies in Circumcision

Michael Sheehan

INTRODUCTION

According to Merriam-Webster (Circumcise, n.d.) circumcision is defined as the procedure to remove the "foreskin of a male" and the literal meaning is "to cut around." "It is one of the oldest surgical operations known to have been performed by ancient people" (Medical Definition of Circumcision, n.d.). Although it is an ancient procedure and is practiced across many cultures, Owings, Uddin, and Williams (2013) with the Centers for Disease Control and Prevention (CDC) estimate that the peak rate of circumcision in the United States was 64.9% in 1981 and its lowest was 55.4% in 2007. However, these percentages do not reflect circumcisions performed outside a hospital or clinic setting, or those performed at any age following discharge from the birth hospitalization (Figure 9.1) The World Health Organization (WHO) estimates that worldwide, one third of males aged 15 years or older are circumcised (Figure 9.2). There are many theories about how circumcision arose, but

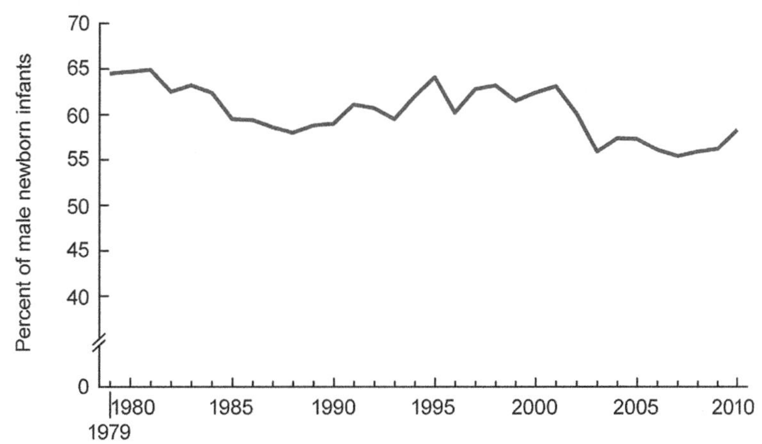

FIGURE 9.1 Rates of circumcision performed on male newborn infants discharged from short-stay hospitals: United States, 1979–2010.

Note: Rates represent circumcisions performed during birth hospitalization. Circumcision is identified by *International Classification of Diseases, Ninth Revision, Clinical Modification* (ICD-9-CM) Procedure Code 64.0.

Source: Centers for Disease Control and Prevention, National Center for Health Statistics. (2013). Trends in circumcision for male newborns in U.S. hospitals: 1979–2010. Retrieved from https://www.cdc.gov/nchs/data/hestat/circumcision_2013/circumcision_2013.htm

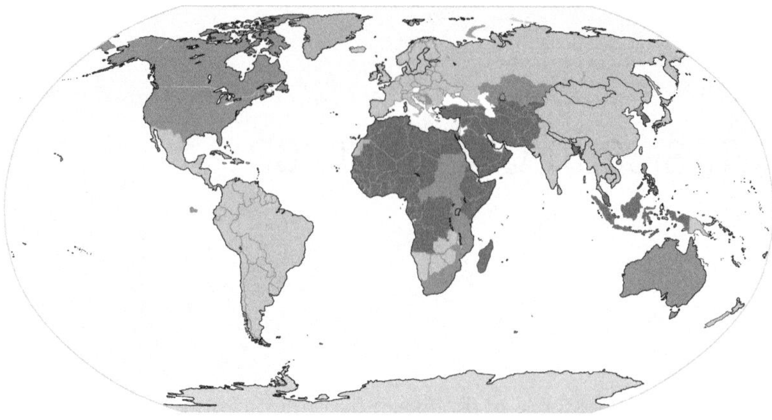

FIGURE 9.2 Male circumcision prevalence (not rate) by country according to the World Health organization's 2007 review of the global trends and determinants of prevalence, safety, and acceptability of circumcision.

Source: Reprinted with permission from WHO, UNAIDS. (2007). *Male circumcision global trends and determinants of prevalence, safety and acceptability* (p. 9). Geneva, Switzerland: WHO, UNAIDS. Copyright 2007 by World Health Organization and Joint United Nations Programme on HIV/AIDS.

the rationale, the historical data, and cultural studies have shown that "these practices are obscure and contested, as are the environmental conditions prevailing when and where such customs emerged" (Controversy and Debate: The Circumcision Experiment, n.d.).

"None of the ancient cultures which practiced circumcision have … claimed that the ritual was introduced as a hygiene measure … [they] explain it [in] different ways, but divine command, tribal identification … family obligation, respect for ancestors and promotion of chastity" are important themes (Controversy and Debate: The Circumcision Experiment, n.d.). In August 2012, the American Academy of Pediatrics (AAP) issued a statement that "the health benefits of … male circumcision outweigh the risks and … justify access to the procedure for [those] who choose it" (p. 1). The AAP charged clinicians of any discipline with the responsibility of providing factually correct information that communicates the risks and benefits of infant circumcision in a nonbiased manner to anyone considering pediatric circumcision. Specifically, the AAP demands that clinicians provide information regarding the alternatives, risks, and benefits in a culturally sensitive and patient-centered effort to help each pediatric patient and legal guardian make an informed decision regarding circumcision.

CIRCUMCISION IN THE ADULT MALE

Adult circumcision can be performed under any number of anesthetic options; local, regional, or general. There are very real indications for this procedure in an adult male, including phimosis, paraphimosis, recurrent balanitis, balanitis xerotica obliterans (BXO), and posthitis. Alternatives to circumcision vary based on the pathophysiology of the patient; if the patient fails conservative therapy (Box 9.1) and chooses to proceed with a surgical intervention, risks and benefits must be reviewed in as much detail as possible. Risks of an adult circumcision include postoperative pain, bleeding, infection, wound disruption, swelling, and cosmetic issues (i.e., scarring). Men may also seek this procedure on an elective basis for nonmedical

BOX 9.1 POSSIBLE MEDICAL TREATMENT ALTERNATIVES TO ADULT CIRCUMCISION

Phimosis: trial of topical steroid creams and a retraction regimen

Balanitis or balanoposthitis: hygiene changes, appropriate antibiotic or antifungal therapy, screen for undiagnosed diabetes or appropriate diabetes control, especially in the context of recurrent or refractory presentation

indications that may be social, cultural, personal, or religious. Benefits of circumcision include a decreased risk of sexually transmitted infections (STIs) and a decreased risk of penile cancer; some men report delayed orgasm.

There are recognized risks for certain subpopulations of men who remain uncircumcised: men in sexual relationships with HIV-infected female partners, men with multiple partners (female and/or male), and men in relationships with women who are at high risk for HIV infection (such as commercial sex workers). These groups should be counseled that while there are inherent risks with any surgical procedure such as circumcision, this procedure may help prevent HIV infection, human papillomavirus (HPV) infection, penile cancer, and STI incidence. Circumcision may also be instrumental in the prevention of cervical cancer and recurrent urinary tract infections in female partners when poor hygiene (in the uncircumcised male) is a contributing factor.

Complications after a circumcision in the adult male are uncommon and have been outlined in a large meta-analysis incorporating more than 500,000 patients by Krill, Palmer, and Palmer (2011), who found a bleeding complication rate of 1%, an infection rate of 0.4%, and one reported death due to an incorrectly placed Plastibell device.

The CDC guidelines (CDC, 2014) demonstrated a 50% to 60% risk reduction for contracting HIV infection and a 30% reduced risk of contracting herpes simplex virus (HSV) infection and HPV infection as a result of circumcising adult men. However, circumcision has only been proved to prevent HIV and sexually transmitted disease transmission *in men* during vaginal sex; it has not been proved to reduce the risk of HIV transmission to female partners. Circumcision has not been conclusively shown to reduce the risk of HIV infection through oral or anal sex.

Circumcision can also "reduce the risk of urinary tract infections (UTIs) [in men]" (CDC, 2014). Critics of these guidelines point out that the recommendations have been based on studies in sub-Saharan Africa where disease transmission and risks are dramatically different than in North America.

CIRCUMCISION IN MALE INFANTS AND CHILDREN

Pediatric circumcision can be done with various forms of anesthesia and, in some instances, without anesthesia. It can also be accomplished via numerous techniques (Table 9.1). Though techniques vary, the overall risks of pediatric circumcision remain low, including bleeding, concealed penis, recurrent phimosis, skin bridge(s), infection, urinary retention, fistulas, and necrosis. As pointed out by Abdulwahab-Ahmed and Mungadi "a meta-analysis reported a median frequency of 1.5% (range 0–16%) for any complication arising from circumcision" (Weiss, Larke, Halperin, & Schenker, 2010, p.1). Abdulwahab-Ahmed and Mungadi (2013) also argued that the primary benefit of pediatric circumcision, like vaccinations, "is to have a technique that can be deployed for mass rollout of circumcision in

TABLE 9.1 Circumcision Devices

Device	Description
Gomco clamp	Invented 1935; in continuous use for more than 70 years Consists of a steel bell which protects the glans and does not leave a foreign body at the site after the procedure
Shield and clamp (Mogen clamp)	Designed by Rabbi Harry Bronstein in 1954; most commonly used by mohels for ceremonial circumcision, does not protect the glans during the procedure or leave a foreign body at the site after the procedure
Plastibell	Introduced in the mid 1950s; widely used, as it is a single-use plastic device that yields consistent cosmetic results, provides hemostasis with a retained suture but more likely to have postprocedural infection owing to a retained foreign body at the site of the procedure
Zhenxi ring	Prominent in Korea and China; a tourniquet-type device
Tara Klamp	Malaysian invention; a tourniquet-type device similar to the Plastibell and Zhenxi ring but instead of suture or a band it uses the pressure of two locking "arms" to constrict the foreskin
SmartKlamp	Released in 2004; two-piece design with a polycarbonate tube to protect the glans during circumcision; foreskin is removed surgically with excellent hemostasis as the clamp remains in place for 5 days postoperatively
Shang Ring	Chinese invention; single-use disposable device requiring no special skills for application and is intended for mass marketing in HIV infection prevention programs; does not provide any protection for the glans during the procedure
PrePex	Unique in design and intent; this device is specifically intended for adult male circumcision and does not require any type of anesthesia; since inception, this device has been used extensively in African populations as part of the HIV infection prevention programs by the CDC, WHO, and UNAIDS
Surgical sleeve excision	Surgical excision of the foreskin is accomplished using two circumferential incisions and one longitudinal incision and then suturing the free edges; there are many variations on this procedure

CDC, Centers for Disease Control and Prevention; UNAIDS, United Nations Programme on HIV/AIDS; WHO, World Health Organization.

an attempt to prevent transmission of HIV" (p. 7) as well as HPV to reduce the lifetime risk of penile cancer. Minor benefits of pediatric circumcision include a reduced risk of urinary tract infections and reduced medical costs. Christakis et al. (Christakis et al., 2000) concluded "that 6 [UTIs] could be prevented for every circumcision complication, and 2 complications can be expected for every penile cancer prevented" (p. 1).

EXPLORING THE CONTROVERSY

In his blog, Matthew Tontonoz points out that "various health benefits have been proposed over the years ... [but in] the midst of the latest debate about HIV transmission and other risks, it is easy to forget that circumcision has long been, in America, a cultural practice looking for a medical justification" (Tontonoz, 2014). In the case of adult circumcision, this debate is settled by each individual patient. Every sentient and able adult has the right to decide what to do with his or her physical person; that choice includes piercings, tattoos, pregnancy, prisoners' rights, surgical procedures, "right to die," and abortion. Should an adult choose circumcision, the patient should be given accurate risk statistics and be presented with alternatives, and the realistic benefits should be reviewed. The controversies in circumcision are mostly centered on pediatric circumcision, and there is a spirited debate about the issue of infant/pediatric circumcision that rages in both scholarly literature and the lay press.

Academic Perspective

While every argument against pediatric circumcision cannot be debated in the scope of this chapter, more obvious cases against pediatric circumcision are easily identified. Oxford University PhD student Brian Earp (2015) proposes that:

> Most basically, the CDC's approach runs counter to the conventional bioethical (and legal) view that unnecessary surgeries, and especially those that remove non-diseased, functional tissue from an individual without his consent, are in and of themselves harmful. As a California Appeals Court ... held ... "[I]t seems self-evident that unnecessary surgery is injurious and causes harm to a patient. Even if a surgery is executed flawlessly, if the surgery were unnecessary, the surgery in and of itself constitutes harm."

This position is mirrored by anticircumcision groups such as Intact America ("intactivists"), National Organization of Circumcision Information Resource Centers (NOCIRC), Doctors Opposing Circumcision (DOC), National Organization of Restoring Men (NORM), and UNCircumcising Information and Resources Centers (UNCIRC). Specifically, the concept of informed parental permission allows for medical interventions in situations of clear and immediate medical necessity only, such as disease, trauma, or deformity. The human penis in its normal, uncircumcised state satisfies none of these requirements. To further this point and counter the argument regarding phimosis, anticircumcision groups point out that phimosis "is a convenient pathological label that can be applied to any penis that someone wants to circumcise ... a complex disease category consisting of a pathologized catalogue of both the distinguishing features of the normal juvenile prepuce and the wide spectrum of adult penile variation" (Denniston, Hodges, Mansfield, & Milos, 1999, pp. 57–58). To wit, if only 1 in 3 men in the world are circumcised, how do the other 66% manage to grow, develop normally, urinate normally, and conceive normally with a foreskin? Aside from consent and a debate about normalcy, sexual sensation and satisfaction is a primary concern of intactivists.

In a study of 1,369 men, 1,059 uncircumcised and 310 circumcised, Bronselaer et al. (2013) found that circumcised men reported decreased sexual pleasure and lower orgasm intensity compared to intact males, circumcised men required more effort or stimulus to achieve orgasm, and men circumcised after puberty reported more pain and less sexual pleasure. Broadly speaking, they concluded that the foreskin was important for "penile sensitivity [and] overall sexual satisfaction" (p. 826). Importantly, the authors noted that "before circumcision without a medical indication [or even with a medical indication], adult men should be informed of the importance of the foreskin in male sexuality" (p. 826).

However, a study by Bossio, Pukall, and Steele (2016) examining the penile sensitivity of adult males circumcised as a child found "minimal long-term implications for penile sensitivity ... as a result of the surgical excision of the foreskin during neonatal circumcision" (p. 1853). The study included 62 men, 30 circumcised and 32 intact, who underwent quantitative sensory testing protocols. While the conclusion was that there were minimal implications for penile sensitivity, the study did indicate that the foreskin of intact men was more sensitive to tactile stimulation and that was lacking in circumcised men.

Perspectives from the Lay Literature

"Some people think of neonatal circumcision as a religious duty or a valuable preventive health measure; others think it is the epitome of child abuse" states Harriet Hall, MD (Hall, 2008), in a blog post on the site *Science-Based Medicine.* Hall goes on to state that some of the more fundamental issues with circumcision relate back to hygiene.

Specifically, "the concept of informed parental permission allows for medical interventions in situations of clear and immediate medical necessity only, such as disease, trauma, or deformity. The human penis in its normal, uncircumcised state satisfies none of these requirements" (Fleiss, 1977, n.p.). The previously discussed study by Bossio et al. (2016) was explored further on the Huffington post by blogger Brian Earp (as he is active on this topic in both the academic world and lay press) and he contends that there were numerous sampling and statistical errors in this study and yet, the findings were still in favor of increased sensitivity of tactile stimulation of the intact men. Specifically, Earp contends that following circumcision the penis "loses all of the sensitivity experienced in the foreskin itself, along with all subjective sensations that are unique to having a foreskin ... among these sensations is the feeling of rolling the foreskin back and forth over the head of the penis during [sexual intercourse]" (Earp, 2016).

CONCLUSION

The questions of consent and reduced sensitivity or sexual enjoyment in juxtaposition to medical benefits bring us to the crux of the controversies of circumcision. There "is a growing movement to leave the 'circumcision decision' to the individual who will be affected by it, so that he can decide—when he's old enough to understand what's at stake—if he'd rather experience sex and masturbation with an intact penis (however sensitive his particular foreskin turns out to be), or with a modified one (if he wants to go for [circumcision])" (Earp, 2016). Despite attempts to quantify the sensitivity of *the* foreskin versus *a* foreskin as well as sexual satisfaction, "sexual experience[s are] largely subjective: different people prefer different things [and experience things differently even with similar anatomy] when it comes to sex, and a lot of sexual enjoyment comes down to psychological factors, not penile anatomy" (Earp, 2015).

From a medical or science standpoint, "there [are] no compelling scientific arguments for or against neonatal circumcision. There are small risks and there are small benefits. The decision is not a medical one. Medical organizations [should not be] 'pro' circumcision, but [they should also] not [be] 'con' either" (Fleiss, 1997, n.p.). Each provider should make every attempt to present the risks, benefits, and alternatives in a clear and unbiased manner and should try to avoid any impulse to convince a patient or family of what is right or wrong in regard to the foreskin or circumcision.

REFERENCES

Abdulwahab-Ahmed, A., & Mungadi, I. (2013). Techniques of male circumcision. *Journal of Surgical Technique and Case Report, 5*(1), 1–7. doi:10.4103/2006-8808.118588

Bossio, J., Pukall C., & Steele, S. (2016). Examining penile sensitivity in neonatally circumcised and intact men using quantitative sensory testing. *Journal of Urology, 195*(6), 1848–1853. doi:10.1016/j.juro.2015.12.080

Bronselaer, G., Schober, J., Meyer-Bahlburg, H., T'Sjoen, G., Vlietink, R., & Hoebeke, P. (2013). Male circumcision decreased penile sensitivity as measured in a large cohort. *British Journal of Urology, 111*(5), 820–827. doi:10.1111/j.1464-410X.2012.11761.x

Centers for Disease Control and Prevention. (2014). CDC recommendations for providers counseling male patients and parents regarding male circumcision and the prevention of HIV infection, STIs, and other health outcomes (Draft). Retrieved from https://www.cdc.gov/hiv/pdf/policies/mcpubliccommentnotice.pdf

Christakis, D., Harvey, E., Zerr, D., Feudtner, C., Wright, J., & Connell, F. (2000). A trade-off analysis of routine pediatric circumcision. *Pediatrics, 105*, 246–249. doi:10.1542/peds.105.1.S2.246

Circumcise. (n.d.). Merriam-Webster Dictionary online. Retrieved from https://www.merriam-webster.com/dictionary/circumcise

Controversy and debate: The circumcision experiment. (n.d.). Retrieved from http://www.circinfo.org/controversy.html

Denniston, G., Hodges, G., Mansfield, F., & Milos, M. (1999). *Male and female circumcision. Medical, legal, and ethical considerations in pediatric practice*. New York, NY: Kluwer Academic/Plenum.

Earp, B. (2015). Do the benefits of male circumcision outweigh the risks? A critique of the proposed CDC guidelines. *Frontiers in Pediatrics, 3*, 18. doi:10.3389/fped.2015.00018

Earp, B. (2016). Does circumcision reduce penis sensitivity? The answer is not clear cut. [Web log comment]. Retrieved from http://www.huffingtonpost.com/brian-earp/does-circumcision-reduce-_b_9743242.html

Fleiss, P. (1997). The case against circumcision. In *Mothering: The magazine of natural family living* (pp. 36–45). Retrieved from http://www.cirp.org/news/Mothering1997

Hall, H. (2008). Circumcision: What does science say? Retrieved from https://sciencebasedmedicine.org/circumcision-what-does-science-say

Krill, A., Palmer, L., & Palmer, J. (2011). Complications of circumcision. *Scientific World Journal, 11*(11), 2458–2468. doi:10.1100/2011/373829

Medical definition of circumcision. (n.d.). Retrieved from http://www.medicinenet.com/script/main/art.asp?articlekey=2739

Owings, M., Uddin, S., & Williams, S. (2013). Trends in circumcision for male newborns in U.S. hospitals: 1979-2010. Retrieved from https://www.cdc.gov/nchs/data/hestat/circumcision_2013/circumcision_2013.pdf

Tontonoz, M. (2014, March). Why is circumcision so popular in America? [Web log comment]. Retrieved from https://matthewtontonoz.com/2015/01/05/why-is-circumcision-so-popular-in-america

Weiss, H., Larke, N., Halperin, D., & Schenker, I. (2010). Complications of circumcision in male neonates, infants, and children: A systematic review. *BMC Urology, 10*(2), 1–13. doi:10.1186/1471-2490-10-2

SECTION II

Overview of Special Issues in Men's Health

CHAPTER 10

The State of Men's Health Services in the Veterans Health Administration

Michael Fenstermaker, Sujay Paknikar, Amarnath Rambhatla, Dana A. Ohl, Ted A. Skolarus, and James M. Dupree

INTRODUCTION

For diseases that place a large burden on our healthcare system, such as cardiovascular disease, diabetes, and cancer, there is increasing recognition that men often have poorer outcomes compared with women. Across all age groups, mortality rates are higher for males than for age-matched females—with men having an average life expectancy 6 years less than women (Wang, Schumacher, Levitz, Mokdad, & Murray, 2013). Gender differences in healthcare-seeking behavior often lead to men presenting with more advanced stages of disease. Additionally, men have poorer health expectancy—a term that encompasses quality of life in addition to life expectancy—when compared to age-matched women (World Health Organization, 2010). In recognition of these issues, there has been a renewed nationwide emphasis on providing holistic approaches to improving "men's health."

The Veterans Health Administration (VHA) is uniquely poised to tackle the challenge of delivering integrated men's health services. As of 2013, the total veteran population within the United States was 22 million (Projected Veteran Population, n.d.), and the VHA represents the largest fully integrated healthcare system in the country. The VHA health system's patient population, despite evolving demographics, is approximately 90% male (Projected Veteran Population, n.d.). Additionally, the VHA trains more physicians and medical professionals that any other healthcare institution in the United States—with more than 70% of all U.S. doctors training at a VHA hospital (Projected Veteran Population, n.d.). Thus, the VHA has the ability to be at the forefront of advancing "men's health" by also shaping physician practice patterns.

Urologists play a particularly important role in maintaining men's health. Urologic conditions account for a substantial proportion of medical conditions pertinent to the male VHA patient population. As defined by the Urological Diseases in America project, prostate cancer, benign prostatic hyperplasia (BPH), lower urinary tract symptoms (LUTS), nephrolithiasis, urinary tract infections (UTIs), and urinary incontinence accounted for 7.6% of all chief complaints in VHA patients (Anger, Saigal, Wang, & Yano, 2008). Because men with LUTS or erectile dysfunction may also have concomitant cardiovascular or metabolic disease (Fode, Gratzke, & Sønksen, 2016; Gandaglia et al., 2016), the urologist can play a central role in identifying men's health concerns and connecting patients to other primary healthcare providers.

In this context, we aimed to identify institutional features within the VHA system that seek to advance the goal of providing high-quality men's healthcare. We reviewed federal regulations on available benefits to U.S. veterans and identified programs that seek to integrate

This chapter was reprinted with permission from Fenstermaker, M., Paknikar, S., Rambhatla, A., Ohl, D. A., Skolarus, T. A., & Dupree, J. M. (2017). The state of men's health services in the Veterans Health Administration. *Current Urology Reports, 18*(11), 88. doi:10.1007/s11934-017-0733-4 multidisciplinary men's health services. Understanding men's health efforts at the VHA will inform other healthcare providers, health system leaders, and policy makers interested in implementing services that address the unique needs of a male patient population.

METHODS

Defining the Domains of Men's Health

Defining the appropriate domains of "men's health" can be difficult. All-inclusive definitions should include conditions that are unique to men, diseases more prevalent in men, diseases with male-specific risk factors, and health problems that necessitate gender-specific strategies for patient outreach (Meryn & Young, 2010). For this study, we used a definition of men's health as determined by an expert panel from the American Urologic Association (AUA) Committee on Men's Health. This expert panel created the AUA Men's Health Checklist and categorized the urologic aspects of men's health into four primary domains: (a) voiding health, (b) reproductive health, (c) sexual health, and (d) health measures such as blood pressure, weight, and genitourinary examination. Voiding health comprises LUTS, stricture disease, hematuria, UTI, urolithiasis, genitourinary pain, and dysuria/discharge. Reproductive health includes male infertility, contraception, undescended testes, testis masses, varicoceles and scrotal disorders, sexually transmitted diseases (STDs), and HIV infection. Sexual health includes symptomatic androgen deficiency, ejaculation disorders, sexual activity, erectile function, and Peyronie's disease. Also relevant are cancer screening such as prostate-specific antigen (PSA) testing and testicular examinations (American Urological Association, 2014). The AUA panel also identified key nonurologic care as important aspects for maintaining men's health, such as substance abuse counseling, screening for metabolic diseases, and immunizations.

Identifying Integrated VHA Men's Health Initiatives

In recent decades, significant efforts have been made to improve the quality of healthcare delivered at the VHA through implementation of evidenced-based medicine practices. The Quality Enhancement Research Initiative (QUERI) and Health Services Research and Development (HSR&D) divisions at the VHA have spearheaded many of these efforts. Founded in 1998, QUERI was established to rapidly implement evidence-based medical practices and develop organizational structures to ultimately improve the quality of healthcare within the VHA (Stetler, Mittman, & Francis, 2008). We sought to identify programs within the VHA that were tailored to integrate multiple aspects of the men's health checklist into a single program. As such, we searched the VHA internal database of QUERI and HSR&D projects using AUA Men's Health Checklist domains as keywords to identify integrative men's health initiatives.

Evaluating Financial Access to Men's Healthcare

Financial barriers limiting access to care can widen gender gaps in health outcomes. Lack of perceived time, money, and the prioritization of other tasks, such as full-time employment, often account for delayed presentations among males (Teo, Ng, Booth, & White, 2016). Efforts to develop comprehensive men's health programs should take these factors into account to optimize male service utilization and health outcomes. As such, we also sought to evaluate covered VHA benefits that pertain to the four domains of the AUA Men's Health Checklist. We reviewed the Code of Federal Regulations, Title 38, which outlines the federal laws and regulations pertaining to the Department of Veterans Affairs. Mandated benefits for veterans are outlined in this code of regulations. These benefits were cross-referenced with aspects of men's health deemed important on the AUA Men's Health Checklist. In addition, we reviewed the Pharmacy Benefits Management database to identify VHA prescription benefits, including tiered medications that are indicated for medical treatments for men's health issues.

RESULTS

VHA Initiatives for Implementing Integrated Men's Health Programs

Review of the project summaries of the 15 national QUERI programs did not reveal any active efforts to integrate aspects of urologic, primary care, and mental health as they pertain to AUA men's health objectives. The VHA HSR&D citation database was then queried to identify programs seeking to integrate men's urologic health with primary care aspects of men's health. Of the queried citations, three active projects were identified that sought to unite previously separate entities that individually address men's health issues.

One men's health program developed through the Pittsburgh VHA HSR&D divisions seeks to incorporate care of the urologic and mental health issues that can arise with end-stage renal disease patients on dialysis (Weisbord et al., 2013). Patients were assigned to treatment arms that included regular assessments of pain, depression, and erectile dysfunction. Dialysis staff were then provided with responses to these questionnaires as well as evidenced-based guidelines on how to manage the associated symptoms. These interventions demonstrated small improvements in patient's symptom scores relating to erectile dysfunction and depression.

In a recent project, a clinical trigger system was developed to reduce delays in diagnostic workup for bladder cancer among men undergoing urinalysis in the primary care setting. Using a computerized system, physicians were alerted to patients who had demonstrable microhematuria, yet no follow-up action (i.e., cystoscopy) was detected (Murphy et al., 2017). While still in developmental phases, this clinical support tool seeks to address breakdowns in communication that can occur with multidisciplinary care inherent to comprehensive men's health programs.

Another program in early development phases at the Ann Arbor VHA seeks to direct prostate cancer survivors to appropriate primary or specialty care for treatment-related side effects. Diseases such as metabolic syndrome and depression are seen at disproportionate rates among prostate cancer survivors, requiring management from disparate groups of providers. As such, multidisciplinary collaboration should be investigated as a possible means of improving posttreatment outcomes and quality of life.

Although efforts to integrate urologic health with primary care issues are limited, the AUA Men's Health Checklist also acknowledges the importance of mental healthcare as a key component of comprehensive men's healthcare (American Urological Association, 2014). In this regard, the VHA is actively working to better assimilate these aspects of men's health into a multidisciplinary model of care. One such QUERI initiative seeks to implant mental healthcare professionals at VHA primary care locations to address suicidality and posttraumatic stress disorder (PTSD) among male patients (Post, Metzger, Dumas, & Lehmann, 2010). A randomized controlled trial comparing usual primary care to a model involving psychiatrist support for the management of PTSD demonstrated improved compliance with visits as well as prescription refills (Schnurr et al., 2013). The colocation of mental health professionals has now become standard throughout VHA primary care offices. These mental health programs demonstrate both the feasibility and efficacy of assuming several aspects of men's healthcare into a combined method of healthcare delivery. Future efforts should seek to fold urologic aspects of care into primary care health maintenance.

Covered Benefits and Medications for Men's Healthcare

Our review of the VHA benefit package and the Code of Federal Regulations Title 38 revealed that all of the AUA Men's Health Checklist items composing the domains of "Urologic Health" are covered under VHA regulations. In the voiding dysfunction and sexual health domains, the VHA provides comprehensive medications and procedure benefits. For patient populations in whom medical management has failed, the Code of Federal Regulations allows for the provision of surgical options for voiding dysfunction. The AUA Men's Health Checklist also recognizes management of male sexuality and hypogonadism as important components of men's health. To address these health concerns, the VHA provides access to topical patch and gel testosterone formulations for this purpose as part of their tier 2 formulary listing (VHA Tiered Medication List, n.d.). Erectile dysfunction is also an important component of men's health as defined by the AUA Men's Health Checklist. The VHA offers comprehensive benefits for treating erectile dysfunction. These include medical treatments, such phosphodiesterase-5 inhibitors, injectable medications, and surgical therapies such as inflatable penile prostheses and collagenase for the management of Peyronie's disease (CHAMPVA, n.d.).

Another important aspect of men's health is the provision of cancer screening at regular checkups. Despite controversies surrounding prostate cancer screening, VHA guidelines mandate coverage for prostate cancer screening as part of the standard benefit package. These VHA guidelines suggest screening for men above 50, except African-American males and those with a family history, who can be screened at age 45.

Historically, coverage for male factor infertility has been limited in most insurance plans. However, the Code of Federal Regulations allows for basic counseling, laboratory testing, and certain procedures for the diagnosis and treatment of organic and nonorganic causes for infertility. The benefits cover many common procedures such as vasectomy and varicocelectomy (CHAMPVA, n.d.). Until recently, there were several notable exclusions. Chief among these omissions were sperm retrieval procedures such as testicular sperm extractions as part of in vitro fertilization (IVF), and sperm banking (CHAMPVA, n.d.). Previous legislative efforts have attempted to close these gaps in coverage. Senate legislative efforts to provide access to IVF for veterans (via bills S.3133 in 2012 and S.131 in 2013) were unsuccessful in the House of Representatives (Women Veterans, 2012; 2013). However, under recent legislation passed in 2017, the Congress temporarily authorized VHA medical centers to provide veterans with access to IVF for service-related injuries (Code of Federal Regulations, 2017). There are still many uncertainties as to how funding will be procured for these services, as these provisions are set to expire on September 30, 2017.

DISCUSSION

Review of the Code of Federal Regulations and VHA formulary listings reveals that the VHA covers many health issues that fall under the domains of "men's health." Yet, there have been limited efforts to integrate aspects of primary care, urology, mental health, and social support structures into a comprehensive men's health program, representing a significant missed opportunity. QUERI initiatives that integrate urologic care with other aspects of preventive healthcare could potentially help improve quality of care for men. For example, integrating referrals for cardiovascular risk assessment among men presenting with erectile dysfunction could lead to improvements in several aspects of men's healthcare. Efforts to manage traumatic brain injuries could also include urology input to tackle issues in voiding dysfunction and neurogenic bladder.

Perhaps an integrative approach could take the form of patient-aligned care teams. Research has already shown that patient-aligned care teams—teams of providers, nurses, administrators, and support staff that care for a small core of patients—help reduce costs while improving patient satisfaction and quality of care (Werner, Canamucio, Shea, & True, 2014). Men's health encompasses many urologic issues and involving urologists in these groups may help to better address patient needs.

Creating an integrated men's health program could also help address perceived overutilization of unnecessary testing. For example, despite recommendations against PSA testing in males with limited life expectancy, there still exist high rates of PSA testing among men with limited life expectancy at the VHA (Tang et al., 2016). In a similar study, high rates of inappropriate imaging were found among low-risk prostate cancer patients in the VHA. Yet, these inappropriate rates were lower among high-volume centers (Makarov et al., 2016). One possible explanation is that ready availability of specialists with guideline-specific knowledge at high-volume centers would help curb inappropriate use. If care teams were to integrate multiple disciplines such as urology and primary care in the provision of men's health, perhaps this may limit variations in utilization of important men's health services.

Recent efforts by the VHA in integrating and developing comprehensive women's health programs could provide a model for similar men's health initiatives. Changing veteran demographics have led the VHA to identify (Cordasco et al., 2014; Washington, Farmer, Mor, Canning, & Yano, 2015) and develop (de Kleijn, Lagro-Janssen, Canelo, & Yano, 2015) institutional measures to advance the provision of care to female veterans. For example, efforts are currently underway to evaluate patient-aligned care teams tailored to women's health needs through a multicenter randomized trial (Yano et al., 2016). These implementation studies regarding women's health could provide prototypes for similar efforts to develop inclusive male health programs.

Furthermore, although the Code of Federal Regulations allows for coverage of treatment options for most men's health issues, data are sparse on how accessible these treatment options are to most veterans. In one study analyzing access to infertility care among female veterans, only 22% of women with a service-connected infertility diagnosis received treatment at a VHA facility. Almost 40% of women with an infertility diagnosis elected to receive care outside the VHA (Mattocks et al., 2015). Another related study demonstrated that many rural patients have poorer comprehensive prostate cancer care (Skolarus et al., 2017). Providing coverage for men's health issues may be insufficient in improving health outcomes if access to these services is limited. Future studies will need to evaluate the effect of recent legislation, such as The Veteran's Choice Act of 2014, on access to care issues.

With shifting demographics in the VHA population, certain aspects of men's healthcare, including infertility, will become increasingly important. In the private insurance market, there is great heterogeneity in coverage for male infertility care. Of the 15 states that mandate insurance coverage for infertility services, only 8 states specifically mandate male factor infertility coverage (Dupree, Dickey, Lipshultz, 2016). A lack of insurance coverage for fertility services creates a significant barrier to accessing and utilizing care (Dupree, 2016), and both the World Health Organization and the American Society of Reproductive Medicine define infertility as a disease (Zegers-Hochschild et al., 2009).

Research suggests that 60% of recent veterans prefer to utilize healthcare services within the VHA system (Analysis of VHA Health Care, 2013). By 2023, 45% of the projected veteran population will have been involved in recent conflicts—up from 30% in 2013 (3). These Operation Iraqi Freedom (OIF), Operation Enduring Freedom (OEF), and Operation New Dawn (OND) veterans are a younger patient population with unique men's healthcare needs. In a study of veterans who served in OEF and OIF, 13.8% of men reported that they had experienced infertility, defined as failure to have a pregnancy after at least 12 months, suggesting that the reproductive domain of men's health will be increasingly important in the VHA system (Katon et al., 2014). With younger patient populations, limited coverage for fertility procedures could lead to large gaps in the delivery of comprehensive men's health programs. This is particularly important as male factor infertility may provide a window into a man's overall health status (Hotaling & Walsh, 2009; Kellesarian et al., 2016; Oliveira, Sousa, Silva, Monteiro, & Alves, 2017). Providing infertility coverage will help reduce barriers to accessing services, but systemic changes and referral patterns will also have to adapt as well to ensure that veterans receive the infertility treatments they require. Primary care physicians and other gatekeepers will need to be made aware of these policy changes to ensure that men are properly referred for needed services. The VHA has the opportunity to lead the way in providing access to this important aspect of men's health.

CONCLUSIONS AND FUTURE DIRECTIONS

Advances in men's health are critical for closing gender gaps in health outcomes. Urologists can serve as a cornerstone of holistic men's healthcare through their involvement in prevalent male issues such as voiding dysfunction, sexual medicine, and male fertility. Through programs such as QUERI, some efforts have been made to unify previously disparate aspects of care involving male patients at the VHA. However, there is still significant progress to be made in developing an overarching men's health program with the VHA system.

Our analysis found that the VHA system offers comprehensive coverage of many preventive, medical, and surgical therapies central to AUA-defined key domains of men's health. These benefits, however, have notable gaps that are only recently being addressed, particularly in the area of male infertility. Veterans returning from recent conflicts are younger and expected to be higher utilizers of the VHA health system. Comprehensive efforts to provide infertility-related services may be beneficial in improving care for these men. The findings are relevant to providers and policy makers because, as a large provider of comprehensive health services tailored to a predominantly male population, the VHA can serve as a model for men's health initiatives nationwide.

REFERENCES

American Urological Association. (2014). AUA men's health checklist. Retrieved from https://www.auanet.org/Documents/education/clinical-guidance/Mens-Health-Checklist.pdf

Analysis of VHA health care utilization among Operation Enduring Freedom (OEF), Operation Iraqi Freedom (OIF), and Operation New Dawn (OND) Veterans. (2013). Retrieved from http://www.publichealth.va.gov/docs/epidemiology/healthcare-utilization-report-fy2015-qtr3.pdf

Anger, J. T., Saigal, C., Wang, M., & Yano, E. M. (2008). Urologic disease burden in the United States: Veteran users of VA healthcare. *Urology, 72*, 37–41. doi:10.1016/j.urology.2007.11.163

CHAMPVA policy manual: Male genial system. (n.d.). Retrieved from https://www.va.gov/PURCHASEDCARE/docs/pubfiles/policymanuals/champva/chapter2/1c2s36-1.htm

Code of Federal Regulations. (2017). §17.380 In vitro fertilization treatment. Retrieved from https://www.ecfr.gov/cgi-bin/text-idx?SID=35a7f389ea9f58348d400303e02babc8&mc=true&node=se38.1.17_1380

Cordasco, K. M., Huynh, A. K., Zephyrin, L., Hamilton, A. B., Lau-Herzberg, A. E., Kessler, C. S., & Yano, E. M. (2015). Building capacity in VA to provide emergency gynecology services for women. *Medical Care, 53*, S81–S87. doi:10.1097/MLR.0000000000000320

de Kleijn, M., Lagro-Janssen, A. L. M., Canelo, I., & Yano, E. M. (2015). Creating a roadmap for delivering gender-sensitive comprehensive care for women veterans: Results of a national expert panel. *Medical Care, 53*, S156–S164. doi:10.1097/MLR.0000000000000307

Dupree, J. M. (2016) Insurance coverage for male infertility care in the United States. *Asian Journal of Andrology, 18*, 339–341. doi:10.4103/1008-682X.177838

Dupree, J. M., Dickey, R. M., & Lipshultz, L. I. (2016). Inequity between male and female coverage in state infertility laws. *Fertility and Sterility, 106*, 1519–1522. doi:10.1016/j.fertnstert.2016.02.025

Fode, M., Gratzke, C., & Sønksen, J. (2016). Male lower urinary tract symptoms reveal and predict important cardiovascular disease. *European Urology, 70*, 797–798. doi:10.1016/j.eururo.2016.07.030

Gandaglia, G., Briganti, A., Montorsi, P., Mottrie, A., Salonia, A., & Montorsi, F. (2016). Diagnostic and therapeutic implications of erectile dysfunction in patients with cardiovascular disease. *European Urology, 70*, 219–222. doi:10.1016/j.eururo.2016.01.054

Hotaling, J. M., & Walsh, T. J. (2009). Male infertility: A risk factor for testicular cancer. *Nature Reviews. Urology, 6*, 550–556. doi:10.1038/nrurol.2009.179

Katon, J., Cypel, Y., Raza, M., Zephyrin, L., Reiber, G., Yano, E. M., … Schneiderman, A.. (2014). Self -reported infertility among male and female veterans serving during Operation Enduring Freedom/ Operation Iraqi Freedom. *Journal of Womens Health, 23*, 175–183. doi:10.1089/jwh.2013.4468

Kellesarian, S. V., Yunker, M., Malmstrom, H., Almas, K., Romanos, G. E., & Javed, F. (2016). Male infertility and dental health status: A systematic review. *American Journal of Men's Health*, pii 1557988316655529. doi:10.1177/1557988316655529

Makarov, D. V., Hu, E. Y. C., Walter, D., Braithwaite, R. S., Sherman, S., Gold, H. T., Zhou, X. H., … Zeliadt, S. B. (2016). Appropriateness of prostate cancer imaging among veterans in a delivery system without incentives for overutilization. *Health Services Research, 51*, 1021–1051. doi:10.1111/1475-6773.12395

Mattocks, K., Kroll-Desrosiers, A., Zephyrin, L., Katon, J., Weitlauf, J., Bastian, L., … Brandt, C. (2015). Infertility care among OEF/OIF/OND women veterans in the Department of Veterans Affairs. *Medical Care, 53*, S68–S75. doi:10.1097/MLR.0000000000000301

Meryn, S., & Young, A. (2010). Making the global case for men's health. *Journal of Men's Health, 7*, 2–4. doi:10.1016/j.jomh.2010.01.001

Murphy, D. R., Meyer, A., Fau-Vaghani, V., , Russo, E., Sittig, D. F., Richards, K. A., … Singh, H. (2017). Application of electronic algorithms to improve diagnostic evaluation for bladder cancer. *Applied Clinical Informatics, 22*, 279–290. doi:10.4338/ACI-2016-10-RA-0176

Oliveira, P. F., Sousa, M., Silva, B. M., Monteiro, M. P., & Alves, M. G. (2017). Obesity, energy balance and spermatogenesis. *Reproduction, 156*, R173–R185. doi:10.1530/REP-17-0018

Post, E. P., Metzger, M., Dumas, P., & Lehmann, L. (2010). Integrating mental health into primary care within the Veterans Health Administration. *Family, System, & Health, 28*, 83–90. doi:10.1037/a0020130

Projected veteran population: 2013 to 2043. (n.d.). Retrieved from http://www.va.gov/vetdata/docs/quickfacts/Population_slideshow.pdf

Schnurr, P. P., Friedman, M. J., Oxman, T. E., Dietrich, A. J., Smith, M. W., Shiner, B., … Thurston, V. (2013). RESPECT-PTSD: Reengineering systems for the primary care treatment of PTSD, a randomized controlled trial. *Journal of General Internal Medicine , 28*, 32–40. doi:10.1007/s11606-012-2166-6

Skolarus, T. A., Chan, S., Shelton, J. B., Antonio, A. L., Sales, A. E., Malin, J. L., & Saigal, C. S. (2013). Quality of prostate cancer care among rural men in the Veterans Health Administration. *Cancer, 119*, 3629–3635. doi:10.1002/cncr.28275

Stetler, C. B., Mittman, B. S., & Francis, J. (2008). Overview of the VA Quality Enhancement Research Initiative (QUERI) and QUERI theme articles: QUERI series. *Implementation Science, 3*, 8. doi:10.1186/1748-5908-3-8

Tang, V. L., Shi, Y., Fung, K., Tan, J., Espaldon, R., Sudore, R., … Walter, L. C. (2016). Clinician factors associated with prostate-specific antigen screening in older veterans with limited life expectancy. *JAMA Internal Medical, 176*, 654–661. doi:10.1001/jamainternmed.2016.0695

Teo, C. H., Ng, C. J., Booth, A., & White, A. (2016). Barriers and facilitators to health screening in men: A systematic review. *Social Science & Medicine, 165*, 168–176. doi:10.1016/j.socscimed.2016.07.023

VHA Tiered Medication List. (n.d.). Retrieved from http://www.pbm.va.gov/PBM/Tiered_Copay/Tiered_Copay_Full_Medication_List.xlsx

Wang, H., Schumacher, A. E., Levitz, C. E., Mokdad, A. H., & Murray, C. J. (2013). Left behind: Widening disparities for males and females in US county life expectancy, 1985–2010. *Population Health Metrics, 11*, 8. doi:10.1186/1478-7954-11-8

Washington, D. L., Farmer, M. M., Mor, S. S., Canning, M., & Yano, E. M. (2015). Assessment of the healthcare needs and barriers to VA use experienced by women veterans: Findings from the national survey of women veterans. *Medical Care, 53*, S23–S31. doi:10.1097/MLR.0000000000000312

Weisbord, S. D., Mor, M. K., Green, J. A., Sevick, M. A., Shields, A. M., Zhao, X., … Fine, M. J. (2013). Comparison of symptom management strategies for pain, erectile dysfunction, and depression in patients receiving chronic hemodialysis: A cluster randomized effectiveness trial. *Clinical Journal of the American Society of Nephrology, 8*, 90–99. doi:10.2215/CJN.04450512

Werner, R. M., Canamucio, A., Shea, J. A., & True, G. (2014). The medical home transformation in the Veterans Health Administration: An evaluation of early changes in primary care delivery. *Health Services Research, 49*, 1329–1347. doi:10.1111/1475-6773.12155

Women veterans and other health care improvements act of 2012. (2012). 112th Session of Congress 2012. Retrieved from https://www.govtrack.us/congress/bills/112/s3313

Women veterans and other health care improvements act of 2013. (2013). 113th Session of Congress 2013. Retrieved from https://www.govtrack.us/congress/bills/113/s131

World Health Organization. (2010). *World Health Statistics 2010*. Geneva, Switzerland: Author.

Yano, E. M., Darling, J. E., Hamilton, A. B., Canelo, I., Chuang, E., Meredith, L. S., & Rubenstein, L. V. (2016). Cluster randomized trial of a multilevel evidence-based quality improvement approach to tailoring VA Patient Aligned Care Teams to the needs of women veterans. *Implementation Science, 11*, 101. doi:10.1186/s13012-016-0461-z

Zegers-Hochschild, F., Adamson, G., deMouzon, J., Ishihara, O., Mansour, R., Nygren, K., … Vanderpoel, S. (2009). International Committee for Monitoring Assisted Reproductive Technology (ICMART) and the World Health Organization (WHO) revised glossary of ART terminology. *Fertility and Sterility, 92*, 1520–1524. doi:10.1016/j.fertnstert.2009.09.009

CHAPTER 11

Caring for the Transgender Client

John Phoenix

INTRODUCTION

Provision of care to the transgender client presents challenges that are unique to this population. Transgender clients can be biologically male or have a gender expression of male, even though they are biologically female. Each category presents opportunities for routine biologic health screenings that could be addressed through male sexual health services. Caring for the transgender client includes offering gender-affirming clinical environment, from the front desk staff all the way through the provider and checkout. If any part of the visit is perceived as nonaffirming, it can negatively impact the chance this client will return for ongoing care.

A hallmark of transgender healthcare should be on safety and education. In the era of the Internet there is a plethora of information available, and contrary to what clients may believe, not everything on the Internet is true. We know this as providers, and we need to educate the consumer regarding this fact. Many clients who present for transgender care have "friends" who have experiences that they share openly, and in turn a client will likely use that as a reference point for any care provided. Many transgender clients will have had at least one prior encounter for care that was a negative experience, and history can create bias toward the future care they might receive. According to the National Transgender Discrimination Survey from 2011, 28% reported postponing medical care because of discrimination (Grant et al., 2011). This section will discuss care of the transgender client from the primary care perspective. It will also cover gender-specific care along with treatment and prevention of HIV infection in the transgendered client.

OVERVIEW OF TRANSGENDER HEALTHCARE

The true number of transgender persons is probably not known; currently there is a lack of reliable and consistent ways of capturing this data. The U.S. census data does not capture gender identity as one of its statistical choices and does not allow for other than the traditional binary genders of male and female. Estimates of the number of transgender persons in the Unites States are approximately 0.3% of the U.S. population (Fernandez & Tannock, 2016). Professionals at the Amsterdam Gender Dysphoria Clinic estimate that 1 in 20,000 individuals from the overall population are transgender, with 1 in 15,000 being transgender women and 1 in 40,000 being transgender males (Gupta, Imborek, & Krasowksi, 2016). A more recent study in the United States estimates that 1 in 200 individuals identify as transgender (Gupta et al., 2016). With increases in access to care through programs under the Patient Protection and Affordable Care Act (PPACA) 2010, more transgender persons are seeking care. As processes in electronic medical records (EMRs) are refined to accurately capture gender identity, the incidence of transgender persons in the United States will be better reflected in data. For medical practices using EMRs, the Department of Health and Human Services (HHS) has mandated that as of 2015, all EMRs collect data on gender identity to meet stage 3 meaningful use criteria (Gupta et al., 2016).

Terminology

When caring for the transgender client, a distinction must be made between gender identity, gender expression, and sexual orientation. Added to this is the transgender person's birth gender or sex, which might be different than their identified gender or the gender in which they live or prefer to live. For the purposes of this chapter, the most common terms in use will be defined. A more detailed list of definitions that encompass more terms for the entire lesbian, gay, bisexual, transgender (LGBT) population are included in the resource section of this chapter.

- "*Transgender* is an inclusive term that may include all individuals whose gender identity or expression does not align with their assigned birth sex" (Gupta et al., 2016, p.1). Many cultures around the world recognize transgender people using varied terms such as "kathoeys" in Thailand; "hijras" in India, Bangladesh, and Pakistan; "warias" in Indonesia; "rae rae's" and "mahus" in French Polynesia; and "travestis" in Latin America (Radix, Sevelius, & Deutsch, 2016).
- *Cisgender* is the term for those whose gender identity or expression aligns with their assigned birth sex (Fernandez & Tannock, 2016).
- *Sex* refers to the binary of male and female, assigned at birth and based on external genitalia.
- *Gender* describes how individuals classify themselves as male or female, and may be different from sex which was assigned at birth.
- *Sexual orientation* describes how an individual defines the physical and emotional attraction to a person of a gender.
- *Gender nonconforming behavioral* variation is gender expression that varies from the cultural and social norms that are expected for that gender.
- *Trans female* is a biologic male who identifies as female.
- *Trans male* is a biologic female who identifies as male.
- *Nonbinary* describes the person who does not identify as male or female. This person may identify with both male and female, neither gender, or any combination of male and female. They often prefer to define themselves as gender queer, a gender, or genderfluid (Gupta et al., 2016).

CREATING A GENDER-AFFIRMING CLINICAL ENVIRONMENT

Transgender individuals experience many barriers to care. Being refused healthcare is something that 31% of transgender people report; in other words, at some time they have been refused care by a medical provider specifically related to their identifying as transgender or gender nonconforming (Grant et al., 2011). Twenty-eight percent of transgender clients report being harassed, and 2% report experiencing violence in a medical care setting (Grant et al., 2011). This discrimination can be in the form of disrespect of gender (or as client often state, "mis-gendering"), harassment, denial of services, or physical violence. This discrimination, insensitivity, and widespread lack of knowledge about health issues unique to the transgender client leads to many transgender clients not seeking or receiving care (Grant et al., 2011). Lack of healthcare provider knowledge of and sensitivity to transgender issues and the need to educate their providers who are seeing them have been reported by 50%

of transgender people (Grant et al., 2011). Care of transgender individuals can be based in primary care where a primary care provider is part of a larger team participating in a team collaboration.

The creation of a gender-affirming clinical environment involves everyone in the office, starting with the front desk staff and continuing through the healthcare provider. Gender affirmation is the process by which people feel socially validated in their gender through relations with others (Sevelius, Patouhas, Keatley, & Johnson, 2014). Nondiscriminatory gender-affirming healthcare includes:

- providers and staff who are knowledgeable, culturally competent, and respectful in addressing transgender related issues
- intake forms that provide patients with an opportunity to list their preferred pronoun(s) and preferred name as well as their legal name
- providers and staff who address them by their preferred name and pronoun
- access to safe bathrooms, which may include all-gender or gender-neutral bathrooms
- thorough and respectful sexual, mental, and physical health assessments
- access to comprehensive transition-related healthcare
- gender-affirming medical care that includes hormone therapy and appropriate surgical referrals
- employing transgender individuals when feasible

Many transgender people may have their biologic name and sex on documents, such as insurance and/or identification, which does not match their preferred name, pronouns, or gender. Using biologic information may be necessary for insurance purposes, but care should be taken to use the preferred name and pronouns in conversation with the client. According to the National Transgender Discrimination Survey, 28% of transgender individuals were open with their providers about their gender, and 21% of those surveyed had not disclosed their gender identity to providers (Hopwood & Reisner, 2015).

Healthcare provider competence for caring for transgender individuals is often absent in medical practices purely out of lack of understanding or forethought. Occasionally one encounters a provider and/or staff who refuse to practice in a culturally sensitive way owing to personal bias. One of the hallmarks of providing gender-affirming care is the assessment of your own comfort with this issue and any biases that you may have. If a provider is uncomfortable talking about transgender healthcare issues, patients will be as well. This is no different from any other part of healthcare that addresses issues with areas of the body traditionally considered private or taboo, such as reproductive function or elimination. For example, if taking a sexual history is uncomfortable, patients will be uncomfortable providing that history. A basic way to open a conversation with a transgender client is to introduce yourself and your preferred pronouns, followed by a simple question of what name they prefer as well as what pronouns they use. Not all transgender males will use the pronouns of he/him/his. They may prefer to use the nonbinary pronouns of ze/zir/zirs or hir/his, or ne/nir/nirs or they/them/their (Gupta et al., 2016). Simply asking these questions can help to set a positive tone for the visit and demonstrate a sense of respect for the person.

Physical examinations can be uncomfortable for both the healthcare provider and the client. Conducting only the examination that is necessary for the complaint, as for any nontransgendered client, is the expectation. Physical examinations should be relevant to the complaint the client presents with and done in a gender-confirming manner. Using appropriate terms, or terms the client prefers to use, for specific body parts can help to reduce anxiety associated with the exam (Wesp, 2016). Provide clients with exam-appropriate garments as for a cisgender person; chaperones should be used for transgender examinations based on the client's preference for gender. Keep in mind, for many transgender male clients this may be the very first pelvic exam, and it may also be the first time they have had another person touch this area of the genitalia. For example, a transgender male undergoing a vaginal examination may prefer a cisgender female to be present in the room.

Electronic medical records and paper charts can create unnecessary anxiety and a sense of bias by lacking gender-sensitive terms and questions. Revising paper forms to allow for the identification of preferred name and pronoun along with legal name and pronoun can create a culture and environment of inclusiveness. Having policies and practices in place to capture this preferred information creates and maintains a supportive environment. Front-line staff need to understand the facility policy regarding this area and can set a positive tone for the encounter by simply referring to clients by preferred names. Based on practice setting, alternate appointment times for transgender clients may be facilitated; this could be especially helpful for trans male clients who are presenting to the gynecologist office for evaluation for a hysterectomy, for example.

Evaluate office space and identify opportunities to provide a more gender-affirming environment. Consider the message conveyed in pictures in the waiting area, and consider placing advertisements that represent other than cisgender persons. Take into account the perceptions of transgender clients, and other clients if a trans male client presents to an office with a roomful of cisgender women and/or cisgender pregnant women. Processes as simple as possibly scheduling trans men for the first appointment of the day could be an accommodation that would have little impact on the operation of the practice, but would speak volumes to gender affirmation.

HEALTH MANAGEMENT OF TRANSGENDER CLIENTS

Primary care goals are the same for transgender clients as for the cisgender client. Providers need to be aware that the prevention needs of transgender clients may include items common to both genders. Transgender women will need to have breast cancer screening because of the estrogen hormones, but also prostate cancer screening, as they likely retain the prostate gland even after gender-affirming genital surgeries. Transgender males will need to have breast exams as well as cervical cancer screenings until they undergo breast reduction and/or hysterectomy.

Empower all clients, but especially trans clients to take an active role in their own healthcare. Assess the transgender client for barriers to care and develop strategies to facilitate adherence. When asked about the top five concerns of transgender persons related to healthcare, 59% identify receiving care in a gender-affirming and nondiscriminatory setting as a priority (Transgender Law Center, 2014).

Sexual Health

Sexual health is an important part of any primary care visit and is important in specialty care as well. Creating an environment in which the provider, staff, and client are all comfortable with the sexual history is an important step. Providers and staff need to assess their own comfort level with talking to clients about sexual history; if providers and staff are uncomfortable with this topic, the client's perception of the ability to discuss sexual health needs will be impacted.

- Make clients feel comfortable and establish rapport with them before beginning discussion in this sensitive area.
- Use gender neutral terms such as partner or spouse.
- Avoid making assumptions about patients based on presentation.

- Pay attention to body language with topics that make you feel uncomfortable.
- Ask clients about preferred pronouns and terms they use to describe their anatomy.
- Ask questions if there are terms that clients use with which you are not familiar.
- Take a sexual organ history on transgender clients, as many of them may not have had any gender reassignment surgeries, and may retain biologic sex organs such as uterus and testicles.
- Ask transgender clients about the sex of partners.

Transgender and cisgender clients alike can have partners of both sexes, and may have more than one sexual partner at any given time. Knowing the number and gender of sexual partners is also important for evaluation of risk of sexually transmitted infections (STIs) in clients. Knowing the sex of partners is also helpful for screening for STIs and knowing which anatomic organs transgender clients use for sex is also important for screening for STIs. Transgender and cisgender clients should be queried regarding testing for STIs such as gonorrhea, chlamydia infection, syphilis, and HIV infection. Delivering recommended preventive sexual health services is important for both transgender and cisgender clients.

Transgender men may need access to reliable forms of contraception. Testosterone is not birth control and can lead to serious complications in pregnancy. Pregnancy should be avoided in transgender men who are actively taking testosterone. Birth control options such as an intrauterine device (IUD) can be an acceptable method for transgender men, as it does not contain any form of systemic hormone. Birth control options such as oral contraception and contraceptive injections can be less desirable because of the hormone component and the possible effects of estrogen and/or progesterone on transition and testosterone levels.

HIV and the Transgender Community

HIV infection affects the transgender community more than it does the general population, and transgender women are at disproportional risk for acquisition of HIV infection. In the United States, 20% of transgender women are living with HIV infection (Baral et al., 2013). Transgender women are 34 more times likely to be living with HIV infection, and they have higher HIV-related complications and death (Baral et al., 2013). From 2009 to 2014, 2,351 transgender people were diagnosed with HIV infection in the United States. Eighty-four percent (1,974) were transgender women, 15% (361) were transgender men, and less than 1% (16) had another gender identity (Centers for Disease Control and Prevention [CDC], 2017). Around half of transgender people (43% [844] of transgender women; 54% [193] of transgender men) who received an HIV diagnosis from 2009 to 2014 lived in the South (CDC, 2017). Prevention of HIV infection in the transgender community presents unique challenges to both the transgender female and male community.

- *Multiple factors have put transgender people at risk for HIV infection and transmission* including multiple sexual partners, anal or vaginal sex without condoms or medicines to prevent HIV, injecting hormones or drugs with shared syringes and other drug paraphernalia, commercial sex work, mental health issues, incarceration, homelessness, unemployment, and high levels of substance misuse compared to the general population. Fear of physical violence and lack of family support are often cited by transgender clients as reasons why they participate in these risky behaviors.
- *HIV behavioral interventions* developed for other at-risk groups have been adapted for use with transgender people. However, the effectiveness of these interventions is understudied. Effective behavioral interventions that address the full range of risk factors and health concerns are needed to improve the health of transgender people.

- *Many transgender people face stigma, discrimination, social rejection, and exclusion* that prevent them from fully participating in society, including accessing healthcare, education, employment, and housing. These factors affect the health and well-being of transgender people, placing them at increased risk for HIV infection.
- *Insensitivity to transgender issues by healthcare providers* can be a barrier for transgender people diagnosed with HIV infection and seeking quality treatment and care services. Few healthcare providers receive proper training or are knowledgeable about transgender health issues and their unique needs. This can lead to limited healthcare access and negative healthcare encounters.
- *Transgender-specific data are limited.* Some federal, state, and local agencies do not collect or have complete data on transgender individuals. Using the two-step data collection method of asking for sex assigned at birth and current gender identity can help increase the likelihood that transgender people are correctly identified in HIV surveillance programs. Accurate data on transgender status can lead to more effective public health actions.
- *Transgender men's sexual health has not been well studied.* Over half of transgender men with diagnosed HIV infection had no identified or reported risk. Additional research is needed to understand HIV risk behavior among transgender men, especially those who have sex with other men (CDC, 2017).

HIV Infection Prevention

HIV infection prevention with pre-exposure prophylaxis (PrEP) using the medication emtricitabine/tenofovir disoproxil (Truvada) was approved by the Food and Drug Administration (FDA) in 2013. Two large clinical trials conducted by Grant et al. showed protective benefit from HIV acquisition in over 92% of individuals who take the medication and had measurable levels in their system (Grant et al., 2010). The Centers for Disease Control and Prevention (CDC) (2015) estimates that there are over 1.2 million people living that are at risk of HIV acquisition that could be eligible for Truvada for PrEP. Utilization of PrEP in the transgender community is an effective way to reduce the incidence of new HIV cases and other sexually transmitted infections. Many transgender clients express concerns over possible interactions between emtricitabine/tenofovir disoproxil for PrEP and cross-gender hormones. To date, there has been no published interaction with any of the commonly used medications for hormone therapy. Use of oral contraceptive medications, specifically those containing estrogen, has been shown to affect vaginal pH in biologic vaginal tissue and may increase risk of acquisition of STI in individuals with biologic vaginas. Consideration of the anatomic parts that transgender clients use for sexual experience should be taken into consideration when discussing PrEP and counseling clients about potential risk reduction. In the CDC guidelines regarding PrEP, they note that maximum blood levels sufficient for protection are achieved in 20 days of consistent dosing (CDC, 2014). These same guidelines suggest 7 days of consistent dosing for rectal tissue and 20 days for vaginal tissue (CDC, 2014). There is no mention of consistent dosing for neovaginal tissue, or a vagina that is created surgically in transgender women. Neovaginal tissue does not lubricate in the same manner as biologic vaginal tissue, leaving it drier and possibly more suspectible to infection through tears and injury and may increase risk for acquisition of HIV (Radix, 2017). Little research exists among transgender persons and PrEP. Of the over 2,500 individuals enrolled in the iPREX study, only 339 or 14%, identified as transgender women (Radix, 2017). Screening for STIs in transgender men and women should be done based on the anatomy that is present. PrEP is discussed in a separate chapter of this book (Chapter 17).

HIV Infection Treatment

Many transgender individuals believe that they cannot take both medications to either prevent HIV infection or treat HIV infection along with their cross-gender hormones. Although there is limited data to suggest an interaction between HIV medications and cross-gender hormones, there are very few interactions. Much of the research that has been done on potential interactions has been done on oral contraceptive medications, which are not generally used for hormone management in transgender women. Both HIV medications and cross-gender hormones can be metabolized through the cytochrome P450 system, which does allow for potential drug-drug interactions. Providers should note that many transgender clients will prioritize their hormone management over HIV medications. But there is little data to date that substantiates any significant decrease in either class of medication and/or the need to adjust doses of medications based on significant changes in measured hormone levels (Radix et al., 2016).

HIV impacts bone development, kidney function, and testosterone, meaning transgender women may require lower doses of antiandrogen medications. Antiandrogen medication such as spironolactone, a potassium-sparing diuretic, may lead to dehydration and theoretically could impact renal function. Providing cross-gender hormone therapy with estrogens may have bone loss protection benefits in transgender women living with HIV infection.

Providing transgender clients with culturally competent care for their gender transition and medications to treat HIV infection is currently recommended. When transgender clients feel welcome in care, the success of viral suppression is enhanced as well as their continued engagement in care for treatment of HIV infection. Providers should implement low-barrier, seamless healthcare and linkage services as a method of engaging transgender clients in care (AIDS United, 2017). Treatment of HIV infection in transgender persons should be guided by current national guidelines based on currently accepted standards of care.

HEALTH DISPARITIES AND THE TRANSGENDER COMMUNITY

Braverman describes health disparities as a "particular type of difference in health . . . in which disadvantaged social groups—such as poor, racial/ethnic minorities, women and other groups who have persistently experienced social disadvantage or discrimination-systematically experience worse health or greater health risks than more advantaged social groups" (Hopwood & Reisner, 2014, Slide 24). Transgender clients experience health disparities in mental health, sexual and reproductive health, substance use, violence/victimization, stigma/discrimination, HIV, incarceration, homelessness, and family/peer relationships. Trans women have an even higher likelihood of experiencing these health disparities, and transgender women are 19.3% more likely to have a history of jail/prison according to the National Transgender discrimination survey (Hopwood & Reisner, 2014).

Transgender youth (TY) are more likely than cisgender youth (CY) to experience mental health disparities. Transgender youth are more likely to experience depression (TY 50% vs. CY 20%), anxiety (TY 25% vs. CY 10%), suicidal ideation (TY 30% vs. CY 10%), suicide attempt (TY15% vs. CY 5%), and self-harm (TY 15% vs. CY 5%) and are more likely to utilize outpatient (TY 22% vs. CY 10%) as well as inpatient (TY 45% vs. CY 215%) mental health services (Hopwood & Reisner, 2014). In a survey by the Fenway Institute 55% of transpersons under the age of 15% had experienced some form of abuse, and 74% of the individuals surveyed over the age of 18 had experienced any type of victimization (Hopwood & Reisner, 2014). Transgender individuals had a 3.58% greater likelihood of being the victim of any type of bullying in a 12-month period (Hopwood & Reisner, 2014).

Hopwood and Reisner (2015) surveyed 145 transgender youth regarding sex, housing, depression, and substance use. In this survey, they report findings for male to female (MTF) and female to male (FTM) percentages of being impacted in these areas. In the MTF group 52.4%

reported having condomless anal and/or vaginal sex, compared with 43.9% of FTM. Causal sex partners were reported in 69.8% of MTF and 42.7% in FTM youth. Sex work was reported by 33.5% of MTF and 1.2% of FTM. Depression was reported by 42.9% of MTF and 54.9% of FTM. Alcohol use was reported by 50.8% of MTF and 58.5% of FTM. Current drug use was 39.7% in MTF and 32.9% in FTM. Unstable housing was reported by 25.4% of MTF and 13.45% of FTM (Hopwood & Reisner, 2014). These numbers demonstrate the areas of need in transgender clients and where providers have great opportunities to impact services by providing culturally and gender-affirming care. Providers need to engage transgender clients and work with them in collaboration with community partners to help decrease these health disparities.

TRANSITION TREATMENT GUIDELINES

It is beyond to scope of this chapter to provide a comprehensive guide to treatment of the transgender client with respect to cross-gender hormone therapy. There are published guidelines for treatment by agencies such as the World Professional Association for Transgender Health (World Professional Association for Transgender Health, 2011), the Endocrine Society, and various country-specific guidelines. The goal of transgender hormone therapy is to induce secondary sex characteristics and to reduce the impact of biologic sex characteristics. Cross-gender hormone therapy does not technically reduce the presence of biologic secondary sex characteristics, but it does suppress the impact of these areas.

Transgender Women

Transgender women require treatment of both their naturally occurring testosterone as well as supplementation of estrogen. The testicles are the primary source of testosterone in these clients, so agents designed to suppress secretion of testosterone become a primary mechanism for treatment, and antiandrogen agents, such as spironolactone, are traditionally used for this purpose. Spironolactone is a potassium-sparing diuretic, so its use can lead to dehydration and retention of potassium. Transgender women need education on reducing dehydration, which can cause problems with constipation as well as blood pressure. Transgender women need to be educated about maintaining adequate amounts of fluid intake and the increased frequency, as well as dietary sources of potassium and how to avoid hyperkalemia. Use of spironolactone can slow androgen-induced hair loss, decrease frequency/firmness/duration of erections, and can cause development of gynecomastia.

Use of any antiandrogen agent will result in shrinking of the testicle, decrease the amount of fluid during ejaculation, and cause the fluid of ejaculation to be clearer in color. These agents can also result in flattening and softening of the testicles, and have been associated with intermittent testicular pain (Deutsch, 2016). By lowering the testosterone levels in transwomen, this can make tucking (the process of hiding the penis and scrotum/testicles by placing them between the legs) easier and often less painful.

Transgender women may be at increased risk for complications such as osteopenia and osteoporosis based on lower levels of testosterone and reduced participation in activities that are known to increase muscle mass and bone health (Radix et al., 2016). This risk can be potentially mitigated with the use of estrogens.

Estrogen supplementation is an additional component of medical management of transgender women. Estrogen can be provided in the form of tablets, patches, cremes, or injections generally in the nonconjugated equine forms, such as estradiol. Clients may elect to use one form of estrogen delivery over another based on fear of needles or perceived benefits of one type of delivery or the experiences of other transwomen. Estrogen levels are maintained in biologic female ranges. Benefits of estrogen therapy is development of breast tissue, softening of the skin, and some redistribution of fat. Estrogen will not have an effect on the voice, as it is testosterone that causes thickening and lengthening of the vocal cords. Changes in voice that transwomen experience is a learned behavior, and there are many sources available on line as well as through speech language pathology to assist with this change.

Transgender women may inquire about the use of progesterone, but there is little evidence to support or deny its use in transwomen. Transwomen may report that it helps with skin softening and breast tissue development and softening, but supplementation with progesterone does not cause a measurable increase in measured levels.

With the implementation of the PPACA, there has been a national trend of increased coverage of medications and surgeries for transgender women. But procedures seen as purely elective, such as removal of unwanted body hair, is often a source of frustration for many transwomen. Unlike the advances made in insurance coverage for gender affirmation surgery under PPACA, much of this is still an uncovered expense. Procedures such as laser hair removal and electrolysis are known to help with reduction of facial and body hair. Although considered medically necessary by organizations such as World Professional Association for Transgender Health (WPATH), these remain uncovered benefits for many transgender women.

Not all transwomen desire gender reassignment surgery or gender-affirming/confirming surgeries. Typical male-to-female gender surgeries are as follows:

- Breast/chest surgery: augmentation mammoplasty (implants/lipofilling)
- Genital surgery: penectomy, orchiectomy, vaginoplasty, chloroplasts, vulvoplasty
- Nongenital, nonbreast surgical interventions: facial feminization surgery, liposuction, lipofilling, voice surgery, thyroid cartilage reduction, gluteal augmentation (implants/lipofilling)
- Hair reconstruction and various aesthetic procedures

Reproductive health should also be discussed with transgender women, and preservation of sperm through sperm banking may be an option for some clients. Several transgender women have been successful in being a biologic parent to offspring by allowing their testosterone levels to return to biologic ranges long enough to produce mature sperm capable of impregnating females. Once the pregnancy is confirmed, most clients will resume their estrogen supplementation and blockade of testosterone. Many clients are also interested in alternative ways to build a family such as adoption.

Transgender Men

Transgender men require testosterone therapy for the development of male secondary sexual characteristics. Development of facial and body hair, change in muscle mass development, altered body fat distribution, cessation of menstrual cycles, enlargement of the clitoris, and deepening of the voice are potential expected changes with testosterone. Testosterone supplementation is available through topical applications or injections. In the United States, there are no acceptable oral testosterone supplements. Occasionally suppression of estrogen is necessary through estrogen blocking with agents such as anastrazole.

With testosterone supplementation, transgender males can expect to have development of facial and body hair, changes in body fat distribution, and changes in development of muscle mass. Testosterone levels are generally maintained in the biologic male ranges. Transgender males will typically experience a deepening of the voice due to the structural changes that testosterone has on the vocal cords of thickening and lengthening. Voice changes in trans males is a permanent change. Enlargement of the clitoris is another change that transgender male clients may experience, and this is also considered to be a permanent change. Cessation of menstruation is common while supplementing with testosterone. Once testosterone levels are allowed to return to the biologic female range, menstruation will typically resume. It is not uncommon or generally of physical concern to have occasional menstrual spotting while on testosterone. This can be a very psychologically distressing episode for transgender men, so education about this side effect and development of strategies to cope with the occasional bleeding is very beneficial. Many transgender male clients have already developed strategies to conceal menstruation through years of lived experience. Dysmenorrhea can remain the same, improve, or worsen while on testosterone. Dysmenorrhea and/or menorrhagia can occasionally be used as medical reasons for hysterectomy in transgender male clients.

Like transgender women, not all transgender males will undergo sexual reassignment surgeries. There are several types of surgeries that transgender men can undergo:

- Breast/chest surgery: subcutaneous mastectomy, creation of a male chest
- Genital surgery: hysterectomy/ovariectomy, reconstruction of the fixed part of the urethra, which can be combined with a metoidioplasty or with a phalloplasty (employing a pedicled or free vascularized flap), vaginectomy, scrotoplasty, and implantation of erection and/or testicular prostheses
- Nongenital, nonbreast surgical interventions: voice surgery (rare), liposuction, lipofilling, pectoral implants, and various aesthetic procedures

Reproductive health should also be discussed with transgender males, such as egg banking or embryo freezing. Factors such as the age of the client as well as the overall health are important factors to consider with respect to reproduction. There is documentation of successful pregnancies in transgender males once their testosterone levels have returned to biologic ranges. It is important to remember that testosterone is not birth control, and can be detrimental to the outcome of a pregnancy. Care should be taken to prevent unintended pregnancies in transgender males with high levels of testosterone.

Transgender Youth

Trans youth are another area of developing medical need. Many transgender youth will undergo puberty blocking with synthetic gonadotropin-releasing hormone. There are many unique challenges to management of cross-gender hormones in the adolescent in prepubertal adolescent which should be addressed on an individual basis with their healthcare providers. Cross-gender hormone therapy and puberty blocking may be managed by pediatric endocrinology or another healthcare provider experienced in this area. Consideration of the physical as well as psychological maturation of the youth are both important when assessing the readiness for puberty blocking and/or cross-gender hormone therapy and eventual surgery.

CONCLUSION

Provision of care to the transgender client is often complex and may require the involvement of multiple members of the healthcare team. Transgender clients are at high risk for health disparities and are often subject to obstacles in the acquisition of care and/or discrimination in the care they receive. Providing care in a gender-affirming environment has been shown to increase client engagement in and retention in care. Transgender clients present with health needs of both their biologic person as well as their transgender person.

RESOURCES FOR PROVIDERS AND PATIENTS

Centers for Disease Control and Prevention: www.cdc.gov/lgbthealth/transgender.htm
Centers for Disease Control and Prevention: www.cdc.gov/hiv/group/gender/transgender/index.html
Centers for Disease Control and Prevention: www.cdc.gov/hiv/risk/prep/index.html

Endocrine Society Clinical Practice Guidelines: www.endocrine.org/guidelines-and-clinical-practice/clinical-practice-guidelines
Fenway Health: fenwayhealth.org/the-fenway-institute/education
Transgender Legal Defense and Education Fund: www.transgenderlegal.org
University of San Francisco Transgender Center of Excellence: transhealth.ucsf.edu/protocols
World Professional Association for Transgender Health: www.wpath.org

REFERENCES

AIDS United. (2017). *Steppin Up: Best practices in providing HIV medical care, support services and funding to trans communities.* Washington, DC: AIDunited.org.

Baral, S. D., Poteat, T., Strömdahl, S., Wirtz, A. L., Guadamuz, T. E., & Beyrer, C. (2013). Worldwide burden of HIV in transgender women: a systematic review and meta-analysis. *The Lancet Infectious Diseases, 13*(3), 214–222. doi:10.1016/s1473-3099(12)70315-8

Centers for Disease Control and Prevention. (2014). Preexposure Prophylaxis for the Prevention of HIV Infection in the United States—2014 Clinical Practice Guideline P. Retrieved from https://www.cdc.gov/hiv/pdf/prepguidelines2014.pdf

Centers for Disease Control and Prevention. (2015, November 27). Vital signs: Estimated percentages and numbers of adults with indications for preexposure prophylaxis to prevent HIV acquisition—United States, 2015. Retrieved from Morbidity and Mortality Weekly Report (MMWR): https://www.cdc.gov/mmwr/preview/mmwrhtml/mm6446a4.htm?s_cid=mm6446a4_w

Centers for Disease Control and Prevention. (2017, August 3). HIV among transgender people. Retrieved from https://www.cdc.gov/hiv/group/gender/transgender/index.html

Deutsch, M. B. (2016). Overview of feminizing hormone therapy. In M. B. Deutsch (Ed.), *Guidelines for the primary and gender-affirming care of transgender and gender nonbinary people* (pp. 26–48). San Francisco: University of California.

Fernandez, J. D., & Tannock, L. R. (2016). Metabolic effects of hormone therapy in transgender patients. *Endocrine Practice, 22*, 383–388. doi:10.4158/EP15950.OR

Grant, R. M., Lama, J. R., Anderson, P. L., McMahan, V., Liu, A. Y., Vargas, L., ... Glidden, D. V. (2010). Preexposure chemoprophylaxis for HIV prevention in men who have sex with men. *New England Journal of Medicine, 363*, 2587–2599. doi:10.1056/NEJMoa1011205

Grant, J. M., Mottet, L. A., Tanis, J., Harrison, J., Herman, J. L., & Keisling, M. (2011). *Injustice at every turn. A report of the National Transgender Discrimination Survey.* Washington, DC: National Center for Transgender Equality and National Gay and Lesbian Task Force.

Gupta, S., Imborek, K. L., & Krasowksi, M. D. (2016). Challenges in transgender healthcare: The pathology perspective. *Laboratory Medicine, 47*, 180–188. doi:10.1093/labmed/lmw020

Hopwood, R., & Reisner, S. L. (2015). Gender affirmative health care: Terminology, demographics and epidemiology. Retrieved from National LGBT Health Education Center: https://www.lgbthealtheducation.org/lgbt-education/continuing-education/?y=132

Radix, A. (2017). PrEP and Transgender People Limited data point to similar efficacy; more scale-up is needed. Retrieved from PrEP and Transgender People: https://www.positivelyaware.com/articles/prep-and-transgender-people

Radix, A., Sevelius, J., & Deutsch, M. B. (2016). Transgender women, hormonal therapy and HIV treatment: A comprehensive review of the literature and recommendations for best practice. *Journal of the International AIDS Society, 19*(suppl 2), 208–210. doi:10.7448/IAS.19.3.20810

Sevelius, J. M., Patouhas, E., Keatley, J. G., Johnson, M. O. (2014). Barriers and facilitators to engagement and retention in care among transgender women living with human immunodeficiency virus. *Annals of Behavioral Medicine, 47*(1), pp. 5–16. doi:10.1007/s12160-013-9565-8

Transgender Law Center. (2014, March 24). *Positively trans.* Retrieved from http://transgenderlawcenter.org/wp-content/uploads/2016/02/PositivelyTrans-2015-7-border-FINAL.pdf

Wesp, L. (2016). Transgender patients and the physical examination. In M. B. Deutsch (Ed.), *Guidelines for the primary and gender-affirming care of transgender and gender nonbinary people.* San Franciso: University of California. Retrieved from http://transhealth.ucsf.edu/pdf/Transgender-PGACG-6-17-16.pdf

World Professional Association for Transgender Health. (2011). Standards of Care for the Health of Transsexual, Transgender, and Gender Non conforming People. Retrieved from http://www.wpath.org

CHAPTER 12

Health-Seeking Behaviors and Needs in Young Adult Males

Jo Ann L. Nicoteri

INTRODUCTION

Young adult males are in various states of transition: adolescence to adulthood; dependence to independence; and pediatric to adult healthcare. Even the definition of young adult varies, but 18 to 24 years of age is accepted for official statistical purposes (Federal Interagency Forum on Child and Family Statistics, 2014). The periods of later adolescence and young adulthood overlap and may be termed "emergent adult" (Curtis, 2014). These young adult years represent the entrance into the "individual's physical, cognitive, and behavioral prime" (Oman, Vesely, Aspy, & Tolma, 2015, p. e51). Psychologist Jeffrey Jensen Arnett, PhD, describes the features of this group as the age of identity exploration; the age of instability, the age of self-focus, the age of feeling in-between, and the age of possibilities (Munsey, 2006).

Yet in today's American culture, adolescence may extend beyond the traditional age range. Those who do not attend and/or do not reside at college and choose to live at home because of financial reasons, comfort, parental pressure (not wanting to become empty-nesters), or lack of direction may remain in the child role (Table 12.1) for years. Young adults are able to be covered under parental health insurance until the age of 26 years in the United States, since the 2010 Patient Protection and Affordable Care Act (PPACA, 2010), making the home of origin more inviting as well. Yet there are positive aspects to young adults having health insurance coverage until the age of 26 years. Young adult males are the least likely to have health insurance and this age group also utilizes acute care (reporting at least one emergency room visit in the past year, 2010–2011 data) regardless of insurance status (Cohen & Martinez, 2012). The PPACA may improve the health of young adults through covered preventive services such as tests for sexually transmitted infections, counseling related to alcohol or nicotine use, nutrition, weight loss, emotional health, vaccinations (including seasonal flu vaccine), and prenatal care (Monaghan, 2014).

In terms of parental relationships, Bradley-Geist and Olson-Buchanan (2014) found that overparenting (often informally referred to as "helicopter parents") was more common among college students who lived at home and had fewer siblings. Overparenting but not specifically parental involvement, according to the same authors, was also associated with lower student self-efficacy and maladaptive responses to workplace scenarios (Bradley-Geist & Olson-Buchanan, 2014).

Developmental milestones may be delayed by factors in the family of origin for young adults. For instance, Erikson's stage of psychological crisis for young adults, intimacy vs. isolation or finding oneself in another, may not be achieved while living in the parental home (Burns et al., 2017). Parents may intentionally or unintentionally stunt this developmental growth by viewing it as parental rejection. Piaget's formal operational stage for the young adult has these individuals differentiating between their own thoughts and others'

TABLE 12.1 General Developmental Progression

Life Stage	Age Range	Defining Characteristics/Description
Infancy	Birth to 1 year	Development of trust, give and take
Toddler	1–3 years	Development of autonomy, still dependent, self-control
Preschool	3–5 years	Development of initiative, play, creativity, direction
School Age	6–11 years	Development of industry, gaining self-confidence, competence
Adolescence	12–18 years	Development of identity/role, finding self, devotion
Young Adult	18–24 years	Development of intimacy with another, relationships, love
Adult	25–40 years	
Middle Adult	41–65 years	Development of accomplishment, success/preparing for future
Older Adult	65 years and over	Development of wisdom, reflection/feeling satisfied

Source: Adapted from Burns, C. E., Dunn, A. M., Brady, M. A., Starr, N. B., Blosser, C. G., & Garzon, D. L. (2017). Pediatric primary care. St. Louis, MO: Elsevier; Edelman, C. L., Kudzma, E. C., & Mandle, C. L. (2014). Health promotion across the lifespan. St. Louis, MO: Elsevier.

thoughts (Burns et al., 2017). This may be difficult to accomplish if parents are "hovering." Cultural and ethnic influences may also come into play in the development of the young adult. Assessment may include the use of tools such as the genogram or ecomap to assist in the evaluation of family structure, function, strengths, alliances, health beliefs, resources, and practices (Burns et al., 2017).

If the young adult male does not enter college after high school and goes directly into the workforce and is not successful, he may establish his identity in ways not associated with the family of origin. The military may be an option. Alternatively, he may become socially isolated or turn to peer groups such as gangs instead of the family (Burns et al., 2017).

Moreover, there may be gender differences within the family and/or peer cohort as to health knowledge and awareness, leading to differences in practices. For example, in one study of college students in the northeastern United States, males had a much lower level of awareness of the human papillomavirus (HPV) vaccine and a lower perception of safety than females (Beshers, Murphy, Fix, & Mahoney, 2015). In a study of German adolescents and young adults, females were less likely to transition to riskier states of alcohol use and were more likely to transition back from frequent risky single-occasion drinking (Probst, Moyo, Purshouse, & Rehm, 2015). Rowley, Johnson, and Sbaffi (Rowley, Johnson, & Sbaffi, 2017) found that there are gender differences in health information-seeking online in that women consult more types of sources using tablet computers more often than men, but men search the Internet for more long-standing health complaints. Despite numerous and varied studies of the health of young adults, Tyler and Williams (2014) cite the lack of research "exploring the discourses young men use when discussing aspect of health and their help-seeking behaviors" (p. 460).

HEALTHY PEOPLE 2020

Healthy People 2020 defines adolescents as ages 10 to 19 and young adults as 20 to 24 years of age making up 21% of the population of the United States (Centers for Disease Control and Prevention [CDC], 2014a). The primary goal is to improve the healthy development, health, safety, and well-being of this subset of the population in order to facilitate negotiating their developmental tasks such as increasing independence and normative experimentation (CDC, 2014a). The health issues and causes of death surrounding young adults are largely preventable; therefore, addressing concerns early will assist them to grow into healthy adults.

Young adult males are influenced, as stated previously, by many sources including family, peers, school, media, and adult mentors. Among the emerging issues for this population is the increasing ethnic diversity of the young adult male with significant disparities particularly for the African American, American Indian, and Hispanic living in poverty (CDC, 2014a). Poor outcomes exist for health problems in these young adults such as obesity, teen pregnancy, and dental decay, while educational achievement may not be as high as their Caucasian counterparts as well (CDC, 2014a).

Early youth developmental interventions may have a positive effect on risky health behaviors. Core indicators identified in Healthy People 2020 for this age group include:

- Healthcare
- Healthy development
- Injury and violence prevention
- Mental health
- Prevention of chronic diseases of adulthood
- Sexual health
- Substance abuse

Healthy People 2020 has as one of its objectives increasing the proportion of adolescents and young adults who have had a wellness visit to a healthcare provider in the past 12 months. Some of the revised objectives focus on education and activities, reducing adolescent and young adult participation in crimes and gang activity, and victimization from crimes of violence (CDC, 2014a).

Based on Healthy People 2020, the American College Health Association developed Healthy Campus 2020 to improve the health and well-being of young adult college students with targets established by 10% improvements (American College Health Association [ACHA], 2012). Main student objective categories are directed at the institutional level to address and provide education and increase the proportion of students receiving this education in the past 12 months:

- *Health Impediments to Academic Performance* (stress, sleep difficulties, anxiety, work, cold/flu/sore throat)
- *Health Communication/Health Information Technology/Educational Community Based Programs* (communication with healthcare providers, health information on injury, violence, pregnancy, sexually transmitted infection and suicide prevention, tobacco, alcohol and other drug use, nutrition, and physical activity)
- *Injury and Violence Prevention* (such as wearing safety helmets, night safety, and prevention of physical and sexual assault, as well as intimate partner violence)
- *Mental and Mental Health Disorders* (addressing issues such as increasing the number of reported diagnoses of anxiety, depression, and eating disorders, and reducing suicide attempts)
- *Nutrition and Weight Status* (increasing numbers with healthy weight, reducing numbers with a diagnosis of obesity, healthier eating)
- *Physical Activity and Fitness* (aerobic and muscle strengthening within federal guidelines)
- *Sexually Transmitted Diseases and HIV Infection* (prevention and diagnosis)

- *Family Planning* (reducing unintended pregnancy, contraception, emergency contraception)
- *Substance Abuse* (reduction)
- *Tobacco Use* (reduction)
- *Immunization and Infectious Disease* (such as flu, hepatitis B, meningococcal, varicella, measles, mumps, and rubella [MMR], and HPV vaccines; ACHA, Healthy Campus 2020, Document, 2012).

These topics were selected to align with national datasets for the target population; however, these topics may also be applicable to all young adult males in the general population. Nevertheless, the delivery of such information may need to be amended and barriers may arise, as will be discussed.

UNITED STATES PREVENTIVE SERVICES TASK FORCE (USPSTF) RECOMMENDATIONS

The USPSTF does not break down its preventive recommendations into specific age groups; therefore, no category specifically addresses young adults age 18 to 24 years. Grade A (good evidence to support the recommendation) and Grade B (fair evidence to support the recommendation) are given to recommendations that would extend to the young adult age group. For instance, Obesity Screening for Children and Adolescents (June 2017) overlaps the young adult as screening is recommended (Grade B) for children 6 years and older and Depression screening (February 2016) is recommended (Grade B) for 12- to 18-year-olds (United States Preventive Services Task Force, 2017). Several recommendations for adults and some of those for children may apply to the young adult, depending upon factors such as family history, behavior, and environment.

Other professional organizations have developed guidelines; the American Association of Pediatrics (American Association of Pediatrics, 2017) published their 2017 edition of Bright Futures, which covers birth up to age 21 years. This resource presents the periodicity schedule of preventive screenings, assessments, physical examinations, procedures, and anticipatory guidance for each age group. With so many specialties offering evidence-based guidelines for populations that overlap with the young adult, Ozer and colleagues recommend the establishment of young adult preventive health guidelines (Ozer, Urquhart, Brindis, Park, & Irwin, 2012). These resources suggest that in the near future the emerging adult may be a separate category supported by its own evidence-based recommendations.

HEALTH-SEEKING BEHAVIORS

For the young adult male, access to healthcare is a prime concern. Up until this time in their lives, most young adults were directed by parents or caregivers or by healthcare providers in school-based clinics (Nicoteri & Arnold, 2005). As the young adult emerges, many do not seek healthcare unless illness arises; for young adult men, wellness may be defined in terms of absence of illness. Many may not have a primary care provider, particularly if transitioning from pediatric care, or utilize the services of an urgent care clinic when ill if chronic disease is not an issue. For those with chronic medical conditions, the transition from pediatric to adult care is associated with poor clinical outcomes, increased costs, and low patient and family satisfaction (Hepburn et al., 2015).

Young men may not see the need for continuing preventive care, may not be aware of family history, and may be reluctant or unable to meet copays, deductible fees, or out-of-pocket costs even if covered by their own health insurance. Compared to females, young adult males do not have a regular source of healthcare (Bell, Breland, & Ott, 2013). A small focus group study of traditional-aged college students (18–23 years) found that although individuals in this age group considered themselves "independent" they still relied on parental supervision of healthcare (Nicoteri & Arnold, 2005). The participants also expected healthcare to be available 24/7 and wanted healthcare to be convenient. However, in the decade since the pilot study was conducted, many retail clinics opened and the "drive through" concept of healthcare has responded to a need. Young adults want healthcare available when they need it and many are not patient to wait for an appointment a day or two later.

There may be various reasons males choose not to seek healthcare or delay seeking healthcare. Data collected as part of the 2008 Health Information National Trends Survey were analyzed qualitatively as to why people avoid medical care. Taber, Leyva, and Persoskie (Tabor, Leyva, & Persoskie, 2015) describe "3 categories of reasons for avoidance behavior in relation to health care identified by participants: (a) unfavorable evaluations of seeking medical care including factors related to physicians, health care organizations, and affective concerns; (b) low perceived need to seek care because the illness or symptoms were expected to resolve or get better over time; and (c) traditional barriers such as high cost, no health insurance, and time constraints (p. 291)." Convenience/time is a common factor related in the aforementioned focus group of college students. These findings also relate to not having a regular source of healthcare as described by Bell, Breland, and Ott (Bell et al., 2013).

In a study involving healthcare-seeking behaviors among university students in Lebanon, behaviors were categorized as formal (professional help); informal relational (family/friends); or informal personal (self-help) (El Kahi, Abi Rizk, Hlais, & Adib, 2012). Informal relational help was sought most often for health-related problems (Bell et al., 2013). The question remains as to how to encourage and develop behaviors in young adults to seek professional care.

Tyler and Williams (Tyler & Williams, 2014) conducted online focus groups drawn from Facebook and Twitter accounts of national organizations relating to young men's and men's health in the United Kingdom. Most of the participants (26/28) were from the United Kingdom and identified themselves ethnically as white British. The health strategies used by these young men (18–30 years) in speaking about their health "formed three discursive themes: (a) conceptualizing health: everyday health versus 'cover man' health; (b) health-seeking: the restrictions of masculinity; and (c) using health care: legitimizing help-seeking through masculine identity" (p. 462). The authors note that the participants in this study perceived health as a "holistic mix" of physical, mental, and social factors rather than just physical health as in previous research. Technology also played a vital role in the methodology. The conclusions were that young men are interested in their health and construct their health practices within their masculinity while maintaining independence, autonomy, and control over their bodies (Tyler & Williams, 2014).

As previously discussed, racial and ethnic disparities also influence health-seeking behaviors. Using the data from the National Survey of Adolescent Males (NSAM), Dariotis and colleagues concluded that black and Latino young adult males are differentiated from whites in terms of sexually transmitted disease (STD) prevalence and incidence but not accounted by individual-level risk factors (Dariotis, Sifakis, Pleck, Astone, & Sanenstein, 2011).

Cheatham, Barksdale, and Rodgers (2008) identified barriers faced by African American men to healthcare. These barriers included socioeconomic status, masculinity, racism, lack of awareness of the need for primary care, religious beliefs, peer influences as well as access to care (Cheatham et al., 2008). Therefore, if differences exist in the prevalence and incidence of health issues based on race and ethnicity, different interventions may need to be planned for the young adult male. Specific barriers need to be addressed in planning for the health needs of young adult males including accessibility to care and the willingness to seek out professional healthcare.

PLANNING FOR THE HEALTH NEEDS OF THE YOUNG ADULT MALE

First and foremost, effective communication must occur between the healthcare provider and the young adult male stressing confidentiality and the rules of the Health Insurance Portability and Accountability Act (HIPAA) (Collins-McBride, Saxe, Duderstadt, & Kaplan, 2017). The visit, for whatever reason it was initiated (other than an emergency), should incorporate as much teaching and health promotion as time and the young man's attention allow. Although it is recommended to have a yearly "checkup," compared to females, many young males do not do so (Bell et al., 2013). Every opportunity to interact with the young adult male must be used to its greatest advantage and impart trust and confidence by the healthcare provider. The aim is to develop a mutual relationship with the new "patient" allowing him to return if he has questions, knowing they will be honestly answered. Not all health concerns may be a quick-fix or a one-visit evaluation.

One of the main components of a healthcare visit for young men besides the comprehensive health history and physical examination is the psychosocial assessment. Strengths and weaknesses of the individual can be ascertained and appropriate interventions planned (Collins-McBride et al., 2017). Social and academic competence, emotional well-being, and risk reduction are areas to continue to be addressed with the young adult male progressing from adolescence (Collins-McBride et al., 2017). Employment competence should also be evaluated for those who choose not to further their education.

Mental health screenings for depression are important because young men may not reveal this information on their own. Symptoms such as weight loss or gain, sleep disturbances, anhedonia, fatigue, and lack of motivation all need to be investigated with a psychological basis in the differential diagnosis. Smoking, alcohol and substance abuse, and recent escalation in these behaviors may all be signals of trying to "escape."

The subjective history should include the history of present illness (HPI) and the chief complaint. As in any healthcare visit the past medical history, surgeries (including dates), medications (plus over-the-counter medications) prescribed and not prescribed specifically for the individual, dental history, communicable diseases and immunizations, allergies (food, drug, and environmental and the specific reaction and when exhibited), and family history (including but not limited to cardiovascular disease, hypertension, sudden cardiac death, cerebrovascular accidents, diabetes, obesity, cancer, substance abuse, and mental health problems) should be obtained (Bickley, 2017; Collins-McBride et al., 2017). Many times young adults, particularly males, based on the author's experience in college health, cannot provide this information. Either they never bothered to ask their parents or caregivers or never thought a family or personal history was important. Often the reply is, "I need to call home to find out."

A discussion of specific behaviors/habits should follow. Home (living arrangements, relationship with parents and siblings); education and employment (goals); eating (patterns, body image, meals); activities (peers, physical activities, sports); drug, alcohol, and tobacco use; sexuality; depression and suicide; and safety (seatbelts, helmets, relationships) all need to be covered to be thorough (Collins-McBride et al., 2017).

To be completely thorough, the sexual history should include a nonthreatening question about sexual orientation or gender identity such as, "Do you have sex with females, males, or both?" The healthcare provider must be comfortable in eliciting this important information in order to meet the young adult's healthcare needs and provide culturally competent care to the lesbian, gay, bisexual, and transgender (LGBT) community to reduce health disparities. Young men in the 18- to 24-year-old age group may be in the "questioning" phase and an open forum with the health professional would be a safe place for them to delve into the topic. Disclosure in this setting is associated with better provider-patient communication and planning for healthcare management (Butler et al., 2016). Gay, bisexual, and other men who have sex with men (MSM) are a diverse community disproportionately impacted by syphilis, HIV infection, and other STDs (CDC, 2017). The latter populations have shared unique experiences that may affect both physical and mental health needs as well (CDC, 2016b).

According to the CDC, the top six causes of death in the United States in 2014 in both age groups for men, 15 to 19 years and 20 to 24 years, in descending order are unintentional injuries, suicide, homicide, cancer, heart disease, and birth defects (CDC, 2014). The next four causes of death differ for the two groups. For the 15- to 19-year-olds, the 7 to 10 leading causes of death are influenza and pneumonia, chronic lower respiratory diseases, stroke, and diabetes (CDC, 2014). For the 20- to 24-year-olds, the 7 to 10 leading causes of death are diabetes, influenza and pneumonia, chronic lower respiratory diseases, and stroke (CDC, 2014). Therefore safety and health promotion, including immunizations, are two imperative topic areas to address during the healthcare visit for young adult males (see also Chapter 5).

In a recent longitudinal study, Coronary Artery Risk Development in Young Adults (CARDIA), data extracted indicated if the heart is healthy in the 20s, in those persons the brain may be larger and healthy in the 40s (Bancks et al., 2017). The study scored 518 people (average age 51 years and followed over 30 years) on the American Heart Association's (AHA) Life's Simple 7: maintaining a healthy blood pressure, controlling cholesterol, reducing blood sugar, being active, eating better, losing weight, and stopping smoking. The researchers found that every point increase in the Life's Simple 7 score was roughly equivalent to 1 year of aging in the amount of brain shrinkage that occurred during the time interval (Bancks et al., 2017). A stronger association was noted between current smoking and smaller brain volume than the other variables (Bancks et al., 2017). It is unclear if heart health affects brain size or if brain size at a young age may influence behaviors affecting heart health, according to the authors. Nevertheless, lifestyle issues need to be reviewed by clinicians at each presenting visit by young adult males as their future health may be affected, even 2 to 3 decades later.

Not only must health needs be identified, but motivators to change should be incorporated in the plan. In an Australian study, four themes emerged from the responses motivating young men to eat healthy foods: (a) physical health; (b) sport or performance; (c) physical appearance; and (d) social influences (Ashton et al., 2017). The healthcare provider must ascertain why the young adult male sought healthcare or decided to change health habits at this particular point in time to assist in engaging the person in the plan of care. As indicated, men generally wait longer to present with a long-standing complaint. Perhaps partner encouragement, family encouragement ("my mother made me come"), and/or something they read on the Internet was the primary factor that brought them to seek professional help.

Although there is not much research relating to young men's use of the Internet for health reasons, most providers have heard many times the statement, "I was looking on the Internet," prior to discussing their symptoms. Often the person is worried about the severity of their symptom, "thinking the worst," when given online the possibilities of diagnoses across a continuum and presents to a healthcare provider. Many persons often know how to recognize a reputable site (looking for.org) or use major medical centers' websites such as the Mayo Clinic. With the advent of multitudes of apps and healthcare devices and trackers, young men today are generally savvy when it comes to navigating the Internet. The development of patient portals for those with a regular healthcare provider also makes it easier for someone to ask a question online without an appointment. Social media may also play a role in that posts about someone's illness may lead another to seek care or pique interest in health. Oh and Kim (2014) found when comparing college students in the United States and South Korea that the American students were more active in using social media and for health purposes; however, regardless of the country, those students with a high level of confidence in searching the Internet for health information and those with higher health concerns or lower perceived health status trusted social media more and found it useful.

It is estimated that 1 in 3 adults in the United States uses the Internet to diagnose or find out more information about a health concern; of this 35%, half followed up with a medical professional (Fox & Duggan, 2013). Women use online resources for health information more than men but groups who are also likely to use the Internet are younger persons, Caucasian adults, those who live in households earning $75,000 or more (higher socioeconomic status [SES]), and those with a college or advanced degree (Fox & Duggan, 2013; Jacobs, Amuta, & Jean, 2017). Data from four cycles (2011–2014) of the Health Information National Trends Survey (HINTS) were analyzed regarding health information–seeking behaviors (Jacobs et al., 2017). Trends from the latter study included the following: (a) Only a small percentage of participants reported using family, friends, or coworkers for health information over the four cycles (females, African Americans compared to non–African Americans, those with more education all less likely); (b) a greater percentage reported using the Internet as the first place they go for health information compared to family/friends/coworkers, health professionals, and traditional media, especially in cycle 4; (c) the use of healthcare professionals increased from cycle 1 to cycle 2 but fell in cycles 3 and 4; (white participants, females less likely to use healthcare professionals and Hispanic compared to non-Hispanic participants and those with cancer more likely to use healthcare professionals as sources of health information); and (d) use of traditional media declined for four cycles (Jacobs et al., 2017, pp. 5–8).

When providing healthcare to young adult males, it is very important to ascertain from what source or sources they are obtaining health information in starting any conversation about their concerns. Not only may myths need to be dispelled and misinformation corrected, but education as to how to navigate the online system to gain the most from reputable Internet resources may be needed. If the young adult male comes equipped with some knowledge or potential diagnosis of his health problem or concern, a dialogue can occur with the clinician. Seeking healthcare should not be considered a sign of weakness, femininity, or vulnerability (Rosu, Oliffe, & Kelly, 2016). Partnering with the person to manage their healthcare needs is key to achieving positive outcomes and adherence to healthcare plans.

Rosu et al. (2016) recommend four strategies to engage men in primary healthcare, particularly by nurse practitioners: (a) level the hierarchies, that is, dispel the power differential, particularly if the provider is a female, through open communication and engaging men in effectual health decision making; (b) talking it through, which can be best achieved by motivational interviewing as a counseling style and mapping progress; (c) seeing diversity within patterns that is addressing specific health needs at differing ages with appropriate assessment tools and viewing small incremental health behavior change as a source of strength and autonomy; and (d) augmenting face-to-face primary healthcare with community and/or web programs. Young adult men may benefit from these interventions by the healthcare provider in taking control of their own health behaviors with perceived support by the professional.

HEALTH PROMOTION FOR THE YOUNG ADULT MALE

Because most young adult males are basically healthy, visits to a healthcare professional are generally episodic in nature for acute illness or injury. The yearly "physical examination" may be neglected because of lack of health insurance, lack of regular healthcare provider, or assuming it is not of high importance if the person is feeling well physically and mentally. Quick health questions may be answered by an Internet search, social media, or contact with peers or family. The amount of money for an insurance copay or deductible may be perceived as being better spent on other items of pleasure or necessities. One's personal health may not have as much value as material possessions and certainly the family of origin plays a role in the development of personal values. For instance, dental care may not be sought by young adult males unless it is perceived that their physical appearance is affected which in turn affects social interactions. For example, in a Nigerian study of male and female college students, Azodo and Ogbomo (2014) concluded that ethnicity, tooth arrangement, size, and strength were significant predictors of self-evaluated dental appearance satisfaction. Physical appearance may be directly related to self-esteem, and although not as prevalent in males, disordered eating behaviors may be exhibited.

For the young adult, the nurse or other health professional may become an informal counselor (Edelman, Kudzma, & Mandle, 2014). The health professional must be astute at assessment, although this may be difficult when meeting with the person for the first encounter. The health history of prior behaviors and prior physical characteristics such as weight is of prime importance. Young men may be performing risky behaviors learned during participation in sports as an adolescent such as using diuretics to make a weight class or using anabolic steroids. Open-ended questions may help elicit pertinent information. Simple screening questions may include, "Do you ever restrict what you eat?" or "Do you ever make yourself vomit or take diuretics to control your weight?" These questions should be prefaced with the disclaimer that the provider asks everyone these questions or something similar so the young male does not feel he is being singled out and resist disclosure.

Although eating disorders are less prevalent in young males, the behaviors may begin as an adolescent and surface after high school. The *Diagnostic and Statistical Manual V (DSM-5)* expands categories so more males may be identified by a specific diagnosis and men may present with comorbid conditions (Raevuori, Keski-Rahkonen, & Hoek, 2014). If a young adult male presents with symptoms of anxiety, depression, excessive exercise, substance disorders, weight loss, or weight gain, an eating disorder should be considered in the differential diagnosis. The young adult male's diet and exercise habits should be reviewed. Simple questions such as, "Tell me what you ate yesterday," or "What did you have to eat today," may be a springboard for discussing what types of food the person eats and/or who prepares the food in the household. Exercising and types and length of workouts provide important data, particularly if the person is overweight or obese. According to the CDC (CDC, 2016c), in the year 2013 to 2014, the percentage of persons 20 years of age or older who were overweight including obesity in the United States was 70.7%; 37.9% were obese. The CDC (CDC, 2016a) also reported there was no significant relationship between obesity and education among men, and among non-Hispanic black and Mexican-American men the higher the income, the greater the rate of obesity.

A body mass index (BMI) assessment should be conducted at each visit with an actual height measurement. Although the young adult male should be finished growing by 18 years of age, there are always exceptions and self-reporting may over- or underestimate height. Risk factors for chronic diseases such as diabetes mellitus, heart disease, hypertension, and cancers should be reviewed, especially in relation to weight, diet, and exercise patterns.

As stated, the young adult male's affect and mental state need to be assessed. At this point in their lives, the main stressor is generally relationships (whether they be with partner, family, and/or peer), employment, school, and finances. Physical cues of self-neglect should be noted and suicide risk taken into account, paying particular attention to the following signs and symptoms: "depression and anxiety, saddened face, feelings of hopelessness or helplessness, weight loss, insomnia impaired judgment or decision making, slow gait, slumped shoulders, or lack of energy" (Edelman et al., 2014, pp. 539–540). Insomnia may be either inability to fall asleep (usually associated with anxiety) or waking up and not being able to fall back to sleep, and is often associated with depression. Appropriate referrals should be made if warranted.

Safety should be stressed in all activities such as helmets for bicycles and motorcycles, seat belts in all motor vehicles, sunscreen, and use and storage of firearms. Use of alcohol, prescription and recreational drugs, and tobacco including how often and the amount should be included in the medical record. Accident and injury prevention are topics of concern for this age group.

Immunizations should be current and documented. If the immunization status is unknown, then every attempt should be made by the patient and the provider to find previous records such as from high school or college. If immunizations are not up to date then a plan should be made to keep them current. Tetanus should be given every 10 years and if in contact with babies or young children, a booster of TDaP (tetanus, diphtheria, and pertussis) is recommended to prevent transmission of pertussis. Measles, mumps, and rubella (particularly because of recent outbreaks), hepatitis B, meningococcal (including type B if in group living), HPV, varicella, and the annual flu vaccine are priorities (Chapter 8). The healthcare provider can refer the patient for further information and tables to the CDC website.

A sexual history, as indicated, including number of lifetime partners, use of barrier methods, and treatment for sexually transmitted infections (STIs) should be conducted. The current CDC guidelines (revised 2016) are as follows for men:

- Chlamydia: Consider screening young men for chlamydia in high prevalence clinical settings or in populations with high burden of infection (e.g., MSM).
- Herpes: Type-specific herpes simplex virus (HSV) serologic testing should be considered for men presenting for an STD evaluation (especially men with multiple sex partners).
- HIV: All men aged 13 to 64 years (opt-out). USPSTF recommends screening in adults ages 15 to 65. All men who seek evaluation and treatment for STDs.
- Hepatitis B screenings: Men at increased risk are screened.
- Hepatitis C screenings: Men born between 1945 to 1965 are screened. Other men if risk factors are present (past or current drug use, receipt of blood transfusion before 1992, long-term hemodialysis, born to mother with hepatitis C, intranasal drug use, receipt of an unregulated tattoo, and other percutaneous exposure).

For MSM the following guidelines apply:

- Chlamydia: At least annually for sexually active MSM at sites of contact (urethra, rectum) regardless of condom use. Every 3 to 6 months if at increased risk.
- Gonorrhea: At least annually for sexually active MSM at sites of contact (urethra, rectum, pharynx) regardless of condom use. Every 3 to 6 months if at increased risk.
- Syphilis: At least annually for sexually active MSM. Every 3 to 6 months if at increased risk.
- Herpes: Type-specific serologic tests can be considered if infection status is unknown in MSM with previously undiagnosed genital tract infection.
- HIV: At least annually for sexually active MSM if HIV status is unknown or negative and the patient himself or his sex partner(s) have had more than one sex partner since most recent HIV test.
- Hepatitis B screenings: All MSM should be tested for HBsAg.
- Hepatitis C screenings: MSM born between 1945 and 1965 should be screened; other MSM if risk factors present; annual HCV testing in MSM with HIV infection.

For persons with HIV infection:

- Chlamydia: For sexually active individuals, screen at first HIV evaluation, and at least annually thereafter. More frequent screening might be appropriate depending on individual risk behaviors and the local epidemiology.
- Gonorrhea: For sexually active individuals, screen at first HIV evaluation and at least annually thereafter. More frequent screening might be appropriate depending on individual risk behaviors and the local epidemiology.
- Syphilis: For sexually active individuals, screen at first HIV evaluation, and at least annually thereafter. More frequent screening depending on individual risk behaviors and local epidemiology.
- Herpes: Type-specific HSV serologic testing should be considered for persons presenting for an STD evaluation (especially for those persons with multiple sex partners), persons with HIV infection, and MSM at increased risk for HIV acquisition.
- Hepatitis B screenings: Test for HBsAg and anti-HBc and/or anti-HBs.
- Hepatitis C screenings: Serologic testing at initial evaluation and annual HCV testing in MSM with HIV infection (CDC, 2016d).

Every effort should be made to provide proper education in a nonjudgmental, nonthreatening environment and to encourage prevention.

CONCLUSION

The key to the management of health for the young adult male is prevention. The majority of this population is healthy, therefore, health promotion is imperative. Yet the 18- to 24-year-old male age group is not singled out in most recommendations. It is a stage of transition in many ways, particularly in healthcare, and often young men do not seek health professionals unless there is an acute health need. If a young man has a chronic health issue, transitioning to adult healthcare may also present problems and pediatric providers should be aware of advocating for the person through the healthcare system.

According to Healthy People 2020 (CDC, 2014a), in addition to healthcare, the goals for adolescents and young adults include healthy development, injury and violence prevention, sexual health, substance abuse counseling, and prevention of chronic diseases of adulthood. Mental health evaluations are essential because symptoms may be exhibited initially as the young adult emerges. Suicidal ideation needs to be explored and appropriate referrals to specialists made with follow-up.

Newer health concerns need to be addressed by the healthcare professional and include disordered eating and gender issues. Masculinity beliefs by the young adult male must be considered by the health professional as well as anticipation of any barriers to seeking health, including motivators that need to be taken into account when planning healthcare and/or management. Sociocultural factors may play important roles; the health professional must know this population and incorporate these factors into planning and management.

Health-promoting behaviors such as immunizations, STD screenings, diet, exercise, substance use, tobacco use, mental health, dental health, safety, and healthy relationships should be reviewed regularly or at each encounter. In today's digital age, reputable sources of health information should be encouraged and myths or misinformation dispelled and corrected.

The role of healthcare professional is of prime importance in moving the young adult male forward through life. Trust and confidence must be gained by the young adult male in his relationship with healthcare professionals. Independence needs to be fostered as the young adult male transitions and emerges into adulthood.

RESOURCES FOR BOTH PROVIDERS AND PATIENTS

American College Health Association: www.acha.org/healthycampus
American Academy of Pediatrics and a collaborative of other federally and state funded projects: www.brightfutures.org/
Centers for Disease Control and Prevention: www.cdc.gov/obesity/adult/index.html
Centers for Disease Control and Prevention: www.cdc.gov/msmhealth/index.htm
Centers for Disease Control and Prevention: www.cdc.gov/healthequity/lcod/index.htm
Centers for Disease Control and Prevention: www.cdc.gov/nchs/fastats/obesity-overweight.htm
Centers for Disease Control and Prevention: www.cdc.gov/vaccines/schedules/hcp/adult.html
Centers for Disease Control and Prevention: www.cdc.gov/std/tg2015/screening-recommendations.htm
Office of Disease Prevention and Health Promotion: www.healthypeople.gov/2020/topics-objectives/topic/Adolescent-Health
U.S. Preventive Services Task Force: www.uspreventiveservicestaskforce.org/

REFERENCES

American Association of Pediatrics. (2017). *Bright futures: Guidelines for health supervision of infants, children, and adolescents* (4th ed.). Elk Grove Village, IL: American Academy of Pediatrics.

American College Health Association. (2012, June). Healthy campus 2020. Retrieved from www.acha.org/healthycampus

Ashton, L. M., Hutchesson, M. J., Rollo, M. E., Morgan, P. J., Thompson, D. I., & Collins, C. E. (2015). Young males motivators and perceived barriers towards eating healthily and active. *International Journal of Behavioral Nutrition and Physical Activity, 12*, 93. doi:10.1186/s12966-015-0257-6

Azodo, C. C., & Ogbomo, A. C. (2014). Self-evaluated dental appearance satisfaction among young adults. *Annals of Medical Health Science Research, 4*(4), 603–607. doi:10.4103/2141-9248.139339

Bancks, M. P., Allen, N. B., Dubey, P., Launer, L. J., Lloyd-Jones, D. M., Reis, J. P., … Schreiner, P. J. (2017, July 19). Cardiovascular health in young adulthood Structural brain MRI in midlife. *Neurology, 89*(7), 680–686. doi:10.1212/WNL.0000000000004222

Bell, D. L., Breland, D. J., & Ott, M. A. (2013). Adolescent and young adult male health: A review. *Pediatrics, 132*(3), 535–546. Retrieved from http://pediatrics.aappublications.org/content/132/3/535

Beshers, S. C., Murphy, J. M., Fix, B. V., & Mahoney, M. C. (2015). Sex differences among college students in awareness of the humanpapilloma virus vaccine and vaccine options. *Journal of American College Health, 63*(2), 144–147. doi:10.1080/07448481.2014.975720

Bickley, L. S. (2017). *Bates' guide to physical examination and history taking.* Philadelphia, PA: Lippincott Williams & Wilkins.

Bradley-Geist, J. C., & Olson-Buchanan, J. B. (2014). Helicopter parents; an examination of the correlates of over-parenting of college students. *Education & Training, 56*(4), 314–328. doi:10.1108/ET-10-2012-0096

Burns, C. E., Dunn, A. M., Brady, M. A., Starr, N. B., Blosser, C. G., & Garzon, D. L. (2017). *Pediatric primary care.* St. Louis, MO: Elsevier.

Butler, M., McCreedy, E., Schwer, N., Burgess, D., Call, K., Przedwoski, J., … Kane, R. L. (2016, March). *Improving cultural competence to reduce health disparities* [Internet]. Rockville, MD: Agency for Healthcare Research and Quality (US). Report No. 16-EHC006-EF (Comparative Effectiveness Reviews, No. 170) 3, Lesbian, Gay, Bisexual, and Transgender Populations. Retrieved from https://www.ncbi.nlm.nih.gov/pubmed/27148614

Centers for Disease Control and Prevention. (2014a). Healthy people 2020. Retrieved from https://www.cdc.gov/nchs/healthy_people/hp2020.htm

Centers for Disease Control and Prevention. (2014b). Leading causes of death in males, 2014. Retrieved from https://www.cdc.gov/men/lcod/2014/allmales/index.htm

Centers for Disease Control and Prevention. (2016a). Adult overweight and obesity. Retrieved from https://cdc.gov/obesity/adult/index.html

Centers for Disease Control and Prevention. (2016b). Gay and bisexual men's health. Retrieved from https://www.cdc.gov/msmhealth/index.htm

Centers for Disease Control and Prevention. (2016c). Obesity and overweight, National Center for Health Statistics. Retrieved from https://www.cdc.gov/nchs/fastats/obesity-overweight.htm

Centers for Disease Control and Prevention. (2016d). Screening recommendations and Considerations referenced in the 2015 STD Treatment Guidelines and Original Sources. Retrieved from https://cdc.gov/std/tg2015/screening-recommendations.htm

Centers for Disease Control and Prevention. (2017). Gay, bisexual, and other men who have sex with men (MSM). Retrieved from https://www.cdc.gov/msmhealth/index.htm

Cheatham, C. T., Barksdale, D. J., & Rodgers, S. G. (2008). Barriers to health care and health-seeking behaviors faced by black men. *Journal of the American Academy of Nurse Practitioners, 20*(11), 555–562. doi:10.1111/j.1745-7599.2008.00359.x

Cohen, R., & Martinez, M. (2012). *Health insurance coverage early release of estimates from National Health Interview Survey 2011*. Atlanta, GA: Centers for Disease Control and Prevention.

Collins-McBride, G. M., Saxe, J. M., Duderstadt, K. G., & Kaplan, R. (2017). *Clinical guidelines for advanced practice nursing*. Burlington, MA: Jones & Bartlett.

Curtis, A. C. (2015). Defining adolescence. *Journal of Adolescent and Family Health, 7*(2), Article 2. Retrieved from http://scholar.utc.edu/jafh/vol7/iss2/2

Dariotis, J. K., Sifakis, F., Pleck, J. H., Astone, N. M., & Sanenstein, F. L. (2011). Racial and ethnic disparities in sexual risk behaviors and STDs during young men's transition to adulthood, *Perspectives on Sexual and Reproductive Behavior, 43*(1), 51–59, doi:10.1363/4305111

Edelman, C. L., Kudzma, E. C., & Mandle, C. L. (2014). *Health promotion across the lifespan*. St. Louis, MO: Elsevier.

El Kahi, H. A., Abi Rizk, G. Y., Hlais, S. A., & Adib, S. M. (2012). Health-care-seeking behavior among university students in Lebanon. *Eastern Mediterranean Health Journal, 18*(6), 598–606.

Federal Interagency Forum on Child and Family Statistics. (2014). America's young adults, special report, 2014. Retrieved from https://www.childstats.gov/pdf/ac2014/YA_14.pdf

Fox, S., & Duggan, M. (2013). Health online 2013, Pew internet. Retrieved from http://pewinternet.org/Reports/2013/Health-online.aspx

Healthy People 2020. Washington, DC: U. S. Department of Health and Human Services, Office of Disease Prevention and Health Promotion. Retrieved from https://www.healthyteennetwork.org/wpcontent/uploads/2014/10/Healthy-People-2020-and-Adolescent-Health.pdf

Hepburn, C. M., Cohen, E., Bhawra, J., Weiser, N., Hayeems, & Guttmann, A. (2015). Health system strategies supporting transition to adult care. *Archives of Disease in Childhood, 100*(6), 559–564. doi:10.1136/archdischild-2014-307320

Jacobs, W., Amuta, A. O., & Jean, K. C. (2017). Health information seeking in the digital age: An analysis of health information seeking behavior among US adults. *Cogent Social Sciences, 3* (1), 1302785. doi:10.1080/23311886.2017.1302785

Monaghan, M. (2014). The Affordable Care Act and implications for young adult health. *Translational Behavioral Medicine, 4*(2), 170–174. doi:10.1007/s13142-013-0245-9

Munsey, C. (2006). Emerging adults: The age of in-between. *Monitor, 37*(6), 68. Retrieved from http://www.apa.org/monitor/jun06/emerging.aspx

Nicoteri, J. A., & Arnold, E. C. (2005). The development of health care-seeking behaviors in traditional-age undergraduate college students. *The Journal of the American Academy of Nurse Practitioners, 17*(10), 411–415. doi:10.1111/j.1745-7599.2005.00071.x

Oh, S., & Kim, S. (2014). College students' use of social media for health in the USA and Korea. *Information Research, 19*(4), 643. Retrieved from http://InformationR.net/ir/19-4/paper643.html (Archived by WebCite® at http://www.webcitation.org/6UFdWuK25)

Oman, R. F., Vesely, S. K., Aspy, C. B., & Tolma, E. L. (2015). Prospective associations among assets and successful transition to early adulthood. *American Journal of Public Health, 105*(1), e51–e56. doi:10.2105/AJPN.2014.302310

Ozer, E. M., Urquhart, J. T., Brindis, C. D., Park, M. J., & Irwin, C. E. (2012). Young adult preventive guidelines: There but can't be found. *Archives of Pediatric Adolescent Medicine, 166*(3), 240–247. doi:10.1001/archpediatrics.2011.794

Patient Protection and Affordable Care Act. (2010). 42 U.S. Code § 18001. Retrieved from http://housedocs.house.gov/energycommerce/ppacacon.pdf

Probst, C., Moyo, D., Purshouse, R., & Rehm, J. (2015). Transition probabilities for four states of alcohol use in adolescence and young adulthood: What factors matter when? *Addiction, 110*(8), 1272–1280. doi:10.1111/add.12985

Raevuori, A., Keski-Rahkonen, A., & Hoek, H. W. (2014). A review of eating disorders in males. *Current Opinion Psychiatry, 27*(6), 426–430. doi:10.1097/YCO.0000000000000113

Rosu, M. B., Oliffe, J. L., & Kelly, M. T. (2016). Nurse practitioners and men's primary healthcare. *American Journal of Men's Health, 11*(5), 1501–1511. doi:10.1177/1557988315617721

Rowley, J., Johnson, F., & Sbaffi, L. (2017). Gender as an influencer of online health Information-seeking and evaluation behavior. *Journal of the Association for Information Science and Technology, 68*(1), 36–47. doi:10.1002/asi.23597

Tabor, J. M., Leyva, B., & Persoskie, A. (2015). Why do people avoid medical care? A qualitative study using national data. *Journal of General Internal Medicine, 30*(3), 290–297. doi:10.1007/s11606-014-3089-1

Tyler, R. E., & Williams, S. (2014). Masculinity in young men's health: Exploring health, help-seeking and health service use in an online environment. *Journal of Health Psychology, 19*(4), 457–470. doi:10.1177/1359105312473784

United States Preventive Services Task Force. (2017). Document. Retrieved from https://www.uspreventiveservicestaskforce.org

CHAPTER 13

Novel Nutritional and Dietary Supplement Approaches and Men's Health

Mark A. Moyad

INTRODUCTION: FOREST OVER THE TREE FOR MEN'S HEALTH

Perhaps it is time to triage men's health issues on the basis of past and current statistics that do not whisper but shout. The obesity epidemic is approaching 40% prevalence in the United States, and it is the highest number observed since prevalence began increasing in the 1970s (Hales, Fryar, Carroll, Freedman, & Ogden, 2018). Just 10 years ago, the prevalence of male obesity was 32%. And, when combining the overweight data with the obesity data arguably 7 to 8 out of every 10 men need to prevent further weight gain and/or lose weight. This is an astounding number today when contemplated, and since the association between weight/waist size and unhealthy metabolic and cardiovascular health changes are well accepted, then a transition to the discussion of the sheer impact of cardiovascular disease (CVD) should occur.

CVD has been the primary cause of death in men every year since 1919 (Benjamin et al., 2017). This statistic needs to be reiterated to male patients to impact overall perspective. In fact, these national statistical disease prevalence observations are also mirrored in some of the largest male prevention trials with a pharmaceutical agent or dietary supplement. And, this is what occurs in large prevention studies since they recruit from diverse geographical regions in general and reflect ongoing concerns in the population itself. For example, the Prostate Cancer Prevention Trial (PCPT) has been debated for some time as to whether benefits exceed the risks of taking this drug for men (Kaplan et al., 2009; Scardino, 2003; Thompson et al., 2003; Traish, Mulgaonkar, & Giordano, 2014). More than 18,000 men participated in this randomized trial, and a total of 10 men died from prostate cancer when combining the number of deaths from the intervention and the placebo arm. However, more than 1,100 men died from other causes during this trial, primarily from CVD and other causes (Thompson et al., 2003). Thus, despite being a clinical trial with a prostate cancer prevention focus, less than 1% of the deaths overall were attributable to prostate cancer.

The selenium and vitamin E supplementation randomized trial (SELECT) was arguably the largest prostate cancer prevention study ever conducted using dietary supplements (Lippman et al., 2009). The message from this trial appeared to be the lack of efficacy or harm from these supplements in men, which is understandable to a point. Yet, another focus, similar to the PCPT for clinicians should be on the primary cause of mortality that was unrelated to the intervention or placebo, and, once again, similar to PCPT, it was CVD. Over 500 deaths from CVD were observed versus a single death from prostate cancer in 5 years of follow-up. This again represents a remarkable ratio and helps establish perspective.

Male prevention trials with drugs or supplements are not the only disciplines that reflect statistical disease prevalence in men and the need to triage preventive advice, but large-scale cancer screening studies should be included in this discussion as well. The most recent and the two largest PSA screening randomized trials includes the United States Prostate, Lung, Colorectal, and Ovarian Cancer Screening Trial (PLCO) and the European Randomized Study of Screening for Prostate Cancer (ERSPC; Tsodikov et al., 2017). As the debate over PSA screening from these two trials abound, another significant observation appears to have been less recognized. In these two trials, over 45,000 men died of various causes, but less than 3% died from prostate cancer and 97% from other causes such as CVD. Thus, whether you debate PSA screening, supplement, or pharmaceutical prevention trials, there exists an unfortunate quiet nexus that emerged from all of trials, and that is the dominant role CVD plays in the morbidity and mortality of men. Therefore, redirecting attention back to CVD prevalence and prevention to positively impact overall men's health in general (the forest) should also assist the clinician to potentially help patients concerned about other chronic and specific health situations (the tree). And, the good news is indeed good—most of the research collected in the area of CVD prevention suggests beneficial lifestyle changes that reduce the risk of CVD also simultaneously reduces the risk of other common medical conditions that affect men (Eyre et al., 2004; Moyad, 2015).

HEART HEALTHY = MEN'S HEALTH

Instead of reviewing all of the numerous and diverse aspects of male heart health disease risk or prevention advice, which abounds by this author (Moyad, 2013) and in the general medical literature, a summary of the more recent and novel lifestyle, supplement, and even prescription medicine research should be highlighted. Still, keeping in mind that attempting to improve the lives of men in terms of quality and quantity is tantamount to triaging male CVD prevention as the priority and that how that priority relates to specific men's health issues from prostate cancer, erectile dysfunction, benign prostatic hyperplasia (BPH), and even other physical and mental health conditions.

Alcohol

The literature and numerous media sources appear to be replete with the potential benefits of moderate alcohol consumption and heart health. Still, the idea of "moderation" appears to have been misconstrued in regard to portion sizes, which today are arguably larger than ever recorded in human history (Zupan, Evans, Couturier, & Marteau, 2017). And, at 7 calories per gram, only second in caloric content to fat, and the overproduction of insulin, and appetite stimulation with excessive intake, then arguably alcohol may be one of the least referred to culprits of excessive weight gain (Caton, Ball, Ahem, & Hetherington, 2004; Traversy & Chaput, 2015). Alcohol intake is also generally underestimated by patients, and current and future concerns of excessive intake abound. For example, alcoholic liver disease is expected to surpass ischemic heart disease in terms of working life lost, and it is currently one of the top three preventable causes of death behind smoking and obesity (Williams et al., 2018).

Novel research suggests even more ancillary detriment with alcohol consumption than previously realized. Alcohol is a known carcinogen but the list of cancers including male cancers appear to be expanding. One of the largest meta-analysis conducted on the subject and prostate cancer risk has found a significant dose-response relationship (Xhao, Stockwell, Roemer, & Chikritzhs, 2016). Heavy drinking (four or more drinks daily on 5 or more days a week) has also been associated with a significant increase in the risk of high-grade prostate cancer and appeared to render the drug finasteride ineffective at reducing cancer risk in the PCPT (Fowke, Howard, Andriole, & Freedland, 2014). Additionally, in the REDUCE (Reduction by Dutasteride of Prostate Cancer Events) trial men reporting more than seven drinks per week were 86% ($p = .01$) more likely to be diagnosed with high-grade prostate cancer. Thus, alcohol may negatively impact the prostate cancer prevention ability of 5-alpha-reductase inhibitors (Gong et al., 2009).

Obesity and Dietary Weight Loss Options (End Justifies the Means?)

The impact of weight gain or obesity on men's health is concerning, but less overt examples of this issue should be emphasized (Klaassen et al., 2017). For example, there is evidence to suggest prostate-specific antigen (PSA) experiences hemodilution with larger body size, which could distort the true cancer clinical scenario by producing a false sense of security. Additionally, a true increased prostate volume and reduction in testosterone commonly occurs in obese men. Arguably, weight gain has become one of the most influential lifestyle factors that could acutely and dramatically reduce testosterone production. And, increasing prostate size increases the secretion of PSA from noncancerous prostate tissue, thus providing a more potentially confusing picture for the clinician and patient in addition to the aforementioned hemodilution issue. If preventing weight gain could reduce prostate enlargement and excessive PSA production in some men, then this alone could provide substantial clinical benefits in reducing the potential for overdiagnosis of nonaggressive prostate tumors based on PSA increases/kinetics. The literature supporting the negative impact of obesity on male fertility and erectile function also abounds and a plethora of supporting literature exists for the ability of weight loss to improve these functions (Fullston, McPherson, Zander-Fox, & Lane, 2017; Glina, de Freitas Barboza, Nunes, Glina, & Bernardo, 2017).

The problem of the obesity epidemic was reflected earlier in this chapter in terms of increasing and astounding prevalence. Yet, obesity touches upon the prostate cancer spectrum in virtually every direction. Obese men have a greater probability of being diagnosed with aggressive prostate cancer and a greater risk of disease recurrence after treatment, and thus also dying from this disease (Goto et al., 2017). There is also a concern with the male hormonal imbalance that obesity causes in the long term and its potential to reduce the efficacy of some of the more novel drugs approved for prostate cancer treatment. In the Health Professionals Follow-up Study (HPFS), arguably one of the most methodologically sound ongoing prospective studies being conducted, weight accumulation after a prostate cancer diagnosis was correlated with a higher risk of lethal prostate cancer in nonsmokers (Dickerman et al., 2017). And, this is, of course, extremely concerning given the advances achieved in prostate cancer treatment in the past decade.

Thus, in summary it should be reiterated that artificial reduction in PSA and/or overproduction of PSA from prostate enlargement, reductions in testosterone, fertility, erectile function, and an increased risk of aggressive prostate cancer cumulatively provides one of the more compelling arguments in men's health to emphasize a healthy weight/waist as one the most important lifestyle change that should be pursued throughout life. It would appear that few goals should be more paramount than this.

An exemplary dietary weight loss trial to discuss with men was called "Preventing Overweight Using Novel Dietary Strategies" or POUNDS LOST study (de Souza et al., 2012; Nicklas et al., 2013; Sacks et al., 2009). This was one of the longest and arguably one of the best dietary weight loss randomized trials ever conducted in terms of quality or methodology in the United States. It attempted to answer the question in the long term using imaging studies among other common medical tests, of whether there was a superior weight loss method in terms of altering carbohydrate, fat, and protein intake (macronutrients). Arguably, this trial appeared to advocate for what this author likes to call the "post-bariatric surgery dietary method" where the end (weight loss achieved) justifies the means (caloric restriction diet or method). It is easy to forget that bariatric surgery is not just successful because of the surgery itself per se, but because of the adherence to long-term caloric restriction after surgery, regardless of the dietary approach used. Somewhat similarly, the beneficial cardiovascular markers, including measures of inflammation and imaging changes in terms of visceral fat, were similar in POUNDS LOST, regardless of the dietary approach as long as identical weight loss was achieved. It was for this reason the authors of the study and this author also advocate for a diet-to-fit personality approach. In other words, the diet that allows for the greatest individual adherence is the diet that works best for the individual. So, rather than being consumed by the best type of diet in general, clinicians and patients need to be consumed by the best diet for their specific patient and themselves that can improve cardiovascular markers of health and of course maintain or improve mood.

What should be reiterated to patients is flexible adherence for long-term success. Whether a reduced-calorie, low-fat, higher-fat, moderate-protein, or higher-protein approach is chosen, along with the goal of slow and methodical or even rapid acute weight loss, it should be based on individual preference or personality, knowing that long-term significant weight loss (the end result) substantiates the method chosen (the means).

DIETARY WHOLE DIVERSE FRESH FRUITS, VEGETABLES, AND OTHER FIBER (LEGUMES . . .) OPTIONS

Media attention and many consumers appear to highlight one fruit or vegetable with each passing year. One should just type in "superfood" in any search engine and prepare to be impressed or, in reality, concerned. Clinicians need to be able to remain objective and explain to patients that these social media reports do not necessarily represent any major research breakthrough, but rather support the ongoing and past research that consuming a diversity of whole low-cost fruits and especially vegetables is just one practical and logical approach to improving men's health. Several examples of this controversy exist including the historical attention garnered toward the compound lycopene and tomatoes in preventing prostate and other cancers based on numerous epidemiologic studies and one notable meta-analysis (Giovannucci, 1999). However, this highlighted meta-analysis concluded by reminding readers that this is just additional evidence that a diversity of fruits and vegetables were important for a healthy diet, but this appeared to be grossly misconstrued. Tomatoes were never the only or necessarily the primary source of lycopene. A variety of other healthy products contain this compound such as apricots, guava, and pink grapefruit (Clinton, 1998; Mourvaki, Gizzi, Rossi, & Rufini, 2005). Watermelon is an outstanding source of lycopene, and is the largest source per gram compared to any other nutritional source, including tomato products. Regardless, lycopene has minimal overall beneficial data in and of itself to solve various issues, but at least the compound and products that contain this compound are generally safe and even heart healthy (Burton-Freeman & Sesso, 2014).

The potential impact of emphasizing a single nutrient or one component of a healthy fruit or vegetable, instead of the whole "natural" product, could potentially have profound consequences. There were and continue to be a plethora of examples but the most recent relevant case was the fascination with pomegranate juice or extract for men's health conditions. Preliminary observational evidence on pomegranate juice or extracts hinted at a benefit for prostate cancer prevention, for example, but the data and research needed more time to evolve. This arguably should have again placed the emphasis from the clinicians' standpoint on consuming more whole diverse fruits and vegetables and waiting to see what is garnered from the higher quality clinical trials of the juice or extracts. And, then these higher quality studies eventually became available and they provided another teaching point (Freedland et al., 2013; Pantuck et al., 2015; Stenner-Liewen et al., 2013). Placebo-controlled trials did not demonstrate a consistent impact on prostate cancer over a placebo, however, and pomegranate juice and most juices can contain larger amounts of calories. Thus, the use of this or other fruit juices cannot currently be supported for men's health issues such as prostate cancer. Again, whole fresh diverse dietary sources provide the nutrients and fiber content to offset the "liquid sugar" that can be derived from just drinking the juices. Encourage patients to walk into any grocery store or go on-line to compare the total sugar content of an 8-ounce or 12-ounce cola soda beverage versus a fruit juice and they will be surprised that there is generally little difference in total sugar and caloric content between the perceived unhealthy versus healthy beverage. And, in both cases, again there is little to no fiber in these beverages. Most again are just "liquid sugar."

How much fiber should be consumed daily and what is really novel about fiber consumption today? Daily intakes of total fiber in the United States and many other Western countries is approximately 10 to 15 g, which is approximately only half or even less than half of the total amount consistently recommended by the American Heart Association (AHA) and American Dietetic Association (20–30 g/day) for adequate overall health (approximately 14 g of fiber per 1,000 calories consumed) (Anderson et al., 2009; Han et al., 2017; Slavin, 2008). This gap in the recommended amount and what is actually consumed could be potentially narrowed if a large part of the advertising focus is placed on gut microbiotia or microbiome to improve overall health. Fiber intake is one of the best solutions to improving overall healthy gut flora instead of consuming probiotic pills (Moyad, 2014).

Dietary fiber from food is easily achieved by low-cost sources of soluble and insoluble fiber rather than powders and pills. For example, I often tell patients to just consume a third of a cup of a bran cereal, which is approximately only the size of 1 to 2 liquor shot glasses, with flaxseed and some small fruit, and before they leave the door in the morning approximately 20 g of fiber will have already been ingested toward the goal of approximately 20 to 30 g (Moyad, 2014). Low-cost fiber sources such as flaxseed powder can provide potentially numerous heart healthy and urologic healthy or men's health benefits and outcomes (Demark-Wahnefried et al., 2001, 2004, 2008; Pan et al., 2009; Parikh, Netticadan, & Pierce, 2018; Rodriguez-Leyva, Dupasquier, McCullough, & Pierce, 2010; Zhang et al., 2008). Interestingly, preliminary clinical data for flaxseed and urologic health prevention including BPH and prostate cancer were arguably as strong as any other nutritional item tested in urology to date, especially when considering the benefit-to-risk ratio (Demark-Wahnefried et al., 2001, 2004, 2008; Zhang et al., 2008). Perhaps the low cost and noncommercialization of this product has led to the lack of objective education that this author has observed on this product. Flaxseed is also one of the largest plant sources of heart healthy omega-3 fatty acids, along with fiber, and is low cost (Parikh et al., 2018), and chia seed is arguably the largest plant source of fiber and omega-3 combined (Marcinek & Krejpcio, 2017), and both of these additions to the male diet would be a healthy step forward.

Fiber itself appears to have become overtly commercialized, and in my experience some patients rely primarily on powders and pills to solve their fiber deficiency, but this is costly and difficult. For example, I often ask patients how many fiber capsules/pills are needed to be consumed daily to obtain just 20 to 30 g of fiber? The answer always seems to provide adequate surprising value, which is 30 to 40 pills a day or more depending on the commercial source (Moyad, 2014). A bolus of only soluble fiber from commercial sources without insoluble fiber can also create excessive bloating and other gastrointestinal issues. Research continues to support the overall and heart healthy health benefits of fiber, especially when it is primarily derived from food sources, because these sources not only occupy the majority of the positive clinical research, but also provide a unique and optimal balance of soluble and insoluble fiber for heart healthy and stool healthy benefits.

Past nutrition advice, similar to the superfood movement, appeared to be replete with data on one bean, soy or one of its components, and its potential ability to prevent prostate cancer. Again, as mentioned earlier the larger forest over the tree provides a more holistic probability-based clinical recommendation. The legumes, especially beans and lentils, in general may not harbor health advertisements but collectively they continue to garner positive heart healthy and prostate healthy data (Dinu, Pagliai, & Sofi, 2017; Li, Li, Shen, Wang, & Zhou, 2017; Zhang, Wang, Chen, Yin, & Song, 2016). In other words, again the focus should be on the forest and not a single tree.

POTASSIUM: THE FORGOTTEN CRITICAL MEN'S HEALTH NUTRIENT

Arguably, the one nutrient that could be the so-called "scurvy" of men's and women's health in the sense that almost 95% to 97% of the population is not ingesting adequate amounts for disease prevention is potassium (Appel, 2017; Moyad, 2014; Palmer & Clegg, 2016). The recommended daily amount from the Institute of Medicine (IOM) is 4,700 mg. There are no other major nutrients recommended at this level for disease prevention, ergo the importance of discussing this with patients. Another issue besides achieving the recommend daily amount is the lack of other solutions apart from food sources of potassium. Dietary supplements are not encouraged to contain more than 99 mg of elemental potassium per pill thus making over-the-counter options unrealistic to achieve potassium goals. Additionally, potassium prescription medications are not simple to comply with daily and this difficulty creates its own issues.

Clinicians should embrace this potassium challenge. Countless potential health benefits could be achieved emphasizing more dietary potassium (Cai et al., 2016; Ekmekcioglu, Elmadfa, Meyer, & Moeslinger, 2016; Grimes et al., 2017; Iwahori, Miura, & Ueshima, 2017; Moyad, 2014; Palmer & Clegg, 2016; Sun et al., 2017; Vinceti et al., 2016). First there are numerous medical conditions that could be prevented with adequate potassium, including hypertension, stroke, kidney stones, and preliminary evidence to suggest a reduction in metabolic syndrome and diabetes and an improvement in bone health. Still in all of these cases it is not just cause but consequence of consuming healthier foods when shifting to a potassium-based diet. And, most foods high in potassium additionally harbor higher fiber concentrations and other healthy nutrients such as magnesium. Some of the highest dietary sources of potassium are also low in sodium, thus providing additional benefits. The potassium-to-sodium ratio ideally should be 1 or greater but currently studies suggest it is 0.32. Adults and children are consuming at least two to three times more sodium compared to potassium. Recent laboratory research even suggests higher potassium intake could reduce vascular calcification and arterial stiffness suggesting even more diverse benefits than generally recognized. For example, it would now be of interest to examine the relationship between potassium and erectile function.

There are always concerns in patients with chronic kidney disease (CKD) or on antihypertensives that hyperkalemia could be an issue (Gilligan & Raphael, 2017). This needs to be placed in perspective that the general intake of potassium is so low overall in the general population that even in CKD, in which potassium restriction is approximately 2,000 mg/day (higher or lower depending on CKD severity), this still requires regular moderate ingestion and not necessarily restriction. Additionally, the prevalence of hyperkalemia and hypokalemia are similar in CKD.

NUTRIENTS VERSUS SUPPLEMENTS (MULTIVITAMIN: TO TAKE OR NOT TO TAKE IS THE QUESTION)

All of the dietary nutrients that could improve the health of men are readily available. Whether dietary supplements are advantageous for prevention continues to be investigated. The general consensus is that any nutrient that is contained in food is better for preventive purposes than any dietary supplement, although after being diagnosed with a condition the potential for a dietary supplement to provide benefit is more evidence-based and becoming accepted (Moyad, 2014).

The more recent legitimate concern in a men's health preventive setting is that several dietary supplements that are marketed as beneficial have the potential, if used in excess, to increase the risk and/or progression of prostate cancer (Algotar et al., 2013; Gontero et al., 2015; Kenfield et al., 2015; Kristal et al., 2014; Lippman et al., 2009; Marshall et al., 2011; Moyad, 2013, 2014, 2015; Stratton et al., 2010). No high-quality study has shown that any supplement can significantly reduce the risk for, or progression of, prostate cancer. And, in could be argued, the antithesis is accurate that several supplements in higher dosages such as vitamin E and more specifically selenium could either increase the risk of prostate cancer and/or foster the progression of this disease once it is established.

One dietary supplement that has now received the equivalent of a phase 3 trial in men's health is a daily multivitamin. This was the largest randomized trial ever conducted on generally healthy men taking a single daily multivitamin (Centrum Silver, Pfizer, NY) and was known as the "Physicians' Health Study II" (PHS2) trial and had primary endpoints of CVD and cancer prevention and secondary endpoints such as cataract prevention. This trial followed 14,600 healthy male physicians for over 11 years, and several results were found in this and other clinical trials versus a placebo. In general, the following results should be reviewed with patients that a single multivitamin a day achieved the following (Christen et al., 2014; Gaziano et al., 2012; Sesso et al., 2012; Zhao et al., 2014):

- The supplement significantly (approximately 8%, "modest reduction") reduced the risk of cancer in men, including those with a personal (not family) history of cancer and those with and without an optimal diet and lifestyle, including it appeared beneficial in those getting less than 4 servings of fruits and veggies daily, 4 to 7 servings per day, and 7 or more servings a day (from PHS2).
- It significantly (about 9% or more in PHS2, "modest reduction") reduced the risk of nuclear cataracts—the most common type (up to 34% reduction in another Centrum multivitamin study of men and women)—and potentially reduced the risk of needing cataract surgery in men and women (this result is not as definitive but suggestive in some studies). Again, cataracts were a secondary endpoint, but the reduction in cataract observation has been fairly consistent from other studies overall.
- A multivitamin could correct some important nutritional insufficiencies or deficiencies from blood testing or because of medications (such as vitamin B_{12} and/or magnesium, vitamin D).
- Only one pill was ingested per day in these clinical trials, which makes it generally low cost, and quality control testing has been consistently good with these supplements (in other words, what they report on the label is specifically what is in the pill).
- They have been heart safe (some could argue even somewhat heart healthy) in clinical trials (PHS2 and even the first PHS), but overall there was no increase or decrease risk of CVD with the multivitamin.
- Side effects were similar overall to a placebo, but there were slightly more people who reported rashes while on Centrum Silver versus placebo, but keep in mind that rashes were also reported almost as often with a placebo. In fact, in the PHS2 trial there was a 7% increased risk of reporting a rash in the 2,125 of the 7,317 participants on Centrum Silver (29%), and in 2002 of the 7,324 participants on placebo (27%). Therefore, just ingesting a placebo or multivitamin daily in this latest clinical trial was associated with a potential increased risk of at least

reporting a rash (over the 11-year study). Thus, all pills, especially supplements, should be reviewed whenever a new rash appears for no other explainable reason.

Still, no pill—except this particular multivitamin—has ever been found to reduce the risk of cancer and cataracts in healthy individuals and with the same overall side effects as a placebo. Some critics will argue that these benefits weren't impressive enough to warrant telling most people to ingest a daily multivitamin and they refer to lower quality studies to support this conclusion. In addition, even if Centrum or Centrum Silver works, then many people would have to take it for a decade or more to see just one individual benefit, so this is another reason why it is not worth it for some individuals and critics. It is true that although the reduction in cancer risk and cataract risk was statistically significant over placebo, the clinical significance of this small effect will be debated for years.

Still, others could argue that cancer will soon surpass CVD as the leading global cause of death and cataracts are the most common cause of blindness around the world and one of the biggest government or private health insurance costs because of the large numbers of procedures needed annually to resolve cataracts. If a low-cost multivitamin has the ability to reduce the risk of cancer and cataracts even modestly, and can help prevent numerous minor or major nutritional deficiencies, especially ones caused by some of the fad or specialty diets, prescription drugs, autoimmune conditions, bariatric surgery, then clinicians should consider recommending one. Otherwise, patients will need to take multiple supplements to get similar coverage for a deficiency or insufficiency, for example.

If clinicians are considering recommending a multivitamin, there are other critical items to consider. The Centrum Silver utilized in the PHS2 study (initiated in the 1990s) was similar in dosage to many children's multivitamins sold in the United States today (Moyad, 2014). Over the years, multivitamin dosages have increased despite the lack of scientific validity to suggest the need for these increases in general. It is for this and other reasons this author recommends either the multivitamin that contains the most evidence such as Centrum Silver or Centrum or a children's multivitamin (a children's multivitamin today generally equates to an adult multivitamin used in past adult clinical trials such as PHS2), or a single daily multivitamin that at least closely reflects the clinical trial nutrients and dosages utilized (see Table 13.1).

The final line of the published PHS2 report had an interesting supportive statement, which suggested that despite the primary reason to take multivitamins is to prevent nutritional deficiency the latest results of this clinical trial support its use in the prevention of cancer in middle-aged and older men (Gaziano et al., 2012). Still, one has to reiterate all of the potential factors that could cause a minor nutritional deficiency in some nutrients today, which are the following (Moyad, 2014):

- Aging (e.g., absorption, digestion, illness)
- Alcohol (e.g., B-vitamins, vitamin B_{12})
- Diets (e.g., vegan, vegetarian; and vitamin B_{12}, calcium, iron)
- Genetics (e.g., autoimmune conditions)
- Medical conditions (e.g., autoimmune, diabetes)
- Medications/supplements (e.g., proton pump inhibitors, H_2-blockers, metformin)
- Menstrual cycle status (e.g., iron)
- Pregnancy (e.g., folic acid, iodine, vitamin D)
- Procedures (e.g., bariatric, intestinal resection)
- Tobacco exposure (numerous nutrients such as vitamin C)
- Weight gain (e.g., vitamin B_{12}, folic acid, iron, vitamin D)

TABLE 13.1 Centrum Silver Formulation Utilized in the PHS2 Intervention Arm

Vitamin A = 5,000 IU (50% as beta-carotene)	Vitamin B_{12} = 25 mcg	Copper = 2 mg
Vitamin C = 60 mg	Biotin = 30 mcg	Manganese = 3.5 mg
Vitamin D = 400 IU	Pantothenic acid = 10 mg	Chromium = 130 mcg
Vitamin E = 45 IU	Calcium = 200 mg	Molybdenum = 160 mcg
Vitamin K = 10 mcg	Iron = 4 mg	Chloride = 72.6 mg
Vitamin B_1 = 1.5 mg	Phosphorus = 48 mg	Potassium = 80 mg
Vitamin B_2 = 1.7 mg	Iodine = 150 mcg	Boron = 150 mcg
Niacin = 20 mg	Magnesium = 100 mg	Nickel = 5 mcg
Vitamin B_6 = 3 mg	Zinc = 15 mg	Vanadium = 10 mcg
Folic acid = 400 mcg	Selenium = 20 mcg	Silicon = 2 mg

IU, International Units; mcg, micrograms (also symbolized by "μg" on some supplement containers); mg, milligrams.

NUTRIENT TESTING CONTROVERSIES

Quantifying the amount of nutrients in serum and tissues has been difficult because the entire field is still in an embryonic stage especially in regard to correlating these numbers with solid clinical risk or endpoints (Moyad, 2014). Therefore, the necessary amount of a given supplement needed is unknown in numerous cases, even after testing. Differences in study populations, methodology, and interpretation of data complicate the comparison of studies. The simple reliability of nutrient testing is the largest issue. Countless nutrient or antioxidant tests are offered today to consumers who are concerned about countless medical issues, yet again the validity of many of these tests—especially as they relate to cancer and other "hard endpoints"—is unknown. Unanswered questions include the following:

- Does the quantified level in serum reflect the tissue concentration?
- What is the best form/metabolic byproduct of the nutrient to test for accuracy?
- Does increasing a specific nutrient because of a reduced test result produce any potentially tangible benefit or even detriment?
- How are the assay results impacted by intrinsic and/or extrinsic factors? Do some dietary supplements in higher amounts interfere with other non-nutrient assays? Does chronic inflammation impact nutrient testing accuracy?

Those and other critical questions should be answered before consumers spend their money on these tests. A few examples can help illustrate the complexity of nutrient testing, which has yet to be fully appreciated.

For example, use of dietary supplements containing large amounts of biotin (marketed as promoting healthy hair, skin, and nails) may interfere with a diverse range of laboratory tests that are biotin based (biotinylated assays). High biotin intake may result in artificially low or high results on PSA and testosterone biotinylated-based assays (sandwich/competitive), as well as other cancer marker tests (e.g., CA125, CA15-3, CEA, CA19) (Elston, Sehgal, Du Toit, Yarndley, & Conaglen, 2016; Li et al., 2017). False increases in thyroid function test results and vitamin B_{12} assays have also been reported.

Given the plethora of tests that may be impacted, patients should be advised to stop taking an individual biotin supplement at least 3 days (and perhaps ideally 1 week) before blood testing. One multivitamin pill per day that includes biotin are usually not a cause for concern because they lack mega-doses.

Systemic inflammation may also result in low values on tests for nutrients such as zinc; selenium; and vitamins B_6, C, A, and D (Duncan, Talwar, McMillan, Stefanowicz, & O'Reilly, 2012). This effect may skew interpretation of research observations because it can suggest that a nutrient deficiency increases the risk for a particular disease when in fact the disease itself is decreasing the measured nutrient level. One could argue that the past push for chemoprevention studies on supplements in men's health such as selenium were partially based on the observation that men with lower risk for cancer harbored higher blood levels of selenium compared to men with cancer (Moyad, 2014). Still, in retrospect it appears this was a consequence of the disease and not the cause of this condition. Thus, the potential ability to set in motion a series of costly research events based on an assay that has not been fully construed is indeed remarkable.

Additionally, vitamin D blood measurements, in particular, may be reduced not only by inflammation but by obesity, smoking, depression, cancer, and lack of physical activity (Datta, Pal, & DE, 2014; Duncan et al., 2012; Moyad, 2014; Waldron et al., 2013). This could partly explain the lack of an effect of supplementation in some major clinical trials; that is, the inflammatory state may be creating the appearance of a vitamin D insufficiency or deficiency in individuals with adequate vitamin D intake. This would again set in motion a series of research events based on incomplete knowledge over the benefits and limitations of the assay itself. This should be given ample consideration in future clinical trials utilizing nutrient testing. Thus, given the ongoing popularity of vitamin D, the supplement and assay requires more attention.

Vitamin D Supplement Controversy

The primary source of vitamin D is ultraviolet light intrinsic activation in the human body, but this vitamin is also contained in dairy products, eggs, vitamin D–fortified cereals, mushrooms, and fatty fish such as salmon and tuna (Moyad, 2014). Serum 25-hydroxyvitamin D assays are readily available, and many men test as vitamin-D deficient or insufficient. As discussed above, however, that assay can be influenced by multiple intrinsic and extrinsic factors (e.g., smoking, obesity, inflammation). Consequently, this test should not be widely advocated until further validation with so-called hard clinical endpoints has been accomplished.

Guidelines on vitamin D from the IOM, published in 2011, set the Recommended Dietary Allowance for vitamin D at only 600 IU (800 IU in those age 71 and older), because of the concern for toxicity (e.g., hypercalcemia, hypercalciuria, nephrolithiasis) and the lack of impressive data to advocate for higher intakes (Ross et al., 2011; Slomski, 2011). Admittedly, the IOM recommendations have not been without controversy (Friedman & Brunton, 2011). Still, in this author's opinion the IOM decision is admirable because it relied on data and not on hype.

Vitamin D appears to have some of the same historical embellishment issues that occurred before randomized trials of other dietary supplements for prostate cancer, when some believed that "more is better." In fact, results of studies of vitamin D for prostate cancer prevention have not been consistently impressive, and several studies have found no impact or potential harm at higher blood levels (Barnett & Beer, 2011; Barnett et al., 2010; Michaëlsson et al., 2010).

Vitamin D is important for bone health, but recommendations or requests for larger intakes to support prostate health have not been supported by strong clinical trial evidence.

Vitamin D mimics hormonal function rather than a so-called traditional vitamin function, which is why caution should be followed because the potential for a U-shaped risk curve (similar to that seen with other hormones) does exist for men's health.

Again, the issues with the assay and the history of prostate cancer supplements being discredited and even encouraging tumor growth in large quantities argue for a "first do no harm" approach until larger trials are published that give further insight. Clinical trials such as the VITamin D and OmegA-3 TriaL (VITAL) should be published soon and they will provide further insight into the benefits and limitations of vitamin D (and even fish oil) preventive supplementation to prevent cancer (Pradhan & Manson, 2016).

Statins, Aspirin, Metformin (S.A.M.)

This author has published several manuscripts on shifting the thought process on pill consumption for men's health. The acronym S.A.M. (statins, aspirin, metformin) is a simplistic method of remembering three of the more important off-label products that should be primarily discussed when time is limited with a patient (Moyad, 2015; Moyad & Vogelzang, 2015) as they relate to men's health and overall health. It sends a simultaneous message to patients to always consider the largest source of morbidity and mortality in the world (CVD) and the process of improving overall health. S.A.M. are all low-cost, generic, and derived from "natural" sources (statins from yeast/fungus, aspirin from willow bark, and metformin from the French lilac) and have arguably more preliminary positive data in the area of prostate cancer prevention/men's health compared to any dietary supplement (Dawe & Mahmud, 2017; Deng et al., 2015; Meng, Liao, Xu, Wei, & Wang, 2016; Huang et al., 2014). It is of interest that these three generic medicines have proved themselves to be heart healthy in the appropriate patients, have unique mechanisms of action, and allow for a variety of individuals from those at high risk of diabetes to heart disease to other cancer concerns to potentially reduce their risk.

The acronym S.A.M. is in reality a unisex name and it is not intended to increase the pill count of a patient but to place perspective on the pills that appear to have the best benefit-to-risk ratio in many patients that qualify for one or more of these pills, even after being diagnosed or treated for cancer. There are literally thousands of supplements today that healthcare practitioners can discuss with patients but in order to create a more pithy and efficient consult, S.A.M. allows for this to interaction to occur (Moyad, 2015; Moyad & Vogelzang, 2015). Simple to remember, low cost, generic, and "natural." The evidence continues to accumulate with either or all of these pills and the potential benefits in the areas of men's health. It is also of interest that several dietary supplements are also positioning themselves as alternatives to S.A.M, namely red yeast rice, salicin, and bebeerine dietary supplements, but not just more clinical trials head-to-head are needed but also a profound investment in more quality control especially with these dietary supplements (Moyad, 2014; Moyad & Klotz, 2011; Shara & Stohs, 2015; Wang, Feng, Chai, Cao, & Qiu, 2017). Therefore, prescription S.A.M continues to be the safest and most researched route versus any so-called alternatives to S.A.M.

Additionally, the ability to discuss S.A.M. also opens the discussion of blood pressure medication if needed. Many antihypertensives are low cost today and the alpha-blockers for BPH were actually derived from the traditional antihypertensive drugs (heart healthy = prostate healthy), although the antihypertensives have yet to accumulate the preliminary data on prostate health compared to S.A.M. Regardless, in the future S.A.M. acronym may need to be changed to include remembering to discuss blood pressure interventions (B.S.A.M.?). All suggestions are welcome for this new potential acronym.

EXERCISE AND MENTAL HEALTH

Before the conclusion of this chapter, it would be regretful if this author would not at least provide some commentary on exercise and men's health. There appears to be a perceived intense focus on the physical benefits of exercise. Today, the attention to mental health should arguably receive as much attention from past to present data (Blake, Mo, Malik, & Thomas, 2009; Deslandes et al., 2009). And, given the devastation of stress, anxiety, depression, suicide, and other mental health conditions on men's health the timing of this exercise discussion could not be more paramount.

For example, one referenced trial published over a decade ago included 156 adult volunteers with major depressive disorder (MDD) randomly assigned a 4-month course of aerobic exercise (30 minutes three times/week), sertraline therapy, or a combination of exercise and sertraline (Babyak et al., 2000 & Blumenthal et al., 1999). After 4 months patients in all three groups demonstrated significant mental health improvements; however, after 10 months, individuals in the exercise group had significantly lower recurrence rates compared to individuals in the medication group of the study. Exercising during the follow-up period was associated with a 51% reduction in the risk of a diagnosis of depression at the end of the investigation. Even recent randomized studies of patients with significant comorbid conditions such as heart failure have significant improvements in physical and mental health with regular exercise (Blumenthal et al., 2012). It is important to explain to patients that if the overall results from exercise studies were viewed similar to a specific pharmacologic intervention, then it probably would have already garnered attention worthy of a Nobel prize in arguably multiple categories of medicine. And, the ability of exercise to work synergistically with medication is also notable.

Still, despite the evidence it appears that clinicians are only prescribing exercise to a minority of patients (Barnes & Schoenborn, 2012). This again represents an opportunity to continue to rely more on the mental health improvements to motivate healthcare professionals and patients. For example, stress, anxiety, and depression demonstrate the potential for improvement with exercise (McMahon et al., 2017; Mikkelsen, Stojanovska, Polenakovic, Bosevski, & Apostolopoulos, 2017; Vancampfort et al., 2018). Furthermore, this benefit appears to be equivalent in children and adults, and thus it is not surprising that even suicidal ideation could be attenuated with exercise. Novel research in other aspects of mental health including increases in brain hippocampal size and memory, even in those patients at high risk of cognitive impairment, continues to generate positive data (Bettio, Rajendran, & Gil-Mohapel, 2017). Again, the ongoing benefits of exercise for physical benefits continue to impress (Mustian et al., 2017), but the mental health benefits should be stressed.

Interestingly, preliminary research suggests that large dosages of dietary supplements could negatively impact the benefits of ongoing exercise regimen by interfering and absorbing free radicals that act as signals of improved skeletal muscle remodeling and even nerve activity or regeneration (Merry & Ristow, 2016). Still, the message is the same regardless, which is mental health benefits of exercise are still preliminary but becoming profound.

CONCLUSION

Diet, supplements, and simply lifestyle issues and recommendations need to be more practical and simple to grasp. Some may think this simplistic shift in thinking is just that, much too simplistic, or too folksy to garner the attention needed for clinical and research milieu changes. However, one could argue that it is has been the lack of recognition or motion toward the simplistic that has caused such gross deviation from the forest and such gravitation toward the individual tree. One could even argue that hundreds of millions of dollars would not have been spent over the past 2 decades on adverse pharmacologic and dietary supplement interventions had more deference been paid to more simplistic correlations or innuendo between the CVD and prostate cancer or men's health nexus. Perhaps it is time to realize that after an era of subscribing to a philosophy of "more is better" including the amount of money needed to invest in a novel and costly preventive agent for men's health or high-dose dietary supplements that do not afford CVD protection, it is now time to believe that "less is more" and heart health is tantamount to prostate, men's, and overall health.

Clinicians and patients need to remember that a chronic prevalent disease, at least epidemiologically speaking, has not been found to be isolated or insular in incidence or prevalence. Areas of the world or specific populations with some of the lowest rates of death from CVD simultaneously enjoy lower rates of mortality from a multitude of devastating diseases including various cancers, and even mental health issues, and ultimately this is what assists in increasing their overall life expectancy. It is time to prioritize or triage and simplify preventive health recommendations for men and, in reality, women and children. The public must be constantly distracted and fatigued from a perceived infinity of incoming behavioral recommendations from countless health awareness campaigns and agendas via multimedia sources that are now open 24 hours a day and 365 days a year. How else does one explain the obsession clinicians witness regularly over medical minutiae such as the latest antiaging supplement or medication that can apparently prevent most diseases compared to long-term evidence-based heart healthy interventions. Thus, a table of 10 recommendations from this chapter are proffered and summarized in Table 13.2. One line (recommendation 10) at the end of the table for personalized men's health recommendation based on the clinician's area of practice and the patient population is provided such as tobacco cessation, vaccine compliance, seat belt utilization, processed and refined food utilization (Moyad, 2014).

TABLE 13.2 Summary of 10 Recommendations Proffered for Men's Health in this Chapter

	Dr. Moyad Recommendation	Commentary
1	Heart health = men's health = all health	Reducing the risk of cardiovascular disease to as close to zero as possible also simultaneously contributes to lowering the risk of numerous men's health conditions and is easy to remember for patients.
2	Alcohol intake should be discussed because it is an epidemic issue underestimated and misconstrued by patients.	In excess, alcohol is carcinogenic (aggressive prostate cancer), is a potentially significant contributor to weight gain, causes nutrient deficiency, is a form of self-medication, and interferes with men's health medication efficacy (5-alpha-reductase inhibitors).
3	Obesity, overweight, dieting, and weight loss	Countless diets exist today but the end (weight loss) justifies the means (the method that fits the personality of the patient). Thus, numerous weight loss methods should be researched and supported.
4	Dietary: whole diverse fresh fruits, vegetables, and other fiber (legumes, etc.) options (Note: these are also sources of protein.)	Heart healthy dietary recommendations in general are supported by evidence and have the potential to reduce the risk of numerous men's health issues (especially when maintaining a healthy weight/waist). Fad superfoods, such as certain fruit juices, have recently failed to find benefits above a placebo, a finding that again supports a diverse whole food healthy approach.

(continued)

TABLE 13.2 Summary of 10 Recommendations Proffered for Men's Health in this Chapter (*continued*)

	Dr. Moyad Recommendation	Commentary
5	Potassium: dietary not supplemental (Recommended dietary allowance of 4,700 mg/day!) Note: Recent decision by the U.S. government to include the potassium content on all food labels in the future is a major victory for all individuals looking to consume more of this nutrient.	Clinicians should focus on what patients should ingest more of, in general, compared to what they should avoid (sodium). Increasing potassium intake from heart healthy sources (avocado, fish, vegetables, fruits, legumes, etc.) naturally reduces excessive sodium intake and lowers blood pressure, stroke risk, and kidney stones. Potassium supplements are not advised because one cannot purchase a product with more than 99 mg of elemental potassium per pill.
6	Dietary supplements for men's health should have a "first do no harm" approach until novel data demonstrates otherwise. Arguably, the only supplement with statistically significant evidence in a phase 3 primary prevention trial of men is a daily single pill multivitamin (Centrum Silver). This trial was known as PHS2.	Dietary supplements for men's health, especially for preventing prostate cancer, have demonstrated either neutral effects or more harm than good from phase 3 clinical trials (e.g., vitamin E and selenium). Thus, be careful before recommending anything above moderation without strong consistent clinical research (including vitamin D). Distribute the multivitamin formulation (from Table 13.1) utilized in PHS2 to patients interested in ingesting a multivitamin or mimicking this specific formulation with another low-cost product.
7	Do not rely on nonvalidated nutrient testing for determining risk and potential endpoints.	For example, vitamin B_{12} testing along with other markers are reliable for vitamin B_{12} status, but vitamin D levels could be impacted by numerous lifestyle and medical conditions.
8	S.A.M discussion (Note: this is not intended to encourage pill utilization but to triage the discussion of pills that are more important to the heart health and men's health discussion compared to discussing hundreds of potentially other pills or supplements for men's health prevention that have not been deemed to support heart health and men's health simultaneously.)	Statins, aspirin, and/or metformin qualification? All three were derived from a "natural" source (yeast/fungus, willow bark, and French lilac), and are low-cost, generic, and proven heart healthy, which is arguably why it is receiving countless clinical trials in men's and women's health. Blood pressure medication and diet/lifestyle changes that could replace or lower the dosage of these medications are also paramount.
9	Exercise for mental health	The intense focus on physical health benefits of exercise should shift toward the dramatic accumulation recently in the data to support lower risks of dementia to depression with physical activity. Stress, anxiety, depression, and suicidal ideation attenuation with physical activity is potentially as notable as any other lifestyle intervention.
10	Other overt sensible recommendations from the clinician based on patient population (Note: not discussed in this chapter but should be personalized based on the practice)	Smoking cessation, vaccine compliance, etc. Even vaccines could be deemed heart healthy today.

Regardless, one must ponder a final critical question that is certain to be initiated by critics of the approach in this chapter, which is, what if heart healthy interventions or lifestyle changes ultimately do not prevent prostate cancer or another men's health condition in some notable future randomized trial? Attempting to reduce or compress the impact of the number one cause of morbidity and death in the worst-case scenario is still at least a worst-case scenario with a positive outcome. Isn't this the real translation of "first do no harm" as it relates to preventive medicine?

REFERENCES

Algotar, A. M., Stratton, M. S., Ahmann, F. R., Ranger-Moore, J., Nagle, R. B., Thompson, P. A., ... Stratton, S. P. (2013). Phase 3 clinical trial investigating the effect of selenium supplementation in men at high-risk for prostate cancer. *Prostate, 73*(3), 328–335. doi:10.1002/pros.22573

Anderson, J. W., Baird, P., Davis, R. H. Jr, Ferreri, S., Knudtson, M., Koraym, A., ... Williams, C. L. (2009). Health benefits of dietary fiber. *Nutrition Reviews, 67*, 188–205. doi:10.1111/j.1753-4887.2009.00189.x

Appel, L. J. (2017). The effects of dietary factors on blood pressure. *Cardiology Clinics, 35*(2), 197–212. doi:10.1016/j.ccl.2016.12.002

Babyak, M., Blumenthal, J. A., Herman, S., Khatri, P., Doraiswamy, M., Moore, K., ... Krishnan, K. R. (2000). Exercise treatment for major depression: maintenance of therapeutic benefit at 10 months. *Psychosomatic Medicine, 62*, 633–638. doi:10.1097/00006842-200009000-00006

Barnes, P. M., & Schoenborn, C. A. (2012). Trends in adults receiving a recommendation for exercise or other physical activity from a physician or other health professional. NCHS Data Brief, 86, 1–8.

Barnett, C. M., & Beer, T. M. (2011). Prostate cancer and vitamin D: What does the evidence really suggest? *The Urologic Clinics of North America, 38*(3), 333–342. doi:10.1016/j.ucl.2011.04.007

Barnett, C. M., Nielson, C. M., Shannon, J., Chan, J. M., Shikany, J. M., Bauer, D. C., ... Beer, T. M. (2010). Serum 25-OH vitamin D levels and risk of developing prostate cancer in older men. *Cancer Causes Control, 21*(8), 1297–1303. doi:10.1007/s10552-010-9557-y

Benjamin, E. J., Blaha, M. J., Chiuve, S. E., Cushman, M., Das, S. R., Deo, R., ... Muntner, P. (2017). Heart Disease and Stroke Statistics-2017 update: A report from the American Heart Association. *Circulation, 135*(10), e146–e603. doi:10.1161/CIR.0000000000000485

Bettio, L. E. B., Rajendran, L., & Gil-Mohapel, J. (2017). The effects of aging in the hippocampus and cognitive decline. *Neuroscience & Biobehavioral Reviews, 79*, 66–86. doi:10.1016/j.neubiorev.2017.04.030

Blake, H., Mo, P., Malik, S., & Thomas, S. (2009). How effective are physical activity interventions for alleviating depressive symptoms in older people? A systematic review. *Clinical Rehabilitation, 23*, 873–887. doi:10.1177/0269215509337449

Blumenthal, J. A., Babyak, M. A., Moore, K. A., Craighead, W. E., Herman, S., Khatri, P., ... Krishnan, K. R. (1999). Effects of exercise training on older patients with major depression. *Archives of Internal Medicine, 159*, 2349–2356. doi:10.1001/archinte.159.19.2349

Blumenthal, J. A., Babyak, M. A., O'Connor, C., Keteyian, S., Landzberg, J., Howlett, J., ... Whellan, D. J. (2012). Effects of exercise training on depressive symptoms in patients with chronic heart failure: The HF-ACTION randomized trial. *JAMA, 308*, 465–474. doi:10.1001/jama.2012.8720

Burton-Freeman, B., & Sesso, H. D. (2014). Whole food versus supplement: Comparing the clinical evidence of tomato intake and lycopene supplementation on cardiovascular risk factors. *Advances in Nutrition, 5*(5), 457–485. doi:10.3945/an.114.005231

Cai, X., Li, X., Fan, W., Yu, W., Wang, S., Li, Z., ... Li, X. (2016). Potassium and obesity/metabolic syndrome: A systematic review and meta-analysis of the epidemiological evidence. *Nutrients, 8*(4), 183. doi:10.3390/nu8040183

Cancer Facts & Figures. (2017). American Cancer Society. Retrieved from https://www.cancer.org/content/dam/cancer-org/research/cancer-facts-and-statistics/annual-cancer-facts-and-figures/2017/cancer-facts-and-figures-2017.pdf

Caton, S. J., Ball, M., Ahem, A., & Hetherington, M. M. (2004). Dose-dependent effects of alcohol on appetite and food intake. *Physiology and Behavior, 81*(1), 51–58. doi:10.1016/j.physbeh.2003.12.017

Centers for Disease Control and Prevention. (2015). Heart disease facts. Retrieved form https://www.cdc.gov/heartdisease/facts.htm

Christen, W. G., Glynn, R. J., Manson, J. E., MacFadyen, J., Bubes, V., Schvartz, M., … Gaziano, J. M. (2014). Effects of multivitamin supplement on cataract and age-related macular degeneration in a randomized trial of male physicians. *Ophthalmology, 121*(2), 525–534. doi:10.1016/j.ophtha.2013.09.038

Clinton, S. K. (1998). Lycopene: Chemistry, biology, and implications for human health and disease. *Nutrition Reviews, 56*, 35–51. doi:10.1111/j.1753-4887.1998.tb01691.x

Datta, S., Pal, M., & DE, A. (2014). The dependency of vitamin d status on anthropometric data. *Malaysian Journal of Medical Sciences, 21*(3), 54–61.

Dawe, D. E., & Mahmud, S. (2017). Biologic and epidemiologic evidence assessing if statins prevent prostate cancer. *Canadian Journal of Urology, 24*(6), 9081–9088.

de Souza, R. J., Bray, G. A., Carey, V. J., Hall, K. D., LeBoff, M. S., Loria, C. M., … Smith, S. R. (2012). Effects of 4 weight-loss diets differing in fat, protein, and carbohydrate on fat mass, lean mass, visceral adipose tissue, and hepatic fat: Results from the POUNDS LOST trial. *The American Journal of Clinical Nutrition, 95*(3), 614–625. doi:10.3945/ajcn.111.026328

Demark-Wahnefried, W., Polascik, T. J., George, S. L., Switzer, B. R., Madden, J. F., Ruffin, M. T. 4th, … Vollmer, R. T. (2008). Flaxseed supplementation (not dietary fat restriction) reduces prostate cancer proliferation rates in men presurgery. *Cancer Epidemiology, Biomarkers & Prevention, 17*, 3577–3587. doi:10.1158/1055-9965.EPI-08-0008

Demark-Wahnefried, W., Price, D. T., Polascik, T. J., Robertson, C. N., Anderson, E. E., Paulson, D. F., … Vollmer, R. T. (2001). Pilot study of dietary fat restriction and flaxseed supplementation in men with prostate cancer before surgery: Exploring the effects on hormonal levels, prostate-specific antigen, and histopathologic features. *Urology, 58*, 47–52. doi:10.1016/S0090-4295(01)01014-7

Demark-Wahnefried, W., Robertson, C. N., Walther, P. J., Polascik, T. J, Paulson, D. F., & Vollmer, R. T. (2004). Pilot study to explore effects of low-fat, flaxseed-supplemented diet on proliferation of benign prostatic epithelium and prostate-specific antigen. *Urology, 63*, 900–904. doi:10.1016/j.urology.2003.12.010

Deng, D., Yang, Y., Tang, X., Skrip, L., Qiu, J., Wang, Y., & Zhang, F. (2015). Association between metformin therapy and incidence, recurrence and mortality of prostate cancer: Evidence from a meta-analysis. *Diabetes/Metabolism Research and Reviews, 31*(6), 595–602. doi:10.1002/dmrr.2645

Deslandes, A., Moraes, H., Ferreira, C., Veiga, H., Silveira, H., Mouta, R., … Laks, J. (2009). Exercise and mental health: Many reasons to move. *Neuropsychobiology, 59*, 191–198. doi:10.1159/000223730

Dickerman, B. A., Ahearn, T. U., Giovannucci, E., Stampfer, M. J., Nguyen, P. L., Mucci, L. A., & Wilson, K. M. (2017). Weight change, obesity, and risk of prostate cancer progression among men with clinically localized prostate cancer. *International Journal of Cancer, 141*(5), 933–944. doi:10.1002/ijc.30803

Dinu, M., Pagliai, G., & Sofi, F. (2017). A heart-healthy diet: Recent insights and practical recommendations. *Current Cardiology Reports, 19*(10), 95. doi:10.1007/s11886-017-0908-0

Duncan, A., Talwar, D., McMillan, D. C., Stefanowicz, F., & O'Reilly, D. S. (2012). Quantitative data on the magnitude of the systemic inflammatory response and its effect on micronutrient status based on plasma measurements. *American Journal of Clinical Nutrition, 95*(1), 64–71. doi:10.3945/ajcn.111.023812

Ekmekcioglu, C., Elmadfa, I., Meyer, A. L., & Moeslinger, T. (2016). The role of dietary potassium in hypertension and diabetes. *Journal of Physiology and Biochemistry, 72*(1), 93–106. doi:10.1007/s13105-015-0449-1

Elston, M. S., Sehgal, S., Du Toit, S., Yarndley, T., & Conaglen, J. V. (2016). Factitious graves' disease due to biotin immunoassay interference—A case and review of the literature. *Journal of Clinical Endocrinology and Metabolism, 101*(9), 3251–3255. doi:10.1210/jc.2016-1971

Eyre, H., Kahn, R., Robertson, R. M., Clark, N. G., Doyle, C., Hong, Y., … Thun, M. J. (2004). Preventing cancer, cardiovascular disease, and diabetes: a common agenda for the American Cancer Society, the American Diabetes Association, and the American Heart Association. *Circulation, 109*(25), 3244–3255. doi:10.1161/01.CIR.0000133321.00456.00

Fowke, J. H., Howard, L., Andriole, G. L., & Freedland, S. J. (2014). Alcohol intake increases high-grade prostate cancer risk among men taking dutasteride in the REDUCE trial. *European Urology, 66*, 1133–1138. doi:10.1016/j.eururo.2014.01.037

Freedland, S. J., Carducci, M., Kroeger, N., Partin, A., Rao, J. Y., Jin, Y., … Pantuck, A. J. (2013). A double -blind, randomized, neoadjuvant study of the tissue effects of POMx pills in men with prostate cancer before radical prostatectomy. *Cancer Prevention Research (Phila), 6*(10), 1120–1127. doi:10.1158/1940-6207.CAPR-12-0423

Friedman, P. A., & Brunton, L. L. (2011). Updated vitamin D and calcium recommendations. *Medscape Medical News*. Retrieved from http://www.medscape.com/viewarticle/738275

Fullston, T., McPherson, N. O., Zander-Fox, D., & Lane, M. (2017). The most common vices of men can damage fertility and the health of the next generation. *Journal of Endocrinology, 234*(2), F1–F6. doi:10.1530/JOE-16-0382

Gaziano, J. M., Sesso, H. D., Christen, W. G., Bubes, V., Smith, J. P., MacFadyen, J., ... Buring, J. E. (2012). Multivitamins in the prevention of cancer in men: The Physicians' Health Study II randomized controlled trial. *JAMA, 308*, 1871–1880. doi:10.1001/jama.2012.14641

Gilligan, S., & Raphael, K. L. (2017). Hyperkalemia and hypokalemia in CKD: Prevalence, risk factors, and clinical outcomes. *Advances in Chronic Kidney Disease, 24*(5), 315–318. doi:10.1053/j.ackd.2017.06.004

Giovannucci, E. (1999). Tomatoes, tomato-based products, lycopene, and cancer: Review of the epidemiologic literature. *Journal of the National Cancer Institute, 91*, 317–331. doi:10.1093/jnci/91.4.317

Glina, F. P. A., de Freitas Barboza, J. W., Nunes, V. M., Glina, S., & Bernardo, W. M. (2017). What is the impact of bariatric surgery on erectile function? A systematic review and meta-analysis. *Sexual Medicine Reviews, 5*(3), 393–402. doi:10.1016/j.sxmr.2017.03.008

Gong, Z., Kristal, A. R., Schenk, J. M., Tangen, C. M., Goodman, P. J., & Thompson, I. M. (2009). Alcohol consumption, finasteride, and prostate cancer risk: Results from the Prostate Cancer Prevention Trial. *Cancer, 115*, 3661–3669. doi:10.1002/cncr.24423

Gontero, P., Marra, G., Soria, F., Oderda, M., Zitella, A., Baratta, F., ... Brusa, P. (2015). A randomized double-blind placebo controlled phase I-II study on clinical and molecular effects of dietary supplements in men with precancerous prostatic lesions. Chemoprevention or "chemopromotion"? *Prostate, 75*(11), 1177–1186. doi:10.1002/pros.22999

Goto, K., Nagamatsu, H., Teishima, J., Kohada, Y., Fujii, S., Kurimura, Y., ... Matsubara, A. (2017). Body mass index as a classifier to predict biochemical recurrence after radical prostatectomy in patients with lower prostate-specific antigen levels. *Molecular and Clinical Oncology, 6*, 748–752. doi:10.3892/mco.2017.1223

Grimes, C. A., Riddell, L. J., Campbell, K. J., Beckford, K., Baxter, J. R., He, F. J., & Nowson, C. A. (2017). Dietary intake and sources of sodium and potassium among Australian schoolchildren: results from the cross-sectional Salt and Other Nutrients in Children (SONIC) study. *BMJ Open, 7*(10), e016639. doi:10.1136/bmjopen-2017-016639

Hales, C. M., Fryar, C. D., Carroll, M. D., Freedman, D. S., & Ogden, C. L. (2017). Trends in obesity and severe obesity prevalence in US youth and adults by sex and age, 2007–2008 to 2015–2016. *Journal of the American Medical Association, 319*(16), 1723–1725. doi:10.1001/jama.2018.3060

Han, M., Wang, C., Liu, P., Li, D., Li, Y., & Ma, X. (2017). Dietary fiber gap and host gut microbiota. *Protein and Peptide Letters, 24*(5), 388–396. doi:10.2174/0929866524666170220113312

Huang, T. B., Yan, Y., Guo, Z. F., Zhang, X. L., Liu, H., Geng, J., ... Zheng, J. H. (2014). Aspirin use and the risk of prostate cancer: A meta-analysis of 24 epidemiologic studies. *International Urology and Nephrology, 46*(9), 1715–1728. doi:10.1007/s11255-014-0703-4

Iwahori, T., Miura, K., & Ueshima, H. (2017). Time to consider use of the sodium-to-potassium ratio for practical sodium reduction and potassium increase. *Nutrients, 9*(7), pii: E700. doi:10.3390/nu9070700

Kaplan. S. A., Roehrborn, C. G., Meehan, A. G., Liu, K. S, Carides, A. D., Binkowitz, B. S., ... Vaughan, E. D. Jr. (2009). PCPT: Evidence that finasteride reduces risk of most frequently detected intermediate -and high-grade (Gleason score 6 and 7) cancer. *Urology, 73*(5), 935–939. doi:10.1016/j.urology.2008.09.079

Kenfield, S. A., Van Blarigan, E. L., DuPre, N., Stampfer, M. J., L Giovannucci, E., & Chan, J. M. (2015). Selenium supplementation and prostate cancer mortality. *Journal of the National Cancer Institute, 107*(1), 360. doi:10.1093/jnci/dju360

Klaassen, Z., Howard, L. E., Moreira, D. M., Andriole, G. L. Jr, Terris, M. K., & Freedland, S. J. (2017). Association of obesity-related hemodilution of prostate-specific antigen, dihydrotestosterone, and testosterone. *Prostate, 77*(5), 466–470. doi:10.1002/pros.23285

Kristal, A. R., Darke, A. K., Morris, S., Tangen, C. M., Goodman, P. J., Thompson, I. M., ... Klein, E. A. (2014). Baseline selenium status and effects of selenium and vitamin E supplementation on prostate cancer risk. *Journal of the National Cancer Institute, 106*(3), djt456. doi:10.1093/jnci/djt456

Li, D., Radulescu, A., Shrestha, R. T., Root, M., Karger, A. B., Killeen, A. A., ... Burmeister, L. A. (2017). Association of biotin ingestion with performance of hormone and nonhormone assays in healthy adults. *JAMA, 318*(12), 1150–1160. doi:10.1001/jama.2017.13705

Li, H., Li, J., Shen, Y., Wang, J., & Zhou, D. (2017). Legume consumption and all-cause and cardiovascular disease mortality. *BioMed Research International, 2017*, 8450618. doi:10.1155/2017/8450618

Lippman, S. M., Klein, E. A., Goodman, P. J., Lucia, M. S., Thompson, I. M., Ford, L. G., ... Coltman, C. A. Jr. (2009). Effect of selenium and vitamin E on risk of prostate cancer and other cancers: The Selenium and Vitamin E Cancer Prevention Trial (SELECT). *JAMA, 301*(1), 39–51. doi:10.1001/jama.2008.864

Marcinek, K., & Krejpcio, Z. (2017). Chia seeds (Salvia hispanica): Health promoting properties and therapeutic applications—A review. *Roczniki Państwowego Zakładu Higieny*, 68(2), 123–129.

Marshall, J. R., Tangen, C. M., Sakr, W. A., Wood, D. P. Jr, Berry, D. L., Klein, E. A., ... Thompson, I. M. Jr. (2011). Phase III trial of selenium to prevent prostate cancer in men with high-grade prostatic intraepithelial neoplasia: SWOG S9917. *Cancer Prevention Research (Phila), 4*(11), 1761–1769. doi:10.1158/1940-6207.CAPR-10-0343

McMahon, E. M., Corcoran, P., O'Regan, G., Keeley, H., Cannon, M., Caril, V., ... Wasserman, D. (2017). Physical activity in European adolescents and associations with anxiety, depression and well-being. *European Child and Adolescent Psychiatry, 26*(1), 111–122. doi:10.1007/s00787-016-0875-9

Meng, Y., Liao, Y. B., Xu, P., Wei, W. R., & Wang, J. (2016). Statin use and mortality of patients with prostate cancer: A meta-analysis. *Onco Targets and Therapy, 9*, 1689–1696. doi:10.2147/OTT.S97993

Merry, T. L., & Ristow, M. (2016). Do antioxidant supplements interfere with skeletal muscle adaptation to exercise training? *The Journal of Physiology, 594*(18), 5135–5147. doi:10.1113/JP270654

Michaëlsson, K., Baron, J. A., Snellman, G., Gedeborg, R., Byberg, L., Sundström, J., ... Melhus, H. (2010). Plasma vitamin D and mortality in older men: A community-based prospective cohort study. *The American Journal of Clinical Nutrition, 92*(4), 841–848. doi:10.3945/ajcn.2010.29749

Mikkelsen, K., Stojanovska, L., Polenakovic, M., Bosevski, M., & Apostolopoulos, V. (2017). Exercise and mental health. *Maturitas, 106*, 48–56. doi:10.1016/j.maturitas.2017.09.003

Mourvaki, E., Gizzi, S., Rossi, R., & Rufini, S. (2005). Passionflower fruit-a "new" source of lycopene? *Journal of Medicinal Food, 8*, 104–106. doi:10.1089/jmf.2005.8.104

Moyad, M. A. (2013). *Complementary and alternative medicine for prostate and urologic health*. New York, NY: Springer Publishing Company.

Moyad, M. A. (2014). *The supplement handbook*. New York, NY: Rodale Publishing.

Moyad, M. A. (2015). Preventing aggressive prostate cancer with proven cardiovascular disease preventive methods. *Asian Journal of Andrology, 17*(6), 874–897; discussion 876. doi:10.4103/1008-682X.156854

Moyad, M. A., & Klotz, L. H. (2011). Statin clinical trial (REALITY) for prostate cancer: An over 15-year wait is finally over thanks to a dietary supplement. *The Urologic Clinics of North America, 38*(3), 325–331. doi:10.1016/j.ucl.2011.05.002

Moyad, M. A., & Vogelzang, N. J. (2015). Heart healthy equals prostate healthy and statins, aspirin, and/or metformin (S.A.M.) are the ideal recommendations for prostate cancer prevention. *Asian Journal of Andrology, 17*(5), 783–791. doi:10.4103/1008-682X.148070

Mustian, K. M., Alfano, C. M., Heckler, C., Kleckner, A. S., Kleckner, I. R., Leach, C. R., ... Miller, S. M. (2017). Comparison of pharmaceutical, psychological, and exercise treatments for cancer-related fatigue: A meta-analysis. *JAMA Oncology, 3*(7), 961–968. doi:10.1001/jamaoncol.2016.6914

Nicklas, J. M., Sacks, F. M., Smith, S. R., LeBoff, M. S., Rood, J. C., Bray, G. A., ... Ridker, P. M. (2013). Effect of dietary composition of weight loss diets on high-sensitivity c-reactive protein: The Randomized POUNDS LOST trial. *Obesity (Silver Spring), 21*(4), 681–689. doi:10.1002/oby.20072

Palmer, B. F., & Clegg, D. J. (2016). Achieving the benefits of a high-potassium, Paleolithic diet, without the toxicity. *Mayo Clinic Proceedings, 91*(4), 496–508. doi:10.1016/j.mayocp.2016.01.012

Pan, A., Yu, D., Demark-Wahnefried, W., Franco, O. H., & Lin, X. (2009). Meta-analysis of the effects of flaxseed interventions on blood lipids. *The American Journal of Clinical Nutrition, 90*, 288–297. doi:10.3945/ajcn.2009.27469

Pantuck, A. J., Pettaway, C. A., Dreicer, R., Corman, J., Katz, A., Ho, A., ... Heber, D. (2015). A randomized, double-blind, placebo-controlled study of the effects of pomegranate extract on rising PSA levels in men following primary therapy for prostate cancer. *Prostate Cancer and Prostatic Diseases*, 18(3), 242–248. doi:10.1038/pcan.2015.32

Parikh, M., Netticadan, T., & Pierce, G. N. (2018). Flaxseed: Its bioactive components and their cardiovascular benefits. *American Journal of Physiology. Heart and Circulatory Physiology, 314*(2), H146–H159. doi:10.1152/ajpheart.00400.2017

Pradhan, A. D., & Manson, J. E. (2016). Update on the vitamin D and OmegA-3 trial (VITAL). *Journal of Steroid Biochemistry and Molecular Biology, 155*(Pt B), 252–256. doi:10.1016/j.jsbmb.2015.04.006

Rodriguez-Leyva, D., Dupasquier, C. M., McCullough, R., & Pierce, G. N. (2010). The cardiovascular effects of flaxseed and its omega-3 fatty acid, alpha-linolenic acid. *Canadian Journal of Cardiology, 26*, 489–496. doi:10.1016/S0828-282X(10)70455-4

Ross, A. C., Taylor, C. L., Yaktine, A. L., Del Valle, H. B. (Eds.); Institute of Medicine (US) Committee to Review Dietary Reference Intakes for Vitamin D and Calcium. (2011). Dietary reference intakes for calcium and vitamin D. Washington, DC: National Academies Press.

Sacks, F. M., Bray, G. A., Carey, V. J., Smith, S. R., Ryan, D. H., Anton, S. D., … Williamson, D. A. (2009). Comparison of weight-loss diets with different compositions of fat, protein, and carbohydrates. *New England Journal of Medicine, 360*(9), 859–873. doi:10.1056/NEJMoa0804748

Scardino, P. T. (2003). The prevention of prostate cancer—the dilemma continues. *New England Journal of Medicine, 349*(3), 297–299. doi:10.1056/NEJMe038109

Sesso, H. D., Christen, W. G., Bubes, V., Smith, J. P., MacFadyen, J., Schvartz, M., … Gaziano, J. M. (2012). Multivitamins in the prevention of cardiovascular disease in men: The Physicians' Health Study II randomized controlled trial. *JAMA, 308*(17), 1751–1760. doi:10.1001/jama.2012.14805

Shara, M., & Stohs, S. J. (2015). Efficacy and safety of white willow bark (Salix Alba) extracts. *Phytotherapy Research, 29*(8), 1112–1116. doi:10.1002/ptr.5377

Slavin, J. L. (2008). Position of the American Dietetic Association: Health implications of dietary fiber. *Journal of the American Dietetic Association, 108*, 1716–1731. doi:10.1016/j.jada.2008.08.007

Slomski, A. (2011). IOM endorses vitamin D, calcium only for bone health, dispels deficiency claims. *JAMA, 305*(5), 453–454, 456. doi:10.1001/jama.2011.50

Stenner-Liewen, F., Liewen, H., Cathomas, R., Renner, C., Petrausch, U., Sulser, T., … Müntener, M.(2013). Daily pomegranate intake has no impact on PSA levels in patients with advanced prostate cancer-results of a Phase IIb randomized controlled trial. *Journal of Cancer, 4*(7), 597–596. doi:10.7150/jca.7123

Stratton, M. S., Algotar, A. M., Ranger-Moore, J., Stratton, S. P., Slate, E. H., Hsu, C. H., … Ahmann, F. R. (2010). Oral selenium supplementation has no effect on prostate-specific antigen velocity in men undergoing active surveillance for localized prostate cancer. *Cancer Prevention Research (Phila), 3*(8), 1035–1043. doi:10.1158/1940-6207.CAPR-09-0143

Sun, Y., Byon, C. H., Yang, Y., Bradley, W. E., Dell'talla, L. J., Sanders, P. W., … Chen, Y. (2017). Dietary potassium regulates vascular calcification and arterial stiffness. *JCI Insight, 2*(19). pii: 94920. doi:10.1172/jci.insight.94920

Thompson, I. M., Goodman, P. J., Tangen, C. M., Lucia, M. S., Miller, G. J., Ford, L. G., … Coltman, C. A. Jr. (2003). The influence of finasteride on the development of prostate cancer. *New England Journal of Medicine, 349*(3), 215–224. doi:10.1056/NEJMoa030660

Traish, A. M., Mulgaonkar, A., & Giordano, N. (2014). The dark side of 5α-reductase inhibitors' therapy: Sexual dysfunction, high Gleason grade prostate cancer and depression. *Korean Journal of Urology, 55*(6), 367–379. doi:10.4111/kju.2014.55.6.367

Traversy, G., & Chaput, J. P. (2015). Alcohol consumption and obesity: An update. *Current Obesity Reports, 4*(1), 122–130. doi:10.1007/s13679-014-0129-4

Tsodikov, A., Gulati, R., Heijnsdijk, E. A. M., Pinsky, P. F., Moss, S. M., Qiu, S., … Etzioni, R. (2017). Reconciling the effects of screening on prostate cancer mortality in the ERSPC and PLCO trials. *Annals of Internal Medicine, 167*(7), 449–455. doi:10.7326/M16-2586

Vancampfort, D., Hallgren, M., Firth, J., Rosenbaum, S., Schuch, F. B., Mugisha, J., … Stubbs, B. (2018). Physical activity and suicidal ideation: A systematic review and meta-analysis. *Journal of Affective Disorders, 225*, 438–448. doi:10.1016/j.jad.2017.08.070

Vinceti, M., Fillippini, T., Crippa, A., de Sesmaisons, A., Wise, L. A., & Orsini, N. (2016). Meta-analysis of potassium intake and the risk of stroke. *Journal of the American Heart Association, 5*(10), E004210. doi:10.1161/JAHA.116.004210

Waldron, J. L., Ashby, H. L., Cornes, M. P., Bechervaise, J., Razavi, C., Thomas, O. L., … Gama, R. (2013). Vitamin D: A negative acute phase reactant. *Journal of Clinical Pathology, 66*(7), 620–622. doi:10.1136/jclinpath-2012-201301

Wang, K., Feng, X., Chai, L., Cao, S., & Qiu, F. (2017). The metabolism of berberine and its contribution to the pharmacological effects. *Drug Metabolism Reviews, 49*(2), 139–157. doi:10.1080/03602532.2017.1306544

Williams, R., Alexander, G., Armstrong, I., Baker, A., Bhala, N., Camps-Walsh, G., ... Yeoman, A. (2018). Disease burden and costs from excess alcohol consumption, obesity, and viral hepatitis: Fourth report of the Lancet Standing Commission on Liver Disease in the UK. *Lancet, 391*(10125), 1097–1107. doi:10.1016/S0140-6736(17)32866-0

Xhao, J., Stockwell, T., Roemer, A., & Chikritzhs, T. (2016). Is alcohol consumption a risk factor for prostate cancer? A systematic review and meta-analysis. *BMC Cancer, 16*(1), 845. doi:10.1186/s12885-016-2891-z

Zhang, M., Wang, K., Chen, L., Yin, B., & Song, Y. (2016). Is phytoestrogen intake associated with decreased risk of prostate cancer? A systematic review of epidemiological studies based on 17,546 cases. *Andrology, 4*(4), 745–756. doi:10.1111/andr.12196

Zhang, W., Wang, X., Liu, Y., Tian, H., Flickinger, B., Empie, M. W., & Sun, S. Z. (2008). Effects of dietary flaxseed lignan extract on symptoms of benign prostatic hyperplasia. *Journal of Medical Food, 11*, 207–214. doi:10.1089/jmf.2007.602

Zhao, L. Q., Li, L. M., & Zhu, H.; For the Epidemiological Evidence-Based Eye Disease Study Research Group EY. (2014). The effect of multivitamin/mineral supplements on age-related cataracts: A systematic review and meta-analysis. *Nutrients, 6*(3), 931–949. doi:10.3390/nu6030931

Zupan, Z., Evans, A., Couturier, D.-L., & Marteau, T. M. (2017). Wine glass size in England from 1700 to 2017: A measure of our time. *BMJ, 359*, j5623. doi:10.1136/bmj.j5623

CHAPTER 14

Mental Health Issues and Men: A Primer

George Byron Peraza-Smith and Yolanda Bone

INTRODUCTION

"It is a man's world" is a common refrain heard and in many respects, it remains true. However, the world is changing with there being less inequality between the genders. For the past few decades, there has been a transition from a male-dominated world view to a more equal, gender neutral world view. With these changes men have had to think of themselves differently, to purport themselves differently, and to evolve their thinking and attitudes about their roles and their place in world. These changes have caused dissonance for many men as they strive to fulfill these shifting male roles. Societal expectations have placed demands on men that are many times contradictory and conflicting with the shifting expectation with their jobs, in their relationships, and within their families. Society continues to expect men to function in outdated stereotypical traditional mindsets while expecting evolved, enlightened social norms. These often-incompatible demands challenge men as they balance the inconsistent emotional and social expectations with their own views of themselves in the world as men, fathers, partners, and citizens.

Men are less likely than women to seek medical care and even more less likely to seek help for mental health problems (WHO, 2016a). Men account for only 36% of referrals for psychological counseling. There is a debate on the accuracy of the reported inequalities between men and women with regards to using mental health services. This is due in part to the numbers only representing mental health problems that have been identified and reported. It is believed that men underreport and are underrepresented in the data. Mental illness stigma has a significant negative impact on a man's perception of having a mental disorder (Moss-Racusin & Miller, 2016). Men encounter perceived or real backlash when they violate well-established male gender stereotypes calling for autonomy, self-reliance, and problem-solving abilities (Moss-Racusin, 2015). A full discussion of mental health issues and men is well beyond the scope of this chapter, but we will introduce several concepts that are relevant for consideration, no matter what an individual's presenting complaint might be.

MEN'S HEALTH-SEEKING BEHAVIORS

Medical Care

Men as a group do not like going to see a provider. Men are more reluctant than women to routinely obtain primary or medical care (Lucas & Benson, 2017). Men proudly will brag "I haven't seen a doctor in years" or "I haven't been to the doctor since I was a boy" or "I don't need a doctor, I am as strong as a mule." These are common slogans that demonstrate less-than-adequate health beliefs or practices by men. According to the Centers for Disease Control and Prevention (CDC, 2017), men are 80% less likely than women to use a regular source of healthcare. From 1970 to 2010 the gap in life expectancy between the genders has widened almost yearly. Women's life expectancy at birth increased from 61.2 to 73.3 years, whereas men's life expectancy rose from 56.4 to 67.5 years. This widened gap in life expectancy at birth lengthened between the sexes, to men's disadvantage, over those 40 years (Baker et al., 2014). This widening discrepancy in life expectancy between the genders is partially explained by men's avoidance attitudes and beliefs about seeking medical care and maintaining preventive practices.

Mental Healthcare

"It's a man's world." No matter how far we have come, generally speaking, men enjoy more opportunities, privileges, and power than women, yet these advantages have not translated into better health outcomes, especially better mental health outcomes (Baker et al., 2014). Mental illness affects all walks of life without regard to gender, age, education or socioeconomic status. However, mental illness may have a more compounded influence in men because men are less likely to discuss their emotional state or feelings and are less likely to seek treatment. When mental health or illness enters the fray, men are even less likely to seek treatment or participate in mental healthcare services.

Men and women experience mental disorders at about the same rate; however, men are less likely to talk about it or to share their feelings. Men are less likely than women to seek treatment for the management of stress, emotional distress, or mental health disorder (American Psychological Association [APA], 2012). Evidence has shown that men are significantly less likely to use mental health services in response to a mental health issue in comparison with women. This is especially so for black, Latino, and Asian men, who have much lower utilization rates than white men, as well as women in general (Whitley, 2017). Men avoid seeking treatment for mental health, optioning instead to go it alone or to self-treat. Many men believe they have to "pull themselves up by their bootstraps" while not showing any emotion and just move on with life. To mask the pain and suffering, this avoidance mindset can lead to self-medicating behaviors. These self-medicating behaviors can take the form of self-destructive behaviors, such as drug abuse, overconsumption or abuse of alcohol, promiscuous sexual encounters, and/or other dangerous and risky activities.

Masculinity and Health

IMAGE OF BEING A MAN

Many men today feel lost; the image of being a man is swiftly evolving and causing men to question who they are and where they fit in the community and society. Men may feel left behind in a society that is rapidly creating new norms and which has placed seismically shifting gender expectations upon them. Men in the U.S. have historically defined masculinity as being strong, authoritarian, and self-reliant, acting as captain, decider, provider, and many other patriarchal roles. Historically, men have held the power in societal roles and dominated females physically, economically, and educationally. As society has evolved and women have demanded more respect and equal rights, the gender roles have significantly transformed. These changes have created a positive influence on society. However, there are downsides for men to these changes as they attempt to appreciate and come to terms with these evolving, ever-fluid social norms.

As women obtain their equal and rightful place in society, some men are experiencing a "masculinity crisis." Women are outpacing men in obtaining college education degrees. Past, reliable male-dominated industrial and manufacturing jobs are being replaced with technological jobs or by a new economy. More men are having to or are choosing to be stay-at-home dads. As society continues to evolve, men are feeling left behind, abandoned, discouraged, and angry (Myers, 2016). While struggling with these old mindsets, men are experiencing high levels of stress, discordance, and emotional distress without having adequate, effective coping skills. For some men, seeking mental health treatment is a sign of a character weakness, a flawed unmasculine trait. This sign of weakness may be avoided at all cost to protect the man's sense of who he is as a man and his masculine identity. Avoidance and ignoring health problems, especially mental health problems, is unsustainable, leading to ineffective coping and self-destructive behaviors in men.

Emotions and Feelings

"Real men don't cry." Men are expected to swallow their feelings or show no emotions. They are expected to be strong and not show vulnerability to others. These unrealistic, biased expectations toward men are prominent in society and even more overt among and between men themselves. Strong emotions may be more detrimental to men than women. An anger response to psychosocial stress has a more negative impact on men's heart rate and cortisol level (Lupis, Lerman, & Wolf, 2014). Men are systematically taught not to feel, not to cry, and not to express emotions. Men often internalize these feelings and many times are numb or non-responsive to those feelings and their surroundings. Men express themselves disconnected from their emotion and feelings. These internalized, unexpressed emotions and feelings can negatively impact a man's health, as well as his mental stability. However, men do not routinely seek positive outlets or treatments in managing these strong, negative emotions and feelings, and choose instead to proceed without social or family support, often suffering in silence.

Gender Differences

Men and women express their feelings and emotions in different ways, based on a variety of cultural, societal, religious, and local expectations and what these expectations both permit and require from the genders. The gender stereotypes regarding expression of feelings and emotions from men and women result from different social expectations and consequences (McCarty, Kelly, & Williams. 2014). Contemporary and/or stereotyped social expectations of men in the United States are that they are tough, self-reliant, physical, and nonemotional; men are expected to be in control of their feelings and emotions. Men are expected to be self-reliant and use their personal power to manage stress, feelings, and emotions. These inequitable social stereotypic expectations unduly cause many men to express feelings and emotions in unhealthy ways. Men are more likely than women to push down or ignore the nature and expression of negative feelings, emotions, and stress. Men are less likely than women to seek out medical advice or treatment for coping and managing stresses. These inadequate coping mechanisms may lead to negative health consequences, such as substance addiction, increased risk-taking behaviors, and medical and psychiatric complications.

The "New Age Man"

The traditional masculine, emotionless image and stereotype of men is juxtaposed with accelerating shifts in societal expectations and roles being imposed on men. Traditional roles held by men in work, family, and community are rapidly changing and becoming more equally distributed among the genders. More men are taking on and working in traditionally female-dominated professions. Men are sharing more active roles in the domestic aspects of family life. Social norms are shifting to allow men to be more expressive of their feelings and emotions.

The emerging new image has permitted some men to become more active and willing participates in their own health and well-being. Men who have embraced this new age image are moving beyond the singular focus of developing physical strength to a more enlightened attitude and commitment to both physical, spiritual, and mental well-being. These "enlightened men" are actively participating and seeking illness prevention and health promotion strategies that have positive impact on the body as well as the mind. More men are looking for opportunities to create positive mental health, spiritual connectedness, and physical well-being. This shift on importance on holistic health creates an opportunity for healthcare providers to develop and market health-related programs that target men's shifting perspectives on mental health.

Social Norms

Social norms exert intensive pressures on men to behave and act in certain ways. Crying is seen as feminine; men are not allowed (by societal norms) and do not let themselves cry. Crying within a social context is a way to relieve distress and to release tension (Kaplan, 2016). However, crying is not an option for many men who must choose other avenues to release and vent stress and painful experiences. Some men will turn the pain into anger and aggression while others will turn it onto themselves in harmful and self-destructive ways. A societal and cultural structure that does not allow men to fully express their emotions and feelings may lead to dysfunctional coping mechanisms and mental distress. Add to this the avoidance of seeking out healthcare or counseling service and this can lead to unhealthy behaviors and negative consequences.

Most boys are born into a social box of expectations that dictate the meaning of being a boy or man. Boys are expected to play with "boy" identified toys and to participate in "boy" identified sports and "boy" identified activities. This early socialization exerts a powerful influence throughout his social, physical, and emotional development. Societal norms have placed preconditions on expectations and roles within society that result in silencing and oppressing the free express of being fully human and actualized man.

"Toxic Masculinity"

Unchecked oppressive views and expectations of men can become toxic. "Toxic masculinity" has been recognized by the World Health Organization (WHO) as leading to men's tendency to die at younger ages that may correlate to the harmful ways that masculinity has been defined in society and the ways that men have been conditioned to be "masculine" (Evans, Frank, Oliffe, & Gregory, 2012). "Socially constructed models of masculinity can have deleterious health consequences for men and boys (e.g., when these models encourage violence or alcohol abuse). Since it is now accepted that gender identities are essentially negotiated, policies are needed which will enable people to shape their own identities and actions in healthier ways" (Commission on Social Determinants of Health, World Health Organization, 2007, pp. 31–32). Toxic masculinity many times leads to unhealthy emotional outlets including angry outburst, aggressive behaviors, and misuse of alcohol or drugs. Men readily experience increased negative health outcomes leading from risky behaviors and lack of willingness to seek healthcare (Baker et al., 2014).

■ MEN AND MENTAL DISORDERS

One in five adults experience a mental illness each year with nearly 5% living with a serious mental illness that interferes with or limits their functioning. Serious mental illness costs

America $193.2 billion in lost earnings per year (National Alliance on Mental Illness, 2015). Mental disorders impact both men and women fairly equally, but men are less likely to talk about their disorder or to seek treatment. Men with mental disorders often experience symptoms differently than women, making recognizing and diagnosing mental illness in men more difficult. For example, men with depression may mask their depressed mood with irritability and anger rather than depressed mood and sadness. Most common mental disorders in men are depression, anxiety, bipolar disorder, psychosis/schizophrenia, and eating disorder. Men are at higher risk than women for substance abuse and suicide.

Suicide Risk

The act of ending one's life is a devastating and harrowing experience; on average there are 121 suicides committed each day. Suicide is the tenth leading cause of death in the United States with 44,193 individuals committing suicide annually, and firearms account for almost half of all these suicides. Men who attempt suicide are more likely to succeed, at a rate three and half times higher than that of women. White men account for 7 out of every 10 suicides, with the suicide rate highest among middle-aged white men (CDC, 2015).

Women attempt suicide three times more often than men; however, when men attempt suicide they are more likely to die than women who attempt suicide. Rates of attempted suicide and suicide deaths vary considerably among demographic groups as well. The ratio of suicide attempts to suicide deaths in youth is estimated to be about 25:1 compared to about 4:1 in the elderly (CDC, 2015). Although suicide attempt data is not tracked, in 2013 there were 494,169 people treated in emergency departments for self-inflicted injuries (CDC, 2015), the closest proxy measure.

There are racial and ethnic disparities with suicides that mirror the same disparate impact on men. Suicide rates vary with subgroups and are affected by factors such as socioeconomic status, employment, occupation, sexual orientation, and gender identity (Substance Abuse and Mental Health Services Administration, 2015). Suicide is the eighth leading cause of death among American Indians/Alaskan Natives across all ages. Suicide rates among Asians and Pacific Islanders and blacks was half that of whites and American Indians/Alaskan Natives. Men in their middle-age years and from low socioeconomic status are more vulnerable to suicide than any other group (Wyllie et al., 2012).

Specific Populations and Mental Health

In practice providers encounter men from all walks of life who are multifaceted with a myriad of different traits and life experiences. It is important to understand the common experiences of men while not projecting stereotypical, preconceived notions onto our expectations and approaches. Treatment effectiveness is enhanced when practitioners take into account the unique life experiences of men.

OLDER MEN

The world's population of older men is growing rapidly, and by 2050, the proportion of the world's older adults is estimated to almost double from about 12% to 22% (WHO, 2016b). The life expectancy for men is 76.4 years, which is nearly 5 years younger than women (Stepler, 2016). Older men are considerably more likely than older women to live with their spouse; in 2014, 67% of older men lived with their spouse (down somewhat from 73% in 1990). Older unmarried men are increasingly likely to live alone (Stepler, 2016), and are at increased risk for loneliness and substance abuse. Over 20% of older adults suffer from a mental or neurological disorder (excluding headache disorders) and 6.6% of all disabilities are attributed to neurological and mental disorders (WHO, 2016b). From the 2000 to 2010 U.S. census, men showed a more rapid growth in the older population than women, noting the largest growth rate for a 10-year age group was for men 85 to 94 years old, indicating that men are living longer (Census Briefs, 2011).

GAY MEN

In 2017 10 million Americans, or 4.1% of the U.S. population, identified as lesbian, gay, bisexual, and transsexual (LGBT), up from 3.2% in 2012 (Gallup, 2017). Mental health issues appear slightly higher among gay men, with incidences of depression, anxiety, and suicidal ideation being two to three times higher than the general population. Many have turned to substances like tobacco, alcohol, and illicit drugs at a higher rate than the general population in order to cope with their emotional issues (King, 2009). For older gay men, many grew up during a time when being gay was ostracized by society. Therefore, they lived a secretive life, isolated from their families, learning to be guarded and living in fear of being exposed. This isolation and fear was even more pronounced for those older gay men who lived in areas that were not accepting of different expressions of sexuality, such as in a rural community, causing them to remain closeted. Many denied their true sexuality and married women and had families, compartmentalizing their real selves and developing skills that allowed them fit into mainstream expectations and society. Because of this lifetime of internal conflict and impulse supression, many older gay men have anxiety and depression (King, 2009).

Today's society is more accepting and open to gay men. More gay men choose to be open about their sexuality, describing a feeling of freedom. LGBT communities throughout the country have flourished, enabling an open lifestyle without fear of rejection. Gay men are at an increased risk of HIV infection, sexually transmitted diseases (STDs or STIs), and hepatitis (CDC, 2012). The practice of safe sex reduces the risk of STDs, so prevention of these infections through safe sex is critical in primary care. The introduction of retroviral medication has made HIV a chronic disease today. Of all the sexually transmitted infections gay men are at risk for, human papillomavirus (HPV), which causes anal and genital warts, is often thought to be a mere inconvenience. However, these infections may play a role in the increased rates of anal cancers in gay men (CDC, 2012). Some health professionals now recommend routine screening with anal Pap smears, similar to the test done on a cervix, to detect early anal cancers.

Gay men's culture in some geographic areas is greatly focused youth and physical fitness. As a result, some gay men have issues with poor body image. There can be abuse of steroids and certain supplements to gain muscle strength, as well as a tendency to exercise excessively. Gay men may be predisposed to eating disorders, such as bulimia or anorexia nervosa.

MENTAL HEALTH: PREVENTION

One of the challenges of any health problem is prevention. With mental health problems, especially in men, prevention is even more challenging because men view mental health as related to feelings, rather than a physical issue. Men have been socialized to not discuss feelings. Feelings are associated with feminity; consequently, men may feel weak or emasculated of sorts. Although this phenomenon is improving, through social media and other outlets seeking to address men's issues, the primary issue is that men do not tend to seek medical attention until there is a problem.

The healthcare community needs to create avenues that address the concerns of men, and educate men that seeking preventive healthcare measures are empowering rather than emasculating. Although most healthcare education programs do not emphasize curricula that introduce the nuances of the LGBT physical, mental, and sexual health needs, providers must recognize their own comfort level when caring for these populations (Chapter 11).

Fitness and Exercise

The benefits of fitness and exercise for overall health has been documented for many years. Exercise improves mental health by reducing anxiety, depression, and negative mood and by improving self-esteem and cognitive function. Exercise has also been found to alleviate symptoms such as low self-esteem and social withdrawal. Exercise can be used as a group social activity to improve health while preventing loneliness.

Diet and Nutrition

There is a growing belief that diet and mental health, both in the short- and long-term, are linked. There is also evolving evidence that specific diseases such as depression, schizophrenia, attention deficit hyperactivity disorder, and Alzheimer's disease may be prevented, controlled, and perhaps avoided with attention to proper nutritional intake. A large proportion of those who eat healthy do not experience as many mental health problems as compared with those that do not consume fresh fruit or vegetables on a daily basis. Primary care providers need to be stressing healthy diets, specifically to men, who tend to "eat conveniently" owing to the pressures of work life. Poor diets contribute not only to poor physical health, but also to affected mental health and overall well-being.

CONCLUSION: MALE-FRIENDLY CLINICAL ENVIRONMENT

It has been suggested that a way to improve men's health is for healthcare practices become "men friendly." What exactly does this mean and/or entail? As discussed previously, men tend to seek medical attention when there is a problem. Consequently, healthcare being stressed and stretched to limits, providers may only focus on the given problem owing to time constraints. What can providers do to improve their practice and make it "men friendly"?

Men need to understand what their reasons are for being in the office. Men respond well to a goal-oriented approach (Spar, 2014). Providers should approach the visit in this fashion, asking men pertinent questions about personal and health goals. The view concerning men's health is largely anything that is not women's health. Men are overrepresented in research studies, but there are conditions that are specific to men that are not even addressed in clinical practice. Addiction, substance abuse, and risk-taking are all more prevalent in men, compared with women, and men die younger than women. This is because men are less likely to seek medical care and because they are more prone to risk-taking and engaging in less healthy lifestyle behaviors. Acknowledging that men's health is a significant field may reach men in seeking medical attention.

Providing mental health services to men can be challenging because of outdated stereotypical views of what it means to be a man. These views are shared by both men themselves as well as society as a whole. Primary care providers and specialty providers alike should consider the man's overall view of self while understanding the impact of the context of the man's personal, work, family, and social life on promoting mental health and preventing mental disease in men. Providers need to understand that men may be less likely to share their emotions and feelings when addressing mental health issues. It is important for the clinical care setting to provide an open and welcoming environment that includes a well-informed attitude on men's mental health.

REFERENCES

American Psychological Association. (2012). Stress in America: Our health at risk. Retrieved from https://www.apa.org/news/press/releases/stress/2011/final-2011.pdf

Baker, P., Dworkin, S. L., Tong S., Banks, I., Shand, T., & Yamey, G. (2014). The men's health gap: Men must be included in the global health equity agenda. *Bulletin of the World Health Organization, 92,* 618–620. doi:10.2471/BLT.13.132795

Census Briefs. (2011). The older population: 2010. Retrieved from https://www.census.gov/prod/cen2010/briefs/c2010br-09.pdf

Centers for Disease Control and Prevention. (2012). Lesbian, gay, bisexual and transgender health. Retrieved from www.cdc.gov/lgbthealth

Centers for Disease Control and Prevention. (2015). Suicides. Retrieved from https://www.cdc.gov/violenceprevention/pdf/suicide-datasheet-a.pdf

Centers for Disease Control and Prevention. (2017). Health care access. Retrieved from https://www.cdc.gov/nchs/fastats/access-to-health-care.htm

Commission on Social Determinants of Health, World Health Organization. (2007). A conceptual framework for action on the social determinants of health. Retrieved from http://www.who.int/social_determinants/resources/csdh_framework_action_05_07.pdf?ua=1

Evans, J., Frank, B., Oliffe, J., & Gregory, D. (2011). Health, illness, men and masculinities (HIMM): A theoretical framework for understanding men and their health. *Journal of Men's Health, 8*(1), 7–15. doi:10.1016/j.jomh.2010.09.227

Gallup. (2017). In U.S., more identifying as LGBT. Retrieved from http://www.gallup.com/poll/201731/lgbt-identification-rises.aspx

Kaplan, S. (2016). Dear science: Why do we cry? *The Washington Post.* Retrieved from https://www.washingtonpost.com/news/speaking-of-science/wp/2016/11/28/dear-science-why-do-we-cry/?utm_term=.251de28eded5

King, M., Semlyen, J., Tai, S., Killaspy, H., Osborn, D., Popelyuk, D., & Nazareth, I. (2009). *Mental disorders, suicide, and deliberate self-harm in lesbian, gay and bisexual people: A systematic review of the literature.* London, UK: Department of Mental Health Sciences, Royal Free and University College Medical School.

Lucas J. W., & Benson, V. (2017). *Tables of summary health statistics for the U.S. population: 2015 National Health Interview Survey.* National Center for Health Statistics. Retrieved from http://www.cdc.gov/nchs/nhis/SHS/tables.htm

Lupis, S. B., Lerman, L., & Wolf, J. M. (2014). Anger responses to psychosocial stress predict heart rate and cortisol stress response in men but not women. *Psychoneuroendocrinology, 49,* 84–95. doi:10.1016/j.psyneuen.2014.07.004

McCarty, M. K., Kelly, J. R., & Williams, K. D. (2014). The cognitive costs of the counter-stereotypic: Gender, emotion and social presence. *The Journal of Social Psychology, 154,* 447–462. doi:10.1080/00224545.2014.933160

Moss-Racusin, C. A. (2015). Male backlash: Organizational penalties for men who violate gender stereotypes. In R. Burke & D. Major (Eds.), *Men in organizations: Allies or adversaries to women's career advancement* (pp. 247–269). London, UK: Edward Elgar Publishing.

Moss-Racusin, C. A., & Miller, H. G. (2016). "Taking charge" of stigma: Treatment seeking alleviates mental illness stigma targeting men. *Journal of Applied Social Psychology, 46,* 319–335. doi:10.1111/jasp.12362

Myers, J. (2016). *The future of men: Masculinity in the twenty-first century.* San Francisco, CA: Inkshares.

National Alliance on Mental Illness. (2015). Mental health by the numbers. Retrieved from http://www.nami.org/Learn-More/Mental-Health-By-the-Numbers

Spar, M. (2014). Addressing the unique needs of men. *Alternative and Complementary Therapies, 20*(4), 176–179. doi:10.1089/act.2014.20401

Stepler, R. (2016). Living arrangements of older Americans by gender. Retrieved from http://www.pewsocialtrends.org/2016/02/18/2-living-arrangements-of-older-americans-by-gender

Substance Abuse and Mental Health Services Administration. (2015). Suicide and race. Retrieved from https://blog.samhsa.gov/2015/07/28/suicide-and-race/#.WYRHZNPyuL8

Whitley, R. (2017). Men's mental health: A silent crisis. *Psychology Today.* Retrieved from https://www.psychologytoday.com/blog/talking-about-men/201702/mens-mental-health-silent-crisis

World Health Organization. (2016a). *Mental health and older adults.* Retrieved from http://www.who.int/mediacentre/factsheets/fs381/en

World Health Organization. (2016b). *World health statistics 2016: Monitoring health for the SDGs.* Geneva, Switzerland: Author.

Wyllie, C., Platt, S., Brownlie, J., Chandler, A., Connolly, S., ... Scourfild, J. (2012). Men, suicide and society: Why disadvantaged men in mid-life die by suicide. Retrieved from https://www.samaritans.org/sites/default/files/kcfinder/files/press/Men%20Suicide%20and%20Society%20Research%20Report%20151112.pdf

CHAPTER 15

Chronic Pain and Men

Susanne A. Quallich and Sallyanne M. Fisher

INTRODUCTION

Pain is a universal challenge and phenomenon that affects all people at some point in their life. One common definition is "Pain is whatever the experiencing person says it is, existing whenever the experiencing person says it does" (McCaffery, 1968). This does allude to the subjectivity of pain and the need to listen and observe the individual experiencing it. Chronic pain affects millions of people each year, and identifying the specifics of its effect on the sexes has been an emerging topic in recent years. Many studies identify that women report pain more frequently and are at higher risk yet have greater adaptability to chronic pain; men will often underreport pain, particularly to female providers. In the case of chronic pain, the importance of understanding how a male patient will experience pain is key to understanding the most efficacious way to help manage and control the pain.

In 1994 The International Association for the Study of Pain (IASP) developed a taxonomy for pain terms and this includes one of the most widely accepted definitions of pain. "Pain is an unpleasant sensory or emotional experience associated with actual or potential tissue damage, or described in terms of such damage" (Mersky & Bogduk, 1994). This group further notes "that pain is always subjective. Every individual learns the application of the word through experiences related to injury in early life. It is unquestionably a sensation in a part or parts of the body, but it is also always unpleasant and therefore also an emotional experience ... If they regard their experience as pain and if they report it in the same ways as pain caused by tissue damage, it should be accepted as pain" (International Association for the Study of Pain, 1994, para. 5). Inherent in the IASP definition is the multifactorial nature of pain, and acceptance of this IASP definition suggests that management of any chronic pain occurs within the larger social and healthcare context, must include quality of life, and must address psychosocial components (Rosenquist et al., 2010). One of the difficulties providers are confronted with is that there is often a report of pain without evidence of tissue damage or pathophysiological causes.

This introduces an important concept. Pain comprises several dimensions: sensory—where and how much it hurts; emotional—the unpleasantness of it; and cognitive—the interpretation based upon past experiences, fears, anxieties, and the threat it poses (Crofford, 2015). This multidimensional aspect of pain can adversely affect a patient's function, quality of life, emotional state, social and vocational status, and general well-being (Duenas, Ojeda, Salazar, Mico, & Failde, 2016). Accordingly, healthcare providers are challenged to provide optimal treatment while attempting to identify the type and source of pain and its severity and impact on the individual experiencing it.

INCIDENCE

Identifying the level and amount of pain experienced by the general population is a difficult task. Most information is the result of surveys of people who chronicle their pain. As always, the subjectivity of pain makes understanding the true extent of the problem challenging.

Data from the United States 2012 National Health Interview Survey reveals that 25.3 million adults (11.2%) are suffering from daily (chronic) pain and 23.4 million (10.3%) are reporting "a lot" of pain (Nahin, 2015; Stanos et al., 2016). There was also evidence that females had a higher incidence of category 3 and 4 pain (0–10 scale), particularly non-Hispanic, English preferred, African American, and Caucasian females. In Britain, Price, Lee, Taylor and Baranowski (2014) noted that 67% of the people in an English health survey with long-term pain identified having anxiety or depression as well. Chronic pain affects employment, access to housing, and high healthcare use (Price et al., 2014). A study done recently by Kawai, Kawai, Wollan, and Yawn (Kawai, Kawai, Wollan, & Yawn, 2017) identified in one county in Minnesota that chronic pain, particularly multisite pain and neuropathic pain, significantly affected physical and psychological health. The report further notes this included depression, reduced activities of daily living, and reduced work performance but not loss of work hours (Kawai et al., 2017). Murphy et al. (Murphy et al., 2017) report the economic cost in the United States alone is as high as $635 billion.

PATHOPHYSIOLOGY OF PAIN

There are two major classes in pain physiology: Normal or nociceptive and abnormal or pathophysiological. The central nervous system (CNS) is responsible for carrying signals from the spinal cord to the brain, the nerves, and finally the body. As described by Zelick (2015) this involves the afferent pathway (nerves that receive information or stimuli) and the efferent pathway (nerves that carry sensation to muscles and stimulate responses). The afferent portion includes pain receptors (nociceptors), afferent nerve fibers, and the spinal cord network. The afferent pathways terminate in the dorsal horn of the spinal cord (first afferent neuron). The second afferent neuron creates the spinal part of the afferent system. The limbic system, reticular formation, thalamus, hypothalamus, and cortex are the components of the CNS involved in the interpretation of pain signals. The efferent pathways are responsible for modulating pain sensation. They are composed of the fibers connecting the reticular formation, midbrain, and substantia gelatinosa (SG). Pain, and the science behind it, is continuously evolving. In 1965, Melzack and Wall introduced the gate control theory of pain management that has revolutionized the world's understanding of pain mechanisms and management (Katz & Rosenbloom, 2017). According to this theory, as explained by Zelick (2015), nociceptive impulses are transmitted to the spinal cord through large A-delta and small C fibers The cells in the spinal cord function as a gate, regulating transmission of impulses to the CNS. The stimulation of larger nerve fibers (A-alpha, A-beta) causes the cells in SG to "close the gate." A closed gate decreases stimulation of T cells (the second afferent neuron), which decreases transmission of impulses, and diminishes pain perception.

The communication of pain occurs by transduction, transmission, modulation, and perception. Transduction is a physiological process whereby a noxious mechanical, chemical, or thermal stimulus is converted (transduced) via specialized receptors on primary afferents into nociceptive impulses. Once transduced and generated, transmission occurs, whereby action potentials (nerve impulses) are conducted to the CNS primarily via two types of primary afferent neurons: thinly myelinated, faster conducting A-delta fibers and unmyelinated, slowly conducting C fibers, both termed primary afferents. These impulses are then sent to the dorsal horn of the spinal cord and then along the sensory tracts to the brain.

Action potentials result from activation of specific sodium channels. Nociceptive impulses travel along these peripheral nerve fibers (peripheral transmission) to the dorsal horn of the spinal cord where they synapse with the second-order neurons (synaptic transmission). Here, the impulse is further transmitted via neurons that cross the spinal cord and ascend to the thalamus and branches to the brainstem nuclei (central transmission). The nociceptive impulses are then relayed to multiple areas of the brain including the somatosensory cortex, the insula, frontal lobes, and limbic system. At this point, modulation occurs, which is the

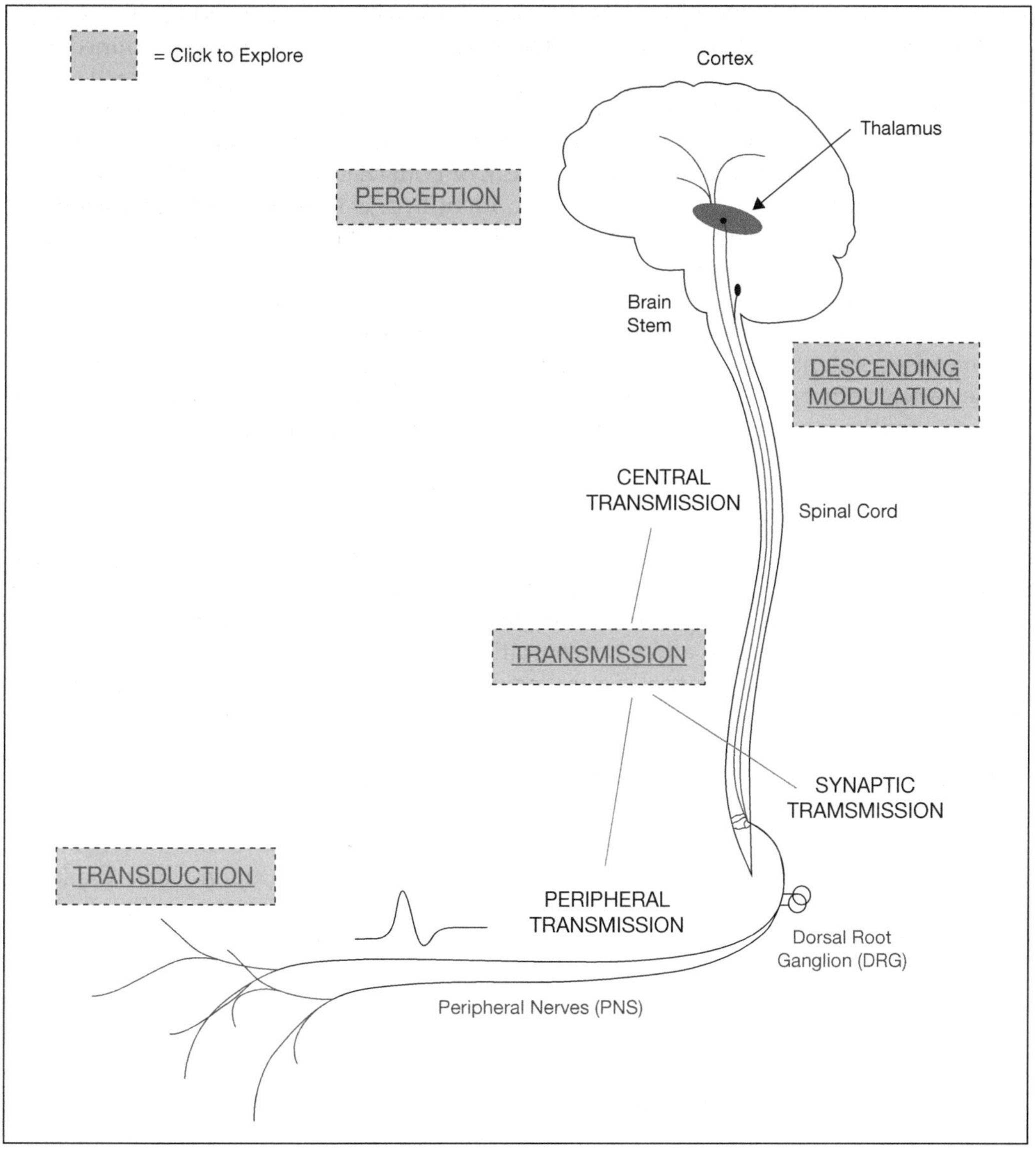

FIGURE 15.1 Representation of Pain Pathway.

Source: Reprinted with permission from University of Wisconsin School of Medicine and Public Health. (2010). Principles of pain assessment—pain management. Retrieved from http://projects.hsl.wisc.edu/GME/PainManagement/session3.1.html

process of dampening or amplifying pain-related neural signals, primarily in the dorsal horn of the spinal cord, but also elsewhere, with input from ascending and descending pathways. Finally, perception, the subjective experience of feeling pain that results from the interaction of transduction, transmission, modulation, and psychological aspects of the individual, ensues (Figure 15.1).

TYPES OF PAIN

In the broadest of terms, pain is classified as acute and chronic. Zacharoff, Pujol, and Corsini (2010) identify acute pain as sudden onset; often it has an identifiable cause (surgery, disease, injury), is of short duration (<1 month), and can be characterized by moaning, crying, or rubbing or holding the affected area. Chronic pain, on the other hand, may have an undetermined onset or may be a pain that continues beyond the period of expected healing (Price et al., 2014). Conventional definitions offer that pain becomes persistent pain beyond 3 to 6 months; it is usually a result of a chronic condition or disease and the functional impairment is prolonged. This impairment can be physical, psychological, or both (Zacharoff et al., 2010). Price et al. (2014) note that the term "chronic" has been identified as suggestive of depression and futility so in the pathway it is recommended to use the term "persistent." Additionally, they indicate that the label "chronic pain patient" may lead to a failure to assess and reassess the causes of pain, whereas the term "persistent" recognizes the presence of a pain condition but does not lessen the imperative to reach an appropriative diagnosis. Those affected by chronic or persistent pain, which develops over time, may also succumb to hopelessness. These patients often develop significant behavioral and psychological comorbid conditions such as depression, preoccupation with pain, insomnia, and irritability.

Contributors to pain are superficial (arising from skin and mucous membranes), deep (somatic) in skin, tissues and muscles arising from nerves in the skin and deep tissue and visceral, originating in internal organs or viscera (Table 15.1). Zacharoff et al. (2010) further identified that pain is also categorized as nociceptive, inflammatory, neurogenic, neuropathic, cutaneous, somatic, and visceral. Nociceptive can be a "normal" pain, such as stepping on a nail. This is usually very short lived. Somatic nociceptors, located in bones, blood vessels, and ligaments, have a low concentration of nerve endings. This pain is dull and poorly localized, and lasts longer. Visceral pain stems from the organs or visceral cavities; these nociceptors are even fewer in number, resulting in longer duration of a diffuse aching sensation. Inflammatory pain occurs when skin, muscle, or bone become injured and an inflammatory reaction sets in. After the tissue heals, the pain resolves. But this pain can progress to a chronic pain state due to changes in the local neuroanatomy and eventually remodeling of the CNS. Neuropathic pain arises from damaged or dysfunctional nerves. It is further broken down in to peripheral or central pain depending upon where the lesion is located. An injury to skin or superficial tissues is cutaneous. These injuries produce well-localized pain due to an abundance of nerve endings from the cutaneous nociceptors that end just under the skin (Zacharoff et al., 2014).

As pain goes, perhaps the most feared version is chronic pain. Acute and end-of-life pain follow a predictable and linear trajectory, are short lived, and generally respond well to opioids (Ballantyne, Kalso, & Stannard, 2016). The World Health Organization's (WHO) analgesic stepladder provides a simple, easy to follow format for cancer pain that has been adapted for use in acute pain as well. Unfortunately, many providers have erred in using this concept to attempt to treat chronic pain in a similar fashion. Chronic pain is not predictable, is persistent or intermittent, and usually defined as lasting at least 6 months. The cause is often unknown, often develops insidiously, and very often is associated with a sense of hopelessness and helplessness so that depression often results.

TABLE 15.1 Types of Pain

Pain Type	Descriptors Used by Patients	Etiology	Examination Findings	Treatment
Neuropathic (pain signal can be felt at site distant from sensory ending affected; may be result of inflammation, infection, nerve entrapment, metabolic derangements, malnutrition, radiation, autoimmune disease)	Burning Shooting Stabbing Cramping Shock-like Tingling Numbness Radiating Cold/hot	Nerve involvement • Tumor • Postherpetic neuralgia • Diabetic neuropathy • Post stroke pain Co-analgesics • Anticonvulsants • Antidepressants • SSNRIs • Local anesthetics	Hypoesthesia Numbness Paresthesias Dysesthesias Pain Stabbing or shock-like sensations with mechanical force over injured nerve	Use of medications that act as membrane stabilizers • Antidepressants ▪ Tricyclics ▪ SSRI ▪ SNRI • Anticonvulsants • Antiarrhythmics • Local anesthetics Anxiolytics Opioids as last resort
Nociceptive (neurons that detect potentially noxious stimuli, such as pressure, heat, cold, tissue acidification)				
Visceral (poorly localized, diffuse pain)	Squeezing Cramping Pressure Distention Deep pain Referred pain can be shaper and better localized	Tumors occupying the liver, pancreas, spleen Postoperative (abdominal surgery) Ascites Irritable bowel syndrome	Secondary hyperalgesia of superficial or deep body wall tissues Can be accompanied by *autonomic symptoms*: profuse sweating, nausea, GI disturbances, alternations to in body temperature, blood pressure, heart rate Strong affective component: anxiety, depression	Opioids Non-opioids • Acetaminophen • NSAIDs • paracetomol
Somatic (well localized)	Gnawing Prickling Sharp Dull Achy Squeezing throbbing sore	Muscle or joint injury Bone metastases Mucositis, Skin lesions (e.g., sunburn)	Reflex muscle spasm Tenderness to palpation Allodynia Sympathetic nervous system hyperactivity (e.g., pallor, dilated pupils, increased muscle tension) Hyperalgesia	Non-opioids • Acetaminophen • NSAIDs • Paracetomol Co-analgesics • Corticosteroids • Local anesthetics • Bisphosphonates • Radioisotopes

SNRI, serotonin and norepinephrine reuptake inhibitors; SSRI, selective serotonin reuptake inhibitors.

TYPES OF CHRONIC PAIN

Chronic pain is the result of the aberrant functioning of the peripheral or central nervous system that has been pathologically modified, due to one or more abnormal cellular signaling mechanisms. Chronic pain can be the result of poorly treated or improperly identified pain that gradually becomes more complex than what the original injury or insult would suggest. There can be both structural and functional alterations in both central and peripheral nervous systems, resulting in a pain condition that is entirely separate from any other pathology. Chronic pain, however, is far more complex than simple biology; inappropriate inputs from nerve endings, the hypothalamic-pituitary-axis, psychology, socioeconomics, cognition, and influences from the healthcare system work to create and sustain an individual's chronic pain experience (Gatchel, McGeary, McGeary, & Lippe, 2014; Turk & Melzack, 2011).

Chronic pain can be described in many ways. Nociceptive pain is produced by primary afferent neurons, including unmyelinated C fibers and myelinated Adelta fibers that are activated by chemical, thermal, and high threshold mechanical signals that indicate damage or danger (Melzack & Wall, 2008). Inflammatory pain results from the interaction of the nervous system and inflammatory mediators that can cause peripheral sensitization and result in a triad of hallmark symptoms: allodynia, hyperalgesia, and spontaneous pain. Inflammatory pain is generally considered adaptive because it does have an important role in tissue protection (Woolf, 2011); however, it becomes maladaptive in the context of chronic inflammation. Inflammation and tissue damage can work together to cause the release of substances that activate peripheral nociceptors and cause a reduction in their activation threshold. This results in nerve endings that are much more responsive to any stimulation. Neuropathic pain, on the other hand, is a clinical description and a condition that may result from trauma or infection, or after other damage to tissue that leads to a sensitization and proliferation of nerve fibers. Neuropathic pain is of neural origin; it can be used generally to encompass a dysfunctional type of pain, or more specifically to refer to pain from peripheral nerve injury (Woolf, 2010). This type of pain is often characterized as shooting, stabbing, or electric pain and does not serve a protective purpose.

Pain that occurs without a history of a specific injury has also been considered be neuropathic pain, given that CNS factors are posited to be involved. This specific type of neuropathic pain is also known as central pain. Central pain is thought to be associated with the concept of central sensitization, which is not meant to exclude contributions from peripheral sensory input, and indicates that CNS factors alone can increase pain levels (Clauw, 2014). Central sensitization results after a process similar to peripheral sensitization but at the level between the primary and parent neuron and secondary projecting neurons in the dorsal horn of the spinal cord. This process involves neuronal remodeling from damage, or overstimulated peripheral nerves, and results in effects at multiple levels including the synapse, the spinal cord, and the neuronal transmission pathways in the CNS. This remodeling process is believed to be vital in chronic pain conditions, and results in amplification of impulses from nonstimulated nerve fibers after input from a separate set of nociceptive fibers (Woolf, 2011). Clinically this presents as pain that is not representative of actual noxious stimuli, representing the ability of the CNS to both remodel and amplify pain. Indicators of central sensitization include pain sensitivity in areas without pathology; pain at the end of the stimulus; and maintenance of pain by low-intensity stimuli that typically do not provoke pain (Woolf, 2011).

Advances in the knowledge of brain chemistry have added to the present understanding of chronic pain. There are measurable differences in brain chemistry with the use of varying verbal descriptors of pain, and this extends to the concentrations of neurotransmitters in various areas of the brain when imaged with a functional MRI scan (Apkarian, Baliki, & Geha, 2009). This is important because there is no distinct pain center of the brain (Jensen,

2010; Jensen & Turk, 2014) meaning that the processing of pain requires the synchronization of nonlocalized brain areas involved in sensory, emotional, motivational, and cognitive processes (Tracey & John, 2010). This provides evidence for the "pain matrix" first described by Melzack (1999) but also demonstrated that this collection of brain regions coordinate to create a multidimensional perception of pain. As additional brain regions are recruited in response to a pain sensation, a distinct and individual perception of pain emerges (Tracey & John, 2010). But many chronic pain conditions may have a similar underlying mechanism: aberrant processing of somatosensory input (Gereau et al., 2014).

Advances in the understanding of pain from brain imaging do not alleviate difficulties in pain assessment within a clinical context. Pain experience and its appraisal are subjective and may not be consistent with objectively gathered data (e.g., heart rate, blood pressure, medication refills). Reports are limited by the unidimensional nature (i.e., pain intensity) of typically employed instruments (Tait & Chibnall, 2014) meaning that within the context of a typical clinic visit a full perspective is not investigated; different pain patients may have different pain trajectories and needs for clinical management.

Comorbid Conditions

Considered from a utilitarian perspective, the most basic function of acute pain is to command one's attention to possible injury that might threaten survival. However, in the absence of acute tissue damage or injury, such as with chronic pain, prolonged pain is largely maladaptive. Chronic pain impacts many domains, not solely psychological or physical (Jensen & Turk, 2014; Institute of Medicine, 2011; Molton & Terrill, 2014). Full description of this illness burden is complex, and must acknowledge age-related differences. Duenas et al. (2016) reviewed numerous studies that reported the negative impact that pain has on these domains, including

- Quality of life
- Functional capacity/limited activity
- Fatigue
- Sleep disturbance/sleep deprivation
- Mood (depression/anxiety/anger)
- Dyscognition (memory/attention)
- Coping mechanisms
- Gender-specific issues

Chronic pain is associated with numerous comorbid conditions that directly influence quality of life and overall health; it increases one's risk for other health issues, while simultaneously decreasing quality of life and creating financial strain (Institute of Medicine, 2011).

Positive or negative moods and expectations also influence outcomes and decrease or increase reports of pain (Bushnell, čeko, & Low, 2013). Both emotion and distraction influence pain perception; more pronounced baseline psychological issues or difficulty coping will have a direct impact on an individual's response to pain (Bushnell et al., 2013). Pain itself provokes an emotional response, and it is this unique reaction that sets the stage for treatment successes and failures as well as potential disability (Watson & Kendall, 2013). Depression, for example, is both a normal reaction to pain and decreased activity, but can also become pathological in chronic pain states (Watson & Kendall, 2013). Pain is an independent risk factor for depression, and depression is also a sequalea of recovery from pain, one that is influenced by biological, behavioral, cognitive, and social factors (Pakpour, Nikoobakht, & Campbell, 2015), highlighting the value of the biopsychosocial approach.

Psychological and social beliefs and behaviors can both create and perpetuate maladaptive coping. Pain behaviors alone can sustain pain and create disability that is not a function of the pain itself, such as a lack of movement leading to muscle weakness (Jensen & Turk, 2014). Clinics and researchers that have adopted the biopsychosocial model (BPSM) have gradually moved from a purely biological model to one that includes important functional and psychological aspects, in addition to the biology of nociception.

Because chronic pain is also subject to the individual's interpretation, it may be possible to predict poor adaptation to chronic pain based on the evaluation of emotional states or attitudes toward pain. Scott, Kroenke, Wu, and Yu (2016) note that depression, pain catastrophizing, and anxiety commonly co-occur with chronic pain. Anxiety, depression, and anger/frustration can predict functional limitations, appraisals of control over pain, and variations in pain intensity. Gatchel, Peng, Peters, Fuchs, and Turk (2007) detailed multiple studies linking emotional states to chronic pain, and suggested that pain and emotions interact in a variety of ways to promote and sustain comorbid symptoms. For example, anxiety has been implicated in increased affective pain responses and maladaptive pain behaviors because it represents uncertainty about the future and uncertainty about the meaning of the pain (Gatchel et al., 2007; Serbic, D., Pincus, T., Fife-Schaw, C., & Dawson, 2016). Pain-related anxiety can result in avoidance of activities that promote recovery and may have a role in amplification of somatosensory input (Lumley et al., 2011).

As a further example, recent studies have evaluated the role of anxiety prospectively to determine risk factors that may predict chronic postoperative pain. Anxiety preoperatively was the primary predictor of chronic postsurgical pain (Jackson, Tian, Wang, Iezzi, & Xie, 2016; Powell et al., 2012), suggesting that patients with higher baseline anxiety may be more prone to develop chronic pain. A recent study of predictors to pain adjustment in spinal cord–injured patients used the BPSM as its theoretical framework, and demonstrated that catastrophizing predicted greater interference due to, or distraction from, pain (Raichle, Hanley, Jensen, & Cardenas, 2007). The authors of both these studies related these responses to the participants' belief about their pain, stating that with chronic pain often came the belief that they were disabled. This is consistent with other authors who have reported that social situations can reinforce these perceptions, contributing to a "disabled" mindset (Flor, 2014; Jensen & Turk, 2014).

Anxiety can become hypervigilence or catastrophizing, both of which predict a low incidence of treatment success (Karoly & Ruehlman, 2007; Sullivan et al., 2001). Patients who catastrophize have difficulty redirecting their attention away from painful stimuli and may suffer even higher decline on activities that require attention, having developed the habit of viewing all sensations as painful stimuli first. Catastrophizing is implicated in increased pain reports, more illness behavior, and both physical and psychological dysfunction across populations (Gatchel et al., 2014; Institute of Medicine, 2011; Lumley et al., 2011; Scott et al., 2016; Seminowicz & Davis, 2006; Sullivan, 2009). Improvement in depression, anxiety, and pain catastrophizing predicts better pain outcomes, with improvement in depression being the most beneficial (Scott et al., 2016;). Outcomes due to this maladaptive behavior are not restricted to chronic pain populations.

ASSESSMENT OF PAIN

Once a patient presents for care, one must always ask if he is currently experiencing pain, or if he has in the last few months. Pain, as noted previously, is a subjective, multidimensional experience. Therefore, it is critical that the provider obtain an accurate and careful assessment of the pain (Stanos et al., 2016). Zacharoff et al. (2010) state that clinicians should reassure patients that their pain is being taken seriously, with an attempt to understand its impact on their overall life and the need for treatment. It is important to believe the patient's reports of pain and be respectful; for example, patients with chronic noncancer pain may have had poor encounters with clinicians in the past and may be hesitant to discuss their concerns. Even if there is a history of addiction or psychological concerns, a careful validation of their distress will lead to improved treatment planning (Zacharoff et al., 2010). Active listening and attention to details of the patient's symptoms will help direct the physical examination and narrow the pain differential diagnosis (University of Wisconsin School of Medicine and Public Health, 2010).

Patient History

Lack of proficient and uniform pain assessment is one of the most challenging barriers in achieving adequate pain control (Glowacki, 2015; Stanos et al., 2016). According to the University of Wisconsin (University of Wisconsin School of Medicine and Public Health, 2010) and Zacharoff et al. (2010) it is of utmost importance to ask specific questions to elicit a full understanding of the patient's pain complaint. It is recommended to ask about the location, quality, and intensity of the pain. Include questions regarding the characteristics of the pain and the aggravating or alleviating factors. Explore how the pain impacts the patient's lifestyle, function, and quality of life. Ask the patient when the pain started and what treatment has been used in the past along with the effectiveness of that treatment. It is also important to ask about the patient's expectations and goals. It is always wise to ask about pain at the initial meeting with a patient and after known pain events. The University of Wisconsin School of Medicine and Public Health developed the mnemonic QISS TAPED to help remember these elements: quality, impact, site, severity, temporal characteristics, aggravating and alleviating factors, impact of pain on function and quality of life, past treatment and response, patient expectations and goals, and then the diagnostics and examination (Table 15.2).

Physical Examination

The physical examination should always include a general physical evaluation as well as a thorough, focused musculoskeletal, neurological, and psychological assessment in order to establish both the potential cause of pain and the likely pathophysiological type(s) of pain (Stanos et al., 2016; Zacharoff et al., 2010). The general appearance of the patient, including attributes of the skin, posture, and demeanor, are important aspects of the general physical examination (University of Wisconsin School of Medicine and Public Health, 2010; Zacharoff et al., 2010).

Any examination for a pain condition needs to include the individual's functional capacity. This includes sexual health. It is crucial to evaluate the site of the reported pain as well as any areas of referred pain to gain a full understanding of the problem. In the case of a musculoskeletal assessment, carefully examine the area in question, including all related areas. Many times knee pain is the complaint, but consider all the structures that affect this, such as the low back, hip, foot, and ankle as well as supporting ligaments, tendons, bones, and muscles (University of Wisconsin School of Medicine and Public Health, 2010; Zacharoff et al., 2010). The neurological screening examination should include standard elements, with testing of the cranial nerves II through XII. Motor and sensory functioning in the limbs and an evaluation of rectal and urinary sphincter function are also recommended. Additionally, if warrented, perform the pathological reflexive signs, such as those of Babinski, Oppenheim, Gordon, Chaddock, Schaefer, and Hoffman (Zacharoff et al., 2010). It is also necessary to do a thorough sensory examination to help establish the causes and possible origins of the pain complaints (Table 15.3).

TABLE 15.2 Pain Assessment Mnemonic (QISS TAPED)

Q	Quality	What were your first symptoms? What words would you use to describe the pain? (achy, sharp, burning, squeezing, dull, icy, etc.) Besides sensations you consider to be "pain," are there other unusual sensations, such as numbness?
I	Impact	How does the pain affect you? How does the pain impact your sleep, activity, mood, appetite (other—work, relationships, exercise, etc.) What does the pain prevent you from doing? (Depression screen) Do you feel sad or blue? Do you cry often? Is there loss of interest in life? Decreased or increased appetite? (Anxiety screen) Do you feel stressed or nervous? Have you been particularly anxious about anything? Do you startle easily?
S	Site	Show me where you feel the pain. Can you put your finger/hand on it? Or show me on a body map? Does the pain move/radiate anywhere? Has the location changed over time?
S	Severity	On a 0–10 scale with 0 = no pain and 10 = the worst pain imaginable, how much pain are you in right now? What is the least pain you have had in the past (24 hours, one week, month)? What is the worst pain you have had in the past (24 hours, one week, month)? How often are you in *severe* pain (hours in a day, days a week you have pain)?
T	Temporal Characteristics	When did the pain start? Was it sudden? Gradual? Was there a clear triggering event? Is the pain constant or intermittent? Does it come spontaneously or is it provoked? Is there a predictable pattern? (e.g., Is it always worst in the morning or in the evening? Does it suddenly flare up?)
A	Aggravating and Alleviating Factors	What makes the pain better? What makes the pain worse? When do you get the best relief? How much relief do you get? How long does it last?
P	Past Response, Preferences	How have you managed your pain in the past? (Ask about both drug and non-drug methods) What helped? What did not help? (Be specific about drug trials—how much and how long?) What medications have you tried? Was the dose increased until you had pain relief or side effects? How long did you take the drug? Are there any pain medicines that have caused you an allergic or other bad reaction? How do you feel about taking medications? Have you tried physical or occupational therapy? What was done? Was it helpful? Have you tried spinal or other injections for pain treatment? What was done? Was it helpful?

(*continued*)

TABLE 15.2 Pain Assessment Mnemonic (QISS TAPED) (*continued*)

E	Expectations, Goals, Meaning	What do you think is causing the pain? How may we help you? What do you think we should do to treat your pain? What do you hope the treatment will accomplish? What do you want to do that the pain keeps you from doing? What are you most afraid of? (Uncovers specific fears, such as fear of cancer, which should be acknowledged and addressed.)
D	Diagnostics and Physical Exam	Examine and inspect site (see below) Perform a systems assessment and examination as indicated Review imaging, laboratory and/or other test results as indicated

Source: Reprinted with permission from University of Wisconsin School of Medicine and Public Health. (2010). Principles of pain assessment—pain management. Retrieved from http://projects.hsl.wisc.edu/GME/PainManagement/session3.1.html

Opioid-Induced Hypogonadism

With the acknowledged epidemic of metrics for both inpatient and outpatient management of patient pain complaints, increasing numbers of men have been tried on or chronically prescribed narcotic pain medications for their pain management. But these medications have a hidden risk with persistent (then chronic) use. Aside from the well-recognized adverse effects including constipation, sedation, and nausea, chronic opioid use can also cause endocrine abnormalities. There is a link between hypogonadism and heightened pain, suggesting that hypogonadal men experience worse pain. Additionally, both men and women with OPIAD/OIH (see below) may suffer from infertility.

A lesser known sequela is opioid-induced androgen deficiency (OPIAD) or opioid-induced hypogonadism (OIH). The primary issue remains that these symptoms and side effects will happen with different duration and doses in each individual, suggesting that any male patient who has been using opioids for pain control be screened for hypogonadism. These alterations in the hypothalamus-pituitary-gonadal (HPG) axis induced by exposure to opioids result in hypogonadotropic hypogonadism. This syndrome is often associated with distressing symptoms such as reduced libido, erectile dysfunction, fatigue, hot flashes, depression, mood alterations, and reduced quality of life (Basaria et al., 2017). Physical findings may include reduced facial and body hair, anemia, decreased muscle mass, weight gain, and osteopenia or osteoporosis (Raheem, Patel, Sisul, Furnish, & Hsieh, 2017). Men taking opioid therapy equivalent to 100 mg of morphine daily should be monitored for development of hypogonadism (Brennan, 2013).

Gudin, Laitman, and Nalamachu (2015) reviewed the available literature regarding OPIAD and noted several relevant factors for men and the opioid prescribing provider. Several studies note that a lesser known side effect of mu opioid analgesics is endocrinopathy, which can contribute to impaired sexual function, decreased libido, and infertility, and be associated long term with osteoporosis and osteopenia (Gudin et al., 2015). In addition most patients do not report these signs to their provider, so it goes unmonitored. It is inherent that many people consider testosterone in men to be strictly related to libido and erectile function, yet testosterone also plays an important role in the prevention of osteopenia and osteoporosis, muscle maintenance, and exercise tolerance. Gudin et al. (2015) also noted that testosterone appears to be involved in endogenous opioid activity. It is fundamental for the binding of opioid receptors, activation of dopamine, and norepinephrine activity, as

TABLE 15.3 Components of a Sensory Examination for Pain Assessment

Sensation	Nerve Fiber Type/ Receptor	Testing Tool	Technique of Testing	Abnormal Findings		Indicates
				↓ (decrease)	↑ (increase)	
Light touch (LT)	Aβ fibers/ Meissner's Pacinian Hair follicle Merkel Ruffini	Brush, cotton wisp/swab/ von Frey hairs	Touch or gentle rub Perpendicular contact with skin surface until fiber bends	Hypoaesthesia or anesthesia	1. Hyperesthesia: increased LT-pain 2. Allodynia: increased LT+ pain Dynamic mechanical (rub); static mechanical (pressure; von Frey)	Sensitization: central and/or peripheral
Sharp (punctuate)	Aδ fibers/ unencapsulated free nerve endings	Pin (safety pin, Medipin, Neuropen)	Perpendicular contact with skin surface without breaching skin integrity	Pinprick hypoalgesia (sharp sensation perceived as dull sensation)	Pinprick hyperalgesia: sharp and excessively painful	Sensitization: central and/or peripheral
Vibration	Aβ fibers/Pacinian	Tuning fork at 128 Hz	Vibrate the tuning fork and place stem on a bony prominence, e.g., malleolus	Hypoesthesia	1. Hyperesthesia: increased without pain 2. Allodynia: increased & painful	Sensitization: central
Cold	Aδ fibers and C fibers/ unencapsulated free nerve endings					

Source: Reprinted with permission from University of Wisconsin School of Medicine and Public Health. Principles of pain assessment—pain management. (2010). Retrieved from http://projects.hsl.wisc.edu/GME/PainManagement/session3.1.html

well as maintenance of blood-brain barrier transport. Deficient testosterone may manifest as poor control of pain, lack of energy, and disturbance of sleep.

Rubenstein and Carpenter (2014) performed a retrospective study of men receiving long-acting opioids versus those on short-acting versions. They concluded that long-acting opioids are associated with a greater odds ratio of androgen deficiency than equivalent doses of short-acting opioids. Additionally, dose was significantly associated with androgen deficiency, but more so for men on short-acting than on long-acting opioids.

Recently, Basaria et al. (2015) evaluated the efficacy of testosterone replacement on pain perception and other androgen-dependent outcomes in men with opioid-induced hypogonadism. In the first randomized, double-blind placebo-controlled trial of testosterone replacement to men with OPIAD, the authors confirmed the antinociceptive role of testosterone. The patients receiving testosterone therapy had improved pain sensitivity to several noxious painful stimuli and enjoyed improved sexual desire and body composition.

Raheem et al. (2017) sought to follow up on this by studying the effect of testosterone therapy on chronic pain as measured subjectively with Numerical Rating Scale (NRS) and objectively with daily morphine equivalent dose (MED). This pilot study demonstrated that testosterone therapy is associated with improvement in the quality of life and reduction of opioid requirements in chronic pain patients. The authors suggest that providers should consider screening of male chronic pain patients undergoing long-term opioid therapy for OIH. Testosterone therapy should be offered to appropriate men with the goal of not only improving hypogonadal symptoms but also decreasing opioid requirements (Raheem et al., 2017). However, this was a small study of only 27 patients, so careful selection of patients is prudent and further study is advised. A prospective observational study by Ajo et al. (2017) was done on a cohort of men receiving chronic pain management and self-reported erectile dysfunction. After treatment in an Andrology Unit with phosphodiesterase type 5 inhibitor (PDE5i) and/or testosterone gel, there was a positive correlation in erectile function, quality of sexual life, and improved anxiety; but there was no significant change in testosterone levels, pain levels, or quality of life.

GENDER GAP REGARDING GENITAL CHRONIC PAIN CONDITIONS

There are clear gender differences in prevalence for some types of chronic pain. It is postulated that there are differences in pain perception between the genders as well. Racine et al. (Racine et al., 2012a) reported that 10 years of experimental data failed to establish a consistent pattern of differences between the genders with *experimental* pain testing. These authors concluded that study results were heavily influenced by the outcome measures chosen and the pain modalities tested, but this has unclear implications clinically. This same group of authors went on to examine the literature regarding possible biopsychosocial factors in pain sensitivity between the genders (Racine et al., 2012b). Their systematic review showed that anxiety was a stronger predictor of pain in men, and may have an increased effect on pain perception in males. This paper also reported that distraction may be an efficient coping style for men faced with pain. Gender expectations seem to have a role in *experimental* pain perceptions, but again this is an unclear relationship to clinical presentation. Racine et al. (2012b) concluded that current data are insufficient to establish a true influence from biopsychosocial factors and pain perception between men and women. Gender differences in pain intensity and pain perception, as this manifests *clinically*, remain poorly described and poorly understood.

Chronic pain is a complex and difficult clinical symptom to understand because of the subjective and personal nature of the complaint and the influence of an individual's perception and past experiences (Crofford, 2015; Gatchel et al., 2014; Turk & Melzack, 2011; Tait &

Chibnall, 2014), meaning that this experience can only be assessed indirectly. Vulvodynia is a chronic pain condition, and ongoing research seeks to evaluate the underlying pain mechanisms while combining specific physiological and psychological interventions (Cox & Neville, 2012; Zhang et al., 2011). Standard evaluation of women with a chronic genital pain condition, such as vulvodynia, follows a process that includes questioning the woman about the personal meaning and attributes of her pain and her sexual function (Bergeron, Rosen, & Morin, 2011; Fall et al., 2010; Haefner et al., 2005; Johansen & Weidner, 2002). This implies a paradigm shift toward understanding this condition as multifactorial, recognizing the subjective nature of pain and the interplay of biological, psychological, and social factors that contribute to and sustain an illness experience (Bergeron, 2011) such as the interplay of their perceptions of their femininity and a desire for validation of their pain. The chronic pain of vulvodynia, as in any chronic pain condition, leads to peripheral processing changes especially with a longer duration of pain (Zhang et al., 2011). This results in more somatic complaints, lower pain thresholds, higher subjective estimation of pain, increased hypervigilance, and higher trait anxiety when compared with both other chronic pain patients and control patients (Cox & Neville, 2012; Haefner, et al., 2005; Turk & Melzack, 2011).

Specifics of Male Genital Pain

Reports of chronic genital pain conditions in men fail to evaluate their experience in a social, sexual, and self-esteem context, and there is no precedent for evaluating genital pain conditions, or specifically testicular/genital pain conditions, as a multifactorial condition in men. Investigations of overall coping, symptom perception, and pain-related disability are vital to understanding the chronic pain experience (Turk & Melzack, 2011) of men with chronic unexplained orchialgia (CUO), and would require a shift in focus away from the present emphasis on questions regarding the presence or absence of pain and coexisting genitourinary symptoms. Ideally this shift would result in assessment that is congruent with the tenets of the BPSM, providing a more inclusive clinical representation of the individual with CUO. More importantly, it would create data that can be compared with other nonmalignant chronic pain conditions and control groups; currently there is no comparable literature base to allow this comparison. For example, the only Cochrane review that discusses nonsurgical options for the treatment of chronic pelvic pain limits its discussion to options for women only (Ballantyne et al., 2016).

The current algorithm for assessment and treatment of CUO neglects psychosocial assessment in favor of medical or surgical intervention, and is designed from a urology perspective (Benson & Levine, 2012). This closely parallels the history of interstitial cystitis (IC) and other urological chronic pelvic pain syndromes (UCPPS), which until recently were evaluated from only a urology perspective, resulting in a record of unpredictable results and poor treatment success (Clemens, 2014). Treating UCPPS from only this single perspective did not take into account the multifactorial nature of what eventually would be identified as a chronic pain, not urological, condition. The shift in focus, due to epidemiological studies, pointed toward the possibility of an underlying chronic pain syndrome in patients with UCPPS. This shift included related disciplines in order to refocus the investigation, to allow for potential systemic syndromes that may have a relationship with UCPPS. The shift toward exploration of UCPPS with application of the principles of chronic pain resulted in progress toward identification of characteristics that UCPPS patients shared with other chronic pain populations, suggesting that more systemically oriented treatments may have increased success. It has also resulted in identification of two phenotypes of UCPPS patients, one with bladder-focused symptoms and one with more systemic, centralized pain (Clemens, 2014).

SEXUALITY, GENDER, AND PAIN

Gender plays in uncertain role in pain perception and pain behaviors, and pain in men may continue to benefit from specialized investigations into their unique experience. The psychosocial factors that are influential in the men's pain behavior have been poorly categorized. Chronic pain is, by definition, a long-term condition that may require management for episodic flares; both the chronicity and acute flares of pain are likely to have significant quality-of-life impacts. Men in the United States already suffer from lower life expectancy and are subject to increased morbidity and mortality rates for some chronic conditions such as heart disease (Centers for Disease Control and Prevention [CDC], 2013). Impact of superimposing chronic pain and its known morbidities on men with their higher rates of "general medical" comorbid conditions has been poorly characterized. Chronic pain interferes with one's self schema of "masculine" in U.S. and Western culture, contributing to shame and perceived weakness; weakness in turn is seen as not masculine.

Other biopsychosocial factors may be influential, such as reports that males minimize symptom reporting, differences in coping styles, and even hormone levels. El-Shormilisy, Strong, and Meredith (2015) performed a systematic review with strict inclusion criteria for evaluating adults with chronic nonmalignant pain and reporting gender-specific outcomes. These authors reported men catastrophize more when in pain, and men manifest increased anxiety leading to increased pain interference. They concluded that gender-specific coping styles influenced the functional status in men and women with nonmalignant chronic pain. Anxiety, especially for men, seems to influence coping and the ability to reinterpret pain sensations.

Pain perception and pain behavior are subject to the influence of gender; one's understanding of men with chronic pain can be augmented by incorporating a men's health view (Keough, 2015). The prevalence of most nonmalignant chronic pain conditions may be higher in women, but this prevalence may be confounded by the fact that men consistently have a lower use of healthcare services and may underreport their pain. Specifically, men have a lower use of pain services and lower use of analgesics (Keough, 2015). Few studies report on men's attempts at self-management of pain or discuss their specific coping strategies.

Because of these factors, clinicians may be evaluating men who have made little effort to self-manage their pain with such modalities as stretching, over-the-counter medications, or exercise. Instead, men with chronic (and particularly unexplained) pain may prefer to travel from provider to provider seeking recommendations, prescriptions, and imaging in an attempt to categorize their pain. Men may prefer distraction to all other methods of self-management, offering a possible rationale for seeking multiple appointments with multidisciplinary providers. But seeking multiple evaluations may also be evidence for use of avoidance by men with chronic pain, as they continue to seek an explanation and diagnosis that is consistent with their self-schema, rather than accepting the diagnosis of "pain" (Hooper & Quallich, 2016; Wenger, 2011). Bernardes and Lima (2010) reported that men who were perceived as less dominant or less masculine by nurses were assumed to have increased dependency issues within the context of chronic low back pain. This lends further support to the documented psychosocial issues for men trying to incorporate chronic pain of any type into their self-schema. It also suggests a role for providers in addressing the identity threat that chronic pain creates for some men.

This perception exposes the prevailing concept among U.S. men (the subjects of this dissertation study) that describes "masculinity" or what it means socially and culturally to be male. Health and masculinity enjoy a parallel relationship: masculinity implies good health and good health permits demonstration of masculinity. Pain, especially chronic *genital* pain, can challenge both the presentation of masculinity and health, and by extension sexual function again, masculine gender and sexual roles, and how this influences the way in which men report pain have been poorly examined within the setting of chronic pain. This impacts the manner in which men choose to answer even well-validated psychometric instruments designed to measure the dimensions of chronic pain and its comorbid conditions. The impact of chronic pain on frequency and quality of sexual activities should be assessed before and after treatment, as pain may be a factor in an individual's pursuit of sexual activity.

The Intersection of Chronic Pain and Sexuality

Chronic pain and sexuality share similarities, given that they both exist at the intersection of biology, psychology, and social factors. Previous studies of chronic pain and sexuality focus primarily on the biology of pain or sexuality, with little attention to the psychological and social contexts influential in maintaining these constructs. Both are sensitive to an individual's overall health, and are heavily influenced by past experience. Chronic pain affects an individual's well-being and quality of life (Gatchel et al., 2007; Jensen & Turk, 2014) and logically could influence sexuality. Certain types of chronic pain, particularly chronic pelvic or genital pain, might also have direct effects on sexuality. Pereira, Olevira, and Nobre (2016) reported that men with genital pain and men with sexual dysfunctions presented significantly more failure anticipation thoughts in comparison to sexually healthy men and may reflect a specific aspect of the contribution of chronic pain to "disordered social relations" (Gatchel et al., 2007, p. 108).

Conceptualization of one's sexuality is a direct influence of class, gender, and education, demonstrating the inextricable relationship between biology and the cultural reality of sexual behavior (Gagnon, 1975; Quallich & Arslanian-Engoren, 2014). Ambler, de C Williams, Hill, Gunary, and Cratchley (2001) reported that pain has a negative impact on sexual function for most patients, but the significance of this statement is limited because the effects of pain on sexual function in the general population are unknown, particularly if they do not seek treatment. Kwan, Roberts, and Swalm (2005) suggested chronic pain can directly impact sexual activity, but this does not imply a lack of satisfaction with sexual activity.

The scarcity of evidence to support evidence for the impact of chronic pain on sexual activity is due to the difficulty with measuring the subjective constructs of chronic pain and sexuality. This is particularly relevant within the context of conditions that affect male genitalia, as the age ranges for some of these conditions vary widely; sexuality is a dynamic construct that can change with age. For instance, an instrument such as the International Index of Erectile Function (IIEF) that has been validated in men over 65 may be a less ideal measure for men who have chronic orchialgia with an average age of 45 (Quallich & Arslanian-Engoren, 2014), but use of this particular instrument allows for comparisons with other populations within urology.

The initial groundwork investigating the relationship between chronic pain and sexuality was reported with chronic back pain patients as study participants (Maruta & Osborne, 1978; Monga, Tan, Ostermann, Monga, & Grabois, 1998; Osborne & Maruta, 1980; Sjogren & Fugl-Meyer, 1981; Vander Kolk, Chubon, & Vander Kolk, 1992). These classic studies demonstrated that chronic pain created complex situations leading to sexual, marital, and psychosocial issues, and that over half of men and women with low back pain had some manner of sexual dysfunction. The retrospective study by Vander Kolk et al. (1992) reported that 72% of their cohort of 100 back injury patients reported some degree of sexual dysfunction, determined by a decrease in the frequency of sexual activity, with a mean reduction of 71.82%. However, these authors noted only a small relationship between reported pain level and reduction in frequency of intercourse, suggesting that other variables that were not measured may have impacted sexual activity. Other authors have reported that subjects report a decreased sexual satisfaction the onset of their pain (Sjogren & Fugl-Meyer, 1981). Back pain patients may have neurological issues that directly create functional issues, most pronounced as erectile dysfunction in men.

Monga et al. (1998) found that a convenience sample of men and women with chronic pain in a variety of sites experienced difficulties in all domains of sexual function except for sexual fantasy. This included difficulties with sexual arousal, sexual behavior, climax, and sexual relationships. They reported that pain patients may be too distracted by their chronic pain to reach a sufficiently high level of sexual arousal, and that greater sexual dysfunction is associated with less successful coping mechanisms, such as catastrophizing and perceptions of decreased control, and fear of pain. Decreased coping mechanisms, on their own, suggest increased sexual function issues for men. Interestingly patients who were employed had overall better sexual function and libido than those who were receiving disability payments, suggesting a role for distraction as a method of coping. In a predominantly male veteran sample, Monga et al. (1998) showed that patients who had positive control appraisals for both pain and life domains had higher scores on the sexual functioning scales.

Chronic pain patients report that sexual activity makes their pain worse, but sex can also act as an anesthetic or distractor, and patients may not notice worsening pain until the following day (Ritchie & Daines, 1992). Patients may report diminished libido, which may be influenced by medications and the fatigue associated with chronic pain. Decreased libido may also be secondary to disappointment with or dislike of their current physical condition, or the depression that is a frequent comorbid condition, which can have the same effect. Richie and Daines (1992) speculated that low libido is exacerbated in men with poor perceptions of their own masculinity. This may be further amplified as their family and social roles are altered, especially if they are forced to stop work or work on a reduced schedule, fueling their search for both explanation for and treatment of their pain.

Kwan et al. (2005) studied a group of women and men with a variety of chronic pain conditions, offering evidence that men and women with chronic pain were highly adaptive, altering their approach to sexual activity based on physical limitations, and that satisfying sexual activity depended more on personal relationships and social support. They also reported that the individual's experience with chronic pain determined their level of sexual function and satisfaction with that function, consistent with the predictions of the BPSM. As their health circumstances changed, their perspective on sexual activity and intimacy also changed. Sexual activity became a less important aspect of overall quality of life than other areas such as sleep and daily activities.

Arabkheradmand et al. (2008) reported that chronic pain and altered erectile dysfunction often coexisted, but that erectile difficulties were not commonly treated in the context of chronic pain. However, this small case series ($n = 3$) demonstrated that treating erectile difficulties improved pain scores and comorbid symptoms.

Studies evaluating the impact of chronic pain have typically failed to evaluate gender as a mediator affecting the extent of any negative impact of chronic pain. Ruehlman, Karoly, and Taylor (2008) reported that in a sample of 2,071 men and women aged 25 to 80 with chronic pain, 37% reported no interference with sexual functioning. However, belief in a cure was a predictor of increased interference with sexual functioning for men, and catastrophizing was a predictor of pain interference on sexual function for both men and women. Their findings are consistent with the scant body of previous research demonstrating men who seek treatment for their pain report higher levels of disability across domains, including sexual function. This study did not clarify whether it is alteration in sexual function or pain itself that drives men to seek treatment.

Men with chronic pain can alter their self-perceptions and health-seeking behaviors (Bernardes & Lima 2010) over time, leading to depression, guilt, and resentment, all of which can decrease desire and augment pain intensity (Arabkheradmand et al. 2008) and which can, in turn, exacerbate erectile function further. There is a clear trend in which discussions of male sexuality become synonymous with, and replaced by, erectile dysfunction in the context of chronic pain. When any aspect of male sexuality has been included in studies of chronic pain, it tends to be a focused measure of erectile function or survey of ejaculatory pain. Decreased physical activity or decreased quality of life is used as a proxy for measures of sexuality or sexual function, a representation of the focus on measurement that the BPSM tries to avoid.

Depression, which is implicated as a comorbid condition in chronic pain, further becomes a surrogate for libido or lack of interest in sexual activity. Bonierbale (2009) and Davis, Bink, and Carrier (2009) reported that assessment instruments are designed to assess sexual function, and generally measure what they were designed to measure, e.g., changes with treatment, as opposed to the dimensions of sexuality. Previous investigations of chronic pain and sexuality suffer from methodological issues, but a definitive association between depression and sexual dysfunction has not been shown for chronic pain patients (Fine, 2011). Although both depression and chronic pain have been consistently shown to influence erectile function and libido, it is unclear if depression within the context of chronic pain creates a scenario in which sexuality become vulnerable, or if a decline in function fuels depression.

Sexuality Related to Chronic Male Genitourinary Pain

Chronic pain may make sexual activity difficult, and men with chronic pain may report a diminished frequency of sexual activity, both alone and partnered, but this should not be taken as an indication that sexual activities are unimportant. Chronic pain may not change all aspects of male sexuality, but a genitourinary location may have a particularly profound impact both on function and well-being. There is disruption of normal social roles and behaviors, which are worsened in the context of intimacy and relationship issues created by chronic pain (Pakpour et al., 2015).

Only two papers to date have discussed the impact of chronic testicular pain on sexual function. Lutz et al. (2005) reported that although the association between generalized urogenital pain and sexual function is unclear, there was an association between testicular pain and libido. Their survey assessed five sexual function domains, demonstrating that the focal nature of testicular pain had a greater negative impact on the sexual function of participants. More recently, Ciftci, Savas, Yeni, Verit, & Topal (2011) administered the International Index of Erectile Function (IIEF) to a small sample of 50 men with orchialgia and 50 control subjects, the only research paper to include a control group, but it was not an intervention study. There was no significant difference in the IIEF scores between these groups for erectile function. Men with orchialgia reported decreased libido and decreased satisfaction related to current sexual activity, and had an overall lower quality of life score, suggesting their chronic pain impacts both daily activities and overall quality of life. This study did not investigate other comorbid pain conditions that influence libido, such as depression or fatigue.

Aubin, Berger, Heiman, and Ciol (2008) reported that if results are adjusted for age and marital status, pain symptoms appear to minimally interfere with dimensions of sexuality for men with chronic pelvic pain syndrome (CPPS), despite previous studies reporting decreased sexual satisfaction and nonsensuality. They concluded that the experience of sexual pleasure and satisfaction is less influenced by pain than previously thought, supporting a multidimensional perspective for sexuality and chronic pain. This is despite reports of significant impairment to quality of life that had been previously proposed as the strongest relationship between erectile dysfunction and CPPS (Müller & Mulhall, 2006). It reinforces the difficulty in establishing the true relationship of sexual dysfunction and pain for this group of men, leaving it open to interpretation as to which symptom presents first. Sexual dysfunction and a decline in libido are a major component of CPPS and result in a decrease in overall quality of life (Anderson, Wise, Sawyer, & Chan, 2006); the relationship of sexual dysfunction to overall quality of life has not been emphasized (Lee et al., 2008) in studies or clinical evaluation.

The majority of CPPS research has ignored sexual dysfunction, and when it is investigated, variable self-report and nonvalidated measures are used (Davis et al., 2009), making comparisons among studies a challenge. Erectile dysfunction is the sexual component most investigated in men with any chronic pelvic pain, and reports of incidence vary widely from 0.6% to 48.3% (Davis et al., 2009), a range reflecting inconsistent measurements and inconsistent sampling methodology. Sexual outcomes in the context of treatment outcomes are rarely evaluated.

Sexuality and pain with sexual acts are not separated in studies; many of these studies evaluate ejaculatory pain but not associated psychological components with sexual well-being beyond quality of life. Davis et al. (2009) reported that the addition of the sexual domain, measured by satisfaction, erection, and ejaculation, better predicted quality of life scores in men with CPPS than assessment without it. But the generalizability of these conclusions was limited by an instrument validated in a male population older than the study population. These authors speculated that the connection with lower quality of life was solely the location of the pain, and that sexual dysfunction and pain synergistically decreased male quality of life.

Men with chronic epididymitis, a condition similar to chronic testicular pain, are also an understudied group regarding sexuality domains. Nickel, Siemens, Nickel, and Downey (2002) reported increased incidence of erectile dysfunction and decreased overall quality of life in men with chronic epididymitis. This is consistent with many other chronic pain patients, but this condition suffers from a lack of clear definition as well as anecdotal data guiding diagnosis. It also overlaps with other syndromes such as chronic orchialgia and CPPS, making conclusions about specific impacts to sexuality difficult.

Chronic scrotal content pain (CSCP) can be interpreted as a blending of the IASP concepts of scrotal/testicular/epididymal pain syndromes. This term began to appear in the literature in 2010 (Quallich & Arslanian-Engoren, 2014), but to date, there has been no investigation into the impact of this particular type of chronic pain on men's sexual behavior or sexual health.

Postvasectomy pain syndrome (PVPS) is a common cause for chronic orchialgia, but is easily identified with the precise history and physical examination. To date, there has been no investigation into the impact of this particular type of chronic pain on men's sexual behavior or sexual health.

SUMMARY OF CHRONIC PAIN COMORBID CONDITIONS IN MEN

Although there is a relatively sparse representation of pain comorbid conditions within discussions of sexuality (that are not centered around sequelae of cancer treatment) pain comorbidities have been reported. The literature offers the most support for gender-specific concerns with the male genitalia. There is support for depression playing a role in male sexual function, and both depression and decreased sexual function contributing to decreased quality of life within the context of chronic nonmalignant pain. Coping issues have been reported: distraction, appraisals of control, and catastrophizing. Physical limitations, either as a result of chronic pain or a condition contributing to chronic pain (e.g., back pain) are also reported as a comorbidity contributing to alterations in sexual function and libido. Fatigue, dyscognition, and sleep disturbances have not been reported to date in reports of men's sexual function and chronic nonmalignant pain.

BARRIERS TO PAIN MANAGEMENT AND MEN'S HEALTH

Pain is the most common reason that patients seek care and the most expensive public health issue in the United States, making pain management, knowledge, and education vital to the role of any healthcare provider. Access to pain management is a basic human right recognized by the United Nations, IASP, and WHO. Poorly treated pain contributes to healthcare resource use, disability, and prescription drug use and abuse. There is a need to acknowledge and invest in specialty populations, such as those within urology, by developing phenotypes and algorithms such as that currently being pursued by the MAPP program. There is a distinct role for categorizing and stratifying patients as a method for cost-effective evaluation and treatment. Pain involves changes to the spinal cord and multiple areas of the brain; this belies the importance of including acknowledgment of the biopsychosocial context of the individual when forming a treatment plan (Borsook, 2012). Chronic pain impacts sensory, emotional, cognitive, modulatory, and autonomic components of the nervous system. Descriptions of these aspects are missing in previous explorations of chronic male genital pain of unexplained orchialgia.

Curricula Issues

Management of pain, and male genital pain, by nurse practitioners (NPs) and physician assistants (PAs) is directly impacted by the absence of urology topics from their curricula, and by the fact that there is no current formal postgraduate training in adult urology. Albaugh (2012) presented the variable educational backgrounds represented across the globe by the title "urology APN [advance practice nurse]," and participants in the survey reported that a lack of urology-specific training represented a barrier to expanding practice into urology environments. Crowe (2014) emphasized in an opinion piece the rapid expansion of APNs as clinicians caring for urology patients is occurring without formal changes to graduate-level nursing curricula.

Didactic components that address men's genital health complaints from a primary care perspective (beyond sexually transmitted infections) are regularly omitted from NP curricula. Men's health remains an afterthought within NP curricula; Auerbach et al. acknowledge that "men's SRH [sexual and reproductive health] ... is largely absent from APRN curricula and clinical training plans" (p. 41). Available literature has very little mention of NP education in men's sexual and reproductive health, and the literature that is available demonstrates a focus toward effective management of previously diagnosed conditions (e.g., prostate cancer, erectile dysfunction).

The Institute of Medicine (IOM) (2011) acknowledges the lack of specific chronic pain management training in *all* healthcare provider curricula. There has been little attention to pain management practices in primary care settings, and the pain management prescribing habits of NPs is neglected further within this sparse body of literature. Droes (2004) reported that NP prescribing habits were heavily influenced by the facility in which they worked. NPs in this study fell into two groups, either focusing on treating the cause of the pain or treating the pain itself, with varied success.

Information in the literature regarding NP prescribing habits for chronic nonmalignant pain is lacking as well. Fontana (2008) interviewed a small number of NPs, reporting that NPs desire to make the best clinical decision based on the cause of pain, as opposed to only treating the pain. This study reported that NPs as a group felt they suffered from a lack of formal education regarding pain management, and felt a "burden of practice" (p. 34) that represented the need to both protect themselves and prevent potential opioid dependence in patients.

Lazarus and Downing (2003) reported that Alabama NPs felt there should be improvements to NP curricula specifically regarding pain management, and thought that a standardized curriculum should be implemented to include pain management principles. A 2013 presentation at the National Organization of Nurse Practitioner Faculty (NONPF) reporting on the results of a national survey of NPs discussed that chronic pain topics are absent from current NP curricula and advanced pharmacology courses (Tyler, Adams, & Sonstein, 2013). The NPs surveyed admitted a knowledge deficit regarding current standards for chronic nonmalignant pain treatment. This further is supported by a 2014 survey from Mongoven, Fishman, Young, and Koebner that reported that both chronic and acute pain management "is inconsistently incorporated into curricula for both nursing and medicine" (p. S38). These reports testify to the fact that a clear barrier to high-quality care for pain management is a lack of education of healthcare professionals regarding pain management. Education should refocus on psychosocial issues of the patients and their families, and move to address barriers and the challenges of clinicians for pain management (Fishman et al., 2013). Current debate centers around curriculum content versus competencies for pain management education (Gereau et al., 2014), but there is a need to define curricula in order to promote effective pain evaluation and management from trained clinicians.

Graduate level programs for NPs include an extensive amount of content in order to prepare students for their certification examination. The argument to include men's health, pain management, and urology within curricula for NPs and PAs is quite clear; it may seem as though providing students with the information to successfully manage chronic diseases that affect men would be sufficient. Curricula content must keep pace with the changing face of the actual clinical population. However, the CDC (2013) reports that over 50% of the deaths seen in men are due to preventable disease; this seemed to indicate that simply teaching disease management is no longer sufficient and that this knowledge must be placed in the context of the prevailing masculine construct. This is further complicated by the fact that there is no defined men's health curriculum for any of the healthcare disciplines and that there is no clear specialty that "owns" men's health (Chapter 1) in a fashion similar to gynecology and obstetrics in their focus on women's health. Providers must acknowledge and recognize the health-seeking behaviors of men are gender-specific (Hooper & Quallich, 2016) and cannot be extrapolated from a more general perception of health seeking.

DETERMINING FUTURE DIRECTIONS

Section 4305 of Patient Protection and Affordable Care Act (PPACA; 111th United States Congress, 2010) mandated the Secretary of Health and Human Services to work with the IOM to raise awareness of chronic pain as a public health issue. This implies that within the tenets of the PPACA, chronic pain is one of the chronic diseases that the act mandates should receive increased support, including care coordination and self-management training for providers (Gereau et al., 2014). The act also mandates increased support for mental health services, which has implications for the treatment of comorbid anxiety and depression, which are common in male chronic pain patients (particularly anxiety) and that may have implications for effective coping in men with chronic pain.

The President's Commission on Combating Drug Addiction and the Opioid Crisis (2017) draft recommended that the Department of Health and Human Services (HHS) develop a national curriculum and standards of care for opioid prescribers, including updated guidelines for specialty practitioners, and including multiple specialties in the guideline development. Additionally, this document recommends that agencies work with stakeholders to develop statutes and regulations and policies to ensure informed patient consent prior to opioid prescribing for chronic pain. The report also recommends that Centers for Medicare and Medicaid Services (CMS) abolish pain assessment as a dimension of patient satisfaction surveys as a way to avoid improper use of these surveys as "savvy providers have figured out that opioids are a way to manipulate satisfaction" (Christie et al., 2017, p. 49). The report encourages clinicians to "identify and describe potential pharmacological and nonpharmacological treatment options, including opioid and nonopioid pharmacological treatments for acute and chronic pain management, along with patient communication and education regarding the risks and benefits associated with each of these available treatment options" (p. 43). Furthermore, the document recommends removal of payer barriers to reimbursement of multimodal and interdisciplinary treatments for chronic pain, such as chiropractors, physical therapy, drug testing during opioid treatment, and behavioral therapy.

Undertreatment of chronic pain creates a risk for decreased quality of life, psychosocial decline, and decreased functional status. A longer wait for evaluation and management can contribute to increased chronicity of chronic pain and decreased outcomes, resulting in higher healthcare costs. In this context it is imperative to treat men with all types of chronic pain more efficiently and more effectively. There should be a drive to offer more both in the sense of a sensitivity to health-seeking behaviors in men (Hooper & Quallich, 2016) and the vernacular cultural beliefs reflected in phrases such as "man up" when dealing with pain.

REFERENCES

111th United States Congress. (2010). Compilation of patient protection and affordable care act. Retrieved from http://housedocs.house.gov/energycommerce/ppacacon.pdf

Ajo, R., Segura, A., Inda, M., Margarit, C., Ballester, P., Martinez, E., ... Peiro, A. M. (2017). Erectile dysfunction in patients with chronic pain treated with opioids. *Medicina Clinica (Barc), 149*(2), 49–54. doi:10.1016/j.medcli.2016.12.038

Albaugh, J. A. (2012). Urology nursing practice educational preparation, titles, training, and job responsibilities around the globe. *Urologic Nursing, 32*(2), 79–85. doi:10.1111/ijun.12007

Ambler, N., de C Williams, A. C., Hill, P., Gunary, R., & Cratchley, G. (2001). Sexual difficulties of chronic pain patients. *The Clinical Journal of Pain, 17*(2), 138–145. doi:10.1097/00002508-200106000-00006

Anderson, R. U., Wise, D., Sawyer, T., & Chan, C. A. (2006). Sexual dysfunction in men with chronic prostatitis/chronic pelvic pain syndrome: Improvement after trigger point release and paradoxical relaxation training. *The Journal of Urology, 176*(4), 1534–1539. doi:10.1016/j.juro.2006.06.010

Apkarian, A. V., Baliki, M. N., & Geha, P. Y. (2009). Towards a theory of chronic pain. *Progress in Neurobiology, 87*, 81–97. doi:10.1016/j.pneurobio.2008.09.018

Arabkheradmand, J., Foroutan, S., Ranjbar, S., Abbasi, T., Hessami, S., & Gorji, A. (2008). Improvement of chronic pain by treatment of erectile dysfunction. *Journal of Sexual Medicine, 5*(12), 2911–2916. doi:10.1111/j.1743-6109.2008.01006.x

Aubin, S., Berger, R. E., Heiman, J. R., & Ciol, M. A. (2008). The association between sexual function, pain, and psychological adaptation of men diagnosed with chronic pelvic pain syndrome type III. *Journal of Sexual Medicine, 5*, 657–667. doi:10.1111/j.1743-6109.2007.00736.x

Ballantyne, J., Kalso, E., & Stannard, C. (2016). Who analgesic ladder: A good concept gone astray. *British Medical Journal, 352*(20), 1–2. doi:10.1136/bmj.i20

Basaria, S., Travison, T. G., Alford, D., Knapp, P. E., Teeter, K., Cahalan, C., ... Edwards, R. R. (2015). Effects of testosterone replacement in men with opioid-induced androgen deficiency: A randomized controlled trial. *Pain, 156*(2), 280–288. doi:10.1097/01.j.pain.0000460308.86819.aa

Benson, J. S., & Levine, L. A. (2012). Evaluation and therapy of chronic scrotal content pain and epididymitis. In Shoskes, D.A. (Ed.), *Urological men's health: A guide for urologists and primary care physicians* (pp. 181–187). New York: Springer.

Bergeron, S., Rosen, N. O., & Morin, M. (2011). Genital pain in women: Beyond interference with intercourse. *Pain, 152*(6), 1223–1225. doi:10.1016/j.pain.2011.01.035

Bernardes, S. F., & Lima, M. L. (2010). Being less of a man or less of a woman: Perceptions of chronic pain patients' gender identities. *European Journal of Pain, 14*(2), 194–199. doi:10.1016/j.ejpain.2009.04.009

Bonierbale, M. (2009). From sexual difficulties to sexual dysfunctions (SD). *Sexologies, 18*(1), 10–13. doi:10.1016/j.sexol.2008.07.005

Borsook, D. (2011). Neurological diseases and pain. *Brain, 135*(2), 320–344. doi:10.1093/brain/awr271

Brennan, M. (2013). The effect of opioid therapy on endocrine function. *The American Journal of Medicine, 126*(3), S12–S18. doi:10.1016/j.amjmed.2012.12.001

Bushnell, M. C., čeko, M., & Low, L. A. (2013). Cognitive and emotional control of pain and its disruption in chronic pain. *Nature Reviews Neuroscience, 14*(7), 502–511. doi:10.1038/nrn3516

Centers for Disease Control and Prevention. (2013). Men and heart disease fact sheet. Retrieved from https://www.cdc.gov/dhdsp/data_statistics/fact_sheets/fs_men_heart.htm

Cheong, Y. C., Smotra, G., & Williams, A. C. (2014). Non-surgical interventions for the management of chronic pelvic pain. *Cochrane Database of Systematic Reviews, 3*, CD008797. doi:10.1002/14651858.CD008797.pub2

Christie, C., Baker, C., Cooper, R., Kennedy, P. J., Madras, B., & Bondi, P. (2017). Final report of the president's commission on combating drug addiction and the opioid crisis. Retrieved from https://www.whitehouse.gov/sites/whitehouse.gov/files/images/Meeting%20Draft%20of%20Final%20Report%20-%20November%201%2C%202017.pdf

Ciftci, H., Savas, M., Gulum, M., Yeni, E., Verit, A., & Topal, U. (2011). Evaluation of sexual function in men with orchialgia. *Archives of Sexual Behavior, 40*(3), 631–634. doi:10.1007/s10508-011-9726-4

Clauw, D. J. (2014). Fibromyalgia: A clinical review. *JAMA, 311*(15), 1547–1555. doi:10.1001/jama.2014.3266

Clemens, J. Q. (2014). Update on the MAPP Project (plenary session May 19). In *American Urologic Association annual conference*, Orlando, FL.

Cox, K. J., & Neville, C. E. (2012). Assessment and management options for women with vulvodynia. *Journal of Midwifery & Women's Health, 57*(3), 231–240. doi:10.1111/j.1542-2011.2012.00162.x

Crofford, L. (2015). Chronic pain: Where the body meets the brain. *Transactions of the American Clinical and Climatological Association, 126*, 167–183.

Crowe, H. (2014). Advanced urology nursing practice. *Nature Reviews Urology, 11*(3), 178–182. doi:10.1038/nrurol.2014.16

Davis, S. N., Binik, Y. M., & Carrier, S. (2009). Sexual dysfunction and pelvic pain in men: A male sexual pain disorder? *Journal of Sex and Marital Therapy, 35*(3), 182–205. doi:10.1080/00926230802716310

Droes, N. S. (2004). Role of the nurse practitioner in managing patients with pain. *Internet Journal of Advanced Nursing Practice, 6*(2), 53–59.

Duenas, M., Ojeda, B., Salazar, A., Mico, J. A., & Failde, I. (2016). A review of chronic pain impact on patients, their social environment and the health care system. *Journal of Pain Research, 9*, 457–467. doi:10.2147/JPR.S105892

El-Shormilisy, N., Strong, J., & Meredith, P. J. (2015). Associations among gender, coping patterns and functioning for individuals with chronic pain: A systematic review. *Pain Research and Management, 20*(1), 48–55. doi:10.1155/2015/490610

Fall, M., Baranowski, A. P., Elneil, S., Engeler, D., Hughes, J., Messelink, E. J., ... de C. Williams, A. C. (2010). EAU guidelines on chronic pelvic pain. *European Urology, 57*(1), 35–48. doi:10.1016/j.eururo.2009.08.020

Fine, P. G. (2011). Long-term consequences of chronic pain: Mounting evidence for pain is a neurological disease and parallels with other chronic disease states. *Pain Medicine, 12*, 996–1004. doi:10.1111/j.1526-4637.2011.01187.x

Fishman, S. M., Young, H. M., Lucas Arwood, E., Chou, R., Herr, K., Murinson, B. B., ... Strassels, S. A. (2013). Core competencies for pain management: Results of an interprofessional consensus summit. *Pain Medicine, 14*(7), 971–981. doi:10.1111/pme.12107

Flor, H. (2014). Psychological pain interventions and neurophysiology: Implications for a mechanism-based approach. *American Psychologist, 69*(2), 188. doi:10.1037/a0035254

Fontana, J. S. (2008). The social and political forces affecting prescribing practices for chronic pain. *Journal of Professional Nursing, 24*(1), 30–35. doi:10.1016/j.profnurs.2007.06.002

Gagnon, J. H. (1975). Sex research and social change. *Archives of Sexual Behavior, 4*(2), 111–141. doi:10.1007/bf01541078

Gatchel, R. J., McGeary, D. D., McGeary, C. A., & Lippe, B. (2014). Interdisciplinary chronic pain management: Past, present, and future. *American Psychologist, 69*(2), 119. doi:10.1037/a0035514

Gatchel, R. J., Peng, Y. B., Peters, M. L., Fuchs, P. N., & Turk, D. C. (2007). The biopsychosocial approach to chronic pain: Scientific advances and future directions. *Psychological Bulletin, 133*(4), 581–624. doi:10.1037/0033-2909.133.4.581

Gereau, R. W., Sluka, K. A., Maixner, W., Savage, S. R., Price, T. J., Murinson, B. B., … Fillingim, R. B. (2014). A pain research agenda for the 21st century. *The Journal of Pain, 15*(12), 1203–1214. doi:10.1016/j.jpain.2014.09.004

Glowacki, D. (2015). Effective pain management and improvement in patients' outcomes and satisfaction. *Critical Care Nurse, 35*(3), 33–41. doi:10.4037/ccn2015440

Gudin, J. A., Laitman, A., & Nalamachu, S. (2015). Opioid related endocrinopathy. *Pain Medicine,* 16, S9–S15. doi:10.1111/pme.12926

Haefner, H. K., Collins, M. E., Davis, G. D., Edwards, L., Foster, D. C., Hartmann, E. (Dee) H., … Wilkinson, E. J. (2005). The vulvodynia guideline. *Journal of Lower Genital Tract Disease, 9*(1), 40–51. doi:10.1097/00128360-200501000-00009

Hooper, G., & Quallich, S. A. (2016). Health seeking in men: A concept analysis. *Urologic Nursing, 36*(4), 163–172.

Institute of Medicine. (2011). *Relieving pain in America: A blueprint for transforming prevention, care, education and research.* Washington, DC: National Academies Press.

International Association for the Study of Pain. (1994). "Part III: Pain terms, a current list with definitions and notes on usage. In H. Merskey & N. Bogduk (Eds.), *Classification of chronic pain, 2nd edition, IASP Task Force on Taxonomy.* Seattle, WA: IASP Press. Retrieved from http://www.iasp-pain.org/AM/Template.cfm?Section=Pain_Definitions&Template=/CM/HTMLDisplay.cfm&ContentID=1728#Pain

Jackson, T., Tian, P., Wang, Y., Iezzi, T., & Xie, W. (2016). Toward identifying moderators of associations between presurgery emotional distress and postoperative pain outcomes: A meta-analysis of longitudinal studies. *The Journal of Pain, 17*(8), 874–888. doi:10.1016/j.jpain.2016.04.003

Jensen, M. P. (2010). A neuropsychological model of pain: Research and clinical implications. *The Journal of Pain, 11*(1), 2–12. doi:10.1016/j.jpain.2009.05.001

Jensen, M. P., & Turk, D. C. (2014). Contributions of psychology to the understanding and treatment of people with chronic pain: Why it matters to ALL psychologists. *American Psychologist, 69*(2), 105. doi:10.1037/a0035641

Johansen, T. E. B., & Weidner, W. (2002). Understanding chronic pelvic pain syndrome. *Current Opinion in Urology, 12*(1), 63–67. doi:10.1097/00042307-200201000-00012

Karoly, P., & Ruehlman, L. S. (2007). Psychosocial aspects of pain-related life task interference: An exploratory analysis in a general population sample. *Pain Medicine, 8*(7), 563–572. doi:10.1111/j.1526-4637.2006.00230.x

Katz, J., & Rosenbloom, B. N. (2015). The golden anniversary of Melzack and Wall's gate control theory of pain: Celebrating 50 years of pain research and management. *Pain Research and Management, 20*(6), 285–286. doi:10.1155/2015/865487

Kawai, K., Kawai, A. T., Wollan, P., & Yawn, B. P. (2017). Adverse impacts of chronic pain on health-related quality of life, work productivity, depression and anxiety in a community-based study. *Family Practice, 34,* 656–661. doi:10.1093/fampra/cmx034

Keogh, E. (2015). Men, masculinity, and pain. *Pain, 156*(12), 2408–2412. doi:10.1097/j.pain.0000000000000328

Kwan, K. H., Roberts, L. J., & Swalm, D. M. (2005). Sexual dysfunction and chronic pain: The role of psychological variables and impact on quality of life. *European Journal of Pain, 9*(6), 643–652. doi:10.1016/j.ejpain.2004.12.008

Lazarus, J. B., & Downing, B. (2003). Monitoring and investigating certified registered nurse practitioners in pain management. *The Journal of Law, Medicine & Ethics, 31*(1), 101–118. doi:10.1111/j.1748-720x.2003.tb00061.x

Lee, D. M., Pye, S. R., Tajar, A., O'Neill, T. W., Finn, J. D., Boonen, S., … Wu, F. C. (2012). Cohort Profile: The European Male Ageing Study. *International Journal of Epidemiology, 42*(2), 391–401. doi:10.1093/ije/dyr234

Lumley, M. A., Cohen, J. L., Borszcz, G. S., Cano, A., Radcliffe, A. M., Porter, L. S., … Keefe, F. J. (2011). Pain and emotion: A biopsychosocial review of recent research. *Journal of Clinical Psychology, 67*(9), 942–968. doi:10.1002/jclp.20816

Lutz, M. C., Roberts, R. O., Jacobson, D. J., McGree, M. E., Lieber. M. M., & Jacobsen, S. J. (2005). Cross-sectional associations of urogenital pain and sexual function in a community based cohort of older men: Olmsted County, Minnesota. *Journal of Urology, 174*(2), 624–628. doi:10.1097/01.ju.0000165386.26542.23

Maruta, T., & Osborne, D. (1978). Sexual activity in chronic pain patients. *Psychosomatics, 19*(9), 531–537. doi:10.1016/S0033-3182(78)70929-1

McCaffery, M. (1968). *Nursing practice theories related t cognition, bodily pain, and man-environment interactions*. Los Angeles, CA: UCLA Students' Store.

Melzack, R. (1999). From the gate to the neuromatrix. Pain, 82, S121–S126. doi:10.1016/s0304-3959(99)00145-1

Melzack, R., & Wall, P. D. (2008). *The challenge of pain*. London, UK: Penguin Books (original work published 1982).

Mersky, H., & Bogduk, N. (1994). *Classification of chronic pain: Descriptions of chronic pain syndromes and definitions of pain terms* (2nd ed.). Seattle, WA: International Association for the Study of Pain (IASP) Press.

Molton, I. R., & Terrill, A. L. (2014). Overview of persistent pain in older adults. *American Psychologist, 69*(2), 197. doi:10.1037/a0035794

Monga, T. N., Tan, G., Ostermann, H. J., Monga, U., & Grabois, M. (1998). Sexuality and sexual adjustment of patients with chronic pain. *Disability and Rehabilitation: An International, Multidisciplinary Journal, 20*(9), 317–329. doi:10.3109/09638289809166089

Müller, A., & Mulhall, J. P. (2006). Sexual dysfunction in the patient with prostatitis. *Current Urology Reports, 7*(4), 307–312. doi:10.1007/s11934-996-0010-4

Nahin, R. (2015). Estimates of pain prevalence and severity in adults: United States, 2012. *The Journal of Pain, 16*(8), 769–780. doi:10.1016/j.pain.2015.05.002

Nickel, J. C., Siemens, D. R., Nickel, K. R., & Downey, J. (2002). The patient with chronic epididymitis: Characterization of an enigmatic syndrome. *The Journal of Urology, 167*(4), 1701–1704. doi:10.1016/S0022-5347(05)65181-6

Osborne, D., & Maruta, T. (1980). Sexual adjustment and chronic back pain. *Medical Aspects of Human Sexuality, 14*, 104–113.

Pakpour, A. H., Nikoobakht, M., & Campbell, P. (2015). Association of pain and depression in those with chronic low back pain: The mediation effect of patient sexual functioning. *The Clinical Journal of Pain, 31*(1), 44–51. doi:10.1097/AJP.0000000000000076

Pereria, R., Oliveira, C. M., & Nobre, P. (2016). Sexual functioning and cognitions during sexual activity in men with genital pain: A comparative study. *Journal of Sex and Marital Therapy, 42*(7), 602–615. doi: 10.1080/0092623X.2015.1113582.

Powell, R., Johnston, M., Smith, W. C., King, P. M., Chambers, W. A., Krukowski, Z., … Bruce, J. (2012). Psychological risk factors for chronic post-surgical pain after inguinal hernia repair surgery: A prospective cohort study. *European Journal of Pain, 16*(4), 600–610. doi:10.1016/j.ejpain.2011.08.010

Price, C., Lee, J., Taylor, A. M., & Baranowski, A. P. (2014). Initial assessment and management of pain: A pathway for care developed by the British pain society. *British Journal of Anaesthesia, 112*(5), 816–823. doi:10.1093/bja/aet589

Quallich, S. A., & Arslanian-Engoren, C. (2014). Chronic unexplained orchialgia: A concept analysis. *Journal of Advanced Nursing, 70*(8), 1717–1726. doi:10.1111/jan.12340

Racine, M., Tousignant-Laflamme, Y., Kloda, L. A., Dion, D., Dupuis, G., & Choinière, M. (2012a). A systematic literature review of 10 years of research on sex/gender and experimental pain perception—Part 1: Are there really differences between women and men? *Pain, 153*(3), 602–618. doi:10.1016/ j.pain.2011.11.025

Racine, M., Tousignant-Laflamme, Y., Kloda, L. A., Dion, D., Dupuis, G., & Choinière, M. (2012b). A systematic literature review of 10 years of research on sex/gender and pain perception—Part 2: Do biopsychosocial factors alter pain sensitivity differently in women and men? *Pain, 153*(3), 619–635. doi:10.1016/j.pain.2011.11.026

Raheem, O. A., Patel, S. H., Sisul, D., Furnish, T. J., & Hsieh, T. (2017). The role of testosterone supplemental therapy in opioid-induced hypogonadism: A retrospective pilot analysis. *American Journal of Men's Health, 11*(4), 1208–1213. doi:10.1177/1557988316672396

Raichle, K. A., Hanley, M., Jensen, M. P., & Cardenas, D. D. (2007). Cognitions, coping, and social environment predict adjustment to pain in spinal cord injury. *The Journal of Pain, 8*(9), 718–729. doi:10.1016/j.jpain.2007.05.006

Ritchie, M. H., & Daines, B. (1992). Sexuality and low back pain: A response to patients' needs. *The British Journal of Occupational Therapy, 55*(9), 347–350. doi:10.1177/030802269205500907

Rosenquist, R. W., Benzon, H. T., Connis, R. T., De Leon-Casasola, O. A., David Glass, D., Korevaar, W. C., ..., Simon, D. L. (2010). Practice guidelines for pain management: An updated report by the American Society of Anesthesiologists Task Force on Chronic Pain Management and the American Society of Regional Anesthesia and Pain Medicine. Anesthesiology, 112, 810–833. doi:10.1097/ALN.0b013e3181c43103

Rubenstein, A., & Carpenter, D. M. (2014). Elucidating risk factors for androgen deficiency associated with daily opioid use. *The American Journal of Medicine, 127*(12), 1195–1201. doi:10.1016/j.amjmed.2014.07.015

Ruehlman, L. S., Karoly, P., & Taylor, A. (2008). Perceptions of chronic pain's interference with sexual functioning: the role of gender, treatment status, and psychosocial factors. *Sexuality and Disability, 26*(3), 123–136. doi:10.1007/s11195-008-9080-1

Scott, E. L., Kroenke, K., Wu, J., & Yu, Z. (2016). Beneficial effects of improvement in depression, pain catastrophizing and anxiety on pain outcomes: A 12-month longitudinal analysis. *The Journal of Pain, 17*(2), 215–222. doi:10.1016/j.jpain.2015.10.011

Seminowicz, D. A., & Davis, K. D. (2006). Cortical responses to pain in healthy individual's depends on pain catastrophizing. *Pain, 120*, 297–306. doi:10.1016/j.pain.2005.11.008

Serbic, D., Pincus, T., Fife-Schaw, C., & Dawson, H. (2016). Diagnostic uncertainty, guilt, mood, and disability in back pain. *Health Psychology, 35*(1), 50–59. doi:10.1037/hea0000272

Sjogren, K., & Fugl-Meyer, A. R. (1981). Chronic back pain and sexuality. *International Rehabilitation Medicine, 3*, 19–25. doi:10.3109/03790798109167110

Stanos, S., Brodsky, M. Argoff, C., Clauw, D. J., D'Arcy, Y., & Donevan, S. (2016). Rethinking chronic pain in a primary care setting. *Journal of Postgraduate Medicine, 128*(5), 502–515. doi:10.1080/00325481.2016.1188319

Sullivan, M. J. (2009). *The Pain Catastrophizing Scale user manual*. Montréal: McGill University.

Sullivan, M. J., Thorn, B., Haythornthwaite, J., Keefe, F., Martin, M., Bradley, L., & Lefebvre, J. (2001). Theoretical perspectives on the relation between catastrophizing and pain. *The Clinical Journal of Pain, 17*(1), 52–64. doi:10.1097/00002508-200103000-00008

Tait, R. C., & Chibnall, J. T. (2014). Racial/ethnic disparities in the assessment and treatment of pain: Psychosocial perspectives. *American Psychologist, 69*(2), 131. doi:10.1037/a0035204

Tracey, I., & Johns, E. (2010). The pain matrix: Reloaded or reborn as we image tonic pain using arterial spin labelling. *Pain, 148*, 359–360. doi:10.1016/j.pain.2009.11.009

Turk, D. C., & Melzack, R. (Eds.). (2011). *The handbook of pain assessment* (3rd ed.). New York, NY: Guilford Press.

Tyler, D. O., Adams, M.L., & Sonstein, F. (2013). Integrating chronic pain assessment and management in nurse practitioner education. (Session April 13). In *NONPF 39th annual meeting*, Pittsburgh, PA.

University of Wisconsin School of Medicine and Public Health. (2010). Principles of pain assessment—Pain management. Retrieved from http://projects.hsl.wisc.edu/GME/PainManagement/session3.1.html

Vander Kolk, C. J., Chubon, R. A., & Vander Kolk, J. K. (1992). The relationship among back injury, pain and sexual functioning. *Sexuality and Disability, 10*(3), 153–161. doi:10.1007/BF01102281

Watson, P., & Kendall, N. (2013). Assessing psychosocial yellow flags. In L. Gifford (Ed.), *Topical issues in pain 2: Biopsychosocial assessment and management, relationships and pain* (pp. 111–129). Bloomington, IN: AuthorHouse UK.

Woolf, C. J. (2010). What is this thing called pain? *The Journal of Clinical Investigation, 120*(11), 3742–3744. doi:10.1172/JCI45178

Woolf, C. J. (2011). Central sensitization: Implications for the diagnosis and treatment of pain. *Pain, 152*(3), S2–S15. doi:10.1016/j.pain.2010.09.030

Zacharoff, K. L., Pujol, L. M., & Corsini, E. (2010). *PainEDU.org manual a pocket guide to pain management*. Newton, MA: Inflexxion.

Zhang, Z., Zolnoun, D. A., Francisco, E. M., Holden, J. K., Dennis, R. G., & Tommerdahl, M. (2011). Altered Central Sensitization in Subgroups of Women With Vulvodynia. *The Clinical Journal of Pain, 27*(9), 755–763. doi:10.1097/ajp.0b013e31821c98ec

CHAPTER 16

Effective Communication Between Men Who Have Sex With Men and Their Providers

Dalmacio D. Flores, Michael Sanchez, and José A. Bauermeister

> *Sexual health is a state of physical, emotional, mental and social well-being in relation to sexuality; it is not merely the absence of disease, dysfunction or infirmity. Sexual health requires a positive and respectful approach to sexuality and sexual relationships, as well as the possibility of having pleasurable and safe sexual experiences. For sexual health to be attained and maintained, rights of all persons must be respected, protected and fulfilled.*
>
> —World Health Organization (2006)

INTRODUCTION

The American Nurses Association (ANA) has enshrined in its Code of Ethics a commitment to nursing practice that recognizes patients' right to self-determination and their inherent dignity, worth, and unique attributes (American Nurses Association, 2001). The American Academy of Physician Assistants' (AAPA) Guidelines for Ethical Conduct also supports and promotes patients' diversity and equal treatment of all persons who seek their care, including a commitment to nondiscrimination based on classes that include gender identity or sexual orientation (American Academy of Physician Assistants, 2013). In tandem, these professions acknowledge a fundamental responsibility for the care of all people, including those who are gay, lesbian, bisexual, or transgender (LGBT). In this chapter, we focus on how providers can communicate with men who have sex with men (MSM) to assist them achieve optimum health.

The goal of this chapter is to enable providers to have meaningful conversations with their MSM patients to help MSM patients open up and receive inclusive care. Achieving communication proficiency entails a three-pronged approach that includes (a) an intrapersonal assessment of providers' knowledge and biases, (b) an interpersonal skill-set that puts MSM patients' needs central in every clinical encounter, and (c) a macrolevel organizational commitment that supports the identified needs of MSM, and ultimately all LGBT patients. This chapter will provide a breakdown of each approach and detail steps that providers can use to communicate effectively with their MSM patients. When successfully executed, these approaches will increase providers' awareness and skills in addressing issues at the intersection of sexual orientation and racial/ethnic minority status, empower patients to be involved in their health, and create a culturally competent clinical environment conducive for shared decision making (Chin, Lopez, Nathan, & Cook, 2016).

Men who have sex with men is the broad term used in the public health literature that includes cisgender males who identify as gay, bisexual, questioning, or queer as well as those who do not identify with those labels but engage in same-sex behaviors. In the United States, around 4.1% of the U.S. adult population identify as LGBT (Gallup, 2017). Additionally, members of this group are identifying and disclosing as LGBT at younger ages (Calzo, Antonucci, Mays, & Cochran, 2011; Martin & D'Augelli, 2009) with Millennials self-identifying more as LGBT compared to members of Generation X and Baby Boomers. This earlier age of disclosure has been attributed to the growing social acceptance of LGBTQ individuals (Gallup, 2017; Pew Research Center, 2017) and the recent recognition of their rights in the federal and state levels. However, previous research has uncovered that earlier self-identification and disclosure as LGBT is associated with greater morbidity, forced sex, harassment, and HIV infection (Friedman, Marshal, Stall, Cheung, & Wright, 2008). The providers' role in ensuring positive health outcomes for this population is therefore imperative given the challenges the population faces in accessing accurate and affirming healthcare.

Health Disparities

Despite advances in LGBT rights in recent years, MSM are still disproportionately affected by poor health outcomes. Although sexual orientation by itself does not cause negative health outcomes, health disparities when compared to their heterosexual peers are well documented (Ranji, Beamesderfer, Kates, & Salganicoff, 2015). Nearly 40 years since the first cases of AIDS were reported, MSM still account for the largest incidence rates of HIV infections in the country (Centers for Disease Control and Prevention [CDC], 2015). MSM also have higher incidence rates for syphilis, herpes, gonorrhea, and chlamydia infection compared to heterosexual men (Operario et al., 2015). MSM are also more likely to experience behavioral and psychosocial challenges, with rates for psychological distress, smoking, cancers, cardiovascular issues, and substance use being higher among MSM (Graham et al., 2011). Among MSM, researchers have noted disparities by sexual identity. For example, men who identify as bisexual and/or who engage in sex with men and women have been shown to have greater disparities in health outcomes compared to gay or heterosexual men (Friedman et al., 2014). In light of these statistics, Healthy People 2020 has prioritized the health needs of sexual minorities in healthcare settings (Graham et al., 2011). For example, more federal guidelines are requiring health systems to collect sexual orientation information (Centers for Medicare and Medicaid Services, 2015; Institute of Medicine (US) Board on the Health of Select Populations, 2013). Other efforts have prioritized the identification of settings providing LGBT inclusive care, such as reporting them in advocacy tools like the Human Rights Campaign's Healthcare Equality Index.

Concerns about stigmatization based on actual experiences or anticipated fears fuels caution among MSM patients when interacting with providers. Historically, members of the LGBT community have had a tumultuous relationship with the U.S. healthcare system. Once considered a mental disorder, the stigmatization of MSM did not disappear after homosexuality was removed from the American Psychiatric Association's Diagnostic and Statistical Manual in 1973. The slow recognition by the government and medical establishment of the AIDS epidemic that ravaged the MSM community in the early 1980s also did not foster trust between the population and providers. Even at present, dubious programs such as reparative therapy to "cure away the gay" perpetuates medical mistrust within the MSM community.

Healthcare providers have multiple opportunities to address these disparities starting with effective communication with MSM patients. Central to the provider's task in addressing the health disparities observed among MSM is their ability to establish caring relationships and address this population's distrust of the medical establishment. The perception by MSM of providers being unsympathetic to sexuality-related issues causes patient discomfort about responding to health screening questions (Mimiaga, Goldhammer, Belanoff, Tetu, &

Mayer, 2007). Ultimately, medical distrust can result in delays in seeking medical care that translate to care complications and worsened outcomes (Galvan, Bogart, Klein, Wagner, & Chen, 2017). Nevertheless, interactions with providers and the entire clinic staff are the salient determinants of patients' perceived safety in the clinical setting, which in turn increases likelihood of sexual orientation disclosure to those professionals (Wilkerson, Rybicki, Barber, & Smolenski, 2011). In the rest of this chapter, we provide a conceptual framework and a series of recommendations that support efforts to increase effective communication between MSM and healthcare providers.

Conceptual Framework: Shared Decision Making and Patient-Centered Care

Shared decision making (SDM) is a model for clinical practice centered around conferring agency to patients where they are able to make autonomous choices (Elwyn et al., 2012). In this model, providers and patients share information, discuss the merits of health-related options, and ultimately agree on a suitable clinical plan (Charles, Gafni, & Whelan, 1997; Peek et al., 2016). Recent federal mandates require healthcare organizations seeking recognition as an accountable care organization (ACO) to meet quality benchmarks such as shared decision making that "takes into account the beneficiaries' unique needs, preferences, values and priorities" (Agency for Healthcare Research and Quality, 2016). The elimination of these barriers are a clinical priority given that SDM is an indicator of patient-centered care (PCC; Barry & Edgman-Levitan, 2012). Further, national accreditation boards such as the National Committee for Quality Assurance, the Accreditation Association for Ambulatory Health Care, and the Joint Commission have included SDM standards in their certification checklists. The Agency for Healthcare Research and Quality (AHRQ; Agency for Healthcare Research and Quality, 2016) has provided a five-step approach to SDM (Table 16.1). These recommendations are consonant with this chapter's goal of enabling providers to have meaningful and patient-directed conversations with MSM patients.

TABLE 16.1 The SHARE Approach and Exemplar Considerations

Step	Action	Exemplar Considerations
1	Seek patient's participation	Using terms that patients use to describe themselves and their partners; instead of "Do you have a girlfriend?" ask, "Are you in a relationship?"
2	Help patient explore and compare treatment options	Providing health information materials in a patient's language or dialect; providing access to culturally competent medical interpreters.
3	Assess patient's values and preferences	Accommodating for patient's use of alternative or complementary medicine when planning care.
4	Reach a decision with the patient	Referring back to patients after a decision is made to verify that plan of care is in accord with their wishes.
5	Evaluate patient's decision	Avoiding passive responses by saying "Any questions?" at the end of patient visits but instead seeking out active engagement. State instead, "I want to make sure that I've helped you understand everything you need to understand about your health. Patients usually have questions because it can be complicated. Could you tell me what you understand, and then I can help clarify. . .?" (Epstein & Street, 2011)

Source: Agency for Healthcare Research and Quality. (2016). The SHARE Approach. Retrieved from https://www.ahrq.gov/professionals/education/curriculum-tools/shareddecisionmaking/index.html

Patient-centered care, with language reminiscent of the professional commitments made by nurses, nurse practitioners, physician assistants, and other care providers, centers on an approach marked by deep respect for all patients as unique individuals and a sense of obligation to care for them on the patients' own terms (Epstein & Street, 2011; Scholl, Zill, Härter, & Dirmaier, 2014). Unlike the biomedical model in which focus has traditionally been on the health concern or problem, PCC focuses on the patient first through patient partnership and individualized care (Robinson, Callister, Berry, & Dearing, 2008). An approach to care that evolved from the informed consent movement, PCC involves a respectful stance at the outset of each clinical encounter and views patients as an expert in the management of their care (Scholl et al., 2014). In this age of protocols and practice guidelines, PCC involves *balancing the art of generalizations and the science of particulars* (McWhinney, 1989). Together with SDM, PCC improves patient-provider communication, care engagement, and treatment fidelity (Agency for Healthcare Research and Quality, 2016).

PROVIDER'S INTRAPERSONAL ASSESSMENT OF SELF

Parallel to creating spaces for dialogue, it is imperative that providers identify their unconscious biases as they may influence care and disrupt opportunities for shared decision making (Peek et al., 2016). Prior to successfully working with MSM, a self-assessment of one's beliefs and knowledge is necessary. Examining biases, which may take the form of overt discrimination or covert attitudes existing just below one's conscious awareness (Szymanski, Kashubeck-West, & Meyer, 2008), and seeking the origins of these beliefs may lead to elimination of biases. The most common sources of homophobia in the United States can be traced to religious beliefs, marital and procreative bias, concern about HIV/AIDS, rigid gender roles, psychiatric labeling, and negative stereotypes (Knox, Schacht, & Whatley, 2014). Acknowledging discomfort with specific topics is also necessary for changing ingrained ways of thinking or behaving (Chin, 2017). There are multiple online resources available to providers to help assess personal biases including the Multicultural Counseling Inventory (Green et al., 2005) and the Implicit Association Test (Project Implicit, 2017). Thus, a key task in the provider's intrapersonal assessment is a recognition of the power differential between patients and providers and the impact of the prevailing heteronormative practice that is the status quo in healthcare (Colpitts & Gahagan, 2016; Stewart & O'Reilly, 2017).

Unconscious bias regarding sexuality can often work alongside stereotypes focused on other identities possessed by a patient (e.g., race/ethnicity, social class, urbanity, gender). For example, compared to white LGBT people, racial/ethnic minority populations tend to lack a regular place of care and more often access public rather than private health facilities (Macapagal, Bhatia, & Greene, 2016). Racial and ethnic sexual minority patients, especially those whose primary language is not English, experience discrimination in healthcare settings that leads to errors and delays in receiving care along with mistrust and discomfort with medical service (Calo et al., 2015). On average, minority populations also appraise that they have less participation during the medical decision-making process (Hawley & Morris, 2017). Thus, when considering the specific needs of MSM of color, caution is advised against subsuming the experiences of racial/ethnic minority MSM within the larger white MSM narrative. For instance, many MSM of color do not openly identify as members of LGBT communities as they perceive that these spaces are predominantly white (Tan et al., 2016). Also, racial/ethnic minority MSM sometimes code switch or engage in behavioral adaptations to conform to specific situations in order to avoid discrimination in their specific racial or ethnic communities (Molinsky, 2007). Posing open-ended questions and asking appropriate probing questions during clinic encounters invites patients to provide detailed responses that will lead to appropriate plans of care. In the next section, we provide insight into the complexity of sexual identities, attractions, and behaviors, as well as highlight strategies to collect these data from patients during a medical encounter.

Navigating Labels and Identities

The components of one's sexuality include attraction (sexual and romantic attractions), expression (actions, dress, and demeanor), identity (how they view themselves and self-identify), behavior (who they engage in sex with), and sex (biological sex characteristics). Each of these components is dynamic and fluid and falls within its own continuum. Gaining full understanding and proficiency in these dimensions takes time. We have found the Genderbread person (Figure 16.1; Killermann, 2017) to be a good way to illustrate these diverse components and is included for the readers' reference.

A general recommendation for providers who are unfamiliar with these concepts includes embracing a reflexive practice, which involves having an awareness of one's emotional responses during and after each encounter that can provide insights for future patient encounters (Scholl et al., 2014). Begin a clinical encounter with new patients by stating your preferred pronouns and asking for theirs (*"My pronouns are he/him/his. Do you have a preferred gender pronoun?"*). Even though the majority of patients will respond with traditional pronoun preferences, seeking their input communicates an inclusive practice.

Providing inclusive care begins with the appropriate asking of patients' sexual orientation and behaviors (Macapagal et al., 2016). LGBT youth have identified negative experiences with providers that include feeling unwelcome, being judged for not being heterosexual, and receiving education about pregnancy even after a female patient disclosed being a lesbian (Snyder, Burack, & Petrova, 2017). Research has indicated that sexual minority individuals endorse the routine collection of sexual orientation data (Cahill et al., 2014). However, some providers are uncomfortable assessing their patients' sexual orientation and sexual behaviors, which can lead to missing crucial information (Cahill et al., 2014). For instance, more than half of providers at the Veteran's Health Administration hospitals thought it was important to assess sexual orientation but admitted that they only rarely collected this information (Sherman, Kauth, Shipherd, & Street, 2014). Similarly, in a study examining providers and potential LGBT patients in emergency room settings, Haider and colleagues (Haider et al., 2017) found that 78% of providers assumed patients would refuse answering inquiries about sexual orientation, whereas only 10% of patients reported that they would refuse when asked. The discrepancy between provider and patient views is an indication of the challenge healthcare professionals and organizations must address to provide meaningful care. Undoubtedly, providers often fear embarrassment and making incorrect assumptions about their patients' sexual orientation and/or behaviors (Baker & Beagan, 2014). Prefacing questions with *"I ask all my patients the following questions..."* eases provider discomfort about perceived intrusiveness (Klein & Nakhai, 2016), and supports the notion that a provider has an openness to creating spaces for dialogue and shared decision making with the patient.

In sum, active listening includes paraphrasing key information offered by patients. Clarifying their responses by respectfully asking them to repeat themselves conveys a provider's commitment to getting information correctly. Remember that keeping heteronormative assumptions in check allows for inclusive care, and thus using inclusive language, such as "partner" instead of "wife," is recommended. This will eliminate the possibility of awkwardness when, for example, a male patient states that his husband has a power of attorney to make health decisions on his behalf after inquiries about a wife is made by a provider. Finally, recognize that mistakes are to be expected in one's journey to proficiently

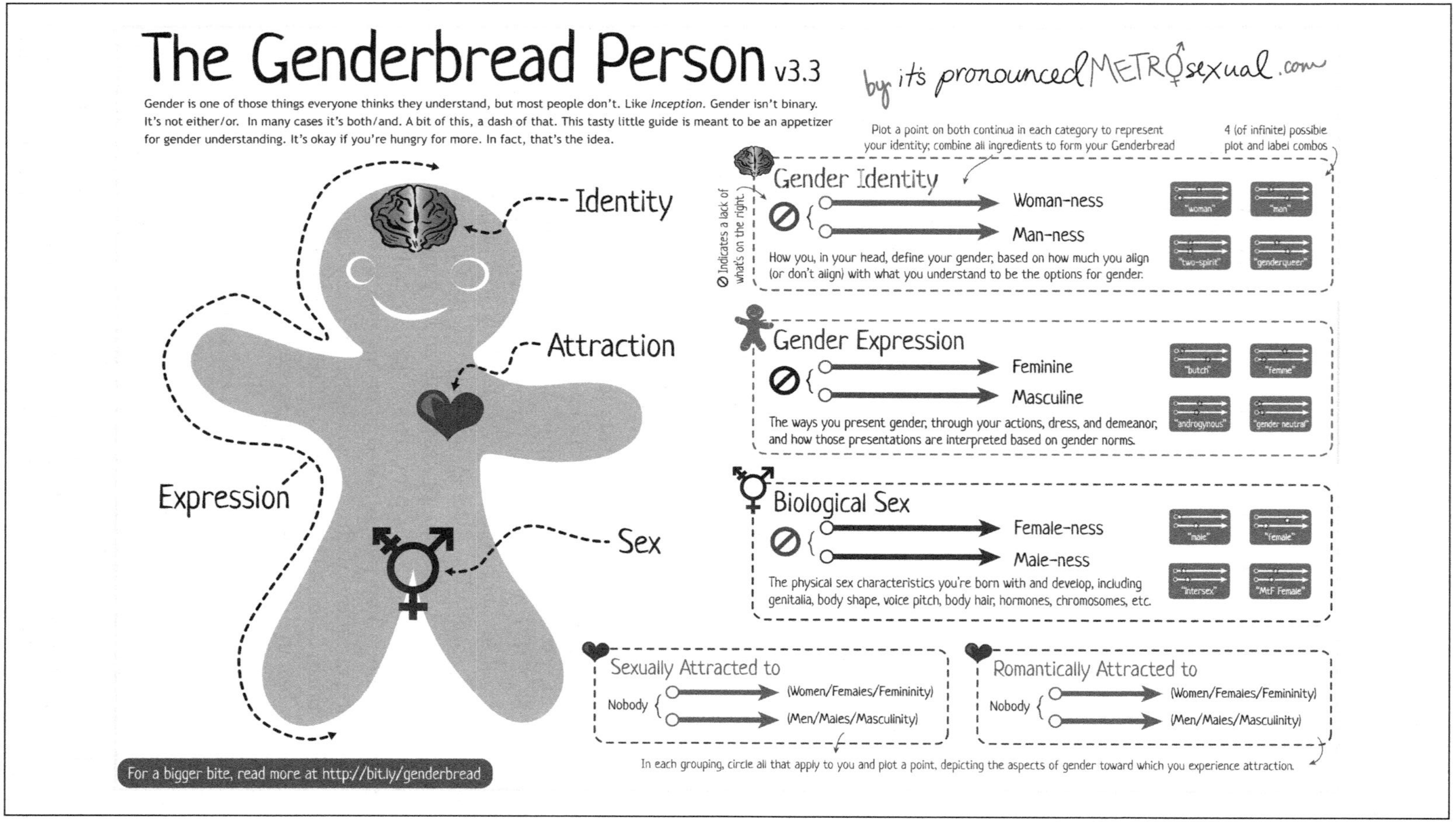

FIGURE 16.1 The genderbread person.

Source: It's Pronounced Metrosexual. Retrieved from http://itspronouncedmetrosexual.com/2015/03/the-genderbread-person-v3

communicate with MSM during clinic visits. The seeming gravity of the error becomes irrelevant if awareness and recognition of misspeaking are immediate. Offering sincere apology after a mistake is prudent.

SHARED DECISION MAKING IN DYADIC COMMUNICATION

Obtaining MSM Sexual History

Obtaining a thorough sexual history and conducting risk assessment of the MSM patient is an essential part of care. MSM are a heterogeneous group of men who have wide-ranging behaviors, characteristics, identities, and healthcare needs. Many men are rarely asked about the gender of sex partners, sexually transmitted infection (STI) risks, sexual behaviors, or symptoms associated with STIs. These types of inquiries are often disregarded owing to provider uneasiness when asking questions as part of the sexual health history (Carter et al., 2014). Despite this, obtaining sexual history should be routinely performed at the initial visit or intake and, at a minimum, on an annual basis because of the increased prevalence of STIs in this population (California Department of Public Health and the California STD/HIV Prevention Training Center, 2015). For patients who are at higher risk for communicable diseases (e.g., HIV, hepatitis, and STIs), more frequent assessments are recommended (Lanier et al., 2014; Oster et al., 2011).

Gathering background information about the patient's sexual history is paramount to providing comprehensive care. Many of the barriers to obtaining a thorough sexual history may be related to the provider's lack of understanding regarding health risks, sexual practices, or terminology used by MSM. However, many of the general principles for obtaining a sexual history also apply to MSM. Using effective techniques to engage patients in dialogue and to gather information requires the use of open-ended questions and using "normalizing" language to help facilitate this discussion and optimize delivery of care. Obtaining a sexual history should be nonjudgmental and provide an opportunity for counseling aimed at minimizing risk-taking behaviors. For some MSM, an open and inclusive discussion with a medical provider may help to ease their own discomfort and/or shame about having sex with other men. For others, an open and inclusive discussion with a provider may circumvent inadequate assumptions (e.g., all MSM are engaging in sex with multiple partners, or exhibit hypersexual characteristics).

Disclosure of sexual orientation often results in greater satisfaction in the delivery of healthcare and increased use of preventive screenings (Quinn et al., 2015). Gathering a thorough sexual history includes asking about the 5 Ps: (a) partners, (b) practices, (c) protection from STIs, (d) past history of STIs, and (e) pregnancy (Figure 16.2; Workowski & Bolan, 2015). Remember that not all MSM identify as gay or only have sex with men (Nagel, Fuld, & Varma, 2014). Therefore, asking about family planning and pregnancy may be included as part of the sexual history.

SEXUAL BEHAVIOR AND PRACTICES

In addition to the standard sexual history questions one would ask any patient, clinicians should assess sexual behaviors and practices MSM might engage in. Some sexual practices have physical risks and must be discussed with patients to identify harm reduction strategies and a SDM risk reduction plan. When discussing these topics, providers should understand the common terminology used by patients. For example, receptive anal intercourse may be commonly referred to as "bottoming" and insertive anal intercourse as "topping."

Inquiring about sexual practices related to anal sex (e.g., lubrication when engaging in anal sex, anal hygiene behaviors such as douching before or after receptive anal sex) should be

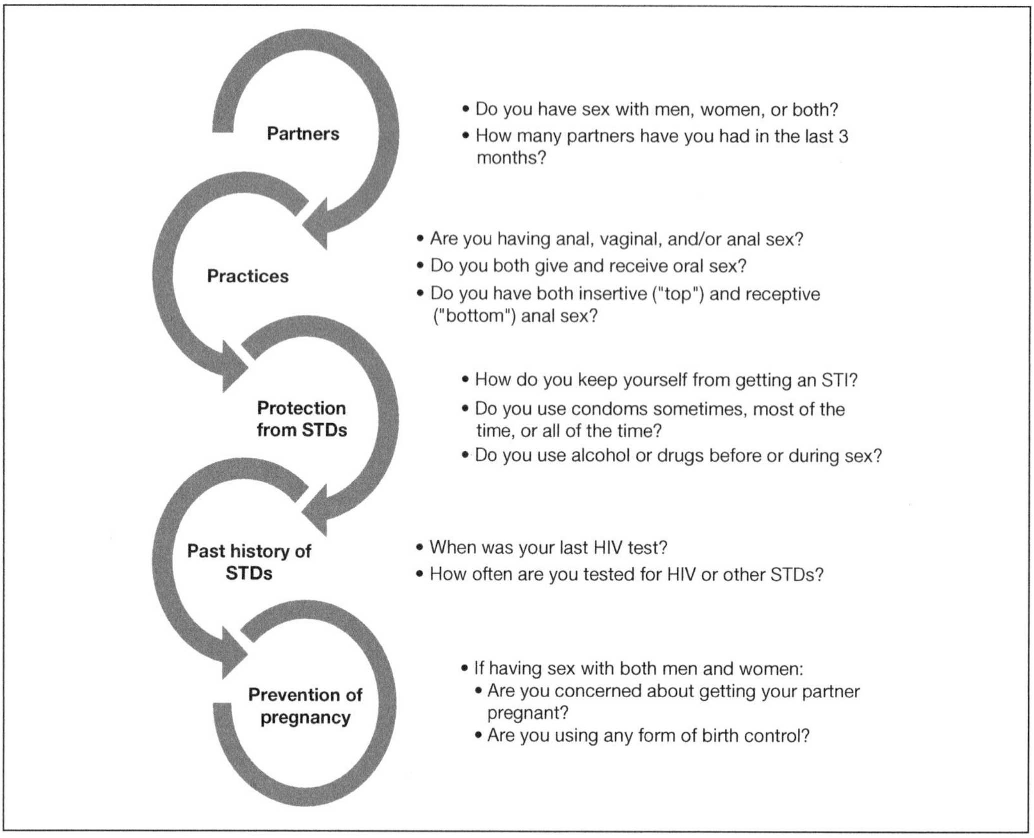

FIGURE 16.2 Five Ps of sexual history.

STDs, sexually transmitted diseases; STI, sexually transmitted infection.

included in the care of the MSM patient. Given that many personal lubricants on the market are formulated with oil or water or are silicone-based, clinicians should educate patients on the appropriate use of these products and potential exposure to STIs, particularly when using oil-based lubricants or petroleum jelly condoms because of the potential for breakage. Similarly, MSM may use products that can cause unintentional harm in an effort to feel clean prior to and/or after sex (Carballo-Diéguez, Bauermeister, Ventuneac, Dolezal, & Mayer, 2010). Often carried out through an enema administration or a hose apparatus, douching products may include water added with soap, salt, and/or antibacterial products, or the use commercially sold solutions (Noor & Rosser, 2014). The widespread practice of douching among MSM is a clinical concern given its association with HIV/STI incidence (Fuchs et al., 2007; Noor & Rosser, 2014). Despite its popular use, unclear guidelines about douching require providers to assess enema use during comprehensive HIV/STI risk assessments and identify less toxic or nontoxic substances (e.g., iso-osmolar products) as alternatives for patients (Noor & Rosser, 2014). Clinicians should also educate patients to avoid anal douching and enemas before colorectal cancer screening via fecal immunochemical test (FIT) as well as prior to anal Pap smears, as they may be more likely to yield inaccurate results.

When completing the sexual health history ask about any additional questions or concerns the patient may have that were not covered. Questions such as, "*What other things about your sexual health and sexual practices should we discuss to help ensure your good health?*" or "*What*

TABLE 16.2 Commonly Reported Sexual Behaviors, Descriptions and Associated Health Risks

Term	Description	Health Risks
Anilingus (also known as rimming, eating ass, rim job, tossing salad)	Sexual stimulation of the anus by use of the mouth, lips, or tongue	Bacterial disease (shigellosis), viral diseases (hepatitis A, B, and C, HPV), STIs
Barebacking	Condomless anal intercourse with a partner of unknown or serodiscordant HIV status	HIV, HPV, STIs
Chemsex (party and play)	Drug and substance use while having sex	HIV, HPV, STIs
Fisting	Insertion of a hand into the rectum	Trauma, laceration, colorectal perforation, increases risks for STIs
Saliva lubrication	Using saliva (spit) as a lubricant	Kaposi sarcoma–associated herpesvirus, HBV, STIs
Sounding (cock-stuffing)	Insertion of a plastic or steel rod into the urethra	Urethritis, STIs, tearing, irritation
Watersports (golden shower)	Sexual activity involving urine	HBV, cytomegalovirus, STIs
		HBV, hepatitis B virus; HPV, human papillomavirus; STI, sexually transmitted infection.

HBV, hepatitis B virus; HPV, human papillomavirus; STI, sexually transmitted infection.

other concerns regarding your sexual health or sexual practices would you like to discuss?" will facilitate dialogue to address any additional concerns that your patient may have (Nusbaum & Hamilton, 2002; Workowski & Bolan, 2015). In addition, developmentally appropriate communication approaches go a long way in facilitating discussions with young MSM. For instance, when engaging with adolescent MSM, giving them ample time to speak shows respectful behavior that earns the trust of youth undergoing developmental transitions. Having private time with youth when parents are asked to step out protects their confidentiality (Snyder et al., 2017) and not sharing all information to parents acknowledges their autonomy.

National data show that condom use among MSM is generally low (Abara et al., 2017). However, aside from focusing on unprotected anal intercourse, providers are also reminded to be on the lookout for a variety of sexual practices that are highly associated with HIV and many other forms of STIs (Rice et al., 2016). Table 16.2 is a compendium of commonly reported sexual behaviors that includes anilingus, barebacking, fisting, saliva lubrication, sounding, substance use, or "chemsex," watersports (Berg, 2009; Breyer & Shindel, 2012; Chow et al., 2016; D'Acunto & Swanson-Biearman, 2015). Not all MSM engage in all of these behaviors; however, it is important for the clinicians to understand these sexual practices to promote appropriate education and counseling for harm reduction (D'Acunto & Swanson-Biearman, 2015).

By relying on SDM and PCC principles while exploring MSM's sexual practices, a provider may create a comfortable space where the patient understands that the assessment is focused on reducing any unanticipated risks rather than seeking to judge or change their sexual practices. In other words, providers should recognize that multiple sexual practices are part of the sexual repertoire for MSM, and focus their efforts in helping MSM to normalize risk-reduction techniques as part of these practices. This is particularly important as prior data has indicated that gay-related rejection sensitivity is associated with condomless anal sex and substance use (Pachankis, Goldfried, & Ramrattan, 2008; Wang & Pachankis, 2016), and may be circumvented if providers can address patients' agency through meaningful clinical conversations (Aholou, Nanin, Drumhiller, & Sutton, 2017). In the section that follows, we discuss the most prevalent health issues experienced by MSM and provide strategies to support SDM and PCC dialogues within the clinical setting.

Common MSM Health Issues

HIV/AIDS

MSM are disproportionally affected by HIV. In 2014, MSM over 13 years of age accounted for nearly 83% of the estimated new HIV diagnoses (Division of HIV/AIDS Prevention, National Center for HIV/AIDS, Viral Hepatitis, Sexual Transmitted Diseases and Tuberculosis Prevention, Centers for Disease Control and Prevention, 2016). Minority groups within the MSM population, particularly blacks and Hispanics, are at even higher risks. Currently, Centers for Disease Control and Prevention (CDC) estimates that 1 in 2 gay/bisexual black men, 1 in 4 gay/bisexual Latino men, and 1 in 6 gay/bisexual men will be diagnosed with HIV if current trends continue (National Center for HIV/AIDS, Viral Hepatitis, STD, and TB Prevention, 2016). Currently, the National HIV/AIDS Strategy has three primary goals: to reduce HIV incidence through testing and linkage to care, to increase access to care and optimize health outcomes, and to reduce HIV-related disparities (White House Office of National AIDS Policy, 2010).

HIV TESTING AND CARE CONTINUUM

The HIV care continuum, also known as the HIV treatment cascade, outlines a sequence of steps for HIV medical care people living with HIV (PLWH) go through. These steps are (a) testing and diagnosis, (b) linkage and retention in medical care, (c) antiretroviral treatment initiation, and (d) viral suppression (Gardner, McLees, Steiner, del Rio, & Burman, 2011). Each of these sequential steps along the HIV care continuum are associated with reduced HIV transmission rates (Skarbinski et al., 2015). Opportunities abound for providers to make sure that MSM receive inclusive care throughout the cascade.

Testing and Diagnosis. It is estimated that approximately 14% to 21% of PLWH are unaware of their diagnosis (Gardner et al., 2011; Hall et al., 2016). This estimate is even higher among MSM and might be as high as 44%. The latest CDC guidelines recommend screening MSM for HIV annually (CDC, 2014). However, more frequent testing may be indicated for MSM who have high-risk exposures such as sexual partners of unknown serostatus, sexual partners who are HIV-infected, and/or recent exposure to STIs (Moyer, 2013; Workowski & Bolan, 2015). Additionally, more frequent HIV screening is recommended for people who inject drugs (PWID) because of the increased risks associated with injection drug use equipment.

Providing ample pre- and post-test counseling to include stigma management (both internalized and anticipated forms of stigma) and dispelling of HIV and testing myths are crucial to encourage collaborative patient-provider conversations about HIV testing (Leblanc, Flores, & Barroso, 2016). Providers may clarify levels of risks associated with specific sexual and drug use behaviors when talking about the benefits of early diagnosis and treatment during clinical encounters. Providing MSM-targeted education about HIV/AIDS symptomology to encourage confirmation of existing medical problems and routinely underscoring the asymptomatic nature of HIV infection is also recommended. Promoting peace of mind is a better option for those who fear an HIV-positive diagnosis, have had risky sex, or choose to live with an unknown HIV status. Framing HIV testing in the context of porous relationship boundaries communicates awareness of realistic relationship concerns. Providers must also counter perception of medical staff as being too busy, which erodes confidence in the accuracy of tests. This may be done by ensuring a consistent manner of communicating HIV test results, emphasizing the accuracy of tests used in the clinic, giving an overview of what the required confirmatory tests would be in the event of an initial positive screen, and reassuring individuals that results are confidential and not reported to law enforcement to criminalize sex work or intravenous drug use. Providers are encouraged to use scripts to routinizing HIV testing across varying clinical settings, including in emergency departments or their private practice.

Risk assessment during an HIV testing visit provides an opportunity for the clinician to provide effective education to minimize the risk of HIV acquisition. HIV prevention education should include need for HIV screening, consistent condoms use, notifying sexual partners of HIV-serostatus, and decreasing the number of sex partners. Pre-exposure prophylaxis, or PrEP, is also an available option to prevent HIV transmission. PrEP refers to the use to antiretrovirals for the prevention of HIV acquisition. Fixed dose tenofovir 300 mg/emtricitabine 200 mg (TDF/FTC, Truvada) was approved by the FDA in 2012. Although awareness of PrEP is low among clinicians (Smith, Mendoza, Stryker, & Rose, 2016), PrEP is safe and effective with a 92% relative risk reduction of HIV transmission in MSM with strong adherence (Grant et al., 2010). Guidelines from the CDC (CDC, 2014) recommend PrEP for MSM who have an HIV-infected sexual partner, had a recent bacterial STI, have a high number of sex partners, have a history of inconsistent or no condom use, or engage in sex work (Box 16.1).

Before starting patients on PrEP, testing should be performed to screen for hepatitis B infection and HIV. Patients should not have signs or symptoms of acute HIV infection. Renal function should also be assessed at baseline and every 6 months while on treatment because tenofovir can cause decreased renal function. PrEP is contraindicated for individuals with an estimated creatinine clearance (eCrCl) of ≤60 mL/min. Renal complications such acute renal failure, and Fanconi's syndrome have occurred. Following the initiation of PrEP clinicians should closely monitor patients. Initially, a 1-month follow-up provides an opportunity to discuss medication adherence and side effects, and answer any questions or concerns the patient may have. Every 3 months, all patients taking PrEP should

BOX 16.1 INDICATIONS FOR PRE-EXPOSURE PROPHYLAXIS AMONG MSM

PrEP is indicated for MSM patients if:

- An adult (18 years or over)
- Without acute or established HIV infection
- Has had a male partner within the past 6 months
- Not in a monogamous relationship with someone who was recently tested and HIV-negative

AND at least one of the following

- Has had condomless anal intercourse (receptive or insertive) in the past 6 months
- Was diagnosed/reported any STI in the past 6 months
- Is in an ongoing relationship with an HIV-positive male partner

MSM, men who have sex with men; PrEP, pre-exposure prophylaxis; STI, sexually transmitted infection.

Source: Centers for Disease Control and Prevention. (2014). Preexposure prophylaxis for the prevention of HIV infection in the United States—2014: A clinical practice guideline. Retrieved from https://www.cdc.gov/hiv/pdf/prepguidelines2014.pdf

receive repeat HIV testing and other STI screening. Renal function should be assessed every 6 months or sooner if other conditions (e.g., diabetes) exist.

Linkage and Retention. Among individuals who tested reactive for HIV in 2013, 73% were linked to HIV medical care within 1 month after diagnosis and 82% were linked to care within 3 months (9). Delays in care are associated with HIV transmission, disease progression, and poor health outcomes (Hall et al., 2016).

Improving provider communication to enhance perception of trustworthiness is crucial when dealing with newly diagnosed patients because the first visits to HIV clinical care has lasting retention implications (Flores, Leblanc, & Barroso, 2016). Provider-patient rapport can be established quicker if patients see the providers as caring. Providers can significantly impact the linkage and retention in care of MSM patients by avoiding paternalistic attitudes and educating them about disclosure strategies to identify support systems to prevent hopelessness and social isolation. Questions such as "Do you have someone you rely on for support who can drive you to appointments?" may reveal an individual's chosen versus birth family. Identify their peer support groups as proxy for family support to decrease loss to follow-up care. Exploring alternative sites for HIV/AIDS care beyond known specialty clinics to curb stigma and address inaccessibility issues is also crucial. Introduce the idea of case management and referrals to patients to ensure access to resources they may not be familiar with. Referring patients to case workers or health navigators is advised for financial assistance, transportation problems, and general assistance to make patients become familiar with healthcare systems and insurance/payment options. Providers as treatment advocates includes educating patients about the benefits of early treatment, emphasizing stigma management, and teaching disclosure skills. For some MSM patients from minority or immigrant communities, respectfully identifying the limitations of traditional healers for the treatment of HIV/AIDS or exploring with patients their beliefs about spirituality can facilitate retention in care.

Secondary prevention efforts are also a crucial area of concern as the unmet needs of newly diagnosed patients with HIV and other comorbid conditions may contribute to further transmission, including the inability to process the shock of diagnosis resulting in unresolved anger and feelings of vulnerability (Heijman, Zuure, Stolte, & Davidovich, 2017). Providers can strengthen patient-provider communication by exploring other correlates that may affect their adherence including assessing longstanding substance use, sexual behaviors, and communication patterns with sex partners.

Antiretroviral Treatment Initiation. Guidelines for the Use of Antiretroviral Agents in HIV-1-Infected Adults and Adolescents (Panel on Antiretroviral Guidelines for Adults and Adolescents, 2016) recommend that antiretroviral therapy (ART) be initiated for all HIV-infected individuals regardless of the CD4 count. When starting ART, patient education should address the benefits of treatment, importance of medication adherence, and strategies to optimize adherence. In certain cases initiation of ART can be deferred owing to structural barriers (e.g., housing instability, cost, insurance coverage), acceptance concerns (e.g., knowledge deficits, readiness, denial, or fear), adherence concerns (e.g., substance use, mental health, lifestyle instability, medical care adherence), and clinical factors, but should be initiated as soon as possible (Beer et al., 2015; Panel on Antiretroviral Guidelines for Adults and Adolescents, 2016). Mistrust of one's physician is negatively associated with ART readiness and adherence among a sample of African American males (Dale et al., 2016; Gwadz et al., 2014).

ART education must be continuous to improve overall health literacy, clarify misconceptions, share strategies about adherence, and highlight ART efficacy (Barroso, Leblanc, &

Flores, 2017). Providers who are knowledgeable, who value patients' input, and who are nonjudgmental, kind, and competent encourage ART initiation. Providers are encouraged to capitalize on individuals' sense of pride, self-efficacy, and personal responsibility to stay healthy and assist them in identifying care resources. Educate about management of HIV/AIDS and strategies for dealing with side effects from ART. Push for collaborative patient-provider relationships geared toward establishing individual independence in care management through open communication. Present ART management as a collaborative pact that is sensitive and nonjudgmental of patients' other healthcare issues (e.g., active drug use, comorbid conditions). Providers must assess motivation and self-efficacy, adapt regimen to patients' lifestyle, initiate trial runs, and consider other sociodemographic issues crucial to ART adherence. Reinforce patients' perceived benefits of free ART and boost optimism about future treatments.

Viral Suppression. Optimal viral suppression is defined generally as a viral load persistently below the level of detection. Current assays can detect HIV RNA levels as low <20 to 75 copies/mL (Panel on Antiretroviral Guidelines for Adults and Adolescents, 2016). HIV treatment goals include the following: (a) maximally and durably suppress plasma HIV RNA, (b) restore and preserve immunological function, (c) reduce HIV-associated morbidity and prolong the duration and quality of survival, and (d) prevent HIV transmission (Panel on Antiretroviral Guidelines for Adults and Adolescents, 2016). Treatment as prevention is a method whereby antiretrovirals are used to minimize the risk of HIV transmission through viral suppression. With the use of ART individuals can decrease their HIV viral load, ideally to undetectable levels, and are therefore less likely to infect their sexual partners (Cohen et al., 2016). Data from the PARTNER study (Rodger et al., 2016) provides evidence that HIV transmission may not occur when viral load is below detectable levels.

Successful and sustained viral suppression not only involves the patient-provider dyad, but other members of the healthcare team. Providers can emphasize patients' active role in their care and the team management/collaborative pact and supportive nature of HIV/AIDS care that includes patients, other trusted providers, pharmacists, social workers, etc.

Effective ART retention strategies include keeping in touch by sending appointment reminders, engaging patients through letters and phone calls in between their medical appointments, celebrating their improved health, and exploring ways patients can incorporate taking ARTs with their daily schedules. Establishing collaborative patient-provider discussions about complementary medicine and the known and unknown effects on ART conveys shared decision making. This includes talks about the pros and cons of local herbal remedies and its pharmacodynamic impact on ARTs. Discuss essential modifications to behavior and coping strategies that would increase likelihood of ART adherence.

SEXUALLY TRANSMITTED INFECTIONS

MSM are at an increased risk of acquiring STIs because of the increased prevalence of STIs in this group. MSM who are sexually active should be screened annually for HIV, *Chlamydia trachomatis*, *Neisseria gonorrhoeae*, syphilis, and hepatitis. Even if MSM do not engage in condomless anal intercourse, they may have unprotected oral sex. The latest STI treatment guidelines from the CDC (Workowski & Bolan, 2015) recommend that clinicians use site-specific screening (regardless of HIV status), which includes oral, urethral, and rectal sites. Nucleic acid amplification test (NAAT) is the preferred approach (Box 16.2). More frequent testing may be indicated, in 3- to 6-month intervals, for those at increased risk or who have multiple sexual partners. Individual risk behaviors, such as number of lifetime sex partners, rate of partner exchange, and frequency of unprotected sex should be assessed (Box 16.3). Many STIs could be asymptomatic in this

BOX 16.2 HIV AND STI SCREENING RECOMMENDATIONS

Chlamydia

- At least annually for sexually active MSM at sites of contact (urethra, rectum) regardless of condom use
- Every 3 to 6 months if at increased risk

Gonorrhea

- At least annually for sexually active MSM at sites of contact (urethra, rectum, pharynx) regardless of condom use
- Every 3 to 6 months if at increased risk

Syphilis

- At least annually for sexually active MSM
- Every 3 to 6 months if at increased risk

Hepatitis B

- All MSM should be tested for HBsAg.

Hepatitis C

- MSM born between 1945 and 1965
- Other MSM if risk factors are present
- Annual HCV testing in MSM with HIV infection

HIV

- At least annually for sexually active MSM if HIV status is unknown or negative and the patient himself or his sex partner(s) have had more than one sex partner since most recent HIV test. Testing should be performed at shorter intervals for those at higher risk.
- All men who seek evaluation and treatment for STDs

HCV, hepatitis C virus; MSM, men who have sex with men; STD, sexually transmitted disease.

Source: Workowski, K. A., & Bolan, G. A. (2015). Sexually transmitted diseases treatment guidelines, 2015. Atlanta, GA: Center for Surveillance, Epidemiology, and Laboratory Services, Centers for Disease Control and Prevention.

BOX 16.3 SEXUALLY TRANSMITTED INFECTION BEHAVIORAL RISK FACTORS

- New sex partner within the past 60 days
- Multiple sex partners
- Sex partner with multiple concurrent sex partners
- Condomless anal intercourse
- Sex work (trading sex for money or drugs)
- Sexual contact (oral, anal, and/or penile) with sex workers
- Encounters with anonymous partners from the Internet or geosocial network apps

TABLE 16.3 STI Treatment Recommendations

Sexually Transmitted Infection	Recommended Treatment
Chlamydia infection	Azithromycin, 1 g orally single dose OR doxycycline, 100 mg orally 2x/day for 7 days
Gonorrhea	Ceftriaxone, 250 mg IM single does PLUS Azithromycin, 1 g oral single dose
Syphilis	Primary: benzathine penicillin G, 2.4 million units IM in a single dose Latent: benzathine penicillin G, 2.4 million units IM, 3 doses at 1-week intervals (7.2 million units total)

IM, intramuscular; STI, sexually transmitted infection.

Source: Workowski, K. A., & Bolan, G. A. (2015). Sexually transmitted diseases treatment guidelines, 2015. Atlanta, GA: Center for Surveillance, Epidemiology, and Laboratory Services, Centers for Disease Control and Prevention.

population. Thus, screening should be based on risk rather than symptoms. MSM-specific factors such as limited or overlapping social and sexual networks are also linked with greater rates of STIs, including HIV among MSM. Therefore, screening for behavioral risk factors is recommended, as these may contribute to the disparities observed in MSM (Table 16.3).

HUMAN PAPILLOMAVIRUS

In men, human papillomavirus (HPV) can lead to the development of oropharyngeal cancer as well as cancer of the penis, anus, and/or rectum. MSM have a high burden of HPV with an estimated prevalence of 65% in gay men and as high as 95% in gay men living with HIV (Moscicki & Palefsky, 2011). The most common site for HPV in MSM is the anal canal (Goldstone et al., 2011), which places MSM at great risk of developing anal cancer. HPV -related disease, specifically high-risk types, account for more than 80% of anal cancers (De Vuyst, Clifford, Nascimento, Madeleine, & Franceschi, 2009).

HPV Screening. Experts recommend performing anal Pap testing in MSM. Through anal Pap smear, a sampling of cells from the anal transition zone can be obtained for cytological detection of HPV-related abnormalities. Results are reported as either negative or normal, atypical squamous cells of undetermined significance (ASCUS), low-grade squamous intraepithelial lesion (LSIL), or high-grade squamous intraepithelial lesion (HSIL). In cases in which abnormal cytological features are present, high-resolution anoscopy is suggested for direct visualization of the lesions and possible biopsy of specimens. Through biopsy anal histopathological examination is performed to grade disease.

HPV Vaccination. The Advisory Committee on Immunization Practices (ACIP) and CDC recommend HPV vaccination for preteens beginning at age 11. Teens and young MSM can also be vaccinated until 27 years of age. The HPV vaccination is available as a quadrivalent HPV vaccine (4vHPV) that protects against HPV types 6, 11, 16, and 18, or nine-valent HPV vaccine (9vHPV) that protects against HPV types 6, 11, 16, 18, 31, 45, 52, and 58. Both of these vaccinations have a two-dose schedule with the administration at 0 and 6-12 months for those between 9 and 14 years of age (Meites, Kempe, & Markowitz, 2017). A three-dose schedule with administration at 0, 1–2, and 6 months is recommended for those between 15 and 26 years of age and those who are immunocompromised at ages 9 through 26 years (Table 16.4).

TABLE 16.4 HPV Vaccine Schedule

Group	Recommended Number of HPV Vaccine Doses	Recommended Interval Between Doses
Persons initiating HPV vaccination at ages 9 through 14 years, except immunocompromised persons	2	0, 6–12 months
Persons initiating HPV vaccination at ages 15 through 26 years and immunocompromised persons initiating HPV vaccination at ages 9 through 26 years	3	0, 1–2, 6 months

Source: Meites, E., Kempe, A., & Markowitz, L. E. (2017). Use of a 2-Dose Schedule for Human Papillomavirus Vaccination—Updated Recommendations of the Advisory Committee on Immunization Practices. American Journal of Transplantation, 17(3), 834–837. doi:10.1111/ajt.14206

MSM are largely unaware of the link between HPV and anal cancers (Fenkl, Jones, Schochet, & Johnson, 2016). Anal cancer and genital warts are viewed as severe conditions by young MSM and yet they do not necessarily see themselves as being at risk for HPV infection (Nadarzynski, Smith, Richardson, Pollard, & Llewellyn, 2017). The HPV vaccine has the ability to prevent anal and oropharyngeal cancers. However, HPV vaccination rates among young MSM 18 to 26 years of age is low. Less than a quarter of providers with high knowledge of HPV and the risk-based recommendations actually do broach this issue with their young MSM patients (Wheldon et al., 2017). Education about the importance of vaccination for the prevention of HPV and HPV-related complications should be discussed with patients.

VIRAL HEPATITIS

The liver has many important functions in the body: it assists in processing nutrients during digestion, fights infection, filters blood, and plays a vital role in the metabolism of medications. All of these processes are affected when the liver is inflamed or damaged due to medications, ingested toxins, heavy alcohol use, or hepatitis. Types of viral hepatitis include hepatitis A, hepatitis B, hepatitis C, hepatitis D, hepatitis E, and hepatitis G. When considering the health of the MSM population, hepatitis A, hepatitis B, and hepatitis C are the most common types.

HEPATITIS A

Approximately 2,500 new hepatitis A virus (HAV) infections occur annually, and it is the most common form of viral hepatitis worldwide. It is estimated that 10% of new HAV infections occur in MSM. Transmission of HAV primarily occurs through the oral-fecal route. This type of transmission most commonly occurs through ingestion of food or water that is contaminated by HAV, or through person-to-person contact exposure to fecal material which includes sexual contact. HAV outbreaks among MSM are also frequently reported.

Clinical Manifestations. The CDC (CDC, 2012) case definition describes HAV infection as an acute illness with a discrete onset of any sign or symptom consistent with acute viral hepatitis and either jaundice or elevated liver function tests (serum alanine aminotransferase or aspartate aminotransferase). Usual signs or symptoms associated with hepatitis include abdominal pain, anorexia, diarrhea, fever, headache, nausea, and vomiting.

Diagnosis. Diagnosis of hepatitis A is confirmed with anti-HAV immunoglobulin M (IgM). Hepatitis IgM antibodies may be detectable 5 to 10 days prior to onset of symptoms.

Prevention. Prevention of hepatitis A can be achieved through proper hand-washing, sanitation, and adequate water and food sources. Immunity in MSM should be assessed prior to administering the vaccination. The Advisory Committee on Immunization Practices (AICP) (Fiore, Wasley, & Bell, 2006) recommends hepatitis A vaccination for MSM. The vaccination is administered as a two-dose series of immunizations through intramuscular injection at 0 and 6 months. Twinrix is also available and should administered at 0, 1, and 6 months to persons aged ≥18 years at risk for both HAV and HBV infections. Assessment of immunity after completing the vaccination series is not indicated.

HEPATITIS B

In 2014 there was an estimated 19,200 new infections of hepatitis B virus (HBV). Approximately 20% of new hepatitis cases occur in MSM. HBV is transmitted by exposure of mucous membranes or percutaneously contact with HBV-infected blood or body fluids. Primary risk factors for MSM include unprotected sex (e.g., condomless anal intercourse), multiple partners, injection drug use, and a history of STI (Thompson, Perz, Moorman, & Holmberg, 2009).

Clinical Manifestations. Symptoms of HBV infection are the same as those with HAV; however, hepatitis B has a longer incubation period between 6 weeks to 6 months.

Diagnosis. Because HBsAg is present in both acute and chronic infection, the presence of IgM antibody to hepatitis B core antigen (IgM anti-HBc) is indicative of either acute or recently acquired HBV infection. Antibody to HBsAg (anti-HBs) is produced after a resolved infection and is the only HBV antibody marker present after vaccination. The presence of HBsAg and total anti-HBc, with a negative test for IgM anti-HBc, indicates chronic HBV infection (Workowski & Bolan, 2015).

Prevention. Because of the higher rates of infection in this population, both ACIP and CDC recommend routine vaccination of MSM against HBV. Currently, three vaccine schedules are approved as monovalent hepatitis B vaccines (Engerix-B and Recombivax), which can be administered at 0, 1, and 6 months; 0, 1, and 4 months; and 0, 2, and 4 months (Table 16.5). Twinrix should be considered as well those at risk for both HAV and HBV infections. Prior to vaccine administration, individuals should be screened for immunity to reduce unnecessary vaccinations. Protection of hepatitis B through vaccination is estimated to last up to 30 years (Bruce et al., 2016).

TABLE 16.5 Hepatitis A and B Vaccination Schedules

Vaccine	Recommended Number of Vaccine Doses	Recommended Interval Between Doses
Hepatitis A vaccination	2	0 and 6–12 months (Havrix) or 0 and 6–18 months (Vaqta)
Hepatitis B vaccination	3	0, 1, and 6 months (Engerix-B, Recombivax HB)
Combined hepatitis A and B vaccination	3	0, 1, and 6 months

HEPATITIS C

Hepatitis C is caused by the hepatitis C virus (HCV). There were approximately 34,000 new HCV infections in the U.S. in 2015 (Campbell et al., 2017). Coinfection of HIV and HCV is increased in MSM and has been reported in major cities across the United States, Asia, and Europe (Chan, Lin, Wong, Wong, & Lee, 2015; Dionne-Odom, Osborn, Radziewicz, Grakoui, & Workowski, 2009; van de Laar et al., 2009; Workowski & Bolan, 2015). HCV transmissions occurs primarily through contact with blood of an infected person, usually through intravenous drug use, and HCV is less commonly transmitted sexually. Within the MSM population, common exposures occur through sexual contact, or sharing of contaminated syringes, needles, or other injection equipment.

Clinical Manifestations. The typical incubation period of HCV is between 14 and 180 days with the most individuals presenting with symptoms around 45 days. Approximately 20% to 30% of newly infected people develop symptoms of acute disease. Symptoms of HCV infection are similar to those with hepatitis A or hepatitis B.

Prevention. HCV screening should be done using a screening assay (either enzyme immune assay [EIA] or chemiluminescence assay [CIA]) for anti-HCV; more specific assays (e.g., nucleic acid testing [NAT] for HCV RNA) provide verification of HCV infection. There is no vaccine against hepatitis C at the present time.

CANCERS

Quality of life may be greatly affected in MSM individuals with cancer. Low rates of health insurance, fear of discrimination, and negative experience with healthcare providers contribute to poor health outcomes in this population. The high incidence of HIV, HPV, and tobacco use among MSM also increase the risk of anal and other types of cancer (Sahasrabuddhe et al., 2013).

ANAL CANCER

Although the incidence of many cancers (lung, prostate, and colorectal) has declined over the past decade, anal cancer incidence has increased over the last 3 decades (van der Zee, Richel, de Vries, & Prins, 2013). MSM have the highest incidence of anal cancer. It is estimated that MSM are 20 times more likely to develop anal cancer than non-MSM/heterosexual men. The risk is even higher among MSM living with HIV, who have a ninefold increase in the incidence over that of HIV-negative MSM (Machalek et al., 2012).

High-risk strains of HPV (type 16 and 11) could progress to anal dysplasia and anal carcinoma similarly to how cervical carcinoma develops in women. Persistent infection by high-risk strains can progress to high-grade intraepithelial lesions (HSILs) (Koskan, LeBlanc, & Rosa-Cunha, 2016). Thus, screening for and early detection of anal dysplasia is critical for early intervention, especially among MSM living with HIV. Clinicians should provide education about HPV and anal cancer to patients because lack of awareness is the greatest barrier to screening. Patients recommend interpersonal education through one-on-one discussion to be provided following the health history (Koskan, LeBlanc, & Rosa-Cunha, 2016). Vaccination against HPV to those under 27 years of age should be encouraged to decrease the incidence of anal cancer and HPV in this population.

PROSTATE CANCER

Prostate cancer is the most common cancer among men (CDC, 2017). Prostate cancer in MSM is an emerging health concern; however, data in this area are limited as sexual orientation is not routinely collected as part of cancer surveillance (Simon Rosser et al., 2016). Currently it is estimated that 5,000 gay men develop prostate cancer each year. Heteronormative assumptions exist particularly around prostate cancer and can be a barrier to quality care. Experiencing social stigma, negative healthcare experiences, and discrimination lead to the isolation that is commonly reported by MSM. The development of prostate cancer can negatively impact emotional and sexual functioning of MSM leading to lower quality of life than that experienced by other men. Awareness of the diversity that exists can minimize inequality in the provision of care and support to MSM.

MENTAL HEALTH

MSM share mental health challenges like their heterosexual counterparts such as affective disorders, sexual trauma, suicidal ideation, and eating disorders. Experiences around their sexuality make these issues all the more complex when considering the marginalization, stigma, and risk of violence this population endures. Nevertheless, MSM patients' positive appraisal of the relationship they have with providers is associated with fewer mental health symptoms (Bankoff, McCullough, & Pantalone, 2013) and underscores the role effective communication has in addressing not just this population's physical health, but their mental health as well.

Internalized Homophobia/Homonegativity. Systemic negativity around a nonheterosexual sexual orientation impacts an individual's view of themselves. When nonaffirming messages are unconsciously internalized, MSM develop negative feelings about themselves (Berg, Munthe-Kaas, & Ross, 2016; Herek, 2000). MSM who suffer from internalized homonegativity report high rates of unsafe sexual behavior, inability to decline unwanted sexual advances, illicit drug use, endorsement of AIDS conspiracy beliefs, depression, and psychological distress (Berg, Weatherburn, Ross, & Schmidt, 2015; Berg et al., 2016; Boone, Cook, & Wilson, 2016; Simon Rosser et al., 2016). Providers are in a position to identify resources that can assist MSM in receiving social support. Whether through direct affirming care or by referring patients to other members of the care team (social workers, counselors, peer navigators, etc.), a more holistic approach is needed to address years of negative messages these individuals have received growing up. Inclusive environments that provide sensitive, supportive, and affirming care to meet the needs of MSM patients will help.

Substance and Drug Abuse. Alcohol and substance use among MSM is higher than their heterosexual counterparts, and can increase the risk for many health problems and safety. Worldwide, the higher prevalence of illicit drug use by MSM compared to their heterosexual peers has been strongly associated with sexually risky behavior (Bourne & Weatherburn, 2017; Scott-Sheldon, Carey, Cunningham, Johnson, & Carey, 2016; Stein et al., 2005). Use of alcohol and/or substances may result in impaired judgment, decreased inhibition, condomless anal intercourse, and experiencing intimate partner violence. Substance use within partnerships or casual sexual relationships is referred to as "chemsex" and is associated with engagement in risk-taking behaviors (Brown, Turner, Hern, & Santos, 2017; Hall, Shoptaw, & Reback, 2015). Substances commonly used within the MSM community that are relatively unfamiliar to clinicians include alkyl nitrates ("poppers"), ketamine ("special K"), crystal methamphetamines, and gamma-hydroxybutyrate ("GHB") and are frequently referred to as "sex drugs."

First, alkyl nitrates, or "poppers" are widely used in the MSM community. Many MSM use "poppers" to enhance sexual experiences and enjoyment due to its psychoactive effects and smooth muscle relaxation. This substance is generally perceived to be harmless among the MSM community (Semple, Patterson, & Grant, 2002). Most commonly, patients may experience headaches when using alkyl nitrates. More serious consequences may occur when combined with phosphodiesterase type 5 inhibitor (PDE5i) such as sildenafil citrate (Viagra) or tadalafil (Cialis). Combining alkyl nitrates with a PDE5i may lead to cognitive impairment, rapid vasodilation, compromised cardiovascular status, or death. Second, ketamines, also known as "club drugs," are used worldwide. Commonly known as K, special K, Vitamin K, and Kitkat, ketamine has both dissociative analgesic and hallucinogenic effects. Ketamine may be used as a powder or in a liquid form that can be added to drinks. Next, Crystal methamphetamine (also known as crystal, meth, and tina) increases sexual urge, and could lead to sexual binges. These prolonged sexual encounters impair the integrity of anal epithelial cells and mucous membranes, increasing the likelihood of HIV transmission and other STIs.

Using crystal meth is called tweaking, and slamming refers to intravenous use. Use of crystal meth is associated with elevation of core body temperature, heart rate, and blood pressure, which increases risk of myocardial infarction and stroke. This stimulant also causes appetite suppression and insomnia in small doses. Sleep deprivation is commonly experienced with use of crystal meth and may lead to exhaustion, paranoia, or aggressive behaviors.

Lastly, gamma-hydroxybutyrate, or GHB, is another frequently used drug in the club scene and with chemsex. GHB is also known as G or liquid ecstasy. Similar to GHB is gamma-butyrolactone, or GBL, which is converted to GHB once in the body. Both of these substances increase libido while producing mildly sedative effects. GHB and GLB are both odorless and undetectable when added to drinks in small amounts. Owing to their high concentration, even small amounts of this substance can lead to nausea and vomiting, as well as seizures, coma, and death. Combining either of these substances with alcohol potentiates their effects.

Combining sex and illicit drugs among MSM is an important public health concern. Individuals may engage in chemsex as a means to increase libido, confidence, and disinhibition. These drugs enhance sexual experiences by increasing physical sensations and intensifying perceptions of intimacy while providing sexual excitement (Weatherburn, Hickson, Reid, Torres-Rueda, & Bourne, 2017). Routinely screening for alcohol and substance use is recommended, as these substances increase the risk for many issues relating to health, employment, relationships, and safety. Club drugs, such as crystal methamphetamine, ketamine, and gamma-hydroxybutyrate, are often used in combination with PDE5i drugs due to difficulty achieving an erection. Combining these substances with inappropriate use of PDE5i drugs may lead to potentially harmful or fatal effects. Screening, brief intervention, and referral to treatment (SBIRT) is an effective approach used to deliver intervention and treatment for those at risk (Bray, Del Boca, McRee, Hayashi, & Babor, 2017).

Body Image. Exploring MSM patients' perceptions about their weight and attractiveness has independent influences on their body image and consequent regard for their overall health. For starters, young gay and bisexual males in high school are more likely than their straight peers to see themselves as being overweight despite being of healthy weight or even underweight (Hadland, Austin, Goodenow, & Calzo, 2014). The same study also showed young gay and bisexual youth to engage more with unhealthy weight control strategies such as using diet pills, fasting, vomiting, or using laxatives. Also, young overweight MSM may engage in more unprotected sex due to perceived inability to negotiate condom use, fat distribution in the abdomen or penis, or low feelings of attractiveness that result in discomfort discussing safer sex practices (Meanley, Hickok, Johns, Pingel, & Bauermeister, 2014; Moskowitz & Seal, 2010). In one study that compared gym exercise patterns (Mor,

Parfionov, Davidovitch, & Grotto, 2014), MSM's desire to conform to accepted standards of male beauty within the MSM community has been associated to more intensive anaerobic training, use of protein powders or supplements or anabolic steroids, and engaging in riskier sexual behavior, compared to heterosexual males. To this end, providers may help patients assess community norms about beauty and empower them with resources to challenge these unrealistic standards. Screening for anorexia or bulimia is warranted.

MANAGEMENT OF COMORBID CONDITIONS

The long-term management of comorbid conditions is crucial to ensuring MSM patients' well-being and quality of life. This is crucial because even with patients who have well-managed HIV infection, for example, long-term antiretroviral therapy is associated with higher levels for cardiovascular disease, myocardial infarctions, and congestive heart failure (Lim, Brown, & Kim, 2014). Further, concomitant use of medications with overlapping and additive toxicities predispose MSM patients to adverse antiretroviral side effects (AIDSinfo, 2017). Having comorbid conditions exacerbates adverse effects as well, such as elevated risks for hepatotoxicity when a patient who suffers from alcoholism is also coinfected with viral hepatitis or when those with psychiatric disorders are prescribed ARTs known to cause CNS-related toxicities (AIDSinfo, 2017).

To counter care fatigue with MSM who have chronic health issues or experience medication side effects, integrating medical with alternative therapies (complementary traditional practices, spiritual dimensions of care, patient support services, etc.) is advised as these also communicates a commitment to patient-centered care (Scholl et al., 2014). Having awareness of patients' social affiliations has implications for their HIV-related outcomes and underscores health access issues beyond typical LGBTQ enclaves (Behler, Cornwell, & Schneider, 2017). Compiling a list of referring agencies and organizations that provide essential services outside metropolitan areas or the local LGBT enclaves communicates a commitment to patients' engagement in care. Asking about their access to centralized clinics and nonprofits may uncover potential threats to uninterrupted receipt of care.

SHARED DECISION MAKING IN THE LARGER CONTEXT

The previous sections have focused on individual and dyadic level factors that affect communication with MSM patients. However, recent scholarship has recognized that individual level factors alone cannot account for health disparities associated with MSM and, in particular, structural inequities fuel the heavy burden of HIV infection in the MSM community (Batchelder, Safren, Mitchell, Ivardic, & O'Cleirigh, 2017; Castel, Magnus, & Greenberg, 2015). The following section will focus on the contextual factors that also have a significant bearing on the patient-provider interaction.

Prior to any clinic visit, the default assumption is that patients are heterosexual; heterosexism is the norm in most clinical encounters and permeates the practices in all levels of the healthcare setting (Baker & Beagan, 2014). Even before MSM patients get a chance to talk to their providers, intake forms in the waiting rooms inquire about one's history of sexual intercourse with the underlying assumption of penile-vaginal penetration (Goins & Pye, 2013). To ensure SDM is fostered beyond the clinical interaction, a macro-level commitment by healthcare organizations has to be in place. DeMeester and colleagues (DeMeester, Lopez, Moore, Cook, & Chin, 2016) have identified SDM organizational drivers that may determine the extent of a practice setting's inclusiveness. We will focus on the following organizational drivers: workflows, health information technology, organizational structure and culture, resources and clinic environment, and staff training and education.

Workflows

Workflow refers to the sequence of administrative and clinical processes that both staff and patients go through during each clinical encounter. Workflow considerations include how appointments are set up or walk-ins are accommodated, procedures for checking in at clinic sites, and patient flow through different members of the care team. Workflow examples for HIV care include accounting for shock and disbelief as barriers to education when delivering seropositive test results. Providers must have awareness that clinical time constraints inhibit understanding of new diagnoses and must be addressed. Providers may offer HIV testing during routine clinic visits or when testing for other STIs and educate patients about their risk levels. A separate precounseling session or a consent form just for HIV may dissuade people from testing as it may be viewed as intimidating, redundant, or time consuming. Institute streamlined clinical operations that reduce waiting times and create efficient clinic flow. Referral systems between central hospitals and community clinics must be efficient and maintain confidential information about patients.

Health Information Technology

Health information technology revolves around the secure application of information technology to healthcare with the goal of information access and exchange across computerized systems. At present, guidelines from the Centers for Medicare and Medicaid Services mandate that health systems with certified electronic health records collect data about sexual orientation (U.S. Department of Health and Human Services, 2016), but only a handful of organizations are complying with this requirement (Alper, Feit, & Sanders, 2013). An example of an adaptive health information system is risk-based screening using electronic medical systems that will prompt providers regarding U.S. Preventive Services Task Force (USPSTF) recommendations such as for HPV vaccine coverage (Wheldon et al., 2017). However, simply adapting electronic health records does not automatically confer PCC unless it leads to patients' meaningful involvement in their care (Epstein & Street, 2011). Providers are reminded to use appropriate and respectful language to address sexual orientation and sexual behaviors in clinic notes that are accessible to other members of the healthcare team (Boone, Cook, & Wilson, 2016).

Organizational Structure and Culture

Leadership and staff commitment to SDM with sexual minority patients is the centerpiece of this third driver. Guaranteeing that care sites are able to recognize and respond to patients' background and context respectfully conveys commitment to patients. Tangible ways to achieve this include having mission statements and policies that spell out a pledge to serve all patients, regardless of sexual orientation and gender identity, having a diverse provider and staff roster that is reflective of the patient population, and developing ongoing relationships with local community organizations that serve diverse LGBT communities (DeMeester, 2016; Peek et al., 2016). Additionally, being cognizant of how racial stereotypes might affect care delivery (e.g., seeing Asian men as members of a model minority or African American men as hypersexual) is one step closer toward unbiased care (Tan et al., 2016). Finally, allowing the use of clinic facilities after hours to local nonprofit organizations or patient groups conveys commitment by providing space for community groups.

Resources and Clinic Environment

The pursuit of SDM with MSM patients may be facilitated by having materials and a physical environment that cater to this population's needs. The availability of tailored educational resources with accessible language assists patients in comprehending their care options and allows the personalization of care offered to them. MSM patients who are not fluent in English would benefit from providers or staff who can communicate with them in their language. If not feasible, making professional medical interpretation services available would also suffice. Unless patients first provide permission, providers are reminded not to use family members or friends as interpreters due to privacy concerns (Baig et al., 2016). To ensure that the clinic environment is welcoming, visual cues that communicate inclusivity (safe zone stickers, rainbow pins, etc.) are recommended. Addressing stigma associated with accessing sexual health services must also be confronted and corrected, such as not labeling community health centers as "family planning clinics" (Formby, 2016).

Staff Training and Education

Providers believe that they do not possess the skills essential to address issues related to the sexual orientation of their LGBT patients. In fact, most of them do not regularly discuss sexual orientation or gender identity when conducting a sexual history from a sexually active adolescent (Kitts, 2010) and they generally feel unprepared to provide competent sexual health services to LGBT youth (Knight, Shoveller, & Carson, 2014). Skills-based training to develop strategies for patient-provider communication around sexual orientation and risk mitigation is recommended (Sexuality Information and Education Council of the United States, 2016; Wheldon et al., 2017). To this end, services and resources from nonprofit groups, such as the Fenway Institute, may be relied on for continuing education of staff. Providers already insist that medical curriculum be inclusive of this population's concerns. This can begin to address communication competency issues during their training (Coleman et al., 2017; Wheldon et al., 2017) or as part of continuing professional education (Stewart & O'Reilly, 2017). On the other hand, providers who are already confident in their knowledge and competency levels in working with LGBT patients are advised to make it known to their patients as this establishes accessibility (Rounds, McGrath, & Walsh, 2014).

CONCLUSION

> *"Two systems of knowledge collide in clinical encounters. Clinicians are experts in biomedicine, patients are experts in their own experience."*
>
> —Carpenter-Song et al., 2007

Beyond expecting provider expertise regarding MSM health needs, this chapter encourages providers to focus on a more achievable goal: the acknowledgment that MSM have shared and unique health concerns. Although this chapter focused on the common health issues that are pertinent for MSM patients, it has to be reiterated that sexual orientation by itself does not cause individuals to be automatically at risk for these conditions. Through an inclusive practice that puts a premium on effective communication, providers can partner with patients to address the behaviors and conditions that may lead to the health issues covered in this chapter. Given the diversity of experiences, identities, behaviors, and characteristics of this patient population, we urge providers to rely on SDM and PCC principles to create and/or support respectful spaces during clinical encounters (Baker & Beagan, 2014). When considering MSM patients' needs providers are cautioned against portraying this population as victims or as a homogeneously vulnerable people. MSM patients have the same need for respectful care to address their physical and mental health concerns. Striking the balance between offering targeted care and not viewing them as mere recipients is achievable when decision-making power is equitable and their concerns are prioritized (Formby, 2016).

We have covered in this chapter the intrapersonal, dyadic, and contextual factors that facilitate or impede effective patient-provider communication. As a recap, we highlight the twofold considerations that providers can use as foundations for a truly patient-centered approach to inclusive MSM healthcare: First, providers have a responsibility to safeguard MSM patients' confidentiality and model respect for their privacy. Second, it is incumbent upon providers to take the lead in challenging entrenched heteronormative assumptions in their practice settings and to correct clinical practice that reinforces sexual and gender binaries. Ultimately, each clinical encounter relies on the mutual respect both parties extend to one another. As nurse practitioners and physician assistants, you have the capacity to set the tone for each patient visit that will ensure the health of your MSM patients.

NATIONAL RESOURCES

Agency for Healthcare Research and Quality: www.ahrq.gov/professionals/education/curriculum-tools/shareddecisionmaking/tools/sharefactsheet/index.html
Centers for Disease Control and Prevention's A Guide to Taking A Sexual History: www.cdc.gov/std/treatment/sexualhistory.pdf
Fenway Institute: fenwayhealth.org/the-fenway-institute
Gay and Lesbian Medical Association: www.glma.org
Lavender Health: lavenderhealth.org
National LGBT Health Education Center: www.lgbthealtheducation.org
National LGBTQ Taskforce: www.thetaskforce.org
Parents, Family, Friends of Lesbians and Gays (PFLAG): www.pflag.org/about
Patient Decision Aids: decisionaid.ohri.ca/AZlist.html
Substance Abuse and Mental Health Services Administration's Top Health Issues for LGBT Populations and Resource Kit: store.samhsa.gov/shin/content/SMA12-4684/SMA12-4684.pdf
U.S. Preventive Services Task Force: www.uspreventiveservicestaskforce.org/BrowseRec/Index

REFERENCES

Abara, W. E., Oraka, E., Jeffries, W. L., Chavez, P., Nasrullah, M., & DiNenno, E. (2017). Prevalence and correlates of condom use among sexually active men who have sex with men in the United States: Findings from the National Survey of Family Growth, 2002, 2006–10 and 2011–13. *Sexual Health, 14*(4), 363–371. doi:10.1071/SH16034

Agency for Healthcare Research and Quality. (2016). The SHARE Approach. Retrieved from https://www.ahrq.gov/professionals/education/curriculum-tools/shareddecisionmaking/index.html

Aholou, T. M., Nanin, J., Drumhiller, K., & Sutton, M. Y. (2017). Opportunities for HIV prevention communication during sexual encounters with black men who have sex with men. *AIDS Patient Care and STDs, 31*(1), 33–40. doi:10.1089/apc.2016.0220

AIDSinfo. (2017). Guidelines for the use of antiretroviral agents in adults and adolescents living with HIV. Retrieved from https://aidsinfo.nih.gov/guidelines/html/1/adult-and-adolescent-arv-guidelines/31/adverse-effects-of-arv

Alper, J., Feit, M. N., & Sanders, J. Q. (2013). *Collecting sexual orientation and gender identity data in electronic health records.* Washington, DC: National Academies Press (US).

American Academy of Physician Assistants. (2013). Guidelines for Ethical Conduct. Retrieved from https://www.aapa.org/wp-content/uploads/2017/02/16-EthicalConduct.pdf

American Nurses Association. (2001). Code of ethics. Retrieved from http://www.nursingworld.org/codeofethics

Baig, A. A., Lopez, F. Y., DeMeester, R. H., Jia, J. L., Peek, M. E., & Vela, M. B. (2016). Addressing barriers to shared decision making among Latino LGBTQ patients and healthcare providers in clinical settings. *LGBT Health, 3*(5), 335–341. doi:10.1089/lgbt.2016.0014

Baker, K., & Beagan, B. (2014). Making assumptions, making space: An anthropological critique of cultural competency and its relevance to queer patients. *Medical Anthropology Quarterly, 28*(4), 578–598. doi:10.1111/maq.12129

Bankoff, S. M., McCullough, M. B., & Pantalone, D. W. (2013). Patient–provider relationship predicts mental and physical health indicators for HIV-positive men who have sex with men. *Journal of Health Psychology, 18*(6), 762–772. doi:10.1177/1359105313475896

Barroso, J., Leblanc, N. M., & Flores, D. (2017). It's not just the pills: A qualitative meta-synthesis of HIV antiretroviral adherence research. *Journal of the Association of Nurses in AIDS Care, 28*(4), 462–478. doi:10.1016/j.jana.2017.02.007

Barry, M. J., & Edgman-Levitan, S. (2012). Shared decision making—The pinnacle of patient-centered care. *New England Journal of Medicine, 366*(9), 780–781. doi:10.1056/NEJMp1109283

Batchelder, A. W., Safren, S., Mitchell, A. D., Ivardic, I., & O'Cleirigh, C. (2017). Mental health in 2020 for men who have sex with men in the United States. *Sexual Health, 14*(1), 59–71. doi:10.1071/SH16083

Beer, L., Valverde, E. E., Raiford, J. L., Weiser, J., White, B. L., & Skarbinski, J. (2015). Clinician perspectives on delaying initiation of antiretroviral therapy for clinically eligible HIV-infected patients. *Journal of the International Association of Providers of AIDS Care (JIAPAC), 14*(3), 245–254. doi:10.1177/2325957414557267

Behler, R. L., Cornwell, B. T., & Schneider, J. A. (2017). Patterns of social affiliations and healthcare engagement among young, black, men who have sex with men. *AIDS and Behavior, 22*(3), 806–818. doi:10.1007/s10461-016-1668-3

Berg, R. C. (2009). Barebacking: A review of the literature. *Archives of Sexual Behavior, 38*(5), 754–764. doi:10.1007/s10508-008-9462-6

Berg, R. C., Weatherburn, P., Ross, M. W., & Schmidt, A. J. (2015). The relationship of internalized homonegativity to sexual health and well-being among men in 38 European countries who have sex with men. *Journal of Gay & Lesbian Mental Health, 19*(3), 285–302. doi:10.1080/19359705.2015.1024375

Berg, R. C., Munthe-Kaas, H. M., & Ross, M. W. (2016). Internalized homonegativity: A systematic mapping review of empirical research. *Journal of Homosexuality, 63*(4), 541–558. doi:10.1080/00918369.2015.1083788

Boone, M. R., Cook, S. H., & Wilson, P. A. (2016). Sexual identity and HIV status influence the relationship between internalized stigma and psychological distress in black gay and bisexual men. *AIDS Care, 28*(6), 764–770. doi:10.1080/09540121.2016.1164801

Bourne, A., & Weatherburn, P. (2017). Substance use among men who have sex with men: Patterns, motivations, impacts and intervention development need. *Sexually Transmitted Infections, 93*(5), 342–346. doi:10.1136/sextrans-2016-052674

Bray, J. W., Del Boca, F. K., McRee, B. G., Hayashi, S. W., & Babor, T. F. (2017). Screening, brief intervention and referral to treatment (SBIRT): Rationale, program overview and cross-site evaluation. *Addiction, 112*, 3–11. doi:10.1111/add.13676

Breyer, B. N., & Shindel, A. W. (2012). Recreational urethral sounding is associated with high risk sexual behaviour and sexually transmitted infections. *BJU International, 110*(5), 720–725. doi:10.1111/j.1464-410X.2011.10810.x

Brown, R. E., Turner, C., Hern, J., & Santos, G. (2017). Partner-level substance use associated with increased sexual risk behaviors among men who have sex with men in San Francisco, CA. *Drug and Alcohol Dependence, 176*, 176–180. doi:10.1016/j.drugalcdep.2017.02.016

Bruce, M. G., Bruden, D., Hurlburt, D., Zanis, C., Thompson, G., Rea, L., … McMahon, B. J. (2016). Antibody levels and protection after hepatitis B vaccine: Results of a 30-year follow-up study and response to a booster dose. *The Journal of Infectious Diseases, 214*(1), 16–22. doi:10.1093/infdis/jiv748

Cahill, S., Singal, R., Grasso, C., King, D., Mayer, K., Baker, K., & Makadon, H. (2014). Do ask, do tell: High levels of acceptability by patients of routine collection of sexual orientation and gender identity data in four diverse American community health centers. *PLoS One, 9*(9), e107104.

California Department of Public Health and the California STD/HIV Prevention Training Center. (2015). A clinician's resource for sexually transmitted diseases (STDs) in gay men and other men who have sex with men (MSM)—The MSM toolkit. Retrieved from https://www.cdph.ca.gov/Programs/CID/DCDC/Pages/STD-MSMToolkit.aspx

Calo, W. A., Cubillos, L., Breen, J., Hall, M., Rojas, K. F., Mooneyham, R., ... Garcia, N. (2015). Experiences of Latinos with limited English proficiency with patient registration systems and their interactions with clinic front office staff: An exploratory study to inform community-based translational research in North Carolina. *BMC Health Services Research, 15*(1), 570. doi:10.1186/s12913-015-1235-z

Calzo, J. P., Antonucci, T. C., Mays, V. M., & Cochran, S. D. (2011). Retrospective recall of sexual orientation identity development among gay, lesbian, and bisexual adults. *Developmental Psychology, 47*(6), 1658–1673. doi:10.1037/a0025508

Campbell, C. A., Canary, L., Smith, N., Teshale, E., Ryerson, A. B., & Ward, J. W. (2017). State HCV incidence and policies related to HCV preventive and treatment services for persons who inject drugs—United States, 2015–2016. *MMWR Morbidity and Mortality Weekly Report, 66*, 465–469. doi:10.15585/mmwr.mm6618a2

Carballo-Diéguez, A., Bauermeister, J., Ventuneac, A., Dolezal, C., & Mayer, K. (2010). Why rectal douches may be acceptable rectal-microbicide delivery vehicles for MSM. *Sexually Transmitted Diseases, 37*(4), 228. doi:10.1097/OLQ.0b013e3181bf9b2d

Carter Jr, J. W., Hart-Cooper, G. D., Butler, M. O., Workowski, K. A., & Hoover, K. W. (2014). Provider barriers prevent recommended sexually transmitted disease screening of HIV-infected men who have sex with men. *Sexually Transmitted Diseases, 41*(2), 137–142. doi:10.1097/OLQ.0000000000000067

Castel, A. D., Magnus, M., & Greenberg, A. E. (2015). Update on the epidemiology and prevention of HIV/AIDS in the USA. *Current Epidemiology Reports, 2*(2), 110–119. doi:10.1007/s40471-015-0042-8

Centers for Disease Control and Prevention. (2012). Hepatitis A, acute 2012 case definition. Retrieved from https://wwwn.cdc.gov/nndss/conditions/hepatitis-a-acute/case-definition/2012

Centers for Disease Control and Prevention. (2014). Preexposure prophylaxis for the prevention of HIV infection in the United States—2014: A clinical practice guideline. Retrieved from https://www.cdc.gov/hiv/pdf/prepguidelines2014.pdf

Centers for Disease Control and Prevention. (2015). Monitoring selected national HIV prevention and care objectives by using HIV surveillance data—United states and 6 dependent areas—2013. Retrieved from https://www.cdc.gov/hiv/pdf/library/reports/surveillance/cdc-hiv-surveillance report_vol20_no2.pdf

Centers for Disease Control and Prevention. (2017b). Prostate Cancer. Retrieved from https://www.cdc.gov/cancer/prostate/index.htm

Centers for Medicare and Medicaid Services. (2015). HHS LGBT Issues Coordinating Committee 2015 Report. Retrieved from https://www.hhs.gov/programs/topic-sites/lgbt/reports/health-objectives-2015.html

Chan, D. P., Lin, A. W., Wong, K. H., Wong, N. S., & Lee, S. S. (2015). Diverse origins of hepatitis C virus in HIV co-infected men who have sex with men in Hong Kong. *Virology Journal, 12*, 120. doi:10.1186/s12985-015-0355-8

Charles, C., Gafni, A., & Whelan, T. (1997). Shared decision-making in the medical encounter: What does it mean? (or it takes at least two to tango). *Social Science & Medicine, 44*(5), 681–692.

Chin, M. H. (2017). Movement advocacy, personal relationships, and ending health care disparities. *Journal of the National Medical Association, 109*(1), 33–35. doi:10.1016/j.jnma.2016.11.003

Chin, M. H., Lopez, F. Y., Nathan, A. G., & Cook, S. C. (2016). Improving shared decision making with LGBT racial and ethnic minority patients. *Journal of General Internal Medicine, 31*(6), 591–593. doi:10.1007/s11606-016-3607-4

Chow, E. P. F., Cornelisse, V. J., Read, T. R. H., Lee, D., Walker, S., Hocking, J. S., ... Fairley, C. K. (2016). Saliva use as a lubricant for anal sex is a risk factor for rectal gonorrhoea among men who have sex with men, a new public health message: A cross-sectional survey. *Sexually Transmitted Infections, 92*(7), 532–536. doi:10.1136/sextrans-2015-052502

Cohen, M. S., Chen, Y. Q., McCauley, M., Gamble, T., Hosseinipour, M. C., Kumarasamy, N., ... Fleming, T. R. (2016). Antiretroviral therapy for the prevention of HIV-1 transmission. *The New England Journal of Medicine, 375*(9), 830. doi:10.1056/NEJMoa1600693

Coleman, T. A., Bauer, G. R., Pugh, D., Aykroyd, G., Powell, L., & Newman, R. (2017). Sexual orientation disclosure in primary care settings by gay, bisexual, and other men who have sex with men in a Canadian City. *LGBT Health, 4*(1), 42–54. doi:10.1089/lgbt.2016.0004

Colpitts, E., & Gahagan, J. (2016). "I feel like I am surviving the health care system": Understanding LGBTQ health in Nova Scotia, Canada. *BMC Public Health, 16*(1), 1005. doi:10.1186/s12889-016-3675-8

D'Acunto, K., & Swanson-Biearman, B. (2015). *Obtaining a sexual history in MSM*. Hawthorne: Haymarket Media, Inc. Retrieved from https://www.clinicaladvisor.com/features/obtaining-a-sexual-history-in-msm/article/435802

Dale, S. K., Bogart, L. M., Wagner, G. J., Galvan, F. H., & Klein, D. J. (2016). Medical mistrust is related to lower longitudinal medication adherence among African-American males with HIV. *Journal of Health Psychology, 21*(7), 1311–1321. doi:10.1177/1359105314551950

DeMeester, R. H., Lopez, F. Y., Moore, J. E., Cook, S. C., & Chin, M. H. (2016). A model of organizational context and shared decision making: Application to LGBT racial and ethnic minority patients. *Journal of General Internal Medicine, 31*(6), 651–662. doi:10.1007/s11606-016-3608-3

De Vuyst, H., Clifford, G. M., Nascimento, M. C., Madeleine, M. M., & Franceschi, S. (2009). Prevalence and type distribution of human papillomavirus in carcinoma and intraepithelial neoplasia of the vulva, vagina and anus: A meta-analysis. *International Journal of Cancer, 124*(7), 1626–1636. doi:10.1002/ijc.24116

Dionne-Odom, J., Osborn, M. K., Radziewicz, H., Grakoui, A., & Workowski, K. (2009). Acute hepatitis C and HIV coinfection. *The Lancet. Infectious Diseases, 9*(12), 775–783. doi:10.1016/S1473-3099(09)70264-6

Division of HIV/AIDS Prevention, National Center for HIV/AIDS, Viral Hepatitis, Sexual Transmitted Diseases and Tuberculosis Prevention, Centers for Disease Control and Prevention. (2016). HIV among gay and bisexual men. Retrieved from https://www.cdc.gov/hiv/group/msm/index.html

Elwyn, G., Frosch, D., Thomson, R., Joseph-Williams, N., Lloyd, A., Kinnersley, P., … Edwards, A. (2012). Shared decision making: A model for clinical practice. *Journal of General Internal Medicine, 27*(10), 1361–1367. doi:10.1007/s11606-012-2077-6

Epstein, R. M., & Street, R. L. (2011). The values and value of patient-centered care. *Annals of Family Medicine, 9*(2), 100–103. doi:10.1370/afm.1239

Fenkl, E. A., Jones, S. G., Schochet, E., & Johnson, P. (2016). HPV and anal cancer knowledge among HIV-infected and non-infected men who have sex with men. *LGBT Health, 3*(1), 42–48. doi:10.1089/lgbt.2015.0086

Fiore, A. E., Wasley, A., & Bell, B. P. (2006). Prevention of hepatitis A through active or passive immunization: Recommendations of the Advisory Committee on Immunization Practices (ACIP). *Morbidity and Mortality Weekly Report: Recommendations and Reports, 55*(7), 1–23.

Flores, D., Leblanc, N., & Barroso, J. (2016). Enroling and retaining human immunodeficiency virus (HIV) patients in their care: A metasynthesis of qualitative studies. *International Journal of Nursing Studies, 62*, 126–136. doi:10.1016/j.ijnurstu.2016.07.016

Formby, E. (2016). Sexuality education with LGBT young people. In J. Ponzetti (Ed.), *Evidence-based approaches to sexuality education* (p. 384). New York, NY: Routledge.

Friedman, M., Marshal, M., Stall, R., Cheung, J., & Wright, E. (2008). Gay-related development, early abuse and adult health outcomes among gay males. *AIDS Behavior, 12*, 891–902. doi:10.1007/s10461-007-9319-3

Friedman, M. R., Dodge, B., Schick, V., Herbenick, D., Hubach, R. D., Bowling, J., … Reece, M. (2014). From bias to bisexual health disparities: Attitudes toward bisexual men and women in the United States. *LGBT Health, 1*(4), 309–318. doi:10.1089/lgbt.2014.0005

Fuchs, E. J., Lee, L. A., Torbenson, M. S., Parsons, T. L., Bakshi, R. P., Guidos, A. M., … Hendrix, C. W. (2007). Hyperosmolar sexual lubricant causes epithelial damage in the distal colon: Potential implication for HIV transmission. *The Journal of Infectious Diseases, 195*(5), 703–710. doi:10.1086/511279

Gallup. (2017). In US, More Adults Identifying as LGBT. Retrieved from http://www.gallup.com/poll/201731/lgbt-identification-rises.aspx

Galvan, F. H., Bogart, L. M., Klein, D. J., Wagner, G. J., & Chen, Y. T. (2017). Medical mistrust as a key mediator in the association between perceived discrimination and adherence to antiretroviral therapy among HIV-positive Latino men. *Journal of Behavioral Medicine, 40*, 784–793. doi:10.1007/s10865-017-9843-1

Gardner, E. M., McLees, M. P., Steiner, J. F., del Rio, C., & Burman, W. J. (2011). The spectrum of engagement in HIV care and its relevance to test-and-treat strategies for prevention of HIV infection. *Clinical Infectious Diseases, 52*(6), 793–800. doi:10.1093/cid/ciq243

Gay and Lesbian Medical Association. (2006). Guidelines for care of lesbian, gay, bisexual, and transgender patients. Retrieved from http://www.rainbowwelcome.org/uploads/pdfs/GLMA%20guidelines%202006%20FINAL.pdf

Goins, E. S., & Pye, D. (2013). Check the box that best describes you: Reflexively managing theory and praxis in LGBTQ health communication research. *Health Communication, 28*(4), 397–407. doi:10.1080/10410236.2012.690505

Goldstone, S., Palefsky, J. M., Giuliano, A. R., Moreira, E. D., Aranda, C., Jessen, H., … Garner, E. I. O. (2011). Prevalence of and risk factors for human papillomavirus (HPV) infection among

HIV-seronegative men who have sex with men. *The Journal of Infectious Diseases, 203*(1), 66–74. doi:10.1093/infdis/jiq016

Graham, R., Berkowitz, B., Blum, R., Bockting, W., Bradford, J., de Vries, B., … Makadon, H. (2011). *The health of lesbian, gay, bisexual, and transgender people: Building a foundation for better understanding*. Washington, DC: Institute of Medicine.

Grant, R. M., Lama, J. R., Anderson, P. L., McMahan, V., Liu, A. Y., Vargas, L., … Glidden, D. V. (2010). Preexposure chemoprophylaxis for HIV prevention in men who have sex with men. *New England Journal of Medicine, 363*(27), 2587–2599. doi:10.1056/NEJMoa1011205

Green, R. G., Kiernan-Stern, M., Bailey, K., Chambers, K., Claridge, R., Jones, G., … Walker, K. (2005). The multicultural counseling inventory: A measure for evaluating social work student and practitioner self-perceptions of their multicultural competencies. *Journal of Social Work Education, 41*(2), 191–208. doi:10.5175/JSWE.2005.200300360

Gwadz, M., Applegate, E., Cleland, C., Leonard, N. R., Wolfe, H., Salomon, N., … Wagner, A. (2014). HIV -infected individuals who delay, decline, or discontinue antiretroviral therapy: Comparing clinic-and peer-recruited cohorts. *Frontiers in Public Health, 2,* 81. doi:10.3389/fpubh.2014.00081

Hadland, S. E., Austin, S. B., Goodenow, C. S., & Calzo, J. P. (2014). Weight misperception and unhealthy weight control behaviors among sexual minorities in the general adolescent population. *Journal of Adolescent Health, 54*(3), 296–303. doi:10.1016/j.jadohealth.2013.08.021

Haider, A. H., Schneider, E. B., Kodadek, L. M., Adler, R. R., Ranjit, A., Torain, M., … German, D. (2017). Emergency department query for patient-centered approaches to sexual orientation and gender identity: The EQUALITY study. *JAMA Internal Medicine, 177*(6):819–828. doi:10.1001/jamainternmed.2017.0906

Hall, I., An, Q., Tang, T., Song, R., Chen, M., Green, T., & Kang, J. (2016). Prevalence of diagnosed and undiagnosed HIV infection—United States, 2008–2012. *Morbidity and Mortality Weekly Report, 65*(24), 613. doi:10.15585/mmwr.mm6524a1

Hall, I., Tang, T., Johnson, A. S., Espinoza, L., Harris, N., & McCray, E. (2016). Timing of linkage to care after HIV diagnosis and time to viral suppression. *JAIDS, 72*(2), e57–e60. doi:10.1097/QAI.0000000000000989

Hall, T. M., Shoptaw, S., & Reback, C. J. (2015). Sometimes poppers are not poppers: Huffing as an emergent health concern among MSM substance users. *Journal of Gay & Lesbian Mental Health, 19*(1), 118–121. doi:10.1080/19359705.2014.973180

Hawley, S. T., & Morris, A. M. (2017). Cultural challenges to engaging patients in shared decision making. *Patient Education and Counseling, 100*(1), 18–24. doi:10.1016/j.pec.2016.07.008

Heijman, T., Zuure, F., Stolte, I., & Davidovich, U. (2017). Motives and barriers to safer sex and regular STI testing among MSM soon after HIV diagnosis. *BMC Infectious Diseases, 17*(1), 194. doi:10.1186/s12879-017-2277-0

Herek, G. M. (2000). The psychology of sexual prejudice. *Current Directions in Psychological Science, 9*(1), 19–22. doi:10.1111/1467-8721.00051

Institute of Medicine (US) Board on the Health of Select Populations. (2013). Collecting Sexual Orientation and Gender Identity Data in Electronic Health Records: Workshop Summary. Washington (DC): National Academies Press (US). 3 Federal Perspective on the Use of Electronic Health Records to Collect Sexual Orientation and Gender Identity Data. Retrieved from https://www.ncbi.nlm.nih.gov/books/NBK154077

Killermann, S. (2017). The Genderbread Person. Retrieved from http://itspronouncedmetrosexual.com/2015/03/the-genderbread-person-v3

Kitts, R. L. (2010). Barriers to optimal care between physicians and lesbian, gay, bisexual, transgender, and questioning adolescent patients. *Journal of Homosexuality, 57*(6), 730–747. doi:10.1080/00918369.2010.485872

Klein, E. W., & Nakhai, M. (2016). Caring for LGBTQ patients: Methods for improving physician cultural competence. *The International Journal of Psychiatry in Medicine, 51*(4), 315–324. doi:10.1177/0091217416659268

Knight, R. E., Shoveller, J. A., Carson, A. M., & Contreras-Whitney, J. G. (2014). Examining clinicians' experiences providing sexual health services for LGBTQ youth: Considering social and structural determinants of health in clinical practice. *Health Education Research, 29*(4), 662–670. doi:10.1093/her/cyt116

Knox, D., Schacht, C., & Whatley, M. (2014). *Human sexuality: Making informed decisions* (4th ed.). Redding, CA: BVT Publishing.

Koskan, A. M., LeBlanc, N., & Rosa-Cunha, I. (2016). Exploring the perceptions of anal cancer screening and behaviors among gay and bisexual men infected with HIV. *Cancer Control: Journal of the Moffitt Cancer Center, 23*(1), 52. doi:10.1177/107327481602300109

Lanier, Y., Castellanos, T., Barrow, R. Y., Jordan, W. C., Caine, V., & Sutton, M. Y. (2014). Brief sexual histories and routine HIV/STD testing by medical providers. *AIDS Patient Care and STDs, 28*(3), 113–120. doi:10.1089/apc.2013.0328

Leblanc, N. M., Flores, D. D., & Barroso, J. (2016). Facilitators and barriers to HIV screening: A qualitative meta-synthesis. *Qualitative Health Research, 26*(3), 294–306. doi:10.1177/1049732315616624

Lim, F. A., Brown Jr, D. V., & Kim, S. M. J. (2014). CE: Addressing health care disparities in the lesbian, gay, bisexual, and transgender population: A review of best practices. *AJN The American Journal of Nursing, 114*(6), 24–34. doi:10.1097/01.NAJ.0000450423.89759.36

Macapagal, K., Bhatia, R., & Greene, G. J. (2016). Differences in healthcare access, use, and experiences within a community sample of racially diverse lesbian, gay, bisexual, transgender, and questioning emerging adults. *LGBT Health, 3*(6), 434–442. doi:10.1089/lgbt.2015.0124

Machalek, D. A., Poynten, M., Jin, F., Fairley, C. K., Farnsworth, A., Garland, S. M., ... Grulich, A. E. (2012). Anal human papillomavirus infection and associated neoplastic lesions in men who have sex with men: A systematic review and meta-analysis. *The Lancet. Oncology, 13*(5), 487–500. doi:10.1016/S1470-2045(12)70080-3

Martin, J., & D'Augelli, A. (2009). Cohort and period effects in research on sexual orientation and gender identity. In W. Meezan & J. Martin (Eds.), *Handbook of research with lesbian, gay, bisexual, and transgender populations* (pp. 191–207). New York, NY: Routledge.

McWhinney, I. R. (1989). 'An acquaintance with particulars...' *Family Medicine, 21*(4), 296–298.

Meanley, S., Hickok, A., Johns, M. M., Pingel, E. S., & Bauermeister, J. A. (2014). Body mass index, body esteem, and unprotected receptive anal intercourse among young men who have sex with men who seek partners online. *Archives of Sexual Behavior, 43*(4), 735–744. doi:10.1007/s10508-013-0159-0

Meites, E., Kempe, A., & Markowitz, L. E. (2017). Use of a 2-Dose Schedule for Human Papillomavirus Vaccination—Updated Recommendations of the Advisory Committee on Immunization Practices. *American Journal of Transplantation, 17*(3), 834–837. doi:10.1111/ajt.14206

Mimiaga, M. J., Goldhammer, H., Belanoff, C., Tetu, A. M., & Mayer, K. H. (2007). Men who have sex with men: Perceptions about sexual risk, HIV and sexually transmitted disease testing, and provider communication. *Sexually Transmitted Diseases, 34*(2), 113–119. doi:10.1097/01.olq.0000225327.13214.bf

Molinsky, A. (2007). Cross-cultural code-switching: The psychological challenges of adapting behavior in foreign cultural interactions. *Academy of Management Review, 32*(2), 622–640. doi:10.5465/amr.2007.24351878

Mor, Z., Parfionov, K., Davidovitch, N., & Grotto, I. (2014). Gym exercising patterns, lifestyle and high-risk sexual behaviour in men who have sex with men and in heterosexual men. *BMJ Open, 4*, e005205. doi:10.1136/bmjopen-2014-005205

Moscicki, A., & Palefsky, J. M. (2011). Human papillomavirus in men: An update. *Journal of Lower Genital Tract Disease, 15*(3), 231–234. doi:10.1097/LGT.0b013e318203ae61

Moskowitz, D. A., & Seal, D. W. (2010). Revisiting obesity and condom use in men who have sex with men. *Archives of Sexual Behavior, 39*(3), 761–765. doi:10.1007/s10508-009-9478-6

Moyer, V. A. (2013). Screening for HIV: U.S. preventive services task force recommendation statement. *Annals of Internal Medicine, 159*(1), 51. doi:10.7326/0003-4819-159-1-201307020-00645

Nadarzynski, T., Smith, H., Richardson, D., Pollard, A., & Llewellyn, C. (2017). Perceptions of HPV and attitudes towards HPV vaccination amongst men who have sex with men: A qualitative analysis. *British Journal of Health Psychology, 22*(2), 345–361. doi:10.1111/bjhp.12233

Nagel, F., W., Fuld, J., & Varma, J. K. (2014). Providing comprehensive health care to men who have sex with men (MSM). *City Health Information, 33*(4), 29–36. Retrieved from http://l.handle.net/2324/1084184

National Center for HIV/AIDS, Viral Hepatitis, STD, and TB Prevention. (2016). Lifetime risk of HIV diagnosis. Retrieved from https://www.cdc.gov/nchhstp/newsroom/2016/croi-press-release-risk.html

National HIV/AIDS Strategy for the United States. (2010). Washington, DC: White House Office of National AIDS Policy. Retrieved from https://www.hiv.gov/federal-response/national-hiv-aids-strategy/overview

Noor, S. W., & Rosser, B. S. (2014). Enema use among men who have sex with men: A behavioral epidemiologic study with implications for HIV/STI prevention. *Archives of Sexual Behavior, 43*(4), 755–769. doi:10.1007/s10508-013-0203-0

Nusbaum, M. R. H., & Hamilton, C. D. (2002). The proactive sexual health history. *American Family Physician, 66*(9), 1705. Retrieved from http://www.ncbi.nlm.nih.gov/pubmed/12449269

Operario, D., Gamarel, K. E., Grin, B. M., Lee, J. H., Kahler, C. W., Marshall, B. D., ... Zaller, N. D. (2015). Sexual minority health disparities in adult men and women in the United States: National Health and Nutrition Examination Survey, 2001–2010. *American Journal of Public Health, 105*(10), e27–e34. doi:10.2105/AJPH.2015.302762.

Oster, A. M., Wiegand, R. E., Sionean, C., Miles, I. J., Thomas, P. E., Melendez-Morales, L., ... Millett, G. A. (2011). Understanding disparities in HIV infection between black and white MSM in the United States. *AIDS, 25*(8), 1103–1112. doi:10.1097/QAD.0b013e3283471efa

Pachankis, J. E., Goldfried, M. R., & Ramrattan, M. E. (2008). Extension of the rejection sensitivity construct to the interpersonal functioning of gay men. *Journal of Consulting and Clinical Psychology, 76*(2), 306. doi:10.1037/0022-006X.76.2.306

Panel on Antiretroviral Guidelines for Adults and Adolescents. (2016). Guidelines for the use of antiretroviral agents in HIV-1-infected adults and adolescents. Department of Health and Human Services. Retrieved from http://www.aidsinfo.nih.gov/ContentFiles/AdultandAdolescentGL.pdf

Peek, M. E., Lopez, F. Y., Williams, H. S., Xu, L. J., McNulty, M. C., Acree, M. E., & Schneider, J. A. (2016). Development of a conceptual framework for understanding shared decision making among African-American LGBT patients and their clinicians. *Journal of General Internal Medicine, 31*(6), 677–687. doi:10.1037/0022-006X.76.2.306

Pew Research Center. (2017). 5 key findings about LGBT Americans. Retrieved from http://www.pewresearch.org/fact-tank/2017/06/13/5-key-findings-about-lgbt-americans

Project Implicit. (2017). Retrieved from https://implicit.harvard.edu/implicit

Quinn, G. P., Schabath, M. B., Sanchez, J. A., Sutton, S. K., & Green, B. L. (2015). The importance of disclosure: Lesbian, gay, bisexual, transgender/transsexual, queer/questioning, and intersex individuals and the cancer continuum. *Cancer, 121*(8), 1160–1163. doi:10.1002/cncr.29203

Quinn, K., Dickson-Gomez, J., DiFranceisco, W., Kelly, J. A., St. Lawrence, J. S., Amirkhanian, Y. A., & Broaddus, M. (2015). Correlates of internalized homonegativity among black men who have sex with men. *AIDS Education and Prevention, 27*(3), 212–226. doi:10.1521/aeap.2015.27.3.212

Ranji, U., Beamesderfer, A., Kates, J., & Salganicoff, A. (2015). *Health and access to care and coverage for lesbian, gay, bisexual, and transgender individuals in the US.* Menlo Park, CA: Kaiser Family Foundation.

Rice, C. E., Maierhofer, C., Fields, K. S., Ervin, M., Lanza, S. T., & Turner, A. N. (2016). Beyond anal sex: Sexual practices of men who have sex with men and associations with hiv and other sexually transmitted infections. *The Journal of Sexual Medicine, 13*(3), 374–382. doi:10.1016/j.jsxm.2016.01.001

Robinson, J. H., Callister, L. C., Berry, J. A., & Dearing, K. A. (2008). Patient-centered care and adherence: Definitions and applications to improve outcomes. *Journal of the American Association of Nurse Practitioners, 20*(12), 600–607. doi:10.1111/j.1745-7599.2008.00360.x

Rodger, A. J., Cambiano, V., Bruun, T., Vernazza, P., Collins, S., van Lunzen, J., ... Lundgren, J. (2016). Sexual activity without condoms and risk of HIV transmission in serodifferent couples when the HIV-positive partner is using suppressive antiretroviral therapy. *JAMA, 316*(2), 171–181. doi:10.1001/jama.2016.5148

Rounds, K. E., McGrath, B. B., & Walsh, E. M. (2014). Perspectives on provider behaviors: A qualitative study of sexual and gender minorities. *Contemporary Nurse, 44*(1), 99–110. doi:10.5172/conu.2013.44.1.99

Sahasrabuddhe, V. V., Castle, P. E., Follansbee, S., Borgonovo, S., Tokugawa, D., Schwartz, L. M., ... Wentzensen, N. (2013). Human papillomavirus genotype attribution and estimation of preventable fraction of anal intraepithelial neoplasia cases among HIV-infected men who have sex with men. *The Journal of Infectious Diseases, 207*(3), 392–401. doi:10.1093/infdis/jis694

Scholl, I., Zill, J. M., Härter, M., & Dirmaier, J. (2014). An integrative model of patient-centeredness–a systematic review and concept analysis. *PloS One, 9*(9), e107828. doi:10.1371/journal.pone.0107828

Scott-Sheldon, L. A., Carey, K. B., Cunningham, K., Johnson, B. T., & Carey, M. P.; MASH Research Team. (2016). Alcohol use predicts sexual decision-making: A systematic review and meta-analysis of the experimental literature. *AIDS and Behavior, 20*(1), 19–39. doi:10.1007/s10461-015-1108-9

Semple, S. J., Patterson, T. L., & Grant, I. (2002). Motivations associated with methamphetamine use among HIV+ men who have sex with men. *Journal of Substance Abuse Treatment, 22*(3), 149–156. doi:10.1016/S0740-5472(02)00223-4

Sexuality Information and Education Council of the United States. (2016). PrEP education for youth-serving primary care providers toolkit. Retrieved from https://www.siecus.org/index.cfm?fuseaction=page.viewPage&pageID=1555

Sherman, M. D., Kauth, M. R., Shipherd, J. C., & Street Jr, R. L. (2014). Provider beliefs and practices about assessing sexual orientation in two veterans health affairs hospitals. *LGBT Health, 1*(3), 185–191. doi:10.1089/lgbt.2014.0008

Simon Rosser, B. R., Merengwa, E., Capistrant, B. D., Iantaffi, A., Kilian, G., Kohli, N., ... West, W. (2016). Prostate cancer in gay, bisexual, and other men who have sex with men: A review. *LGBT Health, 3*(1), 32–41. doi:10.1089/lgbt.2015.0092

Skarbinski, J., Rosenberg, E., Paz-Bailey, G., Hall, H. I., Rose, C. E., Viall, A. H., ... Mermin, J. H. (2015). Human immunodeficiency virus transmission at each step of the care continuum in the United States. *JAMA Internal Medicine, 175*(4), 588–596. doi:10.1001/jamainternmed.2014.8180

Smith, D. K., Mendoza, M. C., Stryker, J. E., & Rose, C. E. (2016). PrEP awareness and attitudes in a national survey of primary care clinicians in the United States, 2009–2015. *PloS One, 11*(6), e0156592. doi:10.1371/journal.pone.0156592

Snyder, B. K., Burack, G. D., & Petrova, A. (2017). LGBTQ youth's perceptions of primary care. *Clinical Pediatrics, 56*(5), 443–450. doi:10.1177/0009922816673306

Stein, M., Herman, D. S., Trisvan, E., Pirraglia, P., Engler, P., & Anderson, B. J. (2005). Alcohol use and sexual risk behavior among human immunodeficiency virus–positive persons. *Alcoholism: Clinical and Experimental Research, 29*(5), 837–843. doi:10.1097/01.ALC.0000164363.40533.E0

Stewart, K., & O'Reilly, P. (2017). Exploring the attitudes, knowledge and beliefs of nurses and midwives of the healthcare needs of the LGBTQ population: An integrative review. *Nurse Education Today, 53*, 67–77. doi:10.1016/j.nedt.2017.04.008

Szymanski, D. M., Kashubeck-West, S., & Meyer, J. (2008). Internalized heterosexism: A historical and theoretical overview. *The Counseling Psychologist, 36*(4), 510–524. doi:10.1177/0011000007309488

Tan, J. Y., Xu, L. J., Lopez, F. Y., Jia, J. L., Pho, M. T., Kim, K. E., & Chin, M. H. (2016). Shared decision making among clinicians and Asian American and Pacific Islander sexual and gender minorities: An intersectional approach to address a critical care gap. *LGBT Health, 3*(5), 327–334. doi:10.1089/lgbt.2015.0143

Thompson, N. D., Perz, J. F., Moorman, A. C., & Holmberg, S. D. (2009). Nonhospital health care-associated hepatitis B and C virus transmission: United states, 1998–2008. *Annals of Internal Medicine, 150*(1), 33–39. doi:10.7326/0003-4819-150-1-200901060-00007

U.S. Department of Health and Human Services. (2016). Health Resources and Services Administration. Program assistance letter. Retrieved from https://bphc.hrsa.gov/datareporting/pdf/pal201602.pdf

van de Laar, T., Pybus, O., Bruisten, S., Brown, D., Nelson, M., Bhagani, S., ... Danta, M. (2009). Evidence of a large, international network of HCV transmission in HIV-positive men who have sex with men. *Gastroenterology, 136*(5), 1609–1617. doi:10.1053/j.gastro.2009.02.006

van der Zee, R. P., Richel, O., de Vries, H. J. C., & Prins, J. M. (2013). The increasing incidence of anal cancer: Can it be explained by trends in risk groups? *The Netherlands Journal of Medicine, 71*(8), 401–411.

Wang, K., & Pachankis, J. E. (2016). Gay-related rejection sensitivity as a risk factor for condomless sex. *AIDS and Behavior, 20*(4), 763–767. doi:10.1007/s10461-015-1224-6

Weatherburn, P., Hickson, F., Reid, D., Torres-Rueda, S., & Bourne, A. (2017). Motivations and values associated with combining sex and illicit drugs ('chemsex') among gay men in South London: Findings from a qualitative study. *Sex Transm Infect, 93*(3), 203–206. doi:10.1136/sextrans-2016-052695

Wheldon, C. W., Sutton, S. K., Fontenot, H. B., Quinn, G. P., Giuliano, A. R., & Vadaparampil, S. T. (2017). Physician communication practices as a barrier to risk-based HPV vaccine uptake among men who have sex with men. *Journal of Cancer Education*, 1–6. doi:10.1007/s13187-017-1223-6

Wilkerson, J. M., Rybicki, S., Barber, C. A., & Smolenski, D. J. (2011). Creating a culturally competent clinical environment for LGBT patients. *Journal of Gay & Lesbian Social Services, 23*(3), 376–394. doi:10.1080/10538720.2011.589254

Workowski, K. A., & Bolan, G. A. (2015). *Sexually transmitted diseases treatment guidelines, 2015*. Atlanta, GA: Center for Surveillance, Epidemiology, and Laboratory Services, Centers for Disease Control and Prevention.

World Health Organization. (2006). Defining sexual heath: Report of a technical consultation on sexual health, 28–31 January, 2002. Retrieved from http://www.who.int/reproductivehealth/publications/sexual_health/defining_sexual_health.pdf

CHAPTER 17

The Itchy, Scratchy, Bumpy, and Burning Truths About Sex, and Pre-exposure Prophylaxis (PrEP)

Rachel Prosser

INTRODUCTION AND THE INTERVIEW

Sex. Getting laid. Shagging. Banging. Screwing. Horizontal mambo. 69. Pitcher or catcher? Top, bottom, or verse? Men, women, or both? Oral, vaginal, or anal? Society has developed a variety of words and phrases to discuss and describe sex. So why is it so difficult to talk about sex with patients? While the act of sex has not changed for hundreds of years, how people arrive at having sex has certainly changed in the last decade. Thanks to the Internet and smart phones, sex is literally at our fingertips; people can find sex partners within minutes. Looking for a quick romp over lunch? Just download an app and "swipe" to find a willing participant. Dating sites, websites that sell things, even sex, and real-time apps make finding sex easy.

If clinicians fail to ask patients relevant questions, we are unlikely to receive accurate answers (Figure 17.1). Using nonmedical terminology and not assuming all men have sex with only women is a start to open dialogue. Cultivate the habit of asking patients if they have sex with men, women, or both. This type of questioning demonstrates that one is open to and aware of a variety of sexual encounters and preferences.

Additional helpful interview questions will include frequency and level of risk associated with the type of sex. Is the sex protected or unprotected or both? Patients may have unprotected sex with a primary partner and then protected sex with nonprimary partners. Level of risk associated with the act(s) of sex may help guide screening.

PHYSICAL EXAMINATION AND IDENTIFICATION OF SUSPECTED STI

To reiterate, if routine sexually transmitted infections (STIs) screening is not part of the plan, you will only be guided to screen based on the specifics of the interview and presenting complaints of an individual patient. Asking the right questions is key; with the exception of genital warts, sexually transmitted infections can be diagnosed with laboratory evaluation and cultures.

Trichomoniasis

The most common STI in the United States is trichomoniasis, commonly referred to as "trich," although as this is not a reportable infection, and the true prevalence is unknown. Trichomoniasis is caused by a protozoan parasite called *Trichomonas vaginalis* and can be spread by oral, anal, and vaginal sex. Its incubation may be from 4 to 28 days, which can complicate identification of partners in some circumstances. According to the Centers for Disease Control and Prevention (CDC), this pesky protozoan has infected upward of 3.7 million people in the United States (CDC, 2017). Approximately only 30% of individuals affected with trichomoniasis

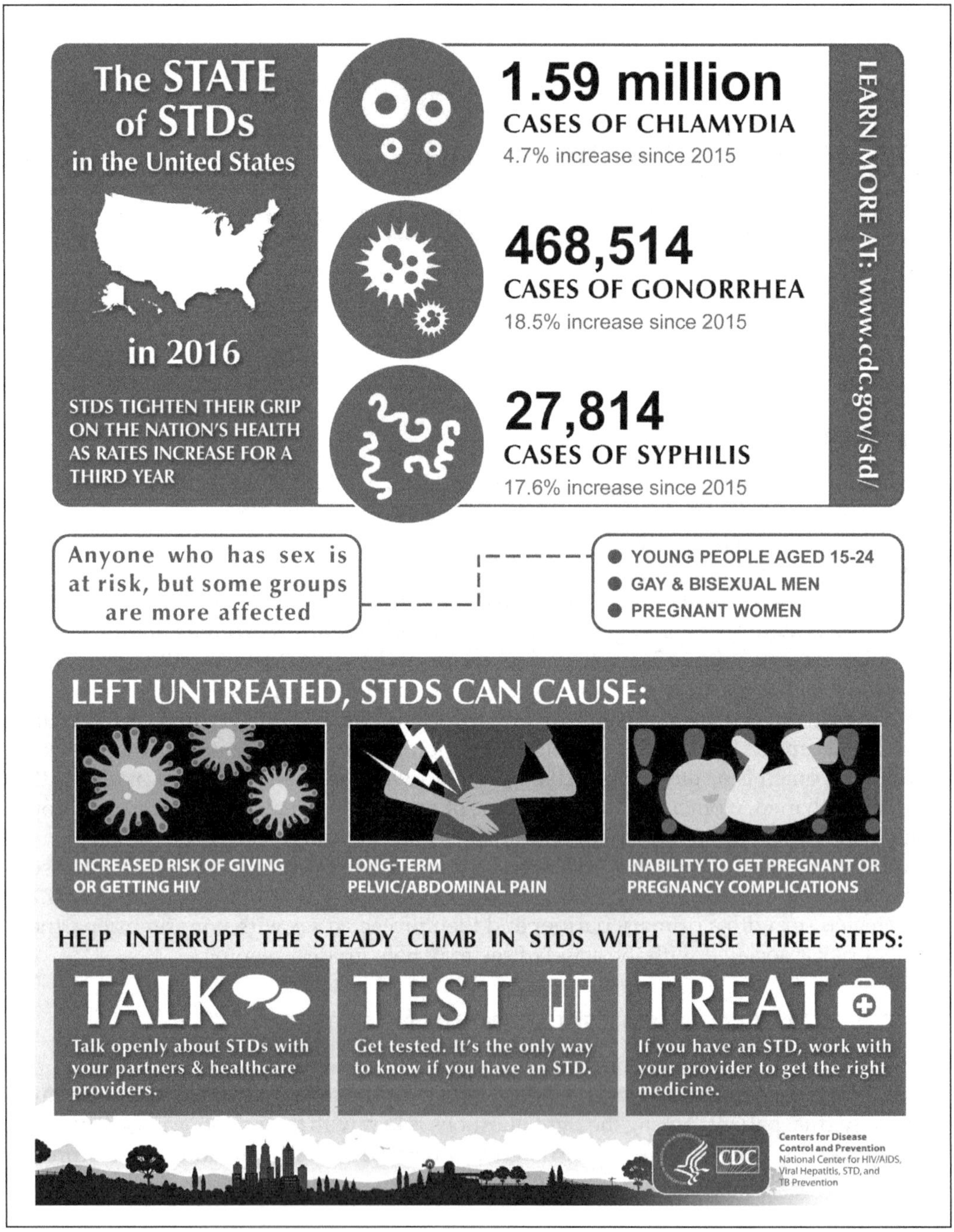

FIGURE 17.1 The State of STDs.

Source: Centers for Disease Control and Prevention. (2016). Sexually Transmitted Diseases Surveillance. Retrieved from https://www.cdc.gov/std/stats16/infographic.htm

will have symptoms. Symptoms range from asymptomatic to itching or irritation inside the urethra, burning after urination or ejaculation, and discharge from the urethra. Men who have been infected will largely be asymptomatic, but may have urethritis, balanitis, epididymitis, complaints of burning to penis after sexual activity, and even infertility if left untreated.

Diagnosing trichomoniasis in men is done with urine or urethral swab culture or a nucleic acid amplification test (NAAT). If considering screening for trichomoniasis, consider screening for other STIs such as chlamydia infection, gonorrhea, syphilis, and HIV infection at the same time. First-line trichomoniasis treatment is either:

Metronidazole (Flagyl) 2 g as a single dose

or

Metronidazole (Flagyl) 500 mg twice a day for 7 days

Men should be counseled to avoid sexual activity for at least 7 days after treatment, and partners should also receive treatment. Approximately 20% of individuals treated will become infected again in the next 3 months. Despite this, test of cure is not recommended, and prevention of trichomoniasis includes abstinence and latex condom use.

Chlamydia Infection

The second most common STI in the United States is chlamydia infection (caused by *Chlamydia trachomatis*), whichis most common in persons under the age of 24. Chlamydia can be transmitted to oral, anal, and vaginal orifices. In 2016, the United States had 1.59 million cases of chlamydia infection, an increase of 4.7% since 2015 (CDC, 2017). Only approximately 50% of men will have symptoms, which may include yellow, watery, thick milky drainage from urethra, painful urination and/or ejaculation, rectal bleeding, pain, and discharge. To a lesser extent, men may exhibit burning and itching around the urethra, pain and swelling in testes, and sore throat (Cunningham, 2017). Men may also be misdiagnosed with epididymitis, prostatitis, or urethritis if not screened appropriately and treated with antibiotic regimens that are not designed to treat chlamydia infection.

Asymptomatic chlamydia infection is common; therefore, clinicians must rely on screening. However, routine screening for men is not recommended. Screening sites include cultures from the throat, anus, and urethra. Urethral swab samples or urine may be obtained to screen for chlamydia. The NAAT is the most sensitive test for urethral swab or first-catch urine specimens. Check with your local laboratory to determine which type of testing is available; if oral and anal screening is not available locally, seek out labs in the area to perform this testing or consider having it evaluated at a sendout lab.

Treatment for uncomplicated urethral and oral chlamydia:

Azithromycin 1 g as single oral dose

or

Doxycyline 100 mg oral twice a day for 7 days

Alternative treatments:

Erythromycin base 500 mg orally four times a day for 7 days

or

Erythromycin ethylsuccinate 800 mg orally four times a day for 7 days

or

Levofloxacin 500 mg orally once a day for 7 days

or

Ofloxacin 300 mg orally twice a day for 7 days

or

Tetracycline 500 mg orally four times a day for 7 days

According to the World Health Organization (2016), the preferred anorectal chlamydia treatment is doxycycline 100 mg orally twice a day for 7 days over azithromycin 1 g orally as a single dose. This recommendation is for individuals with known anorectal infection and those with suspected genital coinfection. Regardless of treatment choice, test of cure for chlamydia after treatment is not recommended unless adherence is questioned or symptoms persist. Prevention of chlamydia infection includes abstinence and latex condom use.

Gonococcal Infection

Another STI on the rise in the United States is gonorrhea, cause by *Neisseria gonorrhoeae*, but it is a worldwide concern as well. According to the CDC (2016a), there are an estimated 820,000 new cases of gonorrhea annually, making gonorrhea the second most common reportable communicable disease and a true public health concern owing to ongoing transmission if regimens are not completed or effective. Gonorrhea is a bacterial infection transmitted via oral, anal, and vaginal sex. Symptoms do not always occur in men; however, in men symptoms may include burning with urination; white, yellow, and/or green discharge from urethra; and less commonly, painful or swollen testicles. Symptoms of rectal gonorrhea infections include discharge, anal itching, soreness, bleeding, and painful bowel movements.

Routine screening for gonorrhea in men is not recommended. However, several screening mechanisms are available. Urine and culture swabs are utilized to detect *N. gonorrhoeae;* check with local labs to determine what testing is being utilized. Treatment for gonorrhea is complicated by local resistance patterns. Data from the national sentinel surveillance system is shown is Figure 17.2. Based on surveillance data, the treatment of uncomplicated urethral, anorectal, or pharyngeal gonorrhea has changed in the past several decades. In an effort to reduce the emergence and spread of drug resistance and to improve treatment efficacy, dual therapy is recommended, with the goal that a therapy is effective at all sites of infection, well-tolerated, and available as a single dose if possible. Current recommendations are for dual therapy to account for increased patterns of resistance:

Ceftriaxone 250 mg IM in a single dose

and

Azithromycin 1 g orally in a single dose

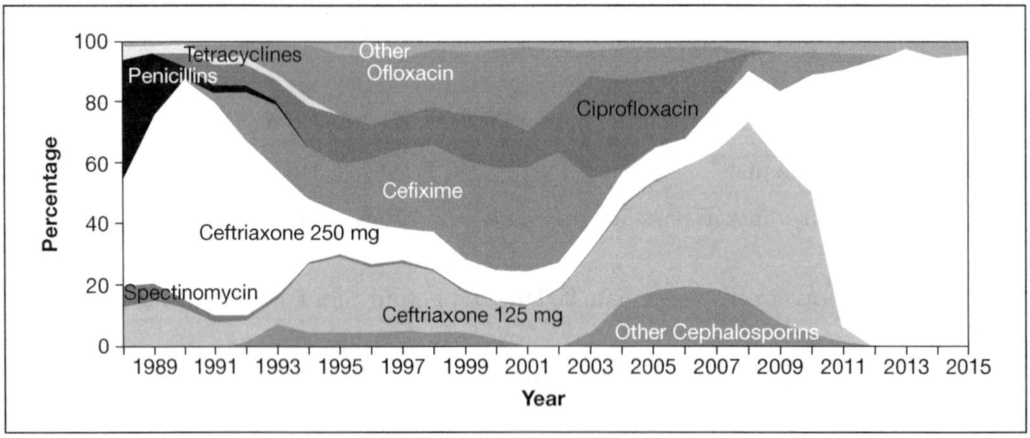

FIGURE 17.2 Gonococcal Isolate Surveillance Project (GISP).

Source: Centers for Disease Control and Prevention. (2016). Gonococcal Isolate Surveillance Project (GISP). Retrieved from https://www.cdc.gov/std/gisp/default.htm

Alternative treatments if ceftriaxone is not available:

Cefodime 400 mg orally in a single dose

and

Azythromycin 1 g orally in a single dose

Test of cure is not recommended if any of the first-line or alternative regimens are utilized. The one exception is to perform test of cure 14 days after treatment if alternative treatment for pharyngeal gonorrhea is utilized. Abstinence and consistent use of latex condoms are recommended to reduce risk for gonococcal infections. Men should be instructed to return for reevaluation if symptoms persist or recur 3 to 5 days after treatment, and this failure rate is higher in men who have sex with men (MSM) (Kirkcaldy et al., 2017).

Syphilis

Syphilis has been a reportable disease in the United States since 1944 and is caused by the bacterium *Treponema pallidum*. Like other STIs, rates of syphilis are on the rise. According to the CDC, between 2015 and 2016, primary and secondary cases of syphilis increased by 18%. There were 27,814 total cases of syphilis reported in 2016, and of these cases, 58% of them were reported in MSM (CDC, 2016b). According to the World Health Organization (WHO) global incidence in men is 1.5 cases per 1,000 males (Newman et al., 2015). Transmission is based on direct contact with a lesion (chancre) during sexual activity, and the bacterium can evade initial host responses, but extensive knowledge of this pathogen remains limited. The initial immune response appears effective as resolution of the primary chancre is observed, but the bacteria spreads widely within the host's system at the same time. The many nonspecific symptoms include rash, adenopathy, fever, headache, generalized malaise, weight loss, sore throat, adenopathy, gastrointestinal abnormalities, and eye involvement (especially in those who are HIV positive).

Unlike other STIs, syphilis has various stages and treatment is based on the stage, ranging from early syphilis and late stages of syphilis, but infected individuals can manifest symptoms of neurologic involvement at any point. The stages of syphilis can be difficult to access and determine (Table 17.1), and individuals are frequently coinfected with HIV. An accurate sexual history and physical examination can help guide the clinician to categorizing the correct stage of syphilis. Sexual partners in the preceding 90 days should be treated presumptively.

Screening for syphilis is completed with blood testing. Nontreponemal test antibody titers may correlate with disease progression. The titers are monitored for fourfold decline after treatment, ideally, 6 months after treatment (e.g., 1:32–1:8). After successful treatment, patients will not transmit syphilis to sexual partners, despite having a reactive nontreponemal test. Future screening for persons previously treated should be quantitative. Screening for syphilis in men should be routine in men with high-risk behaviors. once treated, most people will always have a reactive nontreponemal titer, even after successful treatment. Prevention of acquiring syphilis is abstinence and consistent use of latex condoms.

HIV Infection

HIV itself is not discussed much anymore, but it remains a significant public health concern as men infected acutely have few symptoms and may continue to spread the virus. Persons at risk do not perceive the diagnosis as the death sentence it once was. There are an estimated 1.2 million individuals living with HIV in the United States, in part due to the advancement of combination antiviral therapy. Persons living with HIV can live a normal life

TABLE 17.1 Clinical Overview of Syphilis

Syphilis Stage	Symptoms/Clinical Manifestations	Preferred Treatment	Alternative Treatment (PCN allergy)
Primary	Ulcers or chancre at site of infection	Bicillin L-A 2.4 million units administered in a single dose	Doxycycline 100 mg orally twice daily for 14 d OR tetracycline 500 mg orally four times daily for 14 d
Secondary	Rash, mucocutaneous lesions, and lymphadenopathy	Bicillin L-A 2.4 million units administered in a single dose	Doxycycline 100 mg orally twice daily for 14 d OR tetracycline 500 mg orally four times daily for 14 d
Tertiary	Cardiac problems, gummatous lesions, tabes dorsalis, and general paresis	Bicillin L-A 7.2 million units administered as 2.4 million units in a single dose administered over three doses, one dose a week	Doxycycline 100 mg orally twice daily for 14 d OR tetracycline 500 mg orally four times daily for 28 d
Latent	Contracted in previous year and absence of clinical manifestations	Bicillin L-A 2.4 million units administered in a single dose	Doxycycline 100 mg orally twice daily for 14 days OR tetracycline 500 mg orally four times daily for 14 days
Late latent	All other cases, contracted > 1 y prior	Bicillin L-A 7.2 million units administered as 2.4 million units in a single dose administered over three doses, one dose a week	Doxycycline 100 mg orally twice daily for 14 d OR tetracycline 500 mg orally four times daily for 28 d
Neurologic syphilis	Can manifest during any stage, cranial nerve dysfunction, meningitis, stroke, acute altered mental status, and auditory and/or ophthalmic abnormalities can appear in the first few months or year after infection	Aqueous crystalline penicillin G 18–24 million units per day, administered as 3–4 million units IV every 4 hr or continuous infusion for 10–14 d	

IV, intravenous; PCN, penicillin allergy.

with a life expectancy comparable to their matched gender and ethnicity. More than half of those individuals are over the age of 50. Approximately 300,000 people are unaware of their diagnosis, and fewer than 400,000 are considered in care and have undetectable viral loads.

New HIV infections were steady at approximately 50,000 annually for nearly a decade between 2005 and 2015 (Figure 17.3). Some progress has been made in decreasing new infections, largely by implementing "treatment as prevention." Currently, there are approximately 40,000 new HIV infections annually, but men of color and MSM are disproportionately affected by HIV (Figure 17.4). Acute infection has a variety of nonspecific symptoms, and from 10% to 60% of those infected have no symptoms, and initial symptoms are nonspecific and can resolve with time.

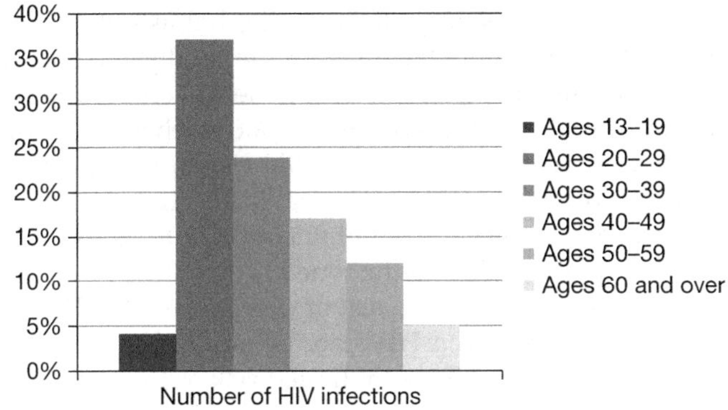

FIGURE 17.3 New HIV infections in 2015 by age.

Source: Data from Centers for Disease Control and Prevention. HIV in the United States: at a glance. Retrieved from https://www.cdc.gov/hiv/statistics/overview/ataglance.html; Centers for Disease Control and Prevention. (2014). Preexposure prophylaxis for the prevention of HIV infection in the United States—2014. Retrieved from https://www.cdc.gov/hiv/pdf/prepguidelines2014.pdf

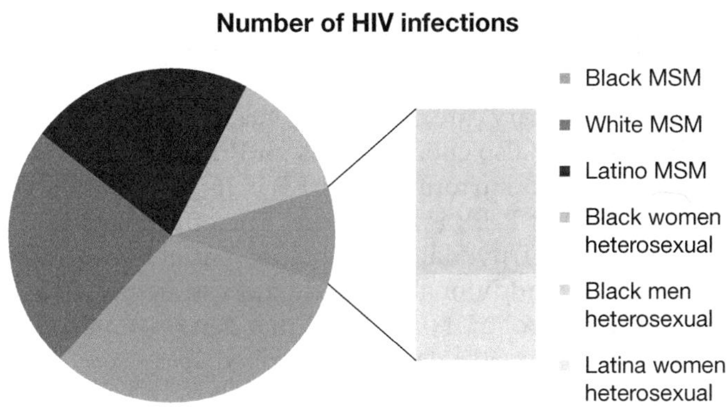

FIGURE 17.4 Number of new HIV infections in 2015.

MSM, men who have sex with men.

Source: Data from Centers for Disease Control and Prevention. HIV in the United States: at a glance. Retrieved from https://www.cdc.gov/hiv/statistics/overview/ataglance.html; Centers for Disease Control and Prevention. (2014). Preexposure prophylaxis for the prevention of HIV infection in the United States—2014. Retrieved from https://www.cdc.gov/hiv/pdf/prepguidelines2014.pdf

The CDC (2014) and United States Preventive Services Task Force (2013) recommend at least one HIV screening in a lifetime for persons aged 13 to 64. More regular screening should be conducted based on risk. MSM, individuals who use intravenous drugs, persons who exchange sex for drugs or money, and incarcerated individuals are at higher risk for acquiring HIV.

The preferred method of HIV screening is the fourth generation HIV antibody and antigen test. This screening method shortens the window of having a reactive test with HIV infection to 4 to 7 days after infection. As with all screening, clinicians should check with their local lab to determine what type of HIV screening is available.

Older HIV screening methods include HIV antibody only. If there is concern that someone has been recently infected, it is possible an antibody has not yet formed. Acute HIV seroconversion refers to the time after HIV infection, generally 4 to 6 weeks after infection. During this time, individuals may present with generalized symptoms of fever, chills, lymphadenopathy, sore throat, flu-like symptoms, body aches, and rash. If combination antibody/antigen tests are not available, this would be an appropriate time to confirm the presence of HIV by ordering an HIV RNA, or viral load. HIV viral loads will be present before an antibody has been produced. It is not uncommon for persons infected with HIV to have extremely high viral loads during the time of seroconversion.

In the event there is a positive screening test or detectable HIV RNA on screening, connecting the individual with specialized HIV care is imperative. For individuals who are being screened frequently for HIV or have continued risk or frequent sexually transmitted infections, they should be offered PrEP. If men are identified early after infection, antiretroviral therapy (ART) should be started as soon as exposure is confirmed and should be continued indefinitely.

PrEP

In 2014, the combination drug, Truvada (emtricitabine-tenofovir disoproxil 200/300 mg) was approved for PrEP. Individuals at risk for acquiring HIV take a drug that was designed for HIV infection treatment daily in an effort to prevent acquiring HIV infection. Patient selection is guided by suspected risk for HIV infection and drug use history, presence/absence of conditions that increase the risk for side effects (e.g., hepatitis B, decreased kidney function), and potential barriers to daily medication (e.g., homelessness). Ideally, PrEP would be administered by primary care/family practice clinicians, but HIV specialists and infectious disease clinicians are also good referrals for PrEP.

The most common question surrounding PrEP is its effectiveness. Like most drug treatments, the Achilles heel of PrEP is adherence. The effectiveness of PrEP is strongly associated with adherence to Truvada, and includes patient counseling regarding the importance of adherence and additional risk reduction strategies. The iPrEX study was the first large randomized control trial (n = 2,470) that demonstrated statically significant results for individuals taking Truvada, daily as prescribed, to decrease risk of HIV infection (Grant et al. 2010).

Men on PrEP should be followed every 3 months with:

- HIV testing
- routine STI screening
- evaluation for medication regimen adherence
- evaluation of risk behaviors
- checking for medication side effects
- assessing possible signs of acute HIV infection

Every 6 months these patients must have their kidney function monitored as well. PrEP should be continued as long as the risk of infection is present, or for 30 days after the last high-risk exposure (Seifert et al., 2015).

Individuals who decide PrEP is something they want to pursue should be screened for HIV. Most clinicians request the patient be abstinent or only have sex with condoms 2 to 4 weeks prior to starting PrEP. The concern is that if someone is started on Truvada when he is seroconverting, drug-resistant HIV strains could develop, because Truvada alone would be considered suboptimal therapy for someone who is HIV positive. The cost effectiveness of PrEP remains a source of debate.

INCARCERATED POPULATIONS

Incarcerated individuals are at greater risk for HIV infection and hepatitis C than the general, nonincarcerated population, and usually have other risk factors for STIs, such as multiple partners and a history of drug use. One third of all hepatitis C cases will walk into a correctional facility. This population should be screened for syphilis, HIV, hepatitis B (HBsAg), hepatitis C (hepatitis C virus antibody), gonorrhea, trichomoniasis, and chlamydia (NAAT for the last three). Screening for HPV infection can also be considered. The routine avenues for reporting and treatment are followed with this population as well, including recommendations for partner treatment and notification.

CONCLUSION

STIs have serious consequences when left unidentified and untreated in men, including ongoing transmission to partners of both genders. Other issues can include male-factor infertility, chronic genital pain, and pain with sexual activity. When there is clinical suspicion, or in the instance of persistent symptoms, men should also be screened for less common pathogens such as *Mycoplasma genitalium*, or *Ureaplasma*.

CASE STUDY

Many years ago, I had a patient who was a known MSM present to my office with complaints of his allergies acting up and he had a rash. I had known this patient for many, many years and by all accounts, we had and have an excellent working relationship. He denied any runny nose, itchy eyes, cough, sore throat, fever, or chills. He was taking an over-the-counter antihistamine without resolution. His rash was diffuse, but mostly on his trunk on his chest, and appeared as slightly raised, red bumps without demarcation. He denied any reason for me to screen him for syphilis stating he hadn't been having any sex. Despite the patient's claim, I deemed it prudent to order a rapid plasma reagin (RPR) screening. His RPR test came back positive. When I called the patient to discuss his results and necessary treatment the conversation went something like this:

Me: Hello. So ... your syphilis test came back positive. You know, it isn't super helpful for you to lie to me when I am trying to take care of you.

Patient: I was not lying to you! I did not have sex!

Me: Well, you obviously had sex or injected drugs (which I knew the patient did not have a history of doing), otherwise your syphilis test would not be positive.

Patient: Well! I didn't know I could get syphilis from oral sex!

The clinical pearls associated with this story are:

1. Follow your gut and screen. It does not hurt anyone to screen for STIs.
2. Educate your patients on how STIs are transmitted.
3. Oral, vaginal, and anal sex are all "real" kinds of sex with "real" risks.

The patient was treated successfully, and we still laugh about this encounter together.

CLINICAL PEARLS

- Identification of acute HIV infection is important; early intervention reduces risk of transmission and may make men eligible for future HIV eradication strategies by reducing latent HIV reservoir.
- Initial clinical manifestations of primary syphilis consist of a painless chancre, which will heal within a few weeks, even untreated.
- *C. trachomatis* is a common cause of nongonococcal urethritis in men.
- Any patient with a gonococcal infection should also be screened for *C. trachomatis*, as they will present simultaneously in many patients.
- Men may be asymptomatic carriers of trichomoniasis for prolonged periods of time, making it difficult to determine when or from whom the infection might have been acquired.
- *N. gonorrhoeae* has developed resistance to the antimicrobial classes most commonly used for therapy, reducing available treatment options.
- Counsel all men with suspected or confirmed acute or early HIV infection to adopt behaviors that include consistent condom use and avoidance of sharing needles, in order to prevent virus transmission.
- Many health departments have embraced Expedited Partner Therapy (EPT), where the partners of infected individuals are treated without the need for a clinician to examine the partner or confirm positive cultures. Check with the laws of your particular state.

RESOURCES FOR CLINICIANS

Centers for Disease Control and Prevention (CDC): Sexually transmitted diseases treatment guidelines (2015). www.cdc.gov/std

The U.S. Preventive Services Task Force (USPSTF) Final Recommendation Statement—Sexually Transmitted Infections: Behavioral Counseling. www.uspreventiveservicestaskforce.org/Page/Document/RecommendationStatementFinal/sexually-transmitted-infections-behavioral-counseling1

REFERENCES

Centers for Disease Control and Prevention. (2016a). Gonococcal Infections. Retrieved from https://www.cdc.gov/std/tg2015/gonorrhea.htm

Centers for Disease Control and Prevention. (2016b). Syphilis and MSM (men who have sex with men). Retrieved from https://www.cdc.gov/std/tg2015/syphilis.htm

Centers for Disease Control and Prevention. (2017). Trichomoniasis—CDC fact sheet. https://www.cdc.gov/std/trichomonas/STDFact-Trichomoniasis.htm

Cunningham, R. (2017). Chlamydia symptoms in men. Retrieved from https://www.stdtestexpress.com/chlamydia-symptoms-men

Grant, R. M., Lama, J. R., Anderson, P. L, McMahan, V., Liu, A. Y., Vargas, L., ... Glidden, D. V. (2010). Preexposure chemoprophylaxis for HIV prevention in men who have sex with men. *New England Journal of Medicine, 363*(27), 2587–2599. doi:10.1056/NEJMoa1011205

Kirkcaldy, R. D., Zaidi, A., Hook, E. W. 3rd, Holmes, K. K., Soge, O., del Rio, C., ... Weinstock, H. S. (2013). Neisseria gonorrhoeae antimicrobial resistance among men who have sex with men and men who have sex exclusively with women: The Gonococcal Isolate Surveillance Project, 2005-2010. *Annals of Internal Medicine, 158*, 321. doi:10.7326/0003-4819-158-5-201303050-00004

Newman, L., Rowley, J., Vander Hoorn, S., Wijesooriya, N. S., Unemo, M., Low, N., ... Temmerman, M. (2015). Global estimates of the prevalence and incidence of Four Curable Sexually Transmitted Infections in 2012 Based on Systematic Review and Global Reporting. *PLoS One, 10*, e0143304. doi:10.1371/journal.pone.0143304

Seifert, S. M., Glidden, D. V., Meditz, A. L., Castillo-Mancilla, J. R., Gardner, E. M., Predhomme, J. A., ... Anderson, P.L. (2015). Dose response for starting and stopping HIV preexposure prophylaxis for men who have sex with men. *Clinical Infectious Diseases, 60*, 804. doi:10.1093/cid/ciu916

United States Preventative Task Force. (2013). Hepatitis C: Screening. Retrieved from https://www.uspreventiveservicestaskforce.org/Page/Document/UpdateSummaryFinal/hepatitis-c-screening

World Health Organization. (2016). WHO guidelines for the treatment of *Chlamydia trachomatis*. Retrieved from http://www.who.int/reproductivehealth/publications/rtis/chlamydia-treatment-guidelines/en

CHAPTER 18

A Men's Health Clinic Exemplar: Experience at the University of Utah

Kelley Taylor and James Hotaling

INTRODUCTION

Patients often have symptoms or topics they would like to discuss with their healthcare providers but are hesitant to voice (King et al., 2015; Scholz, Crabb, & Wittert, 2017). Questions regarding sexual, reproductive, or genital health can weigh heavily on the mind of the patient though various barriers may prevent them from voicing their concerns (Bauer, Haesler, & Fetherstonhaugh, 2016; Teo, Ng, Booth, & White, 2016). Sexual health, for example, is an important part of many adult men's quality of life, and both young and old populations desire this aspect of their health to be addressed more frequently by primary care providers or other clinicians (Bauer et al., 2016; Fuzzell, Fedesco, Alexander, Fortenberry, & Shields, 2016).

Trust between patient and provider is cultivated when the provider shows respect for the patient's concerns and beliefs and, thereby, helps the patient engage in and advocate for his health (Lee King et al., 2015). When men present for care, they may take more time to build trust in a provider and, therefore, feel less comfortable confiding in them at first (Murray & McCrone, 2015; Thompson et al., 2016). Establishing a strong relationship between patient and provider may, then, be even more imperative for male patients, particularly for sensitive questions or concerns (Summers et al., 2016).

Men's health clinics have been established where men with male-specific diagnoses present with the expectation that their sensitive concerns will be discussed in a frank, competent, and respectful manner. Diagnoses addressed include sexual health changes such as erectile or ejaculatory dysfunction; testicular hypofunction and resulting hypogonadism or decreased semen parameters; testicular, penile, or scrotal pain and/or mass; and prostatic changes with or without urinary symptoms (Amano, Earle, & Takemae, 2016; Berger, Messore, Patuszak, & Ramasamy, 2016; Egan, 2016). The University of Utah has had a unique Men's Health Clinic since 2013 that aims not only to treat these particular diagnoses, but also to create an environment where men are willing to seek care, feel comfortable disclosing their symptoms, and develop trusting relationships with their providers.

UNIVERSITY OF UTAH HEALTH

To provide the context for this specialty clinic, University of Utah Health includes 4 hospitals, 12 major multispecialty community clinics, and several individual specialty clinics located primarily in northern Utah along the Wasatch Mountains. This healthcare system receives referrals from Utah and surrounding states, regularly treating patients from 10% of the continental United States (Figure 18.1; University of Utah Health, 2017a). For 7 straight

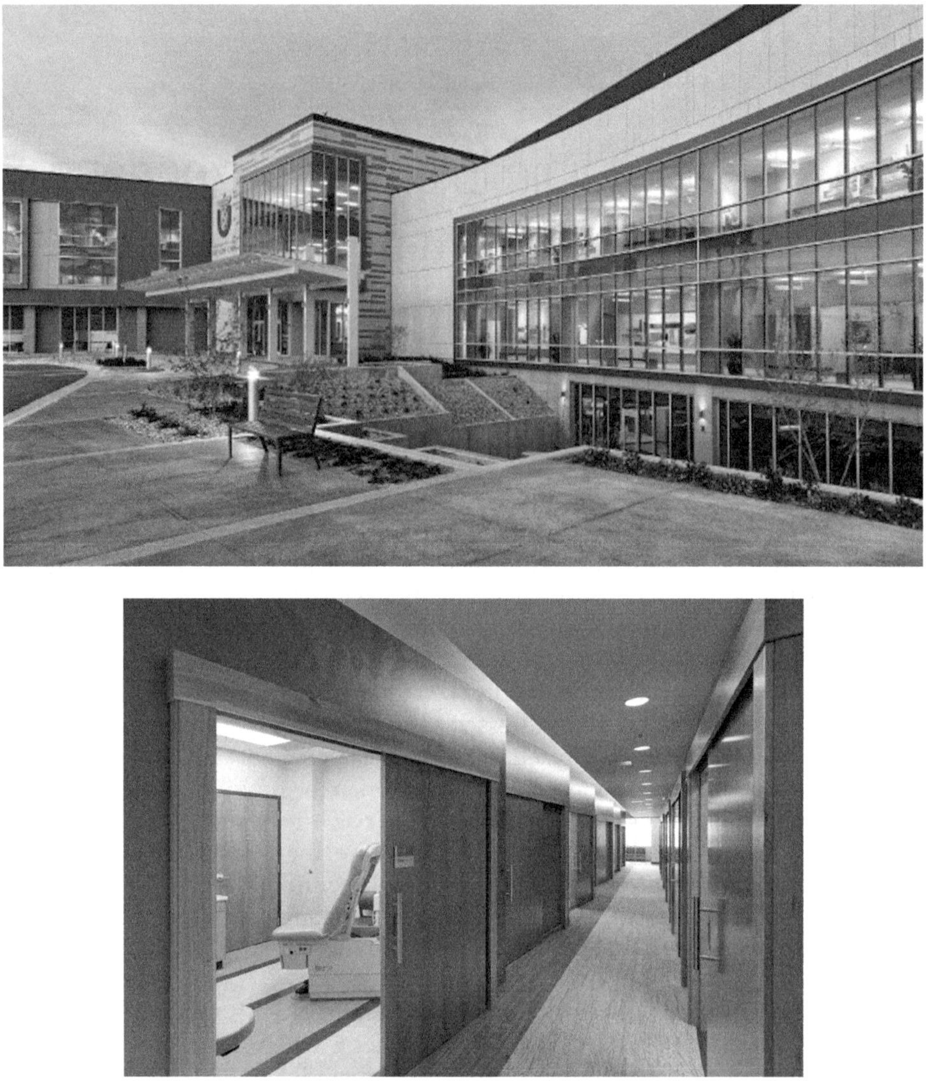

FIGURE 18.1 University of Utah Men's Health Clinic.

Photos courtesy of University of Utah Health.

years, University of Utah Health has ranked in the top 10 of the nation's academic institutions for quality, safety, and accountability (University of Utah Health, 2017b). Referrals to the University of Utah for specialty care include those made to the Men's Health Clinic, a subspecialty of the Division of Urology.

The Men's Health Clinic was established at the University of Utah in 2013 in an effort to better structure care for male patients with urologic and reproductive needs. This clinic integrates the ability to evaluate and treat male-factor infertility, erectile dysfunction, Peyronie's disease, hypogonadism, testicular pain, urinary incontinence, benign prostatic hyperplasia, and other penile and scrotal concerns. The clinic is directly connected to other health specialties, surgical services, and laboratory services, including a nationally recognized Andrology Lab. As part of a larger healthcare system, the University of Utah Men's Health Clinic is committed to the mission of excellence in patient care, education, and research (University of Utah Health, 2017c).

University of Utah men's health providers see patients at four community clinics and via phone consultations when needed. Surgical services for this clinic are provided at three locations, including both outpatient surgical centers and hospitals capable of admitting patients for observation if necessary. Physicians, physician assistants, nurse practitioners, nurses, and clinical support staff work to provide high-quality, patient-centered care at each location. In fiscal year 2017, the University of Utah Men's Health Clinic had nearly 5,000 clinic appointments and over 450 surgical procedures, as well as several community education and outreach events. Patients, upon evaluating their experience, consistently state via online survey responses that they would recommend the clinic to others.

ACCESS TO CLINIC AND CLINIC CAPACITY

Americans have begun to expect value, quality, and increased access to information in their healthcare experience, thereby taking on the roles both of patient and consumer (Hibbard, 2017; Mohammed et al., 2016; Pflueger, 2016). As patients seek to be more involved in their healthcare decisions and expenses, they may access care of their own accord (Mohammed et al., 2016; Pollack et al., 2015). Owing to this growing trend, direct-to-consumer marketing of healthcare and health services has become more prevalent (Carter, Jambulingam, & Chitturi, 2015; Mackey & Liang, 2015). Patient requests for additional information, testing, or prescriptions increase as marketing campaigns for specific diagnoses, laboratory tests, and pharmaceuticals are targeted to particular audiences (Carter et al., 2015; Skeldon, Kozhimannil, Majumdar, & Law, 2015).

Men's health is one area in which both direct-to-consumer marketing and patient inquiries have increased. There has been a profound escalation in advertisements for testosterone replacement therapies, as well as patient requests for testosterone level assessments and interventions (Layton, Kim, & Alexander, 2017). Makers of phosphodiesterase-5 inhibitors for erectile dysfunction have also successfully used marketing to increase demand for their pharmaceuticals (Koo & Yap, 2017; Perelman, 2016). In many cities, independent men's health clinics have been established and, with them, there has been additional marketing to male patients. These clinics and their advertisements purpose to treat erectile dysfunction, low testosterone, male infertility, and benign prostatic hyperplasia (Choy et al., 2015).

The University of Utah Men's Health Clinic is one clinic that employs direct-to-consumer marketing. Social and traditional media campaigns have been used to notify the public of procedures offered at this institution. Community seminars, marketed via targeted mailing lists, have been used to educate interested parties about the prevalence of certain men's health concerns and the available treatment options at the University of Utah Men's Health Clinic. Patient testimonials are employed at times to normalize seeking care for particularly sensitive concerns. At community seminars, for example, existing patients with inflatable penile prostheses or artificial urinary sphincters speak to prospective patients considering these devices.

Whether as a result of marketing campaigns, word of mouth, or a consumer-driven information search, a growing fraction of patients refer themselves to specialty care, though this is more likely to occur if the patient is of higher socioeconomic status (Pollack et al., 2015). While some health institutions limit or prohibit self-referrals, the University of Utah Men's Health Clinic permits patients to schedule an appointment with a specialist without a referral from another provider. This policy can allow men to receive necessary interventions in fewer total visits or lower cost than if they had initially presented elsewhere (Mitchell, Reschovsky, Film, & Franzini, 2017).

Though many patients will self-refer, other healthcare providers remain an indispensable referral source for specialty care. Providers often refer to specialists with whom they are familiar and with whom they have open communication channels, personally and/or professionally (Makaroun et al., 2017; Zuchowski et al., 2015). In fact, primary care providers are more likely to discuss multiple concerns with their patients in one visit if they have peer specialty care providers to whom they can refer less familiar diagnoses or diagnoses that will require specialized interventions (Tuzzio et al., 2017). For a men's health clinic, referring providers frequently include primary care providers, reproductive endocrinologists, surgical or radiation oncologists, and general urologists.

Establishing provider-to-provider relationships can be done through networking opportunities within and without a provider's institution. The University of Utah offers provider lunches both among university providers and between university providers and community providers with whom there are shared patients and shared clinical interests. One way specialty providers can foster open communication with their referring providers is by sending a consultation plan on each referred patient. This, if done in a timely manner, allows continuity of care and engenders trust and learning between providers (Tuot et al., 2017; Vermeir et al., 2015). Another way to preserve communication between providers is to ensure that referring providers have contact information for both the specialty clinic and the specialty providers directly. These provider-to-provider relationships are critical as patients may be willing to accept higher cost and travel time to see a specialist whom their referring provider specifically recommends (Dunlea & Lenert, 2015).

Whether new patients are self-referred or referred from a previous provider, it is important to have appointment availability. Appointments are available in one to three locations of the University of Utah Men's Health Clinic on most weekdays with nurse practitioner, physician assistant, and/or physician. To improve both patient access and clinic utilization, multiple avenues for patient scheduling can be used (Fournier, Rainville, Ingram, & Heale, 2015; Zhao, Yoo, Lavoie, Lavoie, & Simoes, 2017). For many clinics, including most clinics at the University of Utah, new appointments can be scheduled through telephone call centers. The University of Utah Men's Health Clinic has dedicated phone numbers and specific staff members whose responsibility it is to be available for patient calls and scheduling. The University of Utah also uses web-scheduling, where patients can, at any time, select a specialist whom they would like to see and schedule an appointment by selecting from available appointment times as listed online.

When scheduling an appointment via the call center, University of Utah Men's Health Clinic patients are triaged according to chief complaint. This allows each patient to be offered the earliest available appropriate appointment. Clinic templates serve as a guide for all staff members who participate in scheduling. A **clinic template** is an outline of appointment times, appointment lengths, and appointment types for patients to schedule with a particular provider on a given day. Clinic templates, when utilized appropriately, have improved the efficiency of time spent in clinic for both patients and providers (Anderson, Zheng, Yoon, & Khasawneh, 2015; Huang & Marcak, 2015). Clinic templates ensure each patient gets scheduled for an appropriate appointment time, for the appropriate appointment type, with the appropriate provider, and in the appropriate clinic location. Appointment types are classifications that specify the type of care anticipated at a given encounter. Two examples of clinic templates and their corresponding appointment types are shown in Tables 18.1 and 18.2.

The University of Utah Men's Health Clinic has both individual provider clinic days and multiple provider clinic days. On individual provider clinic templates, providers create a schedule that accommodates their own and their patients' needs. While healthcare providers have the prerogative to template their clinics according to their preferences, offering timely appointments, particularly for new patients and urgent concerns, can improve access and outcomes (Liu, Finkelstein, Kruk, & Rosenthal, 2017). Short conversion time from scheduling date to appointment date can limit no-show appointments and prevent patients

TABLE 18.1 Multiprovider Clinic Template

Physician		Nurse Practitioner/Physician Assistant	
Time	**Appointment Type**	**Time**	**Appointment Type**
08:00	Procedure[a]	08:00	New patient visit
08:40	Return patient visit[b]	08:40	Procedure[c]
09:00	New patient visit	09:00	Return patient visit
09:40	New patient visit	09:20	New patient visit
10:20	Return patient visit	10:00	Return patient visit
10:40	New patient visit	10:20	Return patient visit
11:20	Procedure	10:40	Procedure
		11:00	New patient visit
(Lunch)		(Lunch)	
13:00	New patient visit	13:00	Return patient visit
13:40	Return patient visit	13:20	New patient visit
14:00	New patient visit	14:00	Procedure
14:40	New patient visit	14:20	New patient visit
15:20	New patient visit	15:00	Procedure
16:00	Return patient visit	15:20	Return patient visit
16:20	Procedure	15:40	Return patient visit
		16:00	Phone consult
		16:20	Phone consult

[a]Physician procedures (40 minutes): vasectomy, circumcision, penile Doppler ultrasound.
[b]Return patient visits to include preoperative and postoperative appointments.
[c]Nurse practitioner/physician assistant procedures (20 minutes): Peyronie's disease plaque injection, corpora cavernosa injection, testosterone pellet implant, cystoscopy.

from seeking care elsewhere (Osadchiy & KC, 2017). The University of Utah Men's Health Clinic maximizes availability by offering appointments among their providers at multiple locations each day of the week. Extended hour evening clinics and phone consultations are also routinely offered.

At least once weekly there is a joint clinic with physicians, nurse practitioners, and/or physician assistants staffing the same location and same pool of patients. Multiprovider clinic formats are becoming more popular to improve efficient use of resources (El-Sharo, Zheng, Yoon, & Khasawneh, 2015). Placing multiple providers in one location allows an increased number of patients to be seen in a clinic space and makes better use of overlapping appointments. Overlapping appointments reduces clinic cost (Anderson et al., 2015). A model for a multiprovider clinic, with one physician and one nurse practitioner or physician assistant, is shown in Table 18.1 and an individual provider clinic template is shown in Table 18.2.

The University of Utah Men's Health Clinic multiprovider clinics have increased clinic efficiency and clinic capacity while also improving cohesiveness among providers and staff members. While each provider has clinical emphases, all manage similar diagnoses in predictable and uniform ways; a team dynamic and respect between providers can improve their job satisfaction (Poghosyan, Liu, Shang, & D'Aunno, 2017; Song et al., 2017).

TABLE 18.2 Individual Provider Clinic Template

Time	Appointment Type
0800	Procedure[a]
0820	New patient visit
0900	New patient visit
0940	Return patient visit
1000	Return patient visit
1020	Return patient visit
1040	Procedure
1100	New patient visit
1140	Return patient visit
(Lunch)	
1300	New patient visit
1340	Return patient visit
1400	Procedure
1420	Procedure
1440	New patient visit
1500	Return patient visit
1520	Return patient visit
1540	Procedure

[a]Procedures to include Peyronie's disease plaque injection, corpora cavernosa injection, testosterone pellet implant, cystoscopy.

Patients of this clinic often do not hesitate to see a different provider at follow-up visits if more convenient by time or location. In fact, men may favor shorter wait time over seeing their preferred provider (Liu et al., 2017). Patients have rarely expressed a desire for specific-gendered provider or support staff, though this can be accommodated when requested.

When creating a multiprovider clinic, caution should be used to determine that there is enough capacity for the anticipated number of patients. **Clinic capacity** is an evaluation of the maximum number of patients a team of employees can treat effectively in a given amount of time. An appropriate allocation of examination rooms per provider should be established. A clinic that offers procedures will require timely replacement of exam room supplies and prompt sanitizing or sterilizing of equipment. Time with provider tends to be the segment of a clinic visit whose duration is the most difficult to adjust and which is most closely tied to patient satisfaction with their outpatient visit (Bard et al., 2016; Donahue et al., 2017). One way to optimize time providers spend with patients is to employ overlapping visits, whereby one patient can be checked in for or checked out from their appointment while the provider is with another patient (Anderson et al., 2015).

Individual capacity of team members should also be evaluated. Providers will have a personal limitation on the number of patients they can or would like to see in a day. Clinical nurses, medical assistants, administrative assistants, financial advisors, and authorization teams will also each have a capacity for the number of patients they can help each day. For a clinic that offers surgery, available operating room time is a factor in scheduling, as patients may anticipate a short interval from clinic visit to surgical date (Kazemian et al., 2017). A realistic evaluation of both clinic and operating room capacity can help identify how best to format a provider's time to avoid lost time and lost revenue (Martinez, Bernard, Larson, Pasupathy, & Sir, 2016).

CARING FOR THE MEN'S HEALTH PATIENT

Employees of a men's health practice will require specialized training. For example, medical assistants may need to be taught how to clean and drape penises for cystoscopy and penile injections. Given the sensitive nature of many men's health diagnoses, it is imperative to train staff members to remain professional and respectful to these patients and their concerns. Behavior of healthcare providers can be the factor that causes a patient either to voice sensitive concerns or to stay quiet (Bauer et al., 2016). Inquiring about sexual partners and sexual orientation should be done in a tactful, professional manner. One goal of the University of Utah Men's Health Clinic is that patients will feel they can speak frankly and openly about their concerns and expect to receive respectful, informed care in return.

In addition to respecting patients and their concerns, standardizing workflows for particular diagnoses further normalizes the experience for patients of the University of Utah Men's Health Clinic. A **care pathway** is a standard set of assessments and interventions for a particular diagnosis that serves as a guideline for care given by healthcare providers. Care pathways can standardize care so that a patient can experience and even anticipate similar care regardless of which provider he sees within a practice. When a care pathway is followed, it promotes better coordination in patient treatment and improves efficiency (Seys et al., 2017).

Care pathways at the University of Utah Men's Health Clinic begin when a patient schedules an appointment. This clinic has established workflows for new patients, specific to chief complaint, that guide clinic support staff as they help prepare a patient for the visit (Figures 18.2 and 18.3). Diagnoses specific to men's health can require patients to provide unique information either before or at their visit. For example, many insurance plans do not cover infertility treatment (Mehta, Nangia, Dupree, & Smith, 2016). To prevent confusion both at the visit and upon billing, administrative staff members of the University of Utah Men's Health Clinic discuss payment options with a new infertility patient when they schedule the first appointment. The patient then completes an androgen profile laboratory assessment, a semen analysis, and a questionnaire regarding fertility history. The protocol for Peyronie's disease does not specify any lab work or unique billing information. New Peyronie's disease patients are, however, instructed to bring to their first visit a photo of an erection and complete a thorough questionnaire (Figure 18.2).

As shown in Figures 18.2 and 18.3, team members are assigned to obtain previous health records, order and acquire needed laboratory results, and verify that the patient is aware of appointment time and location. Appointment reminders are particularly helpful when an institution like the University of Utah has multiple locations. Phone, email, and text appointment confirmations have been very successful at limiting missed appointments (Boksmati, Butler-Henderson, Anderson, & Sahama, 2016; Perri-Moore et al., 2016). Preparation prior to the appointment helps patients take an active role in their care, which can improve satisfaction for both provider and patient (Pollard, Bansback, & Bryan, 2015; Shay & Lafata, 2015). Though it takes additional time to review this information, patients' first visits are more effective when previous records and data can be evaluated and incorporated into informed clinical judgments (Sinsky et al., 2016).

Care pathways are used before, during, and after clinic appointments. When multiple providers share support staff, care pathways can help direct support staff to answer patient questions. Support staff, including medical assistants and nurses, practice to the fullest extent of their education and training when they are empowered to educate patients in this way

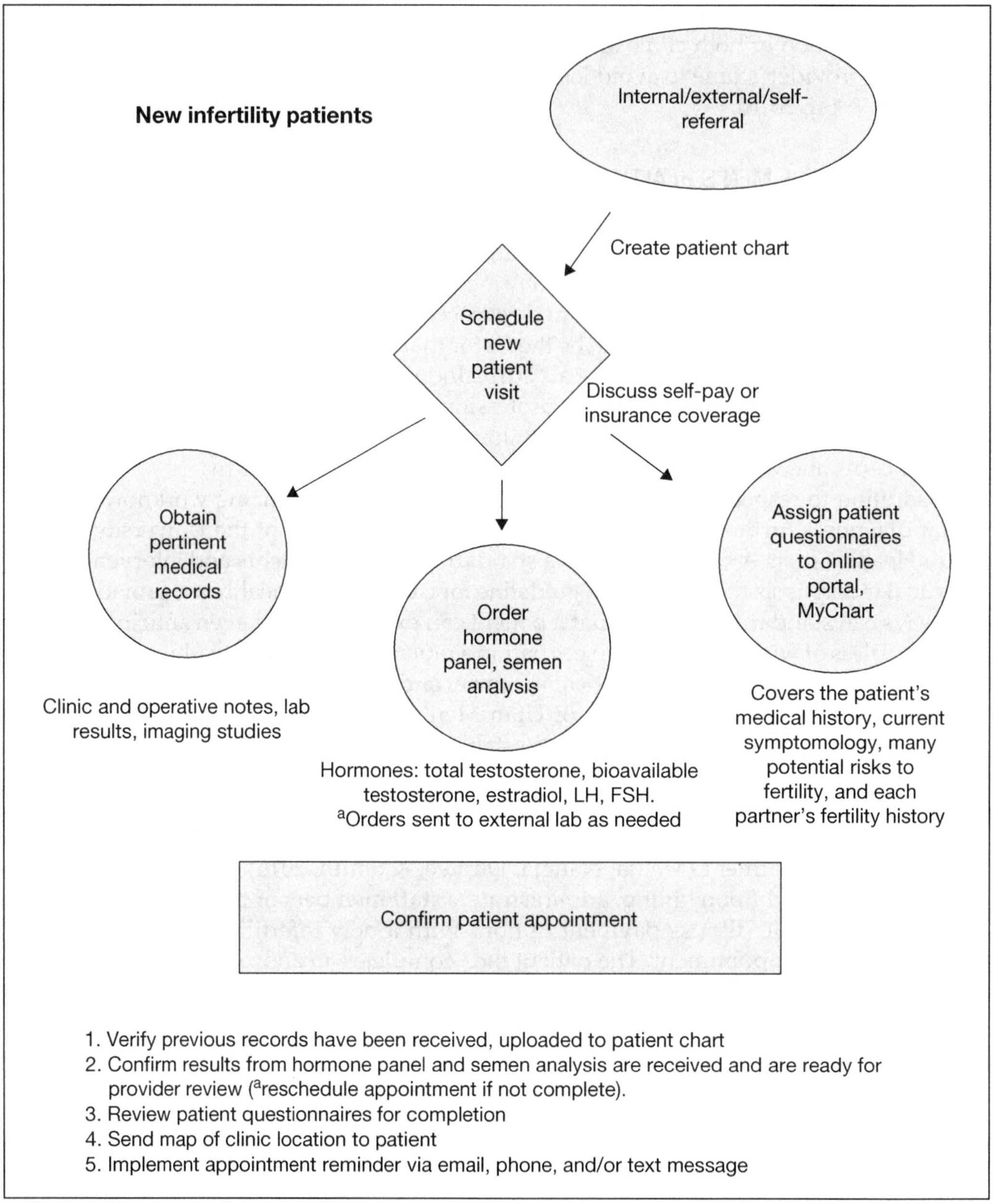

FIGURE 18.2 New infertility patient workflow.

FSH, follicle-stimulating hormone; LH, luteinizing hormone.

(McGough, Kline, & Simpson, 2017). For example, clinical support staff can advise patients on newly prescribed medications or explain upcoming surgeries at the conclusion of a clinic visit, leading to more total time spent with patients. This educational time, whether from clinic support staff or provider, tends to improve patient satisfaction (Martinez, Bernard, Larson, Pasupathy, & Sir, 2016).

Inevitably, patients will need to contact the clinic with questions or concerns between their clinic appointments. Patients who take an active role in their health and in the patient-provider

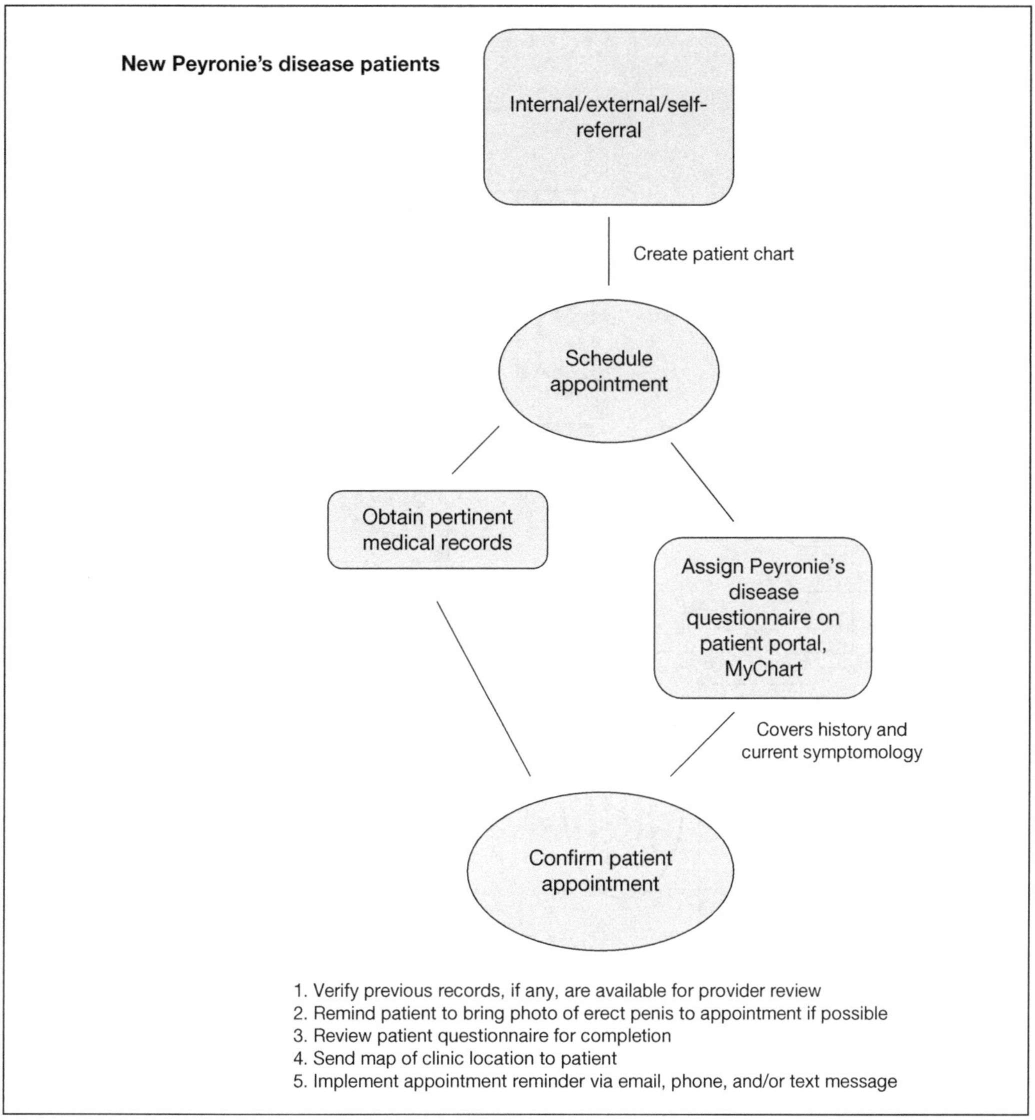

FIGURE 18.3 New Peyronie's disease patient workflow.

relationship are more likely to contact their providers outside of an appointment (Hibbard, 2017). At University of Utah Health, patients can contact any clinic where they have been seen via telephone call, Internet portal, pharmacy, or laboratory. Given the number of methods that patients can contact the clinic, it is vital that providers can manage the influx of patient requests. One way to do this is through care pathways and written protocols that allow clinical support staff to coordinate care for patients without seeking advice from a provider on each individual patient or concern. An example of a care pathway is presented in Figure 18.4. As shown, nurses and medical assistants can assist patients with questions about medication, health symptoms, medication refill requests, laboratory tests, and administrative/scheduling issues. Care pathways have also helped the University of Utah Men's Health Clinic coordinate laboratory work at outside facilities for those patients who live at a distance and acquire these results for the appropriate provider to review.

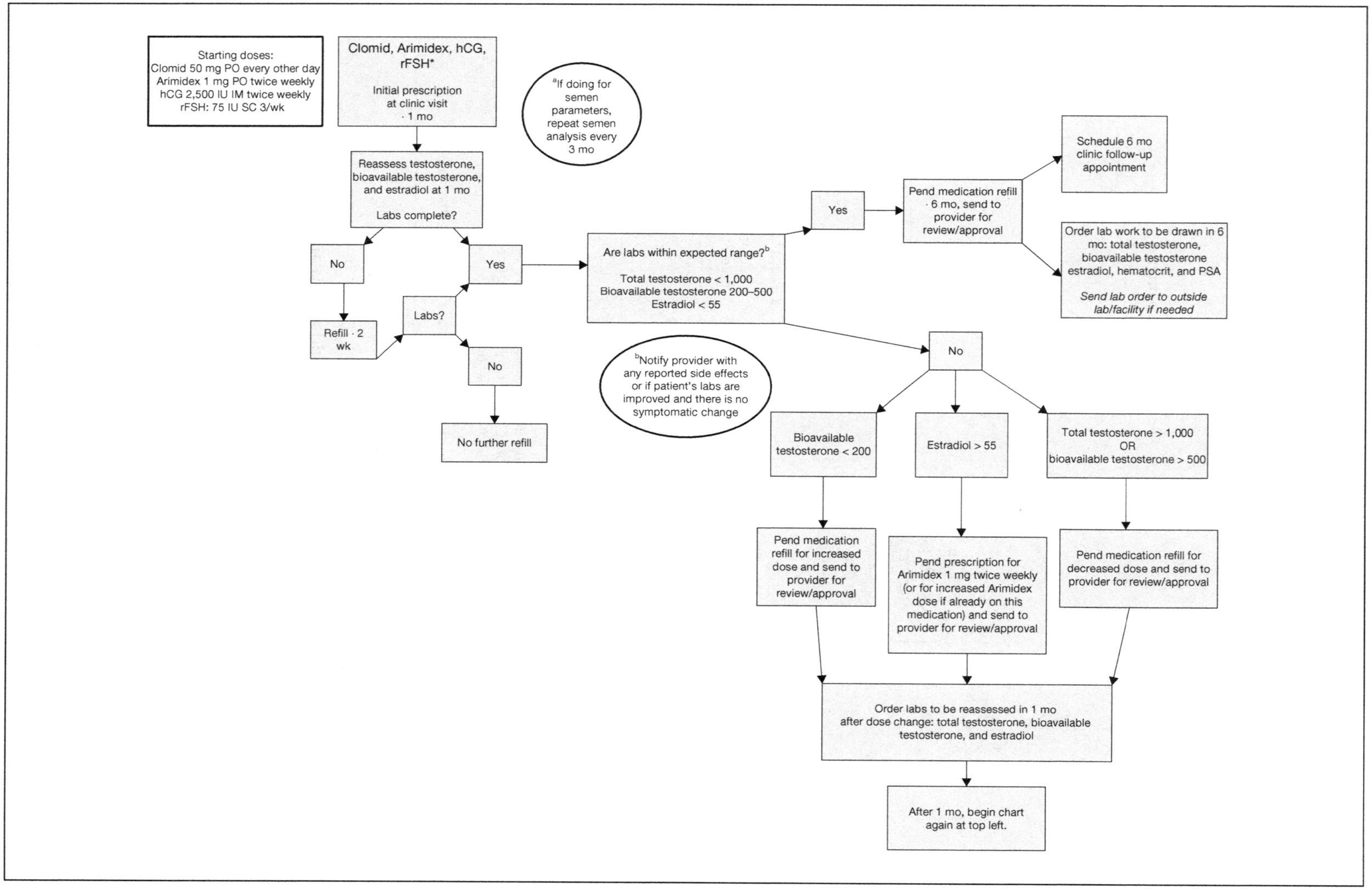

FIGURE 18.4 Medication care pathway.

hCG, human chorionic gonadotropin; IM, intramuscular; PSA, prostate-specific antigen; rFSH, recombinant follicle-stimulating hormone; SC, subcutaneous.

Many institutions have implemented a **patient portal** where patients can view and interact with their medical record electronically. Patient portals are effective tools for patient education and are becoming more commonplace (Ancker et al., 2015). The University of Utah's electronic medical record (EMR) patient portal is entitled *MyChart*. Here, patients can review their clinic notes and instructions, see laboratory results, request medication refills, and ask their providers questions. Patient portals can increase the out-of-clinic work for a provider but can limit the number of clinic visits per patient. Despite reduced or absent reimbursement for care that is not associated with a clinic visit, limiting the number of office visits per patient improves the efficiency of clinical care (Clough, Patel, & Shrank, 2016).

It should not be overlooked that Men's Health patients will often have additional health needs that are not specific to this specialty. Many symptoms treated at a Men's Health Clinic may be a result of systemic diseases and a thorough evaluation for these symptoms will often identify other health concerns or health risks in patients. Of particular concern are those patients who present to a Men's Health Clinic with undiagnosed underlying conditions. This includes erectile or ejaculatory dysfunction as a result of cardiac disease or diabetes mellitus, Peyronie's disease due to tobacco use, and hypogonadism secondary to obesity, sleep apnea, or chronic opiate use. Quality, patient-centered care includes addressing these additional health concerns and referring to other providers when indicated. Table 18.3 lists common referrals made from the University of Utah Men's Health Clinic. As shown, the

TABLE 18.3 Common Referrals From the University of Utah Men's Health Clinic

Referrals From the Men's Health Clinic	
Department	**Reason for Referral**
Anesthesia	Preoperative screening
Cardiology	Erectile dysfunction, cardiac risk factor screening
Endocrinology	Prolactinoma, hypothyroidism
General surgery	Inguinal hernia
General urology	Stone disease, overactive bladder, interstitial cystitis
Genetic counselor	Congenital absence of vas deferens, azoospermia
Hematology	Persistent polycythemia
Infectious disease	Refractory prostatitis, refractory pyospermia
Internal medicine	Chronic disease(s)
Maternal–fetal medicine	Recurrent pregnancy loss
Neurology	Altered penile sensation
Oncology	Elevated/rising PSA, testis mass
Pain management	Refractory orchialgia
Pelvic floor physical therapy	Pelvic pain, pelvic tension
Primary care	General health screening
Psychiatry	Depression
Pulmonology/sleep medicine	Obstructive sleep apnea
Reproductive endocrinology	Female infertility, need for assisted reproduction
Sex therapy	Sexual anxiety, erectile dysfunction, ejaculatory dysfunction

PSA, prostate-specific antigen.

range includes referral to internal medicine to establish care, to pulmonology or hematology for additional screening, sex therapy for psychogenic sexual dysfunction, back to a referring primary care provider, or to general or specialized surgeons for incidental physical findings.

CLINIC POTENTIAL

Clinic access, clinic capacity, and clinical care are all related to clinic potential. Another important factor in clinic potential is the ability to bill and collect for services. As patients have taken on the role of consumer, they have become more interested in the price of health services (Saloner et al., 2017). Prices include both those services that are covered under their insurance plan and those services that are excluded from insurance coverage. Both categories regularly influence University of Utah Men's Health Clinic patients. Male infertility evaluation and intervention is a mandated health insurance benefit in only eight states (California, Connecticut, Massachusetts, Montana, New Jersey, New York, Ohio, and West Virginia) and insurance companies have, historically, had complex requirements to approve erectile dysfunction therapies as well as limited options once treatment is approved (Dupree, Dickey, & Lipshultz, 2016; Le et al., 2017). Men may then end up paying for these interventions out of pocket. With an increasing number of high-deductible plans, patients may also pay out of pocket for typically covered benefits (Catlin, Poisal, & Cowan, 2015). This might include treatment for diagnoses such as hypogonadism, testicular pain, prostatitis, and Peyronie's disease.

The University of Utah employs financial advocates who help patients coordinate cash payment for clinic visits or procedures if these are not covered under their insurance plan. They also assist uninsured patients. While preauthorization teams work to verify insurance approval for covered benefits, the financial advocates communicate directly with the patient to discuss payment options. There is a set cash price for all procedures offered at the University of Utah Men's Health Clinic, both for in-clinic and operating room procedures, with a discount applied for prompt payment. Third-party financing is available for high-cost surgical procedures. Open discussion about cost during a clinic visit is becoming more common and expected (Hunter et al., 2016). Financial advocates have been an invaluable addition to this clinic's team by leading this discussion with patients both during and between clinic appointments.

Proper billing and clinic reimbursement is important for specialty medicine, as it often requires unique coding and billing practices. Table 18.4 shows an example of the clinic

TABLE 18.4 Selected Clinic Procedures

Clinic Procedure	Current Procedural Terminology (CPT) Code
Circumcision (adolescent/adult)	54161
Cystoscopy	52005
Hormone pellet insertion	11980
Inject corpora cavernosa	54235
Inject penile plaque	54200
Irrigate/aspirate corpora cavernosa	54220
Penile Doppler ultrasound	93980 (with 54235 injection)
Spermatic cord nerve block	64450
Vasectomy	52250

TABLE 18.5 Surgical Procedures Scheduled Through the Men's Health Clinic

Surgical Procedure
Epididymectomy
Hydrocelectomy
Inflatable penile prosthesis
Microsurgical denervation of the spermatic cord
Microsurgical testicular sperm extraction
Orchidopexy
Penile plication
Scrotoplasty
Spermatocelectomy
Testicular sperm extraction
Varicocelectomy
Vasectomy reversal

procedures offered at the University of Utah Men's Health Clinic with their appropriate CPT (Current Procedural Terminology) code, while Table 18.5 lists many of the surgical procedures offered at this clinic, many of which have required unique cosmetic coding in order to facilitate billing.

CONCLUSION

Lastly, a clinic must reflect on its processes and identify ways to improve in order to be successful. As healthcare becomes patient or consumer driven, it is important to engage patients when evaluating a clinic's success. The University of Utah has an Exceptional Patient Experience Initiative whereby each patient of the institution has an opportunity to rate many aspects of the care received. After an outpatient clinic visit with the University of Utah Men's Health Clinic, each patient is emailed a survey to evaluate his experience. Questions address, among other topics, ability to contact the clinic office prior to the appointment, privacy protection during the visit, and provider empathy (Lee et al., 2016). Results, including patient comments for each provider and an explanation of the data, are visible on University of Utah Health websites (University of Utah Health, 2017d). Review websites with evaluations for healthcare providers are ubiquitous yet tend to have low numbers of responses and may not provide enough information to help the consumer make an informed judgment about a provider (Lagu et al., 2017). Posting reviews in a centralized, clinic-sponsored location exhibits transparency, trust, and a commitment to patient-centered care. Providers, too, evaluate the changing needs of the clinic. Scheduling, staff allocation, clinic template, and equipment needs may all change over time (Bard et al. 2016).

Patient satisfaction is a growing emphasis for American healthcare systems and is closely tied to the subjective evaluation of the patient-provider relationship (Cobos Haskard-Zolnierek & Howard 2015; Kelley et al., 2015; Price, Elliott, Cleary, Zaslavsky, & Hays, 2015). Satisfaction for both patient and provider is possible by implementing changes based on feedback. The University of Utah Men's Health Clinic has a mission to offer thorough and patient-centered care in an environment where men feel comfortable discussing their concerns.

The clinic also strives to maximize its potential through fine-tuning clinic access and capacity while fostering the development of trusting, lasting patient–provider relationships.

REFERENCES

Amano, T., Earle, C., & Takemae, K. (2016). Are urge incontinence and aging risk factors of erectile dysfunction in patients with male lower urinary tract symptoms? *The Aging Male, 19*(1), 54–57. doi:10.3109/13685538.2015.1103219

Ancker, J. S., Osorio, S. N., Cheriff, A., Cole, C. L., Silver, M., & Kaushal, R. (2015). Patient activation and use of an electronic patient portal. *Informatics for Health and Social Care, 40*(3), 254–266. doi:10.3109/17538157.2014.908200

Anderson, K., Zheng, B., Yoon, S. W., & Khasawneh, M. T. (2015). An analysis of overlapping appointment scheduling model in an outpatient clinic. *Operations Research for Health Care, 4*, 5–14. doi:10.1016/j.orhc.2014.12.001

Bard, J. F., Shu, Z., Morrice, D. J., Wang, D., Poursani, R., & Leykum, L. (2016). Improving patient flow at a family health clinic. *Health Care Management Science, 19*(2), 170–191. doi:10.1007/s10729-014-9294-y

Bauer, M., Haesler, E., & Fetherstonhaugh, D. (2016). Let's talk about sex: Older people's views on the recognition of sexuality and sexual health in the health-care setting. *Health Expectations, 19*(6), 1237–1250. doi: 10.1111/hex.12418

Berger, M. H., Messore, M., Patuszak, A. W., & Ramasamy, R. (2016). Association between infertility and sexual dysfunction in men and women. *Sexual Medicine Reviews, 4*(4), 353–365. doi:10.1016/j.sxmr.2016.05.002

Boksmati, N., Butler-Henderson, K., Anderson, K., & Sahama, T. (2016). The effectiveness of SMS reminders on appointment attendance: A meta-analysis. *Journal of Medical Systems, 40*(4), 90. doi:10.1007/s10916-016-0452-2

Carter, F., Jambulingam, T., & Chitturi, R. (2015). Determinants of perceived value of direct to consumer advertising for prescription drugs: Do they vary by disease condition? *Journal of Marketing Management, 3*(2), 1–20. doi:10.15640/jmm.v3n2a1

Catlin, M. K., Poisal, J. A., & Cowan, C. A. (2015). Out-of-pocket health care expenditures, by insurance status, 2007–10. *Health Affairs, 34*(1), 111–116. doi:10.1377/hlthaff.2014.0422

Choy, J., Kashanian, J. A., Sharman, V., Masson, P., Dupree, J., Le, B., & Brannigan, R. E. (2015). The men's health center: Disparities in gender specific health services among the top 50 "best hospitals" in America. *Asian Journal of Urology, 2*(3), 170–174. doi:10.1016/j.ajur.2015.06.005

Clough, J. D., Patel, K., & Shrank, W. H. (2016). Variation in specialty outpatient care patterns in the Medicare population. *Journal of General Internal Medicine, 31*(11), 1278–1286. doi:10.1007/s11606-016-3745-8

Cobos, B., Haskard-Zolnierek, K., & Howard, K. (2015). White coat hypertension: Improving the patient–health care practitioner relationship. *Psychology Research and Behavior Management, 8*, 133–141. doi:10.2147/PRBM.S61192

Donahue, R., Russell, D., De Riese, C., Smith, C., De Riese, W. T., & Medway, A. (2017). Patients willing to wait: Arrival time, wait time and patient satisfaction in an ambulatory urology clinic. *Urology Practice, 4*(1), 1–6. doi:10.1016/j.urpr.2016.02.003

Dunlea, R., & Lenert, L. (2015). Understanding patients' preferences for referrals to specialists for an asymptomatic condition. *Medical Decision Making, 35*(6), 691–702. doi:10.1177/0272989X14566640

Dupree, J. M., Dickey, R. M., & Lipshultz, L. I. (2016). Inequity between male and female coverage in state infertility laws. *Fertility and Sterility, 105*(6), 1519–1522. doi:10.1016/j.fertnstert.2016.02.025

Egan, K. B. (2016). The epidemiology of benign prostatic hyperplasia associated with lower urinary tract symptoms: Prevalence and incident rates. *Urologic Clinics of North America, 43*(3), 289–297. doi:10.1016/j.ucl.2016.04.001

El-Sharo, M., Zheng, B., Yoon, S. W., & Khasawneh, M. T. (2015). An overbooking scheduling model for outpatient appointments in a multi-provider clinic. *Operations Research for Health Care, 6*, 1–10. doi:10.1016/j.orhc.2015.05.004

Fournier, J., Rainville, A., Ingram, J., & Heale, R. (2015). Implementation of an advanced access scheduling system in primary healthcare: One clinic's experience. *Healthcare Quarterly, 18*(1), 60–64. Retrieved from http://www.longwoods.com/publications/healthcare-quarterly

Fuzzell, L., Fedesco, H. N., Alexander, S. C., Fortenberry, J. D., & Shields, C. G. (2016). "I just think that doctors need to ask more questions": Sexual minority and majority adolescents' experiences talking about sexuality with healthcare providers. *Patient Education and Counseling, 99*(9), 1467–1472. doi:10.1016/j.pec.2016.06.004

Hibbard, J. H. (2017). Patient activation and the use of information to support informed health decisions. *Patient Education and Counseling, 100*(1), 5–7. doi:10.1016/j.pec.2016.07.006

Huang, Y., & Marcak, J. (2015). Grid patient appointment template design to improve scheduling effectiveness. *Journal of Healthcare Engineering, 6*(2), 239–258. doi:10.1260/2040-2295.6.2.239

Hunter, W. G., Hesson, A., Davis, J. K., Kirby, C., Williamson, L. D., Barnett, J. A., & Ubel, P. A. (2016). Patient-physician discussions about costs: Definitions and impact on cost conversation incidence estimates. *BMC Health Services Research, 16*, 108. doi:10.1186/s12913-016-1353-2

Kazemian, P., Sir, M. Y., Van Oyen, M. P., Lovely, J. K., Larson, D. W., & Pasupathy, K. S. (2017). Coordinating clinic and surgery appointments to meet access service levels for elective surgery. *Journal of Biomedical Informatics, 66*, 105–115. doi:10.1016/j.jbi.2016.11.007

Kelley, M., James, C., Kraft, S. A., Korngiebel, D., Wijangco, I., Rosenthal, E., ... Lee, S. S. (2015). Patient perspectives on the learning health system: The importance of trust and shared decision making. *The American Journal of Bioethics, 15*(9), 4–17. doi:10.1080/15265161.2015.1062163

King, A. J., Evans, M., Moore, T. H., Paterson, C., Sharp, D., Persad, R., & Huntley, A. L. (2015). Prostate cancer and supportive care: A systematic review and qualitative synthesis of men's experiences and unmet needs. *European Journal of Cancer Care, 24*(5), 618–634. doi:10.1111/ecc.12286

Koo, K., & Yap, R. L. (2017). Trends in urological direct-to-consumer advertising during prime-time television news programs. *Urology Practice, 4*(1), 7–13. doi:10.1016/j.urpr.2016.03.005

Lagu, T., Metayer, K., Moran, M., Ortiz, L., Priya, A., Goff, S. L., & Lindenauer, P. K. (2017). Website characteristics and physician reviews on commercial physician-rating websites. *Journal of the American Medical Association, 317*(7), 766–768. doi:10.1001/jama.2016.18553

Layton, J. B., Kim, Y., & Alexander, G. C. (2017). association between direct-to-consumer advertising and testosterone testing and initiation in the United States, 2009-2013. *Journal of the American Medical Association, 317*(11), 1159–1166. doi:10.1001/jama.2016.21041

Le, B., McAchran, S., Paolone, D., Gralnek, D., Williams, D., IV, & Bushman, W. (2017). Assessing the variability in insurance coverage transparency for male sexual health conditions in the United States. *Urology, 102*, 126–129. doi:10.1016/j.urology.2016.12.031

Lee, V. S., Miller, T., Daniels, C., Paine, M., Gresh, B., & Betz, A. L. (2016). Creating the exceptional patient experience in one academic health system. *Academic Medicine, 91*(3), 338–344. doi:10.1097/ACM.0000000000001007

Lee King, P. A., Cederbaum, J. A., Kurzban, S., Norton, T., Palmer, S. C., & Coyne, J. C. (2015). Role of patient treatment beliefs and provider characteristics in establishing patient–provider relationships. *Family Practice, 32*(2), 224–231. doi:10.1093/fampra/cmu085

Liu, N., Finkelstein, S. R., Kruk, M. E., & Rosenthal, D. (2017). When waiting to see a doctor is less irritating: Understanding patient preferences and choice behavior in appointment scheduling. *Management Science, Articles in Advance, 64*(5), 1975–1996. doi:10.1287/mnsc.2016.2704

Mackey, T. K., & Liang, B. A. (2015). It's time to shine the light on direct-to-consumer advertising. *Annals of Family Medicine, 13*(1), 82–85. doi:10.1370/afm.1711

Makaroun, L. K., Bowman, C., Duan, K., Handley, N., Wheeler, D. J., Pierluissi, E., & Chen, A. H. (2017). Specialty care access in the safety net—The role of public hospitals and health systems. *Journal of Health Care for the Poor and Underserved, 28*(1), 566–581. doi:10.1353/hpu.2017.0040

Martinez, G., Bernard, B. J., Larson, D. W., Pasupathy, K. S., & Sir, M. Y. (2016). A data-driven approach for better assignment of clinical and surgical capacity in an elective surgical practice. *AMIA Annual Symposium Proceedings, 2016*, 874–883. Retrieved from https://knowledge.amia.org/all-proceedings

Martinez-Gonzalez, N. A., Rosemann, T., Djalali, S., Huber-Geismann, F., & Tandjung, R. (2015). Task-shifting from physicians to nurses in primary care and its impact on resource utilization: A systematic review and meta-analysis of randomized controlled trials. *Medical Care Research and Review, 72*(4), 395–418. doi:10.1177/1077558715586297

McGough, P., Kline, S., & Simpson, L. (2017). Team care approach to population health and care management. *International Journal of Health Governance, 22*(2), 93–103. doi:10.1108/IJHG-11-2016-0048

Mehta, A., Nangia, A. K., Dupree, J. M., & Smith, J. F. (2016). Limitations and barriers in access to care for male factor infertility. *Fertility and Sterility, 105*(5), 1128–1137. doi:10.1016/j.fertnstert.2016.03.023

Mitchell, J., Reschovsky, J. D., Film, R. J., & Franzini, L. (2017). Examining drivers of health care spending: Evidence on self-referral among a privately insured population. *Medical Care, 55*(7), 684–692. doi:10.1097/MLR.0000000000000732

Mohammed, K., Nolan, M. B., Rajjo, T., Shah, N. D., Prokop, L. J., Varkey, P., & Murad, M. H. (2016). Creating a patient-centered health care delivery system: A systematic review of health care quality from the patient perspective. *American Journal of Medical Quality, 31*(1), 12–21. doi:10.1177/1062860614545124

Murray, B., & McCrone, S. (2015). An integrative review of promoting trust in the patient–primary care provider relationship. *Journal of Advanced Nursing, 71*(1), 3–23. doi:10.1111/jan.12502

Osadchiy, N., & KC, D. (2017). Are patients patient? The role of time to appointment in patient flow. *Production and Operations Management, 26*(3), 469–490. doi:10.1111/poms.12659

Perelman, M. A. (2016). What history can teach us about the different response to the launch of addyi versus viagra. *Current Sexual Health Reports, 8*(2), 116–120. doi:10.1007/s11930-016-0075-0

Perri-Moore, S., Kapsandoy, S., Doyon, K., Hill, B., Archer, M., Shana-McWhorter, L., … Zeng-Treitler, Q. (2016). Automated alerts and reminders targeting patients: A review of the literature. *Patient Education and Counseling, 99*(6), 953–959. doi:10.1016/j.pec.2015.12.010

Pflueger, D. (2016). Knowing patients: The customer survey and the changing margins of accounting in healthcare. *Accounting, Organizations and Society, 53*, 17–33. doi:10.1016/j.aos.2016.08.002

Poghosyan, L., Liu, J., Shang, J., & D'Aunno, T. (2017). Practice environments and job satisfaction and turnover intentions of nurse practitioners: Implications for primary care workforce capacity. *Health Care Management Review, 42*(2), 162–171. doi:10.1097/HMR.0000000000000094

Pollack, C. E., Rastegar, A., Keating, N. L., Adams, J. L., Pisu, M., & Kahn, K. L. (2015). Is self-referral associated with higher quality care? *Health Services Research, 50*(5), 1472–1490. doi:10.1111/1475-6773.12289

Pollard, S., Bansback, N., & Bryan, S. (2015). Physician attitudes toward shared decision making: A systematic review. *Patient Education and Counseling, 98*(9), 1046–1057. doi:10.1016/j.pec.2015.05.004

Price, R. A., Elliott, M. N., Cleary, P. D., Zaslavsky, A. M., & Hays, R. D. (2015). Should health care providers be accountable for patients' care experiences? *Journal of General Internal Medicine, 30*(2), 253–256. doi:10.1007%2Fs11606-014-3111-7

Saloner, B., Cope, L. C., Hempstead, K., Rhodes, K. V., Polsky, D., & Kenney, G. M. (2017). Price transparency in primary care: Can patients learn about costs when scheduling an appointment? *Journal of General Internal Medicine, 32*(7), 815–821. doi:10.1007/s11606-017-4003-4

Scholz, B., Crabb, S., & Wittert, G. A. (2017). "Males don't wanna bring anything up to their doctor": Men's discourses of depression. *Qualitative Health Research, 27*(5), 727–737. doi:10.1177/1049732316640294

Seys, D., Bruyneel, L., Deneckere, S., Kul, S., Van der Veken, L., Van Zelm, R., … Vanhaecht, K. (2017). Better organized care via care pathways: A multicenter study. *Public Library of Science One, 12*(7), e0180398. doi:10.1371/journal.pone.0180398

Shay, L. A., & Lafata, J. E. (2015). Where is the evidence? A systematic review of shared decision making and patient outcomes. *Medical Decision Making, 35*(1), 114–131. doi:10.1177/0272989X14551638

Sinsky, C., Colligan, L., Li, L., Prgomet, M., Reynolds, S., Goeders, L., … Blike, G. (2016). Allocation of physician time in ambulatory practice: A time and motion study in 4 specialties. *Annals of Internal Medicine, 165*(11), 753–761. doi:10.7326/M16-0961

Skeldon, S. C., Kozhimannil, K. B., Majumdar, S. R., & Law, M. R. (2015). The effect of competing direct-to-consumer advertising campaigns on the use of drugs for benign prostatic hyperplasia: Time series analysis. *Journal of General Internal Medicine, 30*(4), 514–520. doi:10.1007/s11606-014-3063-y

Song, H., Ryan, M., Tendulkar, S., Fisher, J., Martin, J., Peters, A. S., … Singer, S. J. (2017). Team dynamics, clinical work satisfaction, and patient care coordination between primary care providers: A mixed methods study. *Health Care Management Review, 42*(1), 28–41. doi:10.1097/HMR.0000000000000091

Summers, R. H., Moore, M., Ekberg, S., Chew-Graham, C. A., Little, P., Stevenson, F., … Leydon, G. M. (2016). Soliciting additional concerns in the primary care consultation and the utility of a brief communication intervention to aid solicitation: A qualitative study. *Patient Education and Counseling, 99*(5), 724–732. doi:10.1016/j.pec.2015.12.005

Teo, C. H., Ng, C. J., Booth, A., & White, A. (2016). Barriers and facilitators to health screening in men: A systematic review. *Social Science & Medicine, 165*, 168–176. doi:10.1016/j.socscimed.2016.07.023

Thompson, A. E., Anisimowicz, Y., Miedema, B., Hogg, W., Wodchis, W. P., & Aubrey-Bassler, K. (2016). The influence of gender and other patient characteristics on health care-seeking behaviour: A QUALICOPC study. *BMC Family Practice, 17*(38), 1–7. doi:10.1186/s12875-016-0440-0

Tuot, D. S., Leeds, K., Murphy, E. J., Sarkar, U., Lyles, C. R., Mekonnen, T., & Chen, A. H. (2015). Facilitators and barriers to implementing electronic referral and/or consultation systems: A qualitative study of 16 health organizations. *BMC Health Services Research, 15*, 568. doi:10.1186/s12913-015-1233-1

Tuzzio, L., Ludman, E. J., Chang, E., Palazzo, L., Abbott, T., Wagnar, E. H., & Reid, R. J. (2017). Design and implementation of a physician coaching pilot to promote value-based referrals to specialty care. *The Permanente Journal, 21*, 16–066. doi:10.7812/TPP/16-066

University of Utah Health. (2017a). University of Utah Health: About us. Retrieved from https://healthcare.utah.edu/about

University of Utah Health. (2017b). University of Utah Health: Our rankings. Retrieved from https://healthcare.utah.edu/quality/rankings.php

University of Utah Health. (2017c). About us: Mission and vision. Retrieved from https://healthcare.utah.edu/about/mission.htm

University of Utah Health. (2017d). University of Utah Health: Find a doctor. Retrieved from https://healthcare.utah.edu/fad

Vermeir, P., Vandijck, D., Degroote, S., Peleman, R., Verhaeghe, R., Mortier, E., … Vogelaers, D. (2015). Communication in healthcare: A narrative review of the literature and practical recommendations. *The International Journal of Clinical Practice, 69*(11), 1257–1267. doi:10.1111/ijcp.12686

Zhao, P., Yoo, I., Lavoie, J., Lavoie, B. J., & Simoes, E. (2017). Web-based medical appointment systems: A systematic review. *Journal of Medical Internet Research, 19*(4), E134. doi:10.2196/jmir.6747

Zuchowski, J. L., Rose, D. E., Hamilton, A. B., Stockdale, S. E., Meredith, L. S., Yano, E. M., … Cordasco, K. M. (2015). Challenges in referral communication between VHA primary care and specialty care. *Journal of General Internal Medicine, 30*(3), 305–311. doi:10.1007/s11606-014-3100-x

CHAPTER 19

Urology as a Window to Men's Health

Christian Fuglesang S. Jensen, Mikkel Fode, Mette L. K. Schmidt, Dana A. Ohl, and Jens Sønksen

INTRODUCTION

Urology is a specialty that is relatively specific in its scope, treating diseases in the urinary tract in both men and women, but also genitourinary issues specifically in men. Therefore, the urologist's patient population heavily favors men, and male patients' urological health is a primary concern of the specialty. However, although patients presenting with urological conditions may be straightforward in the specific plan for the condition, the question arises whether this presentation of the urological complaint gives notice of deeper, seemingly unrelated health issues.

There are, in fact, many general health issues that are related to urological complaints. In this chapter we will delve into these relationships, and point out that presentation of urological complaints may represent an opportunity to view what the general health outlook is for the patient. Furthermore, if a man has not practiced regular preventive medicine with a general medical doctor, the visit to the urologist may serve as the impetus for diagnosing these related conditions, advancing to treatment and beneficially altering future health risk, and possibly even increasing life expectancy and quality of life. The urology clinic visit may serve as the reintroduction to the health system and an opportunity for education and screening.

UROLOGICAL CONDITIONS AND GENERAL HEALTH

A specific urological condition has an impact on the man's general health and quality of life as a consequence of the condition itself but may also have an impact through associated health issues. In the past 20 years increasing evidence of a relationship between urological conditions and other seemingly unrelated health issues has emerged. Focus has been on the relationship with lifestyle diseases such as cardiovascular disease, diabetes, and metabolic syndrome. However, urological conditions may also be related to cancers and mental health issues. Accordingly, it has become increasingly evident that urological conditions have a wide impact on the general health of the man and that some of these conditions may serve as a proxy of general health status.

Male Subfertility

Infertility is defined as a failure to conceive after 12 months or more of regular unprotected sexual intercourse (Chapter 27), and is an increasing problem affecting up to 15% of couples. A semen analysis is the cornerstone of male subfertility evaluation and it is well known that impaired semen quality is associated with male subfertility. However, it is less known that semen quality is a marker of general health and that male subfertility is associated with a higher rate of comorbid conditions compared to fertile men. These conditions can be as diverse as obesity, endocrine or genetic issues, and preexisting issues such as previous chemotherapy treatment.

A study on 11,935 American men evaluated for infertility examined the relationship between semen parameters and mortality and found that men with impaired semen quality had significantly higher mortality rates when compared to men with normal semen parameters even after adjustment for comorbid conditions (Eisenberg et al., 2014). Because of the relatively young age of the men (mean age 36.6 years) the absolute risk of mortality was low but the data demonstrate how semen quality might be a marker of general health. Salonia et al. (2009) compared Charlson Comorbidity Index (CCI) scores (Charlson, Pompei, Ales, & MacKenzie, 1987) as a measure of general health between infertile men and fertile men and found a significantly higher rate of comorbid conditions in infertile men. In a cross-sectional study on 2,100 men, the same group also found that with an increasing CCI score the reproductive health of the men declined, measured as reductions in sperm concentration, sperm morphology, and testosterone level and an increase in follicle-stimulating hormone (FSH) (Ventimiglia et al., 2015). Looking further into the comorbid conditions associated with male subfertility, a study on 4,712 men seen for infertility found a dose-response association between poor semen quality and all-cause hospitalizations, especially those due to the lifestyle diseases cardiovascular disease and diabetes (Latif et al., 2015).

Infertility has also been linked to an increased risk of cancer. The best-described link is the association between male subfertility and testicular cancer. Men with infertility have a twofold higher risk of testis cancer compared to fertile men (Eisenberg, Li, Brooks, Cullen, & Baker, 2015). Male infertility has also been associated with an increased risk of other cancers including prostate cancer, colorectal cancer, non-Hodgkin's lymphoma, and melanoma (Eisenberg et al., 2015; Rogers & Walsh, 2017).

In addition to the above somatic conditions, a diagnosis of male subfertility has a negative impact on mental health with manifestations such as isolation, anxiety, and depression. At present, the medical literature very sparsely addresses the impact or feelings men have about fertility, and the discussion about psychosocial impact comes from the disciplines of psychology, sociology, anthropology, and social work. Couples undergoing fertility treatment often describe it as the most upsetting event they have experienced (Greil, 1997; Holley et al., 2015). The depressive symptoms in men undergoing fertility treatment may be negatively affected by an unwillingness of the man to discuss his fertility issues with other people than his partner, as demonstrated in a recent study on 170 infertile men undergoing fertility treatment (Babore, A., Stuppia, Trumello, Candelori, & Antonucci, 2017). As a consequence, men undergoing fertility treatment should be encouraged to share their worries with colleagues and/or friends and they might benefit from having a routine screening for anxiety or depression, or formal referral for these symptoms or indications of potential coping issues as part of their evaluation and treatment for infertility.

Semen quality is a strong biomarker for general health and infertile men are at risk of other seemingly unrelated health problems including lifestyle diseases, cancers, and depression. However, the mechanism behind this is not fully understood. One theory describes a link between male subfertility and testicular cancer explained by the testicular dysgenesis syndrome, whereby exposure to endocrine disrupters during fetal development results in disruptions in testicular development and function (Skakkebaek, Rajpert-De Meyts, & Main, 2001). Both genetics and environmental factors including lifestyle have been proposed as a link between male subfertility and other health issues (Latif et al., 2017; Rogers & Walsh, 2017). Future research will hopefully yield more answers to the mechanism behind these associations to enable a holistic, multidimensional treatment of male subfertility. Until then it is important that urology providers, and those with an interest in men's health, are aware of the potential connection between male factor infertility and overall men's health, and can take proper action to prevent a decline in male general health and diagnose and treat other related health issues.

Erectile Dysfunction

Erectile dysfunction (ED; Chapter 24) is the inability to achieve or maintain an erection sufficient for satisfactory sexual performance (NIH Consensus Conference, 1993). Approximately 30% of men older than 40 years are affected by ED and the prevalence increases with increasing age (Corona et al., 2010). Importantly, ED has been found to be a reliable proxy of a man's general health status predicting future risk of serious cardiovascular disease. This gives the urology provider a unique opportunity to take charge on improving the general health outlook for the man.

Strong evidence supports a significant association between ED and lifestyle-related risk factors and health issues such as smoking, diabetes, hypertension, dyslipidemia, and obesity (Capogrosso, Montorsi, & Salonia, 2016; Saigal, Wessells, Pace, Schonlau, & Wilt, 2006; Tan, Tong, & Ho, 2012). A recent meta-analysis including 12,067 men found that men with metabolic syndrome had a 2.7-fold higher risk of ED compared to men without metabolic syndrome (Besiroglu, Otunctemur, & Ozbek, 2015). As these same factors are important risks for the development of cardiovascular disease it is not surprising that ED is strongly associated with the development of cardiovascular disease. A subgroup analysis from the population-based study "The Prostate Cancer Prevention Trial" (Thompson et al., 2005) followed 8,063 men without cardiovascular disease among whom 3,618 men had ED at baseline and another 2,400 men had ED diagnosed during the study. The risk of cardiovascular disease (angina pectoris, acute myocardial infarction, or stroke) over a period of 5 years was almost 50% higher in men with ED compared to men without ED (Thompson et al., 2005). These findings have been substantiated by a recent meta-analysis (Dong, Zhang, & Qin, 2011) including 12 prospective cohort studies with a total of 36,744 men and a mean follow-up time between 4 and 16 years. In this study the risk of cardiovascular disease among men with ED was 48% higher compared to men without ED. The results remained similar after controlling for conventional cardiovascular risk factors.

These results highlight the strong evidence that ED is associated with cardiovascular disease (Chapter 35) and research has shown that ED predates cardiovascular disease by 3 to 5 years (Hodges, Kirby, Solanki, O'Donnell, & Brodie, 2007; Montorsi et al., 2003). The explanation for this might be due to the smaller diameter of the penile arteries (1–2 mm) compared to the coronary arteries (3–4 mm), suggesting that atherosclerosis may manifest as symptoms of ED before true cardiovascular symptoms become apparent. Another explanation might be that the erectile mechanism is highly dependent on substances produced by the endothelium and thus more susceptible to endothelial dysfunction. No matter the explanation, ED is considered a first sign of systemic vascular disease, making the role of the urology provider important in preventing future cardiovascular manifestations by introducing opportunistic screening and promoting preventive medicine referrals. This becomes even more relevant, considering the fact that ED is a proxy of men's general health even in relatively young men below 40 years of age (Capogrosso et al., 2016).

Besides the risk of future cardiovascular disease, ED is also related to psychological health. Data from the Massachusetts Male Aging Study, a cross-sectional population-based survey of men aged 40 to 70 years, found that the odds ratio for ED among men with depressive symptoms was 1.82, demonstrating a relationship between ED and depression (Araujo, Durante, Feldman, Goldstein, & McKinlay, 1998). Importantly this relationship was independent of a number of confounding variables including medicine use that for several antidepression medications is known to have a negative impact on erectile function. However, the relationship is likely to be bidirectional, meaning that depression can cause ED and ED can be a part of the cause for depression. The important thing for the treating urologist is to be aware of the association so that treatment of depression can be initiated when relevant.

In conclusion, ED functions as a marker of a man's general health predicting future risk of serious cardiovascular disease. It is important that urology providers, and those whose practice may involve men with ED or sexual function complaints, are aware of the connection and initiate a thorough medical assessment to achieve early detection of these potentially life-threatening chronic conditions and thereby alter future health risk and increase life expectancy of the man.

Lower Urinary Tract Symptoms

Male lower urinary tract symptoms (LUTS) are common and include both storage, voiding, and postmicturition symptoms (Abrams et al., 2003). Historically LUTS have been considered a relatively benign problem, although with significant impact on quality of life and risk of more serious complications. However, new evidence suggests that LUTS, similar to ED, is an important predictor of serious cardiovascular disease.

A recent meta-analysis by Gacci et al. (2016) looked at the association between LUTS and cardiovascular disease combining data from 5 longitudinal trials and 10 cross-sectional trials with 32,218 and 25,494 men, respectively. Based on the cross-sectional studies men with moderate to severe LUTS had a significantly increased risk of a reported history of major adverse cardiac events (angina pectoris, acute myocardial infarction, other chronic ischemic heart disease, transient ischemic attack, or cerebrovascular accident). Similarly LUTS was associated with a significant increased incidence of major adverse cardiac events in the longitudinal trials (odds ratio 1.68) (Gacci et al., 2016). Based on these data, LUTS may predict future cardiovascular disease, a notion that should be internalized by *all* practicing clinicians. However, another recent meta-analysis by Bouwman et al. (2015) including five longitudinal trials with 25,020 men found no overall association between LUTS and the development of cardiovascular disease. The primary difference between these two meta-analyses is that the Bouwman study adjusted for confounding variables including obesity, hypertension, and diabetes (Bouwman et al., 2015). As there is no known reason why urinary symptoms themselves should lead to cardiovascular disease it does not seem clinically relevant to adjust for the mentioned confounding variables. In fact, the likely explanation for the association between LUTS and cardiovascular disease is common lifestyle-related risk factors (Pashootan, Ploussard, Cocaul, de Gouvello, & Desgrandchamps, 2015; Raheem & Parsons, 2014). Accordingly, metabolic syndrome may cause LUTS through a pathway involving insulin growth factor resulting in an increased prostate size (Lotti et al., 2014). Furthermore, atherosclerosis in pelvic arteries may lead to functional impairment of the bladder and urinary tract causing LUTS (De Nunzio, Aronson, Freedland, Giovannucci, & Parsons, 2012). As a consequence, it is the responsibility of the provider to initiate a multidisciplinary medical assessment to detect and prevent possible serious cardiovascular disease in the future, or to refer him back to his primary care provider for the necessary evaluation.

Male Hypogonadism

Male hypogonadism is the clinical syndrome caused by androgen deficiency (Dohle, Arver, Bettocchi, Jones, & Kliesch, 2017) (Chapter 29). When hypogonadism occurs after puberty it is defined as late-onset hypogonadism.[1] This diagnosis requires persistent symptoms of

[1] For the purpose of this chapter hypogonadism and late-onset hypogonadism will be used synonymously.

testosterone deficiency and a decreased serum testosterone level. Among the symptoms of androgen deficiency are reduced libido, loss of vigor, mood changes, and ED (Lunenfeld et al., 2015). It is apparent that these symptoms can have an impact on the general health and quality of life of the man, but what about the relationship to other seemingly isolated health issues that might also impact the man's general health status?

Although most likely an impact of the condition itself, poor mental health in relation to hypogonadism deserves mention. In a multinational prospective study including 1,438 hypogonadal men treated with testosterone injections the general mood of the men was assessed both at baseline and after testosterone injections (Zitzmann et al., 2013). At baseline 36%, 45%, and 19% of the men considered their general mood very negative/negative, moderate, and positive/very positive, respectively. After five testosterone injections over a period of 9 to 12 months the distribution changed significantly so that 5%, 19%, and 75% considered their general mood very negative/negative, moderate, and positive/very positive, respectively. This suggests that hypogonadism may have a negative impact on mental health and how testosterone therapy might alleviate symptoms of poor mental health. However, it does not explain whether the negative general mood was caused by testosterone deficiency itself or if it was related to the known symptoms of testosterone deficiency. Regardless, the practicing clinician needs to approach hypogonadal men holistically, keeping in mind the strong association between hypogonadism and poor mental health.

Testosterone has been thought to have a crucial role in the development of prostate cancer since the Nobel prize winner Huggins presented the androgen hypothesis in 1941 (Huggins, 1941). But the relationship between testosterone and prostate cancer appears to be more complicated than originally thought. There is in fact no clear association between intrinsic testosterone levels and prostate cancer, and it does not seem that testosterone treatment in hypogonadal men increases the risk for prostate cancer, nor does testosterone treatment increase the risk for recurrence of prostate cancer after curative treatment (Mirone et al., 2017). *Active* prostate cancer, however, remains a contraindication for testosterone treatment. Older men with hypogonadism should be screened for prostate cancer before treatment with testosterone is initiated.

The relationship between hypogonadism and cardiovascular disease has been a subject of much debate over the past years. Hypogonadism has been shown to be an independent biomarker of cardiovascular disease (Muraleedharan & Jones, 2014). In a prospective population-based study on 2,416 men aged 69 to 81 years baseline testosterone levels were examined in regards to cardiovascular events after a median follow-up time of 5 years (Ohlsson et al., 2011). Men in the highest quartile of testosterone had a lower risk of cardiovascular events (acute myocardial infarction, unstable angina or revascularization, stroke, transient ischemic attack, or death from coronary heart disease or stroke) compared with men in the three lower quartiles. This association remained significant after adjustment for traditional cardiovascular risk factors and was not different in analyses excluding men with known cardiovascular disease at baseline. However, these results do not imply that hypogonadism is a cause for cardiovascular disease. In fact, both cardiovascular disease and known risk factors for cardiovascular disease (obesity, metabolic syndrome and type 2 diabetes) are associated with an increased prevalence of hypogonadism possibly due to increased production of inflammatory cytokines resulting in a decreased production of testosterone (Muraleedharan & Jones, 2014). Available studies linking low testosterone to death from cardiovascular disease represent weak scientific evidence and the causality behind the relationship is not determined. However, screening for cardiovascular disease and risk factors and possible referral to cardiology is advised in older men with hypogonadism and should be initiated by the treating urologists. This highlights the important role of the urologist in the care of men's health.

Even more controversial is the possible relationship between testosterone replacement therapy and increased risk of cardiovascular disease. Two observational studies (Finkle et al., 2014; Vigen et al., 2013) and one placebo-controlled study (Basaria et al., 2010) found that testosterone treatment may be associated with an increased risk of cardiovascular events. However, the studies have major limitations both in design and statistical analyses. Together, these limitations make it difficult to draw conclusions based on these studies. A recent multinational cohort study found that age and prior cardiovascular history, but not testosterone treatment, were predictors of new-onset cardiovascular events (Maggi et al., 2016). These data are supported by a well-performed meta-analysis on randomized placebo-controlled trials that did not find an increased risk of cardiovascular events in men receiving testosterone treatment for hypogonadism (Corona et al., 2014). In fact, there was a cardioprotective effect of testosterone treatment in men with metabolic derangements. However, in general, studies showing safety of testosterone therapy also represent weak scientific evidence due to short duration of follow-up and lack of a randomized design. As a consequence larger randomized trials with longer follow-up are needed before final conclusions on the safety of testosterone treatment can be made, and current guidelines recommend that cardiovascular assessment including assessment of risk factors should be performed before treatment initiation and that testosterone therapy should not be given in men with severe chronic cardiac failure (Dohle et al., 2017).

Metabolic syndrome and diabetes are well-known risk factors for cardiovascular disease and these conditions have been briefly mentioned in the above discussion. However, their relationship to hypogonadism requires further discussion. An American study of 2,162 men above 45 years of age found that the prevalence of hypertension, hyperlipidemia, obesity, and diabetes was significantly higher in men with hypogonadism compared to nonhypogonadal men (Mulligan, Frick, Zuraw, Stemhagen, & McWhirter, 2006). Similarly it has been reported that the risk of hypogonadism increases with increasing body mass index and number of components of the metabolic syndrome (Corona et al., 2006; 2008). It seems that hypogonadism is both the consequence of and cause for metabolic syndrome. This illustrates the common pathophysiological pathways that exist for urological conditions and their related health issues. No matter the direction of causality, it is important for the urologist to advise the patient on the connection between hypogonadism and lifestyle diseases and to initiate screening for lifestyle diseases and in collaboration with other medical specialties initiate proper prevention and treatment to alter the future health risk of the patient.

UROLOGICAL CONDITIONS, GENERAL HEALTH, AND LIFESTYLE—A COMMON PATHOPHYSIOLOGY

There is a strong interconnective relationship among male subfertility, ED, LUTS, and male hypogonadism. What is unique about this relationship is that all these urological conditions share the same associated health issues, namely lifestyle-related diseases including cardiovascular disease, diabetes, and metabolic syndrome. The implication for the treating provider is that quite often the urology provider or men's health provider will serve as a gate-keeper for initiating a multidisciplinary evaluation, prevention, lifestyle intervention, and treatment of these related health issues. This makes the role of the urologist in relation to men's health unique, as illustrated in Figure 19.1. As the described urological conditions share similar associated health issues, we will delve more into the connection and the common pathophysiological pathways explaining this.

Considering male infertility, semen quality has a dose–response association with all-cause hospitalizations especially those due to cardiovascular disease and diabetes

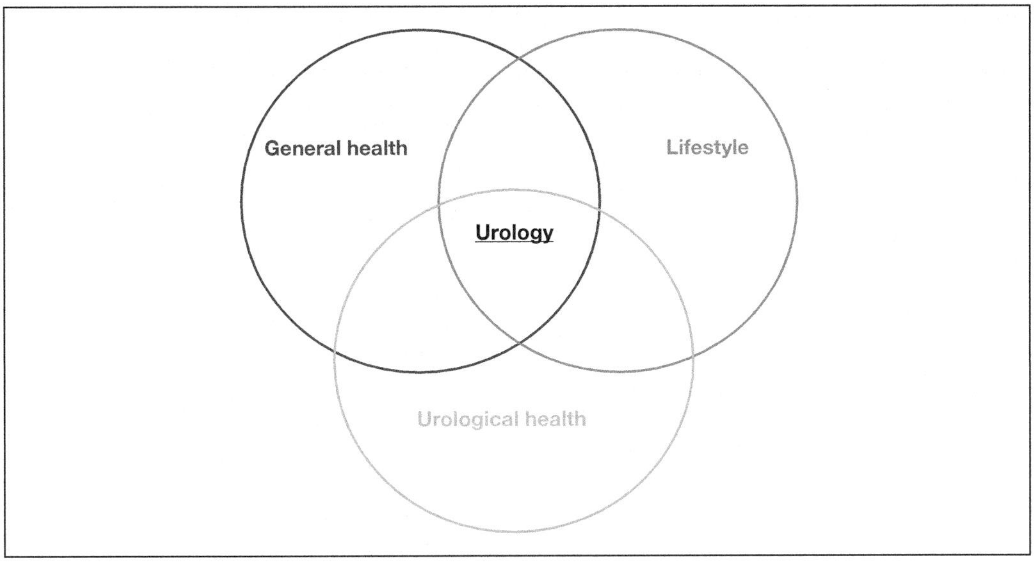

FIGURE 19.1 Venn diagram of the unique role of urology in men's health, illustrated by the overlap of general health, urological health, and lifestyle.

mellitus (Latif et al., 2017). This is possibly due to the impact of lifestyle on both semen quality and risk for cardiovascular disease and diabetes. Moreover, obesity is linked to hypogonadism and this might also be a part of the explanation as to why lifestyle can have a negative impact on semen quality as testosterone plays an important role in production of spermatozoa.

Considering ED, LUTS, and hypogonadism, there is strong evidence supporting an association with both metabolic syndrome, diabetes, and cardiovascular disease (Shabsigh et al., 2008). These associations have been described throughout the chapter. However, there is also a strong interaction between ED, LUTS, and hypogonadism themselves. As an example, the prevalence of ED increases significantly with the severity of LUTS (Rosen et al., 2003) and the risk of ED increases with decreasing testosterone levels (Lunenfeld et al., 2015). There are several proposed mechanisms to explain what seems to be a common pathophysiological pathway. One of the most leading theories is that systemic endothelial dysfunction and atherosclerosis caused by an unhealthy lifestyle affects penile arteries causing ED and pelvic arteries causing LUTS. Another possible explanation is that metabolic syndrome, diabetes, and cardiovascular disease can result in an increased production of inflammatory cytokines leading to a systemic low-grade inflammation. This low-grade inflammation can result in a decreased bioavailability of nitric oxide leading to ED and a decreased production of testosterone leading to hypogonadism (Maiorino, Bellastella, & Esposito, 2015; Muraleedharan & Jones, 2014). In addition, fat tissue contains aromatase that converts testosterone to estradiol, thus contributing to a decrease in testosterone. The common cause and pathophysiological pathway behind ED, LUTS, and hypogonadism may be explained by an unhealthy lifestyle.

This theory is substantiated by evidence of an improvement in symptoms of ED (Maiorino et al., 2015), LUTS (Raheem & Parsons, 2014), and hypogonadism (Camacho et al., 2013) after lifestyle modification including diet and exercise. Table 19.1 describes the association between urological conditions, associated health issues, and recommended actions by the provider.

TABLE 19.1 Urological Conditions, Associated Health Issues, and Recommended Action

Urological Condition	Associated Health Issues	Recommended Action
Male infertility	• Cardiovascular disease • Diabetes • Metabolic syndrome	Consider a basic cardiovascular and metabolic workup including blood pressure, pulse, HbA_{1c}, and lipid profile.
	• Cancer	Consider evaluation for testicular cancer.
	• Poor mental health	Address mental health issues and consider screening for depression and/or anxiety. Involve the female partner and encourage the man to share his worries with friends and/or colleagues.
Erectile dysfunction	• Cardiovascular disease • Diabetes • Metabolic syndrome	Always perform a basic cardiovascular and metabolic workup including blood pressure, pulse, HbA_{1c}, and lipid profile and consider referral to a cardiologist or general practitioner. Inform the patient on possible benefits of lifestyle modifications including diet and exercise and encourage these modifications. If needed, refer the patient to relevant and available lifestyle modification programs.
	Poor mental health	Address mental health issues and consider screening for depression and/or anxiety.
Lower urinary tract symptoms	Cardiovascular disease Diabetes Metabolic syndrome	Consider a basic cardiovascular and metabolic workup including blood pressure, pulse, HbA_{1c}, and lipid profile and consider referral to a cardiologist or general practitioner. Inform the patient on possible benefits of lifestyle modifications including diet and exercise and encourage these modifications. If needed, refer the patient to relevant and available lifestyle modification programs.
	• Poor mental health	Address mental health issues and consider screening for depression and/or anxiety.
Hypogonadism	• Cardiovascular disease • Diabetes • Metabolic syndrome	Perform a basic cardiovascular and metabolic workup including blood pressure, pulse, HbA_{1c}, and lipid profile before treatment initiation with testosterone and consider referral to a cardiologist or general practitioner to optimize secondary prevention in men with preexisting cardiovascular disease. Inform the patient on possible benefits of lifestyle modifications including diet and exercise and encourage these modifications. If needed, refer the patient to relevant and available lifestyle modification programs.
	• Prostate cancer	Perform assessment of prostatic cancer before initiating treatment with testosterone.
	• Poor mental health	Address mental health issues and consider screening for depression and/or anxiety.

CONCLUSIONS

Male subfertility, ED, LUTS, and male hypogonadism are interconnected conditions and share the same associated health issues namely cardiovascular disease, diabetes, and metabolic syndrome. The connection is explained by a common pathophysiological pathway caused by an unhealthy lifestyle.

Male subfertility, ED, LUTS, and male hypogonadism all have a significant impact on the mental health status of the man. This impact is most likely due to the urological condition itself. Infertility is associated with an increased risk of testicular cancer possibly due to exposure to endocrine disrupters during fetal development. Male subfertility, ED, LUTS, and male hypogonadism have a significant impact on the general health of the man and serve as important indicators and predictors of men's general health.

This places a clinician addressing a urology concern in a unique position with the ability, through a multidisciplinary holistic approach, to diagnose, prevent, and treat related conditions and thereby alter future health risk, and possibly increase life expectancy and quality of life of the patient. The clinician functions as a gate-keeper, initiating a multidisciplinary evaluation, prevention, lifestyle intervention, and treatment of possible life-threatening conditions including cardiovascular disease and cancers. This role provides an opportunity to alter the future health risk of the man, and possibly even increasing life expectancy and quality of life.

REFERENCES

Abrams, P., Cardozo, L., Fall, M., Griffiths, D., Rosier, P., Ulmsten, U., … Wein, A. (2003). The standardisation of terminology in lower urinary tract function: Report from the standardisation sub-committee of the International Continence Society. *Urology, 61*(1), 37–49. doi:10.1016/S0090-4295(02)02243-4

Araujo, A. B., Durante, R., Feldman, H. A., Goldstein, I., & McKinlay, J. B. (1998). The relationship between depressive symptoms and male erectile dysfunction: Cross-sectional results from the Massachusetts Male Aging Study. *Psychosomatic Medicine, 60*(4), 458–465. doi:10.1097/00006842-199807000-00011

Babore, A., Stuppia, L., Trumello, C., Candelori, C., & Antonucci, I. (2017). Male factor infertility and lack of openness about infertility as risk factors for depressive symptoms in males undergoing assisted reproductive technology treatment in Italy. *Fertility and Sterility, 107*(4), 1041–1047. doi:10.1016/j.fertnstert.2016.12.031

Basaria, S., Coviello, A. D., Travison, T. G., Storer, T. W., Farwell, W. R., Jette, A. M., … Bhasin, S. (2010). Adverse events associated with testosterone administration. *The New England Journal of Medicine, 363*(2), 109–122. doi:10.1056/NEJMoa1000485

Besiroglu, H., Otunctemur, A., & Ozbek, E. (2015). The relationship between metabolic syndrome, its components, and erectile dysfunction: A systematic review and a meta-analysis of observational studies. *The Journal of Sexual Medicine, 12*(6), 1309–1318. doi:10.1111/jsm.12885

Bouwman, I. I., Voskamp, M. J., Kollen, B. J., Nijman, R. J., van der Heide W. K., & Blanker, M. H. (2015). Do lower urinary tract symptoms predict cardiovascular diseases in older men? A systematic review and meta-analysis. *World Journal of Urology, 33*(12), 1911–1920. doi:10.1007/s00345-015-1560-1

Camacho, E. M., Huhtaniemi, I. T., O'Neill, T. W., Finn, J. D., Pye, S. R., Lee, D. M., … Wu, F. C. (2013). Age-associated changes in hypothalamic-pituitary-testicular function in middle-aged and older men are modified by weight change and lifestyle factors: Longitudinal results from the European Male Ageing Study. *European Journal of Endocrinology, 168*(3), 445–455. doi:10.1530/EJE-12-0890

Capogrosso, P., Montorsi, F., & Salonia, A. (2016). Erectile dysfunction in young patients is a proxy of overall men's health status. *Current Opinion in Urology, 26*(2), 140–145. doi:10.1097/MOU.0000000000000257

Charlson, M. E., Pompei, P., Ales, K. L., & MacKenzie, C. R. (1987). A new method of classifying prognostic comorbidity in longitudinal studies: Development and validation. *Journal of Chronic Diseases, 40*(5), 373–383. doi:10.1016/0021-9681(87)90171-8

Corona, G., Lee, D. M., Forti. G., O'Connor, D. B., Maggi, M., O'Neill TW, … Wu, F. C. (2010). Age-related changes in general and sexual health in middle-aged and older men: Results from the European Male Ageing Study (EMAS). *The Journal of Sexual Medicine, 7*(4 Pt 1), 1362–1380. doi:10.1111/j.1743-6109.2009.01601.x

Corona, G., Mannucci, E., Fisher, A. D., Lotti, F., Petrone, L., Balercia, G., … Maggi, M. (2008). Low levels of androgens in men with erectile dysfunction and obesity. *The Journal of Sexual Medicine, 5*(10), 2454–2463. doi:10.1111/j.1743-6109.2008.00856.x

Corona, G., Mannucci, E., Schulman, C., Petrone, L., Mansani, R., Cilotti, A., … Maggi, M. (2006). Psychobiologic correlates of the metabolic syndrome and associated sexual dysfunction. *European Urology, 50*(3), 595–604; discussion. doi:10.1016/j.eururo.2006.02.053

Corona, G., Maseroli, E., Rastrelli, G., Isidori, A. M., Sforza, A., Mannucci, E., … Maggi, M. (2014). Cardiovascular risk associated with testosterone-boosting medications: A systematic review and meta-analysis. *Expert Opinion on Drug Safety, 13*(10), 1327–1351. doi:10.1517/14740338.2014.950653

De Nunzio, C., Aronson, W., Freedland, S. J., Giovannucci, E., & Parsons, J. K. (2012). The correlation between metabolic syndrome and prostatic diseases. *European Urology, 61*(3), 560–570. doi:10.1016/j.eururo.2011.11.013

Dohle, G. R., Arver, S., Bettocchi, C., Jones, T. H., & Kliesch, S. (2017). *EAU guidelines on male hypogonadism.* Arnhem, The Netherlands: EAU Guidelines Office.

Dong, J. Y., Zhang, Y. H., & Qin, L. Q. (2011). Erectile dysfunction and risk of cardiovascular disease: Meta-analysis of prospective cohort studies. *Journal of the American College of Cardiology, 58*(13), 1378–1385. doi:10.1016/j.jacc.2011.06.024

Eisenberg, M. L., Li, S., Behr, B., Cullen, M. R., Galusha, D., Lamb, D. J., … Lipshultz, L. I. (2014). Semen quality, infertility and mortality in the USA. *Human Reproduction, 29*(7), 1567–1574. doi:10.1093/humrep/deu106

Eisenberg, M. L., Li, S., Brooks, J. D., Cullen, M. R., & Baker, L. C. (2015). Increased risk of cancer in infertile men: Analysis of U.S. claims data. *The Journal of Urology, 193*(5), 1596–1601. doi:10.1016/j.juro.2014.11.080

Finkle, W. D., Greenland, S., Ridgeway, G. K., Adams, J. L., Frasco, M. A., Cook, M. B., … Hoover, R. N. (2014). Increased risk of non-fatal myocardial infarction following testosterone therapy prescription in men. *PloS One, 9*(1), e85805. doi:10.1371/journal.pone.0085805

Gacci, M., Corona, G., Sebastianelli, A., Serni, S., De Nunzio, C., Maggi, M., … Chapple, C. (2016). Male lower urinary tract symptoms and cardiovascular events: A systematic review and meta-analysis. *European Urology, 70*(5), 788–796. doi:10.1016/j.eururo.2016.07.007

Greil, A. L. (1997). Infertility and psychological distress: A critical review of the literature. *Social Science & Medicine (1982), 45*(11), 1679–1704. doi:10.1016/S0277-9536(97)00102-0

Hodges, L. D., Kirby, M., Solanki, J., O'Donnell, J., & Brodie, D. A. (2007). The temporal relationship between erectile dysfunction and cardiovascular disease. *International Journal of Clinical Practice, 61*(12), 2019–2025. doi:10.1111/j.1742-1241.2007.01629.x

Holley, S. R., Pasch, L. A., Bleil, M. E., Gregorich, S., Katz, P. K., & Adler, N. E. (2015). Prevalence and predictors of major depressive disorder for fertility treatment patients and their partners. *Fertility and Sterility, 103*(5), 1332–1339. doi:10.1016/j.fertnstert.2015.02.018

Huggins, C. H. C. (1941). The effect of castration, of estrogen and of androgen injection on serum phosphatase on metastatic carcinoma of the prostate. *Cancer Research, 1*, 293–297.

Latif, T., Kold Jensen, T., Mehlsen, J., Holmboe, S. A., Brinth, L., Pors, K., … Lindahl-Jacobsen, R. (2017). Semen quality as a predictor of subsequent morbidity: A Danish Cohort Study of 4,712 men with long-term follow-up. *American Journal of Epidemiology, 186*(8), 910–917. doi:10.1093/aje/kwx067

Lotti, F., Corona, G., Vignozzi, L., Rossi, M., Maseroli, E., Cipriani, S., … Maggi, M. (2014). Metabolic syndrome and prostate abnormalities in male subjects of infertile couples. *Asian Journal of Andrology, 16*(2), 295–304. doi:10.4103/1008-682X.122341

Lunenfeld, B., Mskhalaya, G., Zitzmann, M., Arver, S., Kalinchenko, S., Tishova, Y., … Morgentaler, A. (2015). Recommendations on the diagnosis, treatment and monitoring of hypogonadism in men. *The Aging Male, 18*(1), 5–15. doi:10.3109/13685538.2015.1004049

Maggi, M., Wu, F. C., Jones, T. H., Jackson, G., Behre, H. M., Hackett, G., … Rosen, R. C. (2016). Testosterone treatment is not associated with increased risk of adverse cardiovascular events: Results from the Registry of Hypogonadism in Men (RHYME). *International Journal of Clinical Practice, 70*(10), 843–852. doi:10.1111/ijcp.12876

Maiorino, M. I., Bellastella, G., & Esposito, K. (2015). Lifestyle modifications and erectile dysfunction: What can be expected? *Asian Journal of Andrology, 17*(1), 5–10. doi:10.4103/1008-682X.137687

Mirone, V., Debruyne, F., Dohle, G., Salonia, A., Sofikitis, N., Verze, P., … Chapple, C. (2017). European association of urology position statement on the role of the urologist in the management of male hypogonadism and testosterone therapy. *European Urology, 72*(2), 164–167. doi:10.1016/j.eururo.2017.02.022

Montorsi, F., Briganti, A., Salonia, A., Rigatti, P., Margonato, A., Macchi, A., … Montorsi, P. (2003). Erectile dysfunction prevalence, time of onset and association with risk factors in 300 consecutive patients with acute chest pain and angiographically documented coronary artery disease. *European Urology, 44*(3), 360–364; discussion 4-5. doi:10.1016/S0302-2838(03)00305-1

Mulligan, T., Frick, M. F., Zuraw, Q. C., Stemhagen, A., & McWhirter, C. (2006). Prevalence of hypogonadism in males aged at least 45 years: The HIM study. *International Journal of Clinical Practice, 60*(7), 762–769. doi:10.1111/j.1742-1241.2006.00992.x

Muraleedharan, V., & Jones, T. H. (2014). Testosterone and mortality. *Clinical Endocrinology, 81*(4), 477–487. doi:10.1111/cen.12503

NIH Consensus Conference. (1993). Impotence. NIH Consensus Development Panel on Impotence. *JAMA, 270*(1), 83–90. doi:10.1001/jama.1993.03510010089036

Ohlsson, C., Barrett-Connor, E., Bhasin, S., Orwoll, E., Labrie, F., Karlsson, M. K., … Tivesten, A. (2011). High serum testosterone is associated with reduced risk of cardiovascular events in elderly men. The MrOS (Osteoporotic Fractures in Men) study in Sweden. *Journal of the American College of Cardiology, 58*(16), 1674–1681. doi:10.1016/j.jacc.2011.07.019

Pashootan, P., Ploussard, G., Cocaul, A., de Gouvello, A., & Desgrandchamps, F. (2015). Association between metabolic syndrome and severity of lower urinary tract symptoms (LUTS), an observational study in a 4666 European men cohort. *BJU International, 116*(1), 124–130. doi:10.1111/bju.12931

Raheem, O. A., & Parsons, J. K. (2014). Associations of obesity, physical activity and diet with benign prostatic hyperplasia and lower urinary tract symptoms. *Current Opinion in Urology, 24*(1), 10–14. doi:10.1097/MOU.0000000000000004

Rogers, M. J., & Walsh, T. J. (2017). Male infertility and risk of cancer. *Seminars in Reproductive Medicine, 35*(3), 298–303. doi:10.1055/s-0037-1603583

Rosen, R., Altwein, J., Boyle, P., Kirby, R. S., Lukacs, B., Meuleman, E., … Giuliano, F. (2003). Lower urinary tract symptoms and male sexual dysfunction: The multinational survey of the aging male (MSAM-7). *European Urology, 44*(6), 637–649. doi:10.1016/j.eururo.2003.08.015

Saigal, C. S., Wessells, H., Pace, J., Schonlau, M., & Wilt, T. J. (2006). Predictors and prevalence of erectile dysfunction in a racially diverse population. *Archives of Internal Medicine, 166*(2), 207–212. doi:10.1001/archinte.166.2.207

Salonia, A., Matloob, R., Gallina, A., Abdollah, F., Sacca, A., Briganti. A, … Montorsi, F. (2009). Are infertile men less healthy than fertile men? Results of a prospective case-control survey. *European Urology, 56*(6), 1025–1031. doi:10.1016/j.eururo.2009.03.001

Shabsigh, R., Arver, S., Channer, K. S., Eardley, I., Fabbri, A., Gooren, L., … Zitzmann, M. (2008). The triad of erectile dysfunction, hypogonadism and the metabolic syndrome. *International Journal of Clinical Practice, 62*(5), 791–798. doi:10.1111/j.1742-1241.2008.01696.x

Skakkebaek, N. E., Rajpert-De Meyts, E., & Main, K. M. (2001). Testicular dysgenesis syndrome: An increasingly common developmental disorder with environmental aspects. *Human Reproduction, 16*(5), 972–978. doi:10.1093/humrep/16.5.972

Tan, H. M., Tong, S. F., & Ho, C. C. (2012). Men's health: Sexual dysfunction, physical, and psychological health—Is there a link? *The Journal of Sexual Medicine, 9*(3), 663–671. doi:10.1111/j.1743-6109.2011.02582.x

Thompson, I. M., Tangen, C. M., Goodman, P. J., Probstfield, J. L., Moinpour, C. M., & Coltman, C. A. (2005). Erectile dysfunction and subsequent cardiovascular disease. *JAMA, 294*(23), 2996–3002. doi:10.1001/jama.294.23.2996

Ventimiglia, E., Capogrosso, P., Boeri, L., Serino, A., Colicchia, M., Ippolito, S., … Salonia, A. (2015). Infertility as a proxy of general male health: Results of a cross-sectional survey. *Fertility and Sterility, 104*(1), 48–55. doi:10.1016/j.fertnstert.2015.04.020

Vigen, R., O'Donnell, C. I., Baron, A. E., Grunwald, G. K., Maddox, T. M., Bradley, S. M., ... Ho, P. M. (2013). Association of testosterone therapy with mortality, myocardial infarction, and stroke in men with low testosterone levels. *JAMA, 310*(17), 1829–1836. doi:10.1001/jama.2013.280386

Zitzmann, M., Mattern, A., Hanisch, J., Gooren, L., Jones, H., & Maggi, M. (2013). IPASS: A study on the tolerability and effectiveness of injectable testosterone undecanoate for the treatment of male hypogonadism in a worldwide sample of 1,438 men. *The Journal of Sexual Medicine, 10*(2), 579–588. doi:10.1111/j.1743-6109.2012.02853.x

SECTION III

Urology and Preventative Cardiology

CHAPTER 20

Overview of Vasectomy

Michelle Angie

INTRODUCTION

Vasectomy is surgical sterilization of males in which the vas deferens is occluded to inhibit pregnancy. It is most commonly done in an office setting and performed by a urologist (90%) or by general surgeons and primary care physicians (American Urological Association [AUA], 2012).

HISTORY

Vasectomy did not originate as a means of birth control. Sheynkin (2009) describes the origins of vasectomy. In 1885, partial excision of the vas was performed as an alternative to orchiectomy to treat enlarged prostate. This procedure was utilized until the mid-1890s when it was proved to be ineffective at relieving symptoms of the hypertrophied prostate. Vasectomies were later performed for prevention of recurrent epididymitis and orchitis. While the development of antibiotics curbed the use of vasectomy for this purpose, the procedure continued to be utilized in some circles and it was not until 1975 that the last prospective study was done to confirm that a vasectomy did not reduce incidence of epididymitis.

In the early 1900s unilateral vasectomy was used for rejuvenation purposes. Men reported renewed energy and vitality after having vasectomy. Testosterone was discovered in 1935, and the procedure lost favor after the late 1940s. In 1897 vasectomy was suggested as a method to prevent males from passing on genetic birth defects. It was also proposed as mandatory treatment for habitual criminals, perverts, insane, and paupers to protect society without harm to the criminals. The rate of involuntary mandatory sterilization for specific individuals grew from 1910 until the practice was stopped in the 1960s. The first public recommendation of using vasectomy for family planning came in 1909, but it was not until the 1970s that it became socially acceptable in the United States. Prior to U.S. acceptance, vasectomy was being used in several developing Asian countries for population control since the 1950s. Vasectomy camps and festivals were organized to perform thousands of vasectomies, some of which paid the men to be vasectomized. Most of these programs ended in the late 1970s and vasectomy in general fell out of favor in that region (Sheynkin, 2009).

PREVALENCE

The number of reported vasectomy procedures performed in the United States varies between different sources. Eisenberg and Lipshultz (2010) analyzed data from the 2002 National Study of Family Growth. From the data, they were able to estimate that 175,000 to 354,000 vasectomies were performed annually from 1998 to 2002. In contrast, the same study found 546,000 to 789,000 tubal ligations were performed in the same time span. This correlates to 6% of men reporting vasectomy while 16% women reported tubal ligation. In another survey, the Centers for Disease Control and Prevention (CDC, 2016) reported in the years 2011 through 2015 that 4.5% of U.S. women 15 to 44 years of age relied on vasectomy as birth control. Another study of the 2008 National Survey of Family Growth reported 13.1% of married men undergoing vasectomy and 21.1% of married women undergoing tubal ligation as form of birth control (Anderson et al., 2012).

ALTERNATIVE CONTRACEPTIVE METHODS

Vasectomy and condoms are the available contraceptives for men in the United States. Experimental options for male contraception are being researched. According to Armory (Canadian Urologic Association, 2016), hormonal and nonhormonal contraceptive options focus on preventing spermatogenesis by either manipulating hormones or other factors involved in spermatogenesis, or by utilizing antisperm compounds. Research is also being done with antimotility agents (Armory, 2016).

Women have various options for contraception. According to Eisenberg and Lipshultz (2010), data obtained from the National Survey of family 2011–2015 reports of U.S. women aged 15 to 44, 15.9% were using the pill, 14.3% relied on female sterilization, and 6.8% had an intrauterine device (IUD), while only 4.5% relied on vasectomy, and 9.2% counted on a condom (CDC, 2016).

PATIENT CHARACTERISTICS

While selection of surgical sterilization can be the decision of an individual or couple, it is often initiated by the female partner (AUA, 2012). In multiple surveys, various characteristics were noted in patients seeking sterilization procedures. Anderson et al. (2012) reported tubal sterilization more common among minority groups and those with lower income and education levels. Vasectomy was reported more often in white men with higher income and education levels. The AUA reviewed multiple studies and reported that the prevalent characteristics of men seeking vasectomy were older age, white race, married or cohabitating, possessing a bachelor's degree, and increasing number of children.

Although data show tubal ligation has been more prevalent than vasectomy, vasectomy is a safer, more cost effective procedure. The AUA describes vasectomy as equally effective as well as being simpler and faster to perform with lower morbidity and mortality rates. It can be done with local anesthetic in an office setting, compared to general anesthesia in operating suite, which makes it less expensive and safer. Complications from a vasectomy are less serious, and men require less recovery time than is common after a tubal ligation (AUA, 2012).

WORLDVIEW

Worldwide, current use of vasectomy varies from country to country. It was not until the 1970s and 1980s that vasectomy became legal in several Western European countries, and not until 2001 in France (Sheynkin, 2009). According to Jacobstein (2015), countries that tend to utilize vasectomy have high socioeconomic development and gender equality; he reports vasectomy prevalence is 12% in North America and 11% in Oceania and Northern Europe. The United Kingdom, New Zealand, and South Korea have prevalence ranging from 17% to 21%, while Australia, Belgium, Denmark, Spain, Switzerland, and the United States have prevalence ranging from 8% to 11%. In Canada, vasectomy accounts for 31% of all contraceptive method use. In poorly developed countries, only 0.7% of women rely on vasectomy as contraception. Vasectomy prevalence in Africa is less than 1%. In these developing countries, there is poor awareness of the existence of the procedure or misunderstanding of the consequences of having a vasectomy, with patients expressing the concerns of castration and erectile dysfunction as a results of the procedure (Jacobstein, 2015).

CONSULTATION

Vasectomy guidelines are available for the practitioner to prepare for counseling the patient. This chapter focuses on the guideline produced by the AUA, and so the aftercare instructions relate to a procedure performed by a surgeon. Other options for review include the guideline by the European Association of Urology (EAU) (Dohle et al., 2012) or the Canadian Urological Association (CAU) in 2016 (Canadian Urologic Association, 2016), which can be found through the CAU website (www.CUA.org).

The AUA formed a consensus panel in 2008 with the task of producing a clinical guideline for vasectomy. The Guideline for Vasectomy was created in 2012 and updated in 2015 specifically to address the concern of prostate cancer in relation to vasectomy. The guideline is available through the AUA website (www.AUAnet.org). There are 15 guideline statements, which cover various aspects of the entire patient experience.

Guideline statement 1 recommends a consultation visit to occur prior to vasectomy. This visit should include a medical history, physical examination, and thorough discussion of risks, benefits, and alternatives to vasectomy. The patient should have appropriate expectations of the entire procedure. Permanency must be stressed; it is best for this discussion be done in person, if possible, as it requires an examination. If a personal discussion is not possible, a phone conversation may occur and the examination can be conducted prior to the procedure.

PATIENT SELECTION

The AUA Guideline addresses patient selection, recommending that the procedure be offered preferentially to a married man with children, as opposed to an unmarried man who has never fathered a child. A man must be of legal age of consent to have a vasectomy. While spousal consent is not required, it is advised that the partner be agreement as the procedure affects the fertility of the couple. (Note: some practitioners may require the presence of the spouse for the discussion and consent process.) The surgeon performing the vasectomy has the right to refuse to perform the procedure, as he or she is bound to protect the patient and do no harm. If, after the consultation, the provider has concerns that the patient may regret the decision later in life, the provider may decline to do the surgery or put a delay on scheduling. Patients who use federal funds, such as Medicaid, are required to wait 30 days after consult to have the procedure performed.

MEDICAL HISTORY

The medical history prior to vasectomy focuses on urologic concerns, prior scrotal surgeries, and blood disorders. It is not required to discuss prostate or testicular cancer, cardiovascular disease, hypertension, stroke, or dementia as vasectomy is not a risk factor for these disorders. Few studies report a statistically significant correlation between prostate cancer and vasectomy. Multiple studies refute a relationship between prostate cancer and vasectomy.

PHYSICAL EXAMINATION

A testicular examination is done to exclude masses concerning for testicular cancer. Noting how the patient tolerates the scrotal exam may indicate how he will tolerate an office-performed procedure, and may provide insight into the development of pain after the procedure if the exam is poorly tolerated. The scrotum is examined for sensitivity, thickness of skin, and possible scarring from previous surgery (AUA, 2012). Miller et al. (2016) describes the rare occurrence of unilateral absence of the vas deferens (UAVD), which could be congenital or due to a trauma or surgical intervention. Miller and colleagues (2016) did a retrospective qualitative study and found the prevalence of UAVD to be 0.36% (95% confidence interval of 0.28%–0.43%). A congenital UAVD could be associated with ipsilateral renal agenesis or cystic fibrosis mutation. It is advised that if a vasectomy is performed on a patient with suspected UAVD, a greater emphasis should be placed in obtaining a postvasectomy semen analysis (PVSA) to confirm sterility.

■ EXPECTATIONS AND COMPLICATIONS

Providers counseling men/couples prior to vasectomy should include particular points when documenting the discussion, for their own legal protection. These concept points are available in a patient-friendly information page located in Appendix B of the unabridged version of the AUA (2012).

Key Concepts During Counseling

Vasectomy is considered a permanent (but not immediate) form of contraception, and another form of contraception will be required after the procedure until sterility is confirmed. Within the abdominal portion of vas and in the seminal vesicles, there are millions of live sperm, which are capable of producing pregnancy. The time required to clear the vas of sperm will vary from weeks to months depending on various factors such as frequency of ejaculation, patient age, surgical technique, and patient anatomy. The patient can rely on the vasectomy as his form of contraception when a PVSA shows no sperm or rare nonmotile sperm. Even if vas occlusion is confirmed and no sperm are seen on PVSA, the chance of conception is not 0%. Recanalization, occurring early, late, or transiently, has been reported. The reported risk of pregnancy after vasectomy is 1 in 2,000 for men after having a PVSA which reported zero to rare nonmotile sperm (AUA, 2012). There is a ≤1% risk of needing a repeat vasectomy; reasons for repeat vasectomy could be failure of occlusion or that the same vas was partially excised twice (AUA, 2012).

Men should refrain from ejaculation for at least 1 week after vasectomy to allow the surgical site to heal and occlusion to form. The exact length of time may be recommended by the individual surgeon (AUA, 2012).

As with any procedure, discussion of potential surgical complications is essential. The risk of surgical complication such as symptomatic hematoma and infection occurs in 1% to 2% of men. The occurrence is closely related to the experience of the clinician and the criteria used to define the complication. If the patient has a known bleeding disorder or is a hemophiliac, thought must be given to the risk versus benefit and the provider may need to recommend an alternative form of birth control.

Lowe (2016) reported most common complications of vasectomy as bleeding and hematoma. Recommendations to reduce the amount of bleeding include scrotal elevation, compression, and support. Lowe described postvasectomy infections as mostly local and able to be resolved with antibiotics. Standard pre- and/or postprocedure antibiotics are not indicated for vasectomy (Lowe, 2016).

Long-term postoperative complications can include sperm granuloma or epididymitis (AUA, 2012). Sperm granulomas are nodules that can occur as a result of sperm infiltrating into surrounding tissue, causing an inflammatory response, and is more common with open-ended vasectomies. The nodules are often painless and found during vasectomy reversal (Lowe, 2016). Sperm granulomas have occurrence of greater than 5% and are most often asymptomatic. If a granuloma is bothersome, the patient can be counseled that it will usually resolve after 2 to 3 months and can be treated with anti-inflammatories as needed (AUA, 2012).

Some postoperative pain is to be expected, but chronic scrotal/testicular/epididymal pain can occur in 1% to 2% of men (AUA, 2012); postvasectomy pain syndrome (PVPS) may necessitate additional medical treatments or surgery. There is no clear cause for the pain, but in many cases it is secondary to congestion in epididymis, venous stasis, sperm granuloma, or nerve impingement (Lowe, 2016). Initial treatment is conservative with nonsteroidal anti-inflammatory drugs (NSAIDs), scrotal elevation and support, sitz baths, and rest. Medications such as gabapentin may be utilized, but if the conservative route fails, surgical intervention such as vasovasostomy (vasectomy reversal), cord denervation, or epididymectomy may be helpful.

There are options for birth control other than vasectomy. Alternatives include permanent and nonpermanent options, each with their own risks and benefits. If fertility is desired after vasectomy, options to consider would be vasectomy reversal, sperm retrieval, or cryopreservation of sperm prior to vasectomy. The success of these options depends on multiple factors, including the skill of the surgeon, time since vasectomy, age of the patient, and manner in which the original vasectomy was performed (AUA, 2012).

PROCEDURE

Bilateral vasectomy is most often an office procedure done under local anesthesia with option of oral sedation. If necessary, the procedure may be performed with intravenous sedation in an operating room setting. This may be required if the patient's anatomy precludes office procedure or if the patient is unable to tolerate the vasectomy under local anesthetic.

The AUA Guidelines (AUA, 2012) recommend the procedure be done using the no-scalpel vasectomy (NSV) technique, or a minimally invasive vasectomy (MIV) technique as opposed to a traditional open vasectomy. The NSV or MIV utilizes a smaller opening in the scrotum and use of specific instruments to isolate the vas. The opening with a NSV or MIV is generally less than 10 mm and no sutures are required to close the wound. Overall postoperative discomfort and complications have been found to be less using these techniques over the traditional vasectomy, which uses a scalpel to make a greater than 1 cm incision and requires sutures to close the wound. Method of anesthetic used is at the discretion of the clinician, but most patients are given a local anesthetic administered with a small-gauge needle. Another option to decrease injection pain is to apply a topical anesthetic cream to the scrotum before injection. It is recommended this be done by the healthcare professional rather than the patient to reduce potential overapplication or toxicity. In addition to local injection, an oral or intravenous sedative may be used at the discretion of the clinician.

The vasectomy procedure has two key steps: isolation of the vas and occlusion of the vas. The vas is isolated with a specialized ring clamp. During the NSV technique, the vas is clamped prior to making the skin opening. With the MIV, the small opening in the skin is made first and the ring clamp is inserted into the opening to isolate the vas. Once the vas has been isolated and exposed, it is divided with or without a small segment excised (AUA, 2012).

Occlusion can be accomplished in various fashions, each with similar but different success rates. The most common techniques include fascial interposition (FI), ligation, clips, folding back, and mucosal cautery (MC). With FI, a layer of fascia is placed between the two divided ends of the vas and layered over one end. This technique is often used in conjunction with other methods such as excision, ligation, or MC. Ligation uses ligatures to occlude the vas, while clips use small surgical clips to occlude the vas. Both approaches are used with division or partial excision and may or may not be used with FI. MC destroys the vasal mucosa by thermal or electric cautery. This can be done on only one or both cut ends of the vas. MC may be used with folding back or FI. Folding back is simply folding the cut ends of the vas back over themselves so the two ends are not facing each other (AUA, 2012).

POSTPROCEDURE CARE

The patient should receive oral or written instructions for postoperative care. Recommendation include wearing of supportive undergarment immediately after the procedure and until no bothersome discomfort is felt by the patient. This support will reduce tension on the spermatic cord which in turn will reduce pain. Oral pain medication, as determined by provider, will help decrease the expected mild pain and swelling. Many surgeons may provide a very modest supply of schedule narcotic pain medicine for the initial days after the procedure. After the first few days, NSAID medications will be most helpful; ice or other cold application can also be helpful as soon as the local anesthetic block wears off. Although the patient can shower the next day, the surgical site should be kept clean and dry. Avoid tub bathing and swimming for 3 to 5 days. Patients may return to nonphysical work after vasectomy as tolerated. He should also be instructed to call the provider with any concerning complaints, excessive pain or bleeding, excessive bruising or swelling, or fever, as is the recommendation for most procedures. As previously mentioned, the patient should refrain from ejaculation for at least 1 week.

POSTVASECTOMY SEMEN ANALYSIS AND VASECTOMY FAILURE

The postvasectomy semen analysis (PVSA) specimen is needed to confirm success of vasectomy and determine if vas occlusion has occurred. The patient must continue to use other forms contraception until he is cleared by the clinician's office, after viewing the PVSA. Patient instruction for collection of PVSA should be as simple as possible to encourage compliance. It is highly recommended to give the patient an actual appointment to return for the specimen analysis, as rate of return to office is lower if the patient has to call for an appointment. The timing of the PVSA is at the discretion of the surgeon, but recommended timing is 8 to 16 weeks after vasectomy. The specimen should be viewed within 2 hours of collection to ensure accurate motility assessment. Per AUA Guideline, acceptable clearance is azoospermia or rare nonmotile sperm (RNMS), which is equivalent to greater than 100,000 nonmotile sperm per milliliter.

Specimens examined in a lab with high Clinical Laboratory Improvement Act (CLIA) certification are able to give the results in volume of sperm per milliliter, but this option may incur additional cost to the patient unless it is bundled into the total price for the vasectomy. Specimens viewed in the provider's office must be reported in terms of presence or absence of sperm and identification of motility. At least 50 fields must be viewed microscopically under high power. No motile sperm may be present. The specimen is not to be centrifuged, as centrifugation will interfere with sperm motility. Home tests approved by the Food and Drug Administration are sensitive to sperm counts greater than 250,000, but do not test for motility; it is ***not*** recommended that home testing substitute for laboratory or office testing.

The vasectomy is considered a failure if pregnancy occurs, or if the PVSA does not result as azoospermia or RNMS in a reasonable time frame. Motile sperm present at 6 months is considered failure due to possible recanalization, and repeat vasectomy should be offered. Failure of the vasectomy may be technical, but failure of the patient to comply with post-procedure instructions and not use alternative birth control during intercourse prior to acceptable PVSA may also contribute to the failure.

CONCLUSION

Vasectomy offers a safe and effective method of permanent birth control, and is covered by most insurance plans. It is less invasive, more cost effective, and has less associated complications than tubal ligation; it has overall lower morbidity than the tubal ligation procedure, which must be performed in the operating room. A vasectomy can be done with local anesthetic or block in the office setting. It is important that the patient (and partner if present) be counseled regarding expected and potential postprocedure events, other alternatives to vasectomy, risk of potential early or late failure of the vasectomy procedure, and postoperative care. Use of the no-scalpel technique is preferred for minimal complications, and postvasectomy specimens are required to confirm sterility.

CLINICAL PEARLS

- Consider telling the patient to treat the vasectomized scrotum like he would a sprained ankle: rest, ice, support, and NSAIDs.
- A small towel under the scrotum can help keep it elevated while the patient is sitting and will make the cold easier to apply.
- Although crushed ice is often used, he may consider a bag of frozen peas or even a cold canned beverage.
- Avoiding ejaculation for at least 1 week afterward allows the procedure site time to heal.
- Vasectomies are not performed near either any of the nerves or vasculature that contribute to erectile function. Any complaints of sexual or erectile difficulties after a vasectomy are psychogenic or stress-related.

RESOURCES FOR CLINICIANS

The American Urological Association. Vasectomy guidelines (Use the unabridged version to access patient friendly instructions): www.auanet.org/guidelines/vasectomy

The Canadian Urological Association. Vasectomy guidelines: www.cua.org/themes/web/assets/files/vasectomy4017_v4.pdf

RESOURCES FOR PATIENTS

American Family Physician patient handout about vasectomy: familydoctor.org/vasectomy-what-to-expect

The AUA publishes a quarterly magazine (*UrologyHealth extra*), which is an excellent resource for patients to get information that is concise, accurate, and up to date.

Urology Care Foundation (www.urologyhealth.org). Vasectomy information: www.urologyhealth.org/urologic-conditions/vasectomy

REFERENCES

American Urological Association. (2012, edited 2015). *Vasectomy: AUA guideline* No. *188*. Elsevier. Retrieved from http://www.auanet.org/guidelines/vasectomy-(2012-amended-2015)

Armory, J. K. (2016). Male contraception. *Fertility and Sterility, 106*(6), 1303–1309. doi:10.1016/j.fertnstert.2016.08.036

Anderson, J. E., Jamieson, D. J., Warner, L., Kissin, D. M., Nangia, A. K., & Macaluso, M. (2012, June). Contraceptive sterilization among married adults: National data on who chooses vasectomy and tubal sterilization. *Contraception, 85*(6), 552–557. doi:10.1016/j.contraception.2011.10.009

Canadian Urologic Association. (2016). 2016 CUA guideline: Vasectomy. Retrieved from https://www.cua.org/themes/web/assets/files/vasectomy4017_v4.pdf

Centers for Disease Control and Prevention. (2016, June). Key statistics from the national survey of family growth—V listing. Retrieved from https://www.cdc.gov/nchs/nsfg/key_statistics/v.htm

Dohle, G. R., Diemer, T., Kopa, Z., Krausz, C., Giwercman, A., Jungwirth, A., & European Association of Urology Working Group on Male Infertility. (2012). European Association of Urology guidelines on vasectomy. *European Urology, 61*(1), 159–163. doi:10.1016/j.eururo.2011.10.001

Eisenberg, M. L., & Lipshultz, L. I. (2010). Estimating the number of vasectomies performed annually in the United States: Data from the national survey of family growth. *Journal of Urology, 184*(5), 2068–2072. doi:10.1016/j.juro.2010.06.117

Jacobstein, R. (2015). The kindest cut: Global need to increase vasectomy availability. *The Lancet. Global Health, 3*(12), e733–e734. doi:10.1016/S2214-109X(15)00168-0

Lowe, G. (2016). Optimizing outcomes in vasectomy: How to ensure sterility and prevent complications. *Translational Andrology and Urology, 5*(2), 176–180. doi:10.21037/tau.2016.03.04

Miller, S., Couture, S., James, G., Plourde, S., Rioux, J., & Labrecque, M. (2016). Unilateral absence of vas deferens: Prevalence among 23,013 men seeking vasectomy. *International Brazilian Journal of Urology, 42*(5), 1010–1017. doi:10.1590/S1677-5538.IBJU.2015.0717

Sheynkin, Y. R. (2009). History of vasectomy. *The Urologic Clinics of North America, 36*(3), 285–294. doi:10.1016/j.ucl.2009.05.007

CHAPTER 21

Discussion of Premature Ejaculation

Ruby Nzoma

INTRODUCTION

As a primary care provider one of the most common male sexual complaints one may encounter is premature ejaculation (PE). The focus of this chapter will be to provide the reader with an overview of PE and discuss assessment, diagnosis, management, and referral. This promotes the goal of providing clinically and culturally competent care to patients who may or may not be comfortable discussing such a sensitive topic, but whose quality of life and that of their partners can be greatly enhanced by the intervention of a knowledgeable clinician.

OVERVIEW AND INCIDENCE

Survey data highlight the current inconsistencies in reported PE prevalence. Data from the National Health and Social Life Survey as included in the American Urological Association (AUA) clinical guidelines report a prevalence of 21% in men ages 18 to 59 in the United States (AUA, 2010). Data from the Global Study of Sexual Attitudes and Behaviors (GSSAB) report an approximate prevalence of 30% across all age groups (Serefoglu et al., 2014). The disparities in reported prevalence can be attributed to varying definitions of PE, as well as lack of confirmation of PE subtype in self-reports (Serefoglu et al., 2014). Although dissimilarities in prevalence exist, it is accepted that PE may be the most common male sexual disorder (AUA, 2010).

At the present time, there is not a universally accepted definition of PE. Although the term PE will be used throughout this chapter, it is important to be aware that the terms early ejaculation and rapid ejaculation may be encountered in other texts (AUA, 2010). The *Diagnostic and Statistical Manual of Mental Disorders* (*DSM-V*) defines PE as a man's recurrent inability to control orgasm and ejaculation in less than 1 minute of vaginal penetration and before climax is desired (American Psychiatric Association, 2013). PE is classified as a disorder only in the context of vaginal penetration, secondary to lack of establishment of time duration for oral and manual stimulation (American Psychiatric Association, 2013). Additionally, there is a lack of existing data in the literature related to PE in the setting of anal penetration, which would be helpful information for patients who engage in anal intercourse.

Two subtypes of PE have been identified: primary (lifelong) and secondary (acquired) (American Urological Association, 2010). Primary begins with the first sexual encounter and includes early ejaculation at almost every sexual experience with time to ejaculation between 30 and 60 seconds or between 1 and 2 minutes with nearly every or every sexual partner (McMahon, Jannini, Serefoglu, & Hellstrom, 2016). Secondary PE occurs after having normal ejaculatory experiences; it occurs when one develops PE at some point in life and is frequently situational (McMahon et al., 2016). Onset of symptoms and the reduction of previously normal ejaculatory latency in secondary PE are the main distinguishing factors (McMahon et al., 2016). For the purposes of this text the AUA definition of PE will guide the chapter: "premature ejaculation is ejaculation that occurs sooner than desired, either before or shortly after penetration, causing distress to either one or both partners" (AUA, 2010).

PHYSIOLOGY

PE is of unknown exact cause and has been historically explained by diverse psychological and biological theories (McMahon et al., 2016). Most commonly acquired PE can be attributed to relationship or psychological problems, sexual performance anxiety, and/or erectile dysfunction. Less commonly it can be due to prostatitis, hyperthyroidism, or withdrawal/detox from prescribed or recreational drugs (Cooper et al., 2016; McMahon et al., 2016). The literature also suggests that the cause of PE is best considered as a series of psychological, relational, and organic risk factors (McMahon et al., 2016). When a patient presents with complaints of a sexual nature it is imperative that in addition to providing a supportive, comfortable environment with a knowledgeable and compassionate provider a thorough history including a brief sexual history be obtained (Goodwach, 2017).

HISTORY

Clinicians should also include a brief sexual history in addition to the history obtained from each patient; this allows for identification of sexual concerns and the scheduling of a longer appointment for a detailed sexual history and examination if said concerns are identified (Goodwach, 2017). The goal of a sexual history is to begin to distinguish between possible biological causes for sexual function complaints and psychosocial influences, which will be better served by referral to a sex therapist or other specialized clinician. Clinicians should begin by having the patient describe the concern in his own words; men may confuse PE and erectile dysfunction. The detailed sexual history should include the date and mode of the onset of PE, self-estimated intravaginal ejaculatory latency time (IELT) (the time from vaginal intromission to intravaginal ejaculation), perceived control over ejaculation, personal distress and interpersonal difficulty associated with ejaculatory problems, intercourse frequency, and presence of other sexual dysfunctions (Jiann, 2016). Obtaining an in-depth history will elicit the common presentation and symptom of PE, which is the inability to delay ejaculation for more than 1 minute (American Psychiatric Association, 2013). The four main categories of risk factors for the development of PE are psychorelational (anxiety, relational and marital problems), endocrine (hyperthyroidism), urological (prostate inflammation/infection), and other sexual symptoms (comorbid with erectile dysfunction [ED], hypoactive sexual desire) (Jiann, 2016). Clinicians must remain mindful of potential sociocultural considerations that may impact evaluation of PE from both the patient and provider standpoint in order to provide high-quality care for a disorder of such a sensitive nature. The onus is on the provider to overcome any personal knowledge deficits and to be able to provide current evidence-based information.

An integral part of providing holistic care is the assessment and treatment of sexual complaints both related and not related to chronic illness (Goodwach, 2017). Because primary care clinicians manage most stable chronic illnesses, men generally prefer primary care clinicians when seeking treatment for sexual problems (Jiann, 2016). This illustrates the need for these providers to be conscious of their own social and cultural influences on the patient interaction, and to understand the patient by being aware of some of the inhibitors to engagement in conversations regarding sexual difficulties (Table 21.1; Althof, Rosen, Perelman, & Rubio-Aurioles, 2013). Keeping these in mind will help facilitate an office visit in which both the patient and provider are comfortable and respected. Include or exclude the patient's partner when collecting the history based on the patient's preference.

TABLE 21.1 Barriers to Discussion of Sexual Function Concerns

Patient	Provider
Shame or embarrassment	Worry of offending patient
Unaware of possible treatment	Lack of knowledge about certain sexual issues and treatment beyond medication
Sensitivity to clinicians' reluctance to discuss sexual difficulties	Personal untreated sexual difficulties that make it harder to discuss difficulties with patient
Belief that problem is related to age/illness/ medication	Stereotypical belief that patient is too old, sick, or disabled for sex

PHYSICAL EXAMINATION

The physical examination should include performing a focused examination of the genitourinary, neurological, and endocrine systems (Jiann, 2014). Abnormal findings on clinical exam may or may not include evidence of hyperthyroidism, prostatitis, abnormalities in the pulses of legs and feet, penile discharge or unusual anatomical variations, or evidence of neurological deficits (Rhoads & Petersen, 2014). All exam findings should coincide with the information elicited from the history.

DIAGNOSTIC TESTS

Laboratory testing can provide additional information when an organic cause of PE is suspected based on the history and clinical exam findings (Jiann, 2016). Testing may include serum analysis of thyroid-stimulating hormone (TSH), glucose, testosterone, thyrotropin, prolactin, and prostate-specific antigen to provide screening for hyperthyroidism, diabetes, hormonal disorders, and prostate cancer (McMahon et al., 2016). Diagnosis of prostatic infection can be aided by the culturing of prostatic secretions as well as urine and semen (McMahon et al., 2016). In addition to laboratory testing, it is also important evaluate for coexisting erectile dysfunction by the administration of a validated instrument (Althof & McMahon, 2016).

In order to establish an accurate objective assessment of PE a validated multidimensional self-report questionnaire should be administered. Three of the most commonly administered are the Premature Ejaculation Diagnostic Tool, Index of Premature Ejaculation, and the Premature Ejaculation Profile (Althof & McMahon, 2016; McMahon et al., 2016). These tools provide insight into the patient's perceived ejaculatory control, distress and interpersonal difficulty, and level of satisfaction with sex life. Additionally these instruments are brief and can be hand-scored, which can limit patient anxiety as well as sustain provider fidelity. Such data are useful for guiding the treatment of psychological and interpersonal components of PE.

MANAGEMENT

Once a diagnosis of PE has been established there are several modes of management that can be offered. Management of PE can begin simply with recommending use of over-the-counter options such as condoms for penetrative intercourse or implementing a thicker condom. Both LifeStyles and Durex offer a thicker condom (LifeStyles Extra Strength and Durex Extra Safe, respectively). Most large condom manufacturers also provide condoms that contain benzocaine, a local anesthetic, on the inside, such as Trojan Extended Pleasure. K-Y Duration is a lidocaine spray to be applied to the penis prior to intercourse, but it should not be used with a condom. The purpose of these interventions is to decrease sensation to the penetrative partner and prolong intercourse. All options can be purchased at most local drug and grocery stores as well as online. Although these products direct consumers to discuss use with clinicians prior to use, most may not do so, but it is imperative that clinicians are aware of these readily available options and ask if men have previously tried them.

Focused breathing or nonsexual thoughts when signals of impending climax are felt as well as masturbation prior to intercourse are additional options patients can employ on their own. Behavioral management options for treatment of PE have been offered to men since the 1950s (Jern, 2014). The AUA's third guideline statement for the treatment of PE states that "The risks and benefits of all treatment options should be discussed with the patient prior to any intervention. Patient and partner satisfaction is the primary target outcome for the treatment of PE" (AUA, 2010). Clinicians should refer the patient to urology or sex therapy for treatment initiation.

Inclusion of the partner in the assessment and treatment of PE should be routinely suggested in assessment and treatment of sexual disorders unless culturally inappropriate or the patient is not partnered. Men may be more inclined to seek treatment for dissatisfaction with their partnered sexual experiences, indicating that there is another person who may also be experiencing sexual discontent. Partners of men with PE reported less emotional closeness and satisfaction during sex (Rosen, Heiman, Long, Fisher, & Sand, 2014). Rosen et al. also identified that the partner's perspective is significantly important to both the prediction and understanding of the individual's sexual and relationship satisfaction (Rosen et al., 2014). If the provider assesses and treats the patient with the working knowledge that ejaculatory dysfunction has a substantial negative influence on both the man and his partner, and consequently has implications for the couple as a whole, the couple is going to receive the kind of holistic care that is more likely to lead to positive outcomes.

The goals of behavioral treatment for PE include development of sexual skills that enable men to delay ejaculation while diminishing performance anxiety, increasing sexual self-confidence, and broadening their sexual repertoire. The second goal maintains a focus on resolution of psychological and interpersonal issues that may have been a precursor to, may be maintained, or may be the consequence of PE for the man, partner, or couple (Althof & McMahon, 2016). Treatment can be group or individual and integrates psychodynamic, behavioral, system, and cognitive approaches within a short-term psychotherapy model (Althof & McMahon, 2016). Two main classes of behavioral therapies with overlapping elements are available for men living with PE. The first class consists of psychosexual or relationship counseling (psychotherapy) for men and/or couples to address the interpersonal and psychological concerns that may be contributing to PE (Cooper et al., 2015). The second class entails physical techniques to help men develop specific sexual skills to delay ejaculation and improve self-confidence (Cooper et al., 2015). Table 21.2 details selected behavioral techniques, the objective of which is to learn to recognize the feelings of arousal in order to improve control of ejaculation (Cooper et al., 2015).

The literature reveals the increased effectiveness of a combination of pharmacological and psychological therapies, which provide men with both medication and behavioral techniques to delay ejaculation and to address the associated psychological and interpersonal issues. One such combination was dapoxitine 30 mg with a brief psychological intervention results exhibited a fourfold increase in IELT compared to the twofold increase in the dapoxetine only group (McMahon et al., 2016). Pharmacological treatments for PE will be discussed further following a brief introduction to complementary and alternative medicine (CAM) for PE.

Acupuncture, Chinese herbal medicine, Ayurvedic herbal medicine, and topical "severance secret" cream were investigated in a systematic review for the treatment of PE. These treatments are not typically not provided in conventional Western healthcare systems (Cooper

TABLE 21.2 Selected Behavioral Techniques Applied With Premature Ejaculation

Technique	Description
Semans stop–start technique	The man/partner stimulates penis until the urge to ejaculate is felt, then stimulation is withdrawn until the sensation passes. This method is repeated a few times before ejaculation is allowed to occur.
Masters and Johnson squeeze technique	Partner stimulates the penis until the urge to ejaculate is felt, then the glans of the penis is squeezed until the sensation dissipates. This is repeated before allowing ejaculation to occur.
Sensate focus/focusing	The man and partner initially focus on touch excluding breasts, genitals, and intercourse to encourage body awareness while reducing performance anxiety; genital touching is gradually reintroduced followed by full intercourse.
Pelvic floor rehabilitation	Pelvic floor exercises may also assist in ejaculatory control.

et al., 2016). The authors indicated the necessity of further well-designed randomized controlled trials of these treatments to truly evaluate their effectiveness. Limited data illustrated preliminary effectiveness of the CAM therapies: Acupuncture, Ayurvedic medicine, and "severance secret" cream on increasing IELT over placebo, and a combination of Chinese medicine and selective serotonin reuptake inhibitors (SSRIs) improve outcomes over either therapy alone (Cooper et al., 2016). It is vital for the primary care provider to have some basic understanding of these therapies to be able to recognize them when in discussion with patients, to inform them that more study on these options is necessary and ongoing, and to be able to direct patients to evidence-based treatments if they are amenable to them.

Men suffering from PE may be hesitant to seek treatment, meaning that by the time they present they may have been experiencing sexual difficulties for an extended period of time (Jiann, 2016). The provider must take this into account when prescribing a treatment. This is because a more aggressive regimen may be necessary to promptly restore sexual satisfaction (Jiann, 2016). Pharmaceutical treatments of male sexual dysfunction offer a direct and clinically, friendly, time-saving option for the initial treatment of PE. The AUA promotes the use of SSRIs or topical anesthetics (Table 21.3) for the treatment of PE with the optimal choice being based on both provider judgment and provider preference (American Urological Association, 2010). Ideally PE treatment should be an on-demand oral medication with a rapid, well-tolerated action effective from the first dose (American Urological Association, 2010; Jiann, 2016). SSRIs including sertraline, fluoxetine, and citalopram are used to effectively treat PE and are noted to have revolutionized PE treatment (Mcmahon, 2016). Controversy exists over the ideal drug regimen, but men have been reported to prefer the convenience of "on demand" dosing as opposed to daily dosing (American Urological Association, 2010; Mcmahon, 2016). This is especially valuable to men who engage in infrequent intercourse, while those in established relationships may prefer the convenience of a daily medication regimen (Mcmahon, 2016).

An on-demand topical anesthetic for the treatment of PE such as a lidocaine-prilocaine cream/gel/spray is a viable option for PE treatment. That diminishing glans sensitivity may inhibit the spinal reflex arc responsible for ejaculation has been established in the literature (Mcmahon, 2016). Topical treatments may also cause substantial penile hypoanesthesia and possible transvaginal absorption, which can result in vaginal numbness and resultant female anorgasmia if no condom is used (Mcmahon, 2016). In the discussion of risks and benefits, patient education regarding proper application, dry time, and hand hygiene should be emphasized to decrease the incidence of these sequelae.

TABLE 21.3 Medical Management for Premature Ejaculation

Therapy	Recommended Dose
Oral Therapies	
Nonselective Serotonin Reuptake Inhibitor	
Clomipramine	25–50 mg/d *or* 25 mg 4–24 hr pre-intercourse
Selective Serotonin Reuptake Inhibitors	
Fluoxetine	5–20 mg/d
Paroxetine	10/20/40 mg/d *or* 20 mg 3–4 hr pre-intercourse
Sertraline	25–200 mg/d *or* 50 mg 4–8 hr pre-intercourse
Topical Therapies	
OTC lidocaine cream	Lidocaine 1%–4% cream 20–30 minutes pre-intercourse
Lidocaine/prilocaine cream	Lidocaine 2.5%/prilocaine 2.5% 20–30 minutes pre-intercourse
Promescent spray (lidocaine spray)	5–10 minutes pre-intercourse (not FDA approved)

FDA, Food and Drug Administration; OTC, over the counter.

Note: The oral medications are off-label use.

Pharmacologic management of PE may be initiated by the primary care provider, although comanagement with or referral to urology are also prudent alternatives. At this time many investigational trials exist for alternate pharmacological treatments for PE including additional SSRIs, PSD502, PDE5i, tramadol, alpha-1-receptor antagonists, oxytocin antagonists, modafinil, and botulinum A toxin (Mcmahon, 2016). No surgical procedures for treatment of PE are currently utilized in practice.

In treatment of PE, as in the initial assessment, it is necessary to be mindful of the importance of the culture of the patient and the patient's partner, both in treatment seeking and treatment adherence. It is important to understand that sexual dysfunction cross-culturally causes distress in relationships, although discussion of the issue does not. Knowledgeable clinicians who can elicit frank discussion in a respectful comfortable environment are essential to providing sensitive culturally competent care for men with PE. Tips for management of PE can assist both novice and expert clinicians in the provision of care of men with sexual dysfunction.

CONCLUSION

Provision of care for PE is likely to be encountered by primary care clinicians. With a working knowledge of how to assess and treat PE, as well as when to refer cases, many men with PE can be managed in primary care. A culturally aware clinician who values the importance of integrating the partner into the plan of care can increase the quality of life for a couple struggling with a common but treatable sexual disorder.

CLINICAL PEARLS

- Always ask men to detail their specific concern; some men confuse PE and erectile dysfunction.
- Limited studies exist in the literature emphasizing the impact of PE on the partner, but some existing studies do indicate effects of PE on the female partner. This dynamic is essential to explore in order to understand the effects of PE on the sexual relationship as a whole.
- Assessment, evaluation, and physical examination are vital to confirm that a urology referral is correct.
- There is currently no Food and Drug Administration–approved treatment for PE.

RESOURCES FOR THE CLINICIAN

The American Association of Sexuality Educators, Counselors and Therapists (AASECT). www.AASECT.org
American Urological Association. (2010). Pharmacologic management of premature ejaculation. www.auanet.org/guidelines/premature-ejaculation-(2004-reviewed-and-validity-confirmed-2010)
Kinkly. www.kinkly.com
UpToDate. www.uptodate.com (membership required)
Urology Care Alliance (UCA). www.urologycares.com

RESOURCES FOR THE PATIENT

The American Association of Sexuality Educators, Counselors and Therapists (AASECT). www.AASECT.org
The British Association of Urological Surgeons (BAUS). www.baus.org.uk
Kinkly. www.kinkly.com

CONDOM INFORMATION

- The American Association of Sexuality Educators, Counselors and Therapists (AASECT). www.AASECT.org
- Durex. www.durex.com
- K-Y. www.k-y.com/duration
- Lifestyles. www.lifestyles.com
- Trojan. www.trojanbrands.com

REFERENCES

Althof, S. E., & McMahon, C. G. (2016). Contemporary management of disorders of male orgasm and ejaculation. *Urology, 93*, 9–21. doi:10.1016/j.urology.2016.02.018

Althof, S. E., Rosen, R. C., Perelman, M. A., & Rubio-Aurioles, E. (2013). Standard operating procedures for taking a sexual history. *The Journal of Sexual Medicine, 10*(1), 26–35. doi:10.1111/j.1743-6109.2012.02823.x

American Psychiatric Association. (2013). *Diagnostic and statistical manual of mental disorders: DSM-5* (5th ed.). Arlington, VA: American Psychiatric Association Publishing.

American Urological Association. (2010). Pharmacologic management of premature ejaculation. Retrieved from http://www.auanet.org/guidelines/premature-ejaculation-(2004-reviewed-and-validity-confirmed-2010)

Cooper, K., Martyn-St James, M., Kaltenthaler, E., Dickenson, K., Cantrell, A., Wylie, K.,... Hood, C. (2015). Behavioral therapies for management of premature ejaculation: A systematic review. *Sexual Medicine, 3,* 174–188. doi:10.1002/sm2.65

Cooper, K., Martyn-St James, M., Kaltenthaler, E., Dickinson, K., Cantrell, A., Ren, S., ... Hood, C. (2016). Complementary and alternative medicine for management of premature ejaculation: A systematic Review. *Sexual Medicine, 5,* 1–18. doi:10.1016/j.esxm.2016.08.002

Goodwach, R. (2017). Let's talk about sex. *Australian Family Physician, 46*(1), 14–18.

Jern, P. (2014). Evaluation of a behavioral treatment intervention for premature ejaculation using a handheld stimulating device. *Journal of Sex and marital Therapy, 40,* 358–366. doi:10.1080/0092623X.2013.857376

Jiann, B. (2016). The office management of ejaculatory disorders. *Translational Andrology and Urology, 4,* 526–540. doi:10.21037/tau.2016.05.07

McMahon, C. (2016). Emerging and investigational drugs for premature ejaculation. *Translational Andrology and Urology, 5,* 487–501. doi:10.21037/tau.2016.04.02

McMahon, C. G., Jannini, E. A., Serefoglu, E. C., & Hellstrom, W. J. (2016). The pathophysiology of acquired premature ejaculation. *Translational Andrology and Urology, 4,* 434–449. doi:10.21037/tau.2016.07.06

Rhoads, J., & Petersen, S. W. (2014). Male genitourinary disorders. In J. Rhoads & S. W. Petersen (Eds.), *Advanced health assessment and diagnostic reasoning* (2nd ed., pp. 294–319). Burlington, MA: Jones & Bartlett Learning.

Rosen, R. C., Heiman, J. R., Long, J. S., Fisher, W. A., & Sand, M. S. (2015). Men with sexual problems and their partners: Findings from the international survey of relationships. *Archives of Sexual Behavior, 45,* 159–171. doi:10.10007s10508-015-0568-3

Serefoglu, E. C., McMahon, C. G., Waldinger, M. D., Althof, S. E., Shindel, A., Adikan, G.,... Torres, L. O. (2014). An evidence-based unified definition of lifelong and acquired premature ejaculation: Report of the second international society for sexual medicine ad hoc committee for the definition of premature ejaculation. *Sexual Medicine, 2,* 41–59. doi:10.1002/sm2.27

CHAPTER 22

Peyronie's Disease

Nancy Brownlee

INTRODUCTION

Peyronie's disease (PD) was first reported in 1561 by Fallopius and later described by Francois Gigot de la Peyronie in 1743 (Peyronie, 1743). It is a fibrous plaque of the tunica albuginea of the corpus cavernosum and presents as a plaque(s) along the shaft of the penis. The American Urological Association (AUA) defines PD as an acquired penile abnormality characterized by fibrosis of the tunica albuginea, which may be accompanied by pain, deformity, erectile dysfunction (ED), and/or distress (American Urological Association, 2015). This causes the penis to curve or angulate during erection. The patient may or may not have pain and may or may not have difficulty with penetration; therefore, patients may be reluctant to seek treatment if they do not have pain and the curve is not severe enough to cause pain for the partner. Men also may not be aware of treatment options available.

The true incidence of PD in the male population has not been established, in part due to methodological issues and inconsistent definitions. Recent estimates suggest a prevalence of 0.5% to 20.3% within specific populations, and depending on how the condition is defined (American Urological Association, 2015), and suspicion is that the true rate is unknown, as men may not recognize the abnormal presentation.

ANATOMY AND PHYSIOLOGY

The process that eventually leads to PD has been poorly characterized, but is believed to be the result of repetitive microtrauma during sexual activity. This trauma alters the elastin content of the tunica albuginea of the penis and corpora cavernosa, resulting in inelasticity during erection and curvature. The course for each man is in unique, with some noticing pain, followed by scar tissue, some never having pain, and some men reporting pain only with erection.

There are two phases of this inflammatory process injury, the active phase when a patient initially has the injury and has pain on erection (nocturnal or during intercourse) and changes in the shape or curve of the penis. This phase may last 6 to 18 months (Gur, Limin, & Hellstrom, 2011). The second phase is the quiescent phase in which there is stabilization of the curve or deformity and the pain has resolved. Men may also present with a sudden painless curve or plaque, shortening of penis, narrowing or hourglass shape, and hinging, not previously observed. Most plaques are noted to be dorsal penile curvatures palpated on the dorsal surface. Plaques found (less commonly) on the lateral or ventral sides cause greater difficulty with coitus. Median curvature seen is approximately 48 degrees and presents during the middle-age years between 40 and 60 years old, although younger and older ages have been reported (American Urological Association [AUA], 2015; Chilton, Castle, Westwood, & Pryor, 1982). The range of curvature reported is 10 to 90 degrees, although 10 degrees may not be clinically significant. There is no agreed-upon minimum curvature in order to initiate intervention, as this was the range identified by the panel writing the AUA guidelines (AUA, 2015; Chilton et al., 1982), although most authorities agree that curvature less than 30 degrees does not warrant intervention. ED may also precede the time they present to a clinician with PD. There is a strong psychological component that needs to be evaluated because of clinical depression due to PD (Nelson et al., 2008). PD may stabilize and/or improve without treatment (Berookhim, Choi, Alex, & Mulhall, 2014; Levine & Burnett, 2013).

HISTORY AND CLINICAL MANIFESTATIONS

Many men with this condition will tolerate it until it is stable, particularly if they have ED and are unpartnered, and then may decide to seek evaluation. As with all patients, a detailed medical history should include date of onset, whether onset was sudden or gradual, and the course it followed including duration and impact on sexual activity. Ask about previous sexual function, any injuries, or penile surgery as well as any personal or family history of fibromatosis such as Dupuytren or Ledderhose disease. Other associated conditions include Paget's disease and urethral stricture.

Assess for risk factors for ED such as vascular disease, diabetes, smoking history, and any age-related diseases such as hyperlipidemia and any cardiovascular events. A history of prior surgeries, and treatment for ED, with a focus on intracavernosal injection therapy, should be noted. A psychosexual history is imperative and any photographs the patient has taken of his penis demonstrating the curvature are helpful. Patients may be embarrassed to initiate the conversation that they took a picture of themselves in the erect state. Reassure the patient that PD is a real condition and that any additional information is valued (AUA, 2015; Jones, 1997; Levine & Burnett, 2013). Also, including the sexual partner during your evaluation of the patient may help with the partner's role in sexual intimacy and encourage the patient to keep his sexual expression active.

Neither men nor their partners may recall a specific injury, which may mean there is an inherited predisposition for PD (Ralph et al., 1997). PD has been associated with fibrotic diseases such as Dupuytren's palmar fibromatosis, as well as contracture of the plantar fascia known as Ledderhose disease and tympanosclerosis (Jordan & McCammon, 2012). Other causes proposed include various positions of intercourse, such as when the female is in the superior position, that could potentially be traumatic (Pires, Travis, & Ellsworth, 2015).

ETIOLOGY AND RISK FACTORS

Causes of PD include injury due to sports, such as a hit or kick to the penis, straddle injury, sexual trauma such as penile buckling during intercourse, and bumping or hitting the erect penis against the pubic bone. This trauma likely begins when the penis buckles and causes injury to the septal insertion of the tunica albuginea, which causes intravasation of blood and release of fibrinogen. The inflammation process is enacted, causing an increase in the fibrotic response. Growth factors are released, which leads to thrombus formation entrapping the fibrin, causing aberrant wound healing and a plaque to form. Most men do not recall a distinct injury that predates the development of pain, scarring or curvature.

PHYSICAL EXAMINATION

A full male genital examination should be performed (Chapter 4) to ensure there are no other explanations for the penile curvature complaint. The penis should be palpated on gentle stretch to better assess the shaft for any plaques, indurations, or nodules. As noted previously, most plaques are on the dorsal surface of the penis, and may present as a distinct mass or as an "i-beam" that is between the two corpora. Penile length is measured in the flaccid state fully stretched from tip to base. Part of the examination should include looking at his hands and feet to check for any contractures or nodules.

DIAGNOSTIC TESTS

Laboratory evaluation is not indicated, unless there is also an issue with erectile function; in this context, a routine evaluation for causes of ED can be initiated (Chapter 22). In-office penile length measurements and measurement of the curvature can be assessed to establish a baseline and track the progress of any further changes. Photographs provided by men of their erection in the home environment are often helpful as well. Clinicians should refer the patient to urology for an in-office intracavernosal injection (ICI) with or without Doppler ultrasound for accurate measurement of the curve and documentation of the plaque, as well as the degree of arterial inflow disease.

MANAGEMENT AND TREATMENT

Psychosocial effects are present with PD and can include an increased incidence of depression, decreased self-esteem, and a change in relationship dynamics that can often include self-isolation (Nelson et al., 2008; Quallich, 2017), shame, and anger. Men should be screened as needed and referred for additional management of a positive finding. Pain management is appropriate during the active phase by offering nonsteroidal anti-inflammatory medications (NSAIDs). Numerous medications that have been tried to improve penile curvature associated with PD, including vitamin E, potassium aminobenzoate (Potoba), colchicine, and tamoxifen, have not proved reliably successful.

The only Food and Drug Administration–approved medical therapy for PD is intralesional injections with collagenase *Clostridium histolyticum* (CCH). Patients in the CCH study had a curve of at least 30 degrees and saw improvement of up to 34% in penile curvature (Gelbard et al., 2013). This requires patient compliance of receiving two injections at least 24 hours apart (no longer than 1 week apart) every 6 weeks which is considered one treatment cycle. There are four cycles until a total of eight injections have been administered; this process can take up to 6 or 7 months to complete, although the patient is not obligated to complete all four cycles. The patient is instructed in penile modeling and must wait 48 hours after each series of two injections to begin the modeling. He must not have sexual intercourse for at least 2 weeks after each injection. Side effects include allergic reaction, hematoma, edema, pain, ecchymoses, blister, pruritus, painful erection, ED, and procedural pain. It is possible to have a corporal rupture (penile fracture), although this is rare; CCH can only be done by a provider registered with the drug manufacturer's risk evaluation and mitigation strategy (REMS) program. Advanced practice providers can be REMS certified.

Other options that have shown moderate or conditional recommendations include intralesional therapy with verapamil or interferon alpha-2b (AUA, 2015). Penile stretching devices alone or in addition to intralesional therapy may be helpful, but there is no high-level evidence for this intervention.

Surgical intervention is appropriate when patients are refractory to CCH and it is the patient's choice. It can include plication of the plaque, partial excision and grafting, or penile prosthesis. Each of these procedures has the risk of penile shortening, and they are not performed by all urologists.

Algorithms for evaluation and treatment assist the practitioner to educate the patient and provide a plan of care (Pires et al., 2015). The AUA recommends that practitioners should only evaluate and treat a man with PD when they have the experience and diagnostic tools to appropriately evaluate, counsel, and treat the disease (AUA, 2015).

CONCLUSION

Although there have been a variety of modalities (topical, electromotive therapies, shockwave therapy, x-ray treatment) tried to address the deformity seen with PD, there is a paucity of data to support their effectiveness and safety. Men with PD can report significant psychosocial impact, and this perspective should be incorporated into their management. Providers should remember that the presentation of PD can change over time in a particular patient, and should adjust the treatment approach as this disease evolves.

CLINICAL PEARLS

- Although many nonsurgical options for treatment of PD have been suggested, most have very little evidence to support their use.
- Anti-inflammatory medications prior to intercourse may be helpful in moderating pain with erection.
- The key with management of PD is emphasis on keeping expectations of treatment outcomes realistic, and documentation of these discussions.
- In-clinic measurements of flaccid length can prevent patient overestimation of the effects of the condition, and provide a metric for treatment success.
- Advise men to take an antiallergy medication prior to or shortly after CCH (Xiaflex) injection, as this may help reduce local reaction and edema.
- Managing client expectations related to body image is crucial when treating men with PD, because men may not see immediate results after any treatment.

RESOURCES FOR THE CLINICIAN

American Urological Association Guidelines: http://www.auanet.org/guidelines/male-sexual-dysfunction-peyronies-disease-(2015)
National Institute of Health: www.ncbi.nlm.nih.gov/pmc/articles/PMC5027990/
Society of Sexual Medicine: www.jsm.jsexmed.org/article/S1743-6095(16)30160-6/pdf
Society of Urologic Nurses and Associates: SUNA Core Curriculum

RESOURCES FOR THE PATIENT

Association of Peyronie's Disease Advocates (APDA): www.peyroniesassociation.org
Auxilium: peyronies-disease.xiaflex.com/patient/
Men's Health Network (MHN): www.menshealthnetwork.org
The Urology Care Foundation: www.urologyhealth.org/urologic-conditions/peyronies-disease

REFERENCES

American Urological Association. (2015). Guidelines. Retrieved from http://www.auanet.org/guidelines/peyronies-disease-(2015)

Berookhim, B. M., Choi, J., Alex, B., & Mulhall, J. P. (2014). Deformity stabilization and improvement in men with untreated Peyronie's disease. *BJU International, 113*, 133–136. doi:10.1111/bju.12346

Chilton, C. P., Castle, W. M., Westwood, C. A., & Pryor, J. P. (1982). Factors associated in the etiology of Peyronie's disease. *British Journal of Urology, 54*(6), 748–750. doi:10.1111/j.1464-410X.1982.tb13640.x

Gelbard, M., Goldstein, I., Hellstrom, W. J., McMahon, C. G., Smith, T., Tursi, J., & Carson, C. C. (2013). Clinical efficacy, safety and tolerability of collagenase clostridium histolyticum for the treatment of peyronie's disease in 2 large double blind, randomized, placebo controlled phase 3 studies. *Journal of Urology, 190*(1), 199–207. doi:10.1016/j.juro.2013.01.087

Gur, S., Limin, M., & Hellstrom, W. J. (2011). Current status and new developments in Peyronie's disease: Medical, minimally invasive and surgical treatment options. *Expert Opinion Pharmacotherapy, 12*(6), 931–944. doi:10.1517/14656566.2011.544252

Jones, W. J. (1997). Counseling men with sexual dysfunction. *AUA Update Series XVI*(lesson 23):178–184.

Jordan, G. H., & McCammon, K. A. (2012). Peyronie's disease. In A. J. Wein, L. R. Kavoussi, A. C. Novick, A. W. Partin, & C. A. Peters (Eds.), *Campbell-Walsh urology* (10th ed., pp.792–809). Philadelphia, PA: Saunders Elsevier.

Levine, L. A., & Burnett, A. L. (2013). Standard operating procedures for Peyronie's disease. *Journal of Sexual Medicine, 10*(1), 230–244. doi:10.1111/j.1743-6109.2012.03003.x

Nelson, C. J., Diblasio, C., Kendirci, M., Hellstrom, W., Guhring, P., & Muljall, J. P. (2008). The chronology of depression and distress in men with Peyronie's disease. *Journal of Sexual Medicine, 5*(8), 1985–1990. doi:10.1111/j.1743-6109.2008.00895.x

Peyronie, F. (1743). Sur quelques, obstacles qui s'opposent a l' ejaculation naturelle de la semence. *Memoires Academie de Chirurgie*, 1, 425–434.

Pires, J., Travis, M., & Ellsworth, P. (2015). Peyronie's disease: Overview and recent treatment advances. *Urologic Nursing, 24*, 164–178.

Quallich, S. A. (2017). Clostridium histolyticum (Xiaflex®) for the treatment of Peyronie's disease. *Urologic Nursing, 37*(5), 270–272.

Ralph, D. J., Schwartz, G., Moore, W., Pryor, J. P., Ebringer, A., & Bottazzo, G. F. (1997). The genetic and bacteriological aspects of Peyronie's disease. *Journal of Urology, 157*(1), 291–294. doi:10.1016/S0022-5347(01)65362-X

CHAPTER 23

Penile and Scrotal Disorders

Hillary B. Durstein and Sara M. Drummer

INTRODUCTION

There are a variety of common scrotal and penile issues that are certain to drive men to seek evaluation, either with their primary care provider or through direct self-referral to a urology clinic. Many of these issues are benign, but can provoke significant anxiety when they are noticed. Other issues can be more urgent and require additional action on the provider's part to efficiently evaluate them. This suggests the value of both a through and focused history and examination when any male presents with a scrotal or penile complaint. The history needs to be comprehensive, structured, and relevant to the patient's stated chief concern, and must include the pertinent information of location, duration, and pain, preferably all explained in the patient's own words. It is important to listen to the patient and allow him to explain in his own terms. Sexually transmitted infections should always be part of the differential diagnosis with penile and scrotal complaints, but will not be discussed in this chapter. Always consider any complaint of a testicular mass to be a malignancy (Gomella, 2015) until proved otherwise.

HYDROCELE

Incidence

The known incidence of hydrocele is 1% in men (Borgmann, 2014). Hydrocele results secondary to testicular torsion, epididymitis, trauma, tumor, and varicocele operation or as a recurrence after primary repair of a communicating hydrocele. It can also occur spontaneously, with the patient unable to recall any episode of trauma.

Anatomy and Physiology

Hydroceles are generally unilateral and involve the tunica vaginalis, which is the serous membrane surrounding the front and sides of the testicle. Acquired or idiopathic hydrocele is due to defective absorption of fluid by the tunica vaginalis or excessive production of fluid within the scrotal sac, which can be seen with infection, testicular tumor, and trauma (Buckley, 2017).

Hydroceles are categorized as communicating and noncommunicating. Majority of cases of hydrocele in the adult are noncommunicating because the processus vaginalis obliterates during embryonic development (Borgmann, 2014). Communicating hydroceles indicate the that processus vaginalis communicates with the peritoneal cavity and in the adult may have increased risk of incarceration (Lallas & Gomella, 2015).

History

Common presentation of hydrocele in the adult male consists of complaints of unilateral swelling of the testicle. Signs and symptoms include fullness of the involved side. A large hydrocele can cause pain and sensation of heaviness, and if due to infection, preceding symptoms may be queried (Borgmann, 2014). Scrotal swelling may worsen with activity and is not usually painful unless associated with infection (Buckley, 2017).

Risk Factors

Risk factors include a scrotal injury as an adult, infection (including sexually transmitted infection), testicular torsion, epididymitis, and tumor (Borgmann, 2014). Other known risk factors are Ehlers-Danlos syndrome, indirect inguinal hernia, hydrocephalus with ventriculoperitoneal (VP) shunt, peritoneal dialysis, and undescended testicle with patent processus vaginalis (Lallas & Gomella, 2015).

Physical Examination

Aside from noting the size of the scrotum as compared with in nonhydrocele side, there should be an attempt at transillumination (shining a penlight through the scrotum in a darkened room). If the scrotum transilluminates, this favors a simple hydrocele, but this finding is not diagnostic. Palpation of the testes bilaterally should be attempted in order to feel for the testicle itself and any possible testicular mass. Hydroceles may be palpated as small soft collections of fluid or as large, tense, painful collections of fluid. Examine the groin bilaterally for an inguinal hernia. If lymphedema of external genitalia or lower extremities is present, tissue edema can be mistaken for the hydrocele (Lallas & Gomella, 2015). Noncommunicating hydroceles do not vary in size, but a communicating hydrocele may present as small in the morning and progressively become larger during the day (Borgmann, 2014). This may also be true if the scrotal swelling is due to a hernia rather than a hydrocele. It is usually difficult to palpate the testicle through the scrotum in the presence of a hydrocele, while the unaffected testicle is normal in appearance and with palpation.

Diagnostic Tests

Diagnostic tests for hydrocele include urinalysis and urine culture if epididymitis-orchitis is suspected. Tumor markers (beta-human chorionic gonadotropin [beta-hCG], alpha-fetoprotein; see Chapter 30) are tested if a tumor is suspected. The scrotal ultrasound scan is the standard imaging test for diagnosis and detects underlying testicular abnormality such as tumor and epididymitis and confirms actual hydrocele (Lallas & Gomella, 2015).

Medical Management

Aspiration of the hydrocele is not usually recommended, as it can recur in several days, and the procedure creates potential infection risk. Conservative management includes scrotal support (Buckley, 2017) and other symptomatic management such as nonsteroidal anti-inflammatory drugs (NSAIDs) for discomfort. Most hydroceles do not require treatment. There are no complementary alternative medicine recommendations.

Medications are used to treat epididymitis-orchitis, but prescription medications to treat the simple hydrocele are generally not needed. No treatment is necessary for the unbothered patient with a simple hydrocele.

Men should be referred to urology for discomfort and/or cosmetic concern and for any mass/tumor/underlying pathology reported on ultrasound examination (Buckley, 2017).

Urological management of hydrocele is usually a hydrocelectomy, whereby the accumulation of usually clear yellow fluid is drained and the tunica vaginalis is repaired to prevent recurrence of the hydrocele. Prevention includes wearing protective devices during contact sports.

VARICOCELE

Incidence

Varicocele is an abnormal dilatation of the pampiniform plexus of veins situated within the spermatic cord above the testicle (Ohlander & Niederberger, 2015). Varicoceles can be asymptomatic or they can be uncomfortable; they can also impact spermatogenesis (Ohlander & Niederberger, 2015). The incidence of varicocele is 15% to 20% in the adult male population; the majority are left sided (75%–90%) and 33% are bilateral (Crawford & Crop, 2014). Varicoceles are seen in 35% to 40% of men presenting with complaint of primary infertility versus 70% to 80% with secondary infertility, as in having already fathered a child; however, varicoceles are not causative of infertility in the majority of adult males (Ohlander & Niederberger, 2015).

Anatomy and Physiology

Over 90% of varicoceles are found on the left side owing to the anatomy of the left spermatic vein and higher venous pressure as it drains into the left renal vein. Dilatation of veins found in the scrotum due to incompetent venous valves in the spermatic cord cause a varicocele, and rarely varicocele is due to occlusion of the renal vein from a tumor or thrombus of the renal vein (Buckley, 2017). Varicoceles may be congenital or acquired, thought to be due to right-angle insertion of left spermatic vein into left renal vein, resulting in turbulent blood flow and increased intravascular back pressure (Ohlander & Niederberger, 2015). Extrinsic compression would result from a mass causing the varicocele, such as left renal vein compression (Ohlander & Niederberger, 2015).

History

Common presentation of varicoceles is generally asymptomatic, but there may be a history of a dull ache or pulling sensation in the left scrotum (Buckley, 2017). Sensations such as the dull ache, heavy sensation, sense of increased heat, or the presence of tortuous veins increase with activity (including intercourse), standing, and Valsalva maneuver. These symptoms are relieved by recumbence (Ohlander & Niederberger, 2015). Some men come in with only a complaint of infertility as the primary issue.

Risk Factors

There are few actual risk factors for varicocele, as their presence is a function of an individual's anatomy. Potential risks for varicocele include congenital absence of valves in spermatic vein or acquired incompetence of spermatic vein valves and extrinsic compression that increases intravascular pressure (i.e., retroperitoneal pathological process) (Ohlander & Niederberger, 2015).

Physical Examination

The gold standard for diagnosis of a varicocele is to examine the patient in a warm room after he has been standing for 10 minutes; this allows veins of the pampiniform plexus to fill. Examine the patient while he is supine and standing upright with and without performing Valsalva maneuver (Ohlander & Niederberger, 2015). Palpation of a varcocele is

TABLE 23.1 Varicocele Classification

Grading	Explanation
Subclinical	Not visible or palpable; demonstrated in diagnostic testing (i.e., ultrasound) Questionable clinical significance
Grade 1	Varix palpable only with Valsalva maneuver, not visible
Grade 2	Varix palpable without need for Valsalva maneuver, visible at rest
Grade 3	Varix visible on visual inspection and palpable

Note: Varix describes the tortous dilatation of a vein.

best described as a "bag of worms" felt above the testis (Table 23.1), although in reality, the finding is far more subtle. Perform a routine examination of the abdomen for masses as well.

Radiological evaluation of a varicocele can be used when its presence is uncertain on physical examination, recurrence is suspected, or it is present after treatment. Ultrasound imaging is preferred for such diagnosis and helps exclude other intrascrotal pathology (Ohlander & Niederberger, 2015). Bilateral scrotal color flow Doppler study is the preferred ultrasound study to compare both testis and assess blood flow patterns. Abdominal computed tomography imaging is indicated if renal or other retroperitoneal mass is suspected of causing the varicocele, as suggested by unilateral right-sided varicocele or varicoceles that do not empty when supine.

Laboratory testing for semen analysis is indicated for the infertile male with confirmed varicocele; referral should be made to an andrologist or urologist for additional testing and evaluation (Chapter 27).

Medical Management

Initial management of varicocele includes NSAIDs, ice, and scrotal support or athletic support underwear for symptomatic relief (Ohlander & Niederberger, 2015). Referral for surgical management to a urologist is recommended for consistent pain that interferes with activity and for infertile men who are wanting to conceive, especially in the setting of an atrophic testis. Surgical treatment successfully eliminates over 90% of varicoceles; embolization and sclerotherapy are also options to treat varicocele (Ohlander & Niederberger, 2015; Simon, 2014).

SPERMATOCELE

Overview

A spermatocele is a cystic mass, most often in the head of the epididymis, that contains fluid and spermatozoa; it can also be described as an epididymal cyst if less than 2 cm in size (Buckley, 2017). Peak incidence is in the fourth to fifth decade of life, and to date no racial or ethnic predilection has been identified. Spermatoceles are reported in 30% to 70% of adult males undergoing high-resolution scrotal ultrasound examination (Hirsh & Gomella, 2015).

Anatomy and Physiology

The distinction between a spermatocele and an epididymal cyst is based on size; epididymal cysts over 2 cm are spermatoceles. They do not affect fertility, although the potential for some decreased sperm transport is real. Spermatoceles are always located superior to the testis, which differentiates them from hydroceles. Spermatoceles typically range in size 2 to 5 cm (Hirsh & Gomella, 2015).

HISTORY

The typical presentation is a painless, asymptomatic intrascrotal mass found on self-examination or routine office examination and may be described by the patient as "a third testicle." Occasionally it presents with scrotal pain or heaviness without associated urinary symptoms (Hirsh & Gomella, 2015). Palpation reveals a smooth, soft, spherical nontender mass at the head of the epididymis; it lies superior and posterior to the testis and is distinct from the testis. A cystic mass above the testis is often demonstrated on transillumination (Hirsh & Gomella, 2015).

Risk Factors

Risk factors include inflammation and trauma, and a possible source could be extensive bicycling (2 or more hours, 6 days a week) (Buckley, 2017). In general, these structures arise spontaneously in the absence of a history of trauma or infection.

Physical Examination

Palpation of the testis bilaterally should be attempted in order to feel for the testicle itself and any possible testicular mass. Examine the groin bilaterally for an inguinal hernia. Ultrasound will distinguish this from solid mass or other pathology (Buckley, 2107).

Medical Management

Management of a spermatocele initially includes supportive care, which is usually sufficient and consists of scrotal support, heat, NSAIDs, and continued self-examination (Hirsh & Gomella, 2015). Most spermatoceles do not require treatment (Hirsh & Gomella, 2015). Referral to urology for surgical intervention is elective and indicated for progressive enlargement, persistent pain, or interference with work/recreational activities due to its location in the scrotum. Surgery should be deferred in men seeking to preserve their fertility as a spermatocelectomy can cause epididymal obstruction (Hirsh & Gomella, 2015).

TESTICULAR TORSION

Incidence

A testicular torsion occurs when there is a twisting of the spermatic cord, resulting in ischemia to the affected testicle. A torsion is most likely to occur in a younger male, but may occur at any age. It most often occurs in males 12 to 18 years old, with a peak incidence at the age of puberty. Torsion is a true urological emergency; if left untreated, the testicle will suffer ischemia and eventually become nonviable.

Anatomy and Physiology

When torsion in the spermatic cord occurs, it cuts off the arterial blood flow to the testicle, resulting in ischemia to the testicle. If left untreated, the testicle will become necrotic and the tissue will in turn die within 4 to 12 hours of the onset of symptoms.

History

When obtaining the history of the patient with testicular torsion, he will most often complain of a severe, acute onset of pain in the testicle, and this may have occurred after vigorous physical activity or minor trauma. The pain is most likely unilateral in nature, but can occur bilaterally, and he may describe pain that is referred or radiates to the pelvis or the inguinal groin. Men may also complain of nausea and vomiting, due to the severity of pain. There may be irritative voiding symptoms, but these symptoms are not considered common. It is extremely important to obtain the time frame of onset of the symptoms so that prompt diagnosis and treatment may be initiated. Men should be asked if there is a history of any similar episodes in the past that resolved spontaneously; this suggests a pattern of spontaneous torsion and detorsion.

Risk Factors

Definitive risk factors have not been identified, but do include a history of cryptorchidism, a previous contralateral torsion, or previous testicular trauma to that testicle. Patient may have a "bell clapper" deformity, in which the testicle has a true horizontal lie in the scrotum. This deformity increases the likelihood of the patient's testicle to swing, contributing to torsion of the spermatic cord. A patient may also have a very long spermatic cord or increased testicular volume, including masses.

Physical Examination

During the physical examination make sure to perform a full assessment of the scrotum. The testicle may be firm and riding very high into the scrotal sac, and the testis may or may not be palpable if considerable swelling is present. The spermatic cord is not usually palpable, but may be felt as thickened or knotty. Possible scrotal wall erythema and edema may be noted and the cremasteric reflex is often absent (Gomella, 2015). The patient will be very tender on even a gentle scrotal exam and most often will demonstrate guarding due to the pain. It may be very difficult to obtain a thorough assessment but the examination should be attempted to the best of the clinician's ability.

Diagnostic Tests

Men with suspected testicular torsion should be advised to proceed to the nearest emergency room for evaluation, as this is a true emergency, where the urological referral and a scrotal ultrasound examination can be performed concurrently. The most important diagnostic test obtained for a testicular torsion is scrotal ultrasound imaging with Doppler. The Doppler image obtained with scrotal ultrasound will evaluate the arterial blood flow into the testicle itself. This will diagnose if there is true ischemia and the need for emergent treatment. Ultrasound test should be performed emergently, but should not delay urological referral.

Diagnostic tests to evaluate for torsion include urinalysis and urine culture if epididymitis-orchitis is suspected; complete blood count and testing for sexually transmitted infection (STI) may be appropriate, depending on the patient's history and the context of the presentation.

Medical and Surgical Management

Management of a testicular torsion must include emergent urological referral for possible surgical exploration. During the surgical exploration the urologist will examine bilateral testicles. On the affected side the spermatic cord will be unwound; the affected testicle would then be assessed to determine if the testicle is salvageable. If so, the testicle will be fixed to the scrotal wall, along with the unaffected side, to prevent any future recurrences of the torsion. If the testicle is determined to be unsalvageable, due to necrosis, an orchiectomy will be performed to remove the necrotic tissue. Then the unaffected testicle will be fixed to the scrotal wall to prevent a future torsion. Males who have had severe sudden onset of pain, hours prior to evaluation, who were not treated and whose pain has since resolved should still be evaluated for possible necrosis of the testicle.

If urological referral or surgery cannot be performed in a reasonable amount of time, manual detorsion should be considered. Historical thinking is that the testicle usually rotates medially, but there is little reported in the literature to support this claim. If a medial torsion is suspected, the clinician should attempt to rotate the testicle laterally toward the thigh. A successful detorsion may require multiple rotations before the spermatic cord will fully be unwrapped. Alternatively the testicle is twisted laterally, instead of medially, requiring the testicle to be untwisted medially. Even with successful detorsion, the patient will still require surgical intervention in the near future for orchidopexy, owing to the high risk of torsion recurrence.

CRYPTORCHIDISM

Incidence

Cryptorchidism is an undescended testicle; this is caused by the failure of the testes to descend fully into the scrotum during fetal development. This is when the testis/testes neither reside nor can be manipulated in the scrotum, but may be palpated in the inguinal canal or may also reside in the abdomen. Incidence of an undescended testicle is 1% to 4% of full-term infant males. Incidence is significantly increased in premature infants, and up to 30% of premature male infants may be affected (Wood & Elder, 2009). This is the most common congenital abnormality of the urinary tract and demonstrates geographic variability, with a higher incidence seen in Denmark and Finland (Boisen et al., 2004).

Anatomy and Physiology

Cryptorochid testes stop during fetal development and do not descend fully into the scrotum by 4 months of age, or the equivalent for preterm male infants. These mechanisms for descent have not been fully described, but may be androgen-dependent and influenced by mechanical, hormonal, and neurotransmitter influences.

History and Risk Factors

Risk factors for undescended testicle occur in multiple genetic disorders, but most often occur in preterm delivery. Some environmental factors may include low maternal estrogen levels, maternal smoking, and maternal diabetes mellitus. Cryptorchidism is usually an isolated finding without other conditions associated with it; however, neural tube defects, cerebral palsy, genetic issues resulting in lowered testosterone, and other disorders of sexual development can be seen with undescended testicles.

Medical and Surgical Management

Management of the undescended testicle should occur when the child is young, preferably age 6 to 18 months. Preferential treatment would be for the child to have his testis surgically fixed in the scrotal cavity by a procedure called orchidopexy. Hormonal treatment is no longer an approved method of treatment, but has been a recommended treatment in years past. Successful treatment in early age increases the chances of the testicle being viable in adulthood and reduce the potential impact on fertility. It is recommended that young boys be treated before the age of 10 years for the highest chance of optimal testicle performance later in life, relative to both sperm and testosterone production. Even with successful treatment males with undescended testicles will have significant risk factors and concerns in adulthood. Testicular malignancy is 10 to 100 times more common in these men (Lip, Murchison, Cullis, Govan, & Carachi, 2013) than in the general population, and they need serial scrotal ultrasound tests for surveillance.

Successful treatment at an early age will reduce this risk, but will not eliminate the increased risk completely. Risk for malignancy is even higher in men whose testicles never descended or who never obtained treatment. Bilateral testicular involvement equates an even higher risk for malignancy than unilateral involvement. All men with a history of undescended testicles, treated or not, must be educated and taught the importance of monthly testicular self-examinations at the age of puberty. These exams should continue into adulthood.

Other concerns resulting from undescended testicles include risks of hypogonadism, which may be seen as early the teens and early adulthood. Patients may also suffer from infertility, characterized by low sperm count, low sperm quality, and lower fertility rates (van Brakel et al., 2014). The risk of infertility is doubled in untreated unilateral undescended testes (Chapter 27), with occurrence that may be as high as 35% in bilateral undescended testes (van Brakel et al., 2014). Surgical treatment before the age of 2 years may help with decreasing the risk of infertility.

HEMATOSPERMIA

Incidence

Hematospermia is the presence of visible blood in the semen; it is most often self-limiting, and will often resolve on its own. Hematospermia accounts for 0.02% of all new patient visits in urology offices every year; it is also present in 0.5% of men who presented for annual prostate cancer screenings each year. The mean age of men suffering from blood in the semen is 37 years old, with the mean duration of recurrence 1 to 24 months, and in 2.4% to 3.5% of cases yearly, the symptom results in a diagnosis of malignancy (Gomella, 2015).

History and Risk Factors

The most common cause of hematuria is prostatitis, and it may also occur from prostatic calcification or obstructed prostate ducts. Hematuria may occur from vascular abnormalities, including hemangiomas or arteriovenous malformations. It may also be seen in prostate cancer, in bladder cancer, and after invasive procedures including prostate biopsy, cystoscopy, and resections of the prostate. Lastly hematospermia may be seen in coagulation disorders, and possibly if there have been long intervals between ejaculation events.

The blood in the semen could range from streaks of blood to gross, frank blood. The blood may appear pink, bright red, or dark brown. The natural history is for the blood to appear bright red and then progress to maroon or brown. It may occur in a single episode, continuously, or intermittently. Most often men will be asymptomatic, and the ejaculations are painless, but men may complain of pelvic, perineal, scrotal, or penile discomfort. They may also have hematuria, irritative voiding symptoms, dysuria, pain with ejaculation, or urethral discharge.

Physical Examination

On physical examination a general abdominal/pelvic examination should be performed. The scrotum, testes, epididymis, and inguinal groin should be evaluated for tenderness, edema, or masses. The penile meatus should be examined for bloody discharge. A digital rectal examination (DRE) of the prostate should be performed for any masses, nodules, tenderness, or bogginess of the prostate, which may demonstrate an abnormal texture or sponginess due to swelling and inflammation of the prostate.

Diagnostic Tests

Laboratory data should include urinalysis, urine culture/sensitivity, and PSA (prostate-specific antigen) test. Evaluation might also include (depending on presentation and examination) a complete blood count (including white blood cells and platelets), prothrombin time/international normalized ratio (PT/INR), urethral swab/urine studies for STI, and urine cytological test. This is the primary extent of the initial evaluation.

If all diagnostic studies appear to be negative and the patient is not responding to initial treatment of antibiotics, a semen culture and sensitivity test can be very telling. The patient may be suffering from an atypical bacterial infection that requires an specific antibiotic regimen. A semen sample can be obtained by having the patient ejaculate into a sterile cup in the privacy of his own home. He will then take the specimen to an outpatient laboratory, within 1 to 2 hours of obtaining the specimen, with an order for a bodily fluid culture/sensitivity.

However, for some men, the hematospermia may persist or become increasingly painful. Their evaluation can progress to imaging studies, including transrectal ultrasound of the prostate or newer, more advanced imaging studies such an MRI of the prostate, which provides excellent detailed images of the prostate for diagnostic purposes. Further diagnostic evaluation that may be performed by the urologist may include a cystoscopy of the prostate and bladder.

Medical Management

Hematospermia is most often self-limiting; if asymptomatic or only a single occurrence, then no treatment or diagnostic workup is warranted. Behavioral and conservative treatments included ejaculation of three to four times per week, warm soaking baths, anti-inflammatory agents, decreased caffeine intake, and decreasing the patient's overall stress levels.

If symptoms continue, then the patient may require additional medical management. Men younger than 40 years old most often suffer from infectious causes and may have a higher risk of malignancy. A trial of empiric antibiotics may be considered. Recommendations would be to treat with antibiotics with known prostate penetration and treat for a longer duration than that for a typical urinary tract infection. Prostate infections most often require a regimen of 3 to 6 weeks of treatment. Antibiotics most often used for prostate treatment include trimethoprim/sulfamethoxazole, doxycycline, levofloxacin, or ciprofloxacin. Considerations with treatment include careful monitoring with fluoroquinolones for any athletes or patients with history of cardiac abnormalities. Men should be counseled regarding fluoroquinolones and the black box warnings for severe tendinitis and cardiac dysrhythmias.

Criteria for referral to a urological practitioner include any male who does not respond to the initial treatment with antibiotics and any abnormal findings on DRE, laboratory studies, or imaging that may represent possible malignancy. Surgical procedures that the urologist may perform for further evaluation of the patient would include office cystoscopy.

PHIMOSIS

Incidence

Phimosis occurs when the foreskin cannot be retracted past the penile glans because of tightening or narrowing of the foreskin opening. This can occur at any age, and occurs in 2% of all uncircumcised males (Newman, Wyman, & Welch, 2017). Elderly men are at a higher risk owing to loss of skin elasticity and infrequent erections.

Anatomy and Physiology

The tightening of the foreskin can result from scarring or loss of elasticity of the foreskin over time. There may also be adhesions attached to the penile head that tether the foreskin and do not allow for its retraction. Signs and symptoms of the phimosis include erythema, itching, discharge, edema, penile pain, and pain with sexual intercourse.

History and Risk Factors

While obtaining history from the patient it is important to obtain circumcision status, along with noting if the foreskin was previously able to be retracted. At times a male who has undergone a circumcision at an earlier age may still suffer from phimosis, especially if the foreskin was only partially removed. Also important to note is any ballooning of the foreskin while voiding or postvoid dribbling that occurs. This would indicate a partial/near complete obstruction of the urine passage, which is a more serious problem.

Risk factors include poor hygiene, traumatic retraction of the foreskin, indwelling Foley catheters, chronic balanitis, penile carcinoma, genital piercings, and scarring from previous STIs. Risk factors also include other dermatological conditions, such as, for example, lichen sclerosis.

Physical Examination

During the physical examination the clinician must examine the penis, assessing for the degree of retractability and the amount of urethral meatal exposure. Inguinal lymph nodes should be palpated as well to establish that there is no concern for significant infection.

Diagnostic Tests

Laboratory evaluation is not usually performed unless there are concerns for possible STIs or urinary tract infection. If so, the clinician should obtain a urinalysis and urethral swab/urine studies for STI. The clinican may also perform a topical swab of the penile smegma/purulent drainage of the foreskin if there are concerns for bacterial and/or candidal infections. Imaging studies are not usually necessary, but a postvoid residual urine test can establish that this condition is not contributing to bladder-emptying issues.

Medical Management

The most important behavioral conservative management of phimosis is preventive. Minor phimosis can be resolved with good genital hygiene. Gentle retraction of the foreskin during voiding and bathing is beneficial. Aggressive retraction is not recommended owing to risk of making symptoms worse.

Medical management includes topical steroids with or without antifungal treatment. If symptoms are severe, patients may need catheterization for any urological obstruction until surgical procedures can be performed. Severe cases require surgical interventions.

Criteria for referral to a urological practitioner include any patient who does not respond to topical medical treatment or retraction. Also any patients whose foreskin potentially or severely obstruct urine from freely passing must be referred. If the patient is so severely obstructed that urine is prevented from flowing through the opening of the foreskin, which is a urological emergency, the patient should be referred for emergent urological evaluation.

Surgical Management

Circumcision is considered the gold standard of surgical procedures to treat phimosis. Surgical removal of the foreskin can be performed electively to prevent further worsening of the condition or may be performed emergently, if necessary. In situations in which a circumcision cannot be performed then a preputioplasty, also known as dorsal slit, may be performed on an emergent basis. In this case an incision is made on the dorsal aspect of the foreskin, far enough back to allow for easy retraction. This is a very quick and easy procedure, which can be performed at the bedside. It may also be performed on patients wanting to maintain their foreskin for personal reasons.

It is important to consider that some religions/cultures do not support circumcision as a practice. Patients might be reluctant to have any surgical treatment performed because of fear of affecting sexual pleasure or affecting their male ego. The patient must be educated to understand that this situation can become increasingly severe, and may result in severe infections underneath the foreskin. He may eventually be unable to urinate owing to the severity of the tightening of the foreskin.

PARAPHIMOSIS

Incidence

Paraphimosis occurs when the uncircumcised male's foreskin is retracted and becomes trapped behind the penile glans. It occurs in 0.7% of all uncircumcised males. It may occur at any age, but again occurs most often in the elderly who are already affected with some form of phimosis.

Anatomy and Physiology

When the foreskin is retracted and becomes trapped behind the penile glans this causes a constriction of the penile shaft. This compression acts like a tourniquet, causing vascular entrapment of the penile head. The compression also does not allow arterial blood flow into the penis, causing ischemia to the affected area, and necrosis and gangrene if left untreated. Paraphimosis is consider a urological emergency and warrants an emergent urological referral.

History and Risk Factors

Paraphimosis can occur in any male with an uncircumcised penis, mainly after Foley catheter insertion/penile examination when the foreskin is not returned to its natural position. It also may occur in any man with a partial phimosis, penile trauma, or gentle piercings, or during sexual intercourse/masturbation.

Physical Examination

Abnormal findings are penile pain and edema. The patient may have erythema, which may start to turn dark red/purple in later stages, when necrosis may develop.

Diagnostic Tests

No diagnostic testing is usually performed.

Medical and Surgical Management

Men should be directed to go to the nearest emergency room. Medical management includes manual reduction by placing firm, continuous pressure is placed on the distal end of the penis for approximately 5 minutes, to reduce the edema. This may be accompanied by the application of ice as long as there is no evidence of ischemia to the glans. Then place both thumbs on the glans, with the second and third fingers on the foreskin. While pushing forward with the thumbs on the head of the penis, simultaneously pull downward on the foreskin with your fingers. The clinician may administer local anesthesia (ice, lidocaine without epinephrine, or penile block) prior to the procedure for pain control. This procedure must be done with caution in men who are immunocompromised, diabetic, or alcoholic to avoid skin injury, which may provide opportunity for infection.

Most common behavioral conservative treatments are preventive measures and pain control. This includes good genital hygiene and always returning foreskin to the natural position after cleaning.

CLINICAL PEARLS

- Tenderness, fever, or other symptoms such as nausea, vomiting, and abdominal pain associated with acute hydrocele require immediate evaluation to rule out other scrotal pathology.
- The inability to transilluminate a hydrocele could be due to a thick-walled or septated hydrocele or presence of solid mass such as tumor or hernia.
- Hydroceles may spontaneously resolve over time if underlying epididymitis is a factor, this would be considered a "reactive hydrocele" from the underlying epididymitis.
- Majority of varicoceles are left-sided and diagnosed on physical examination; nonpalpable (sublinical) varicoceles have questionable impact on fertility, and repair may not improve fertility.
- Suspect renal or retroperitoneal pathology if the varicocele is acute in onset, only right-sided, or remains engorged in the supine position.
- A common pitfall lies is in distinguishing between hydrocele and spermatocele. Spermatoceles are always located superior to the testis and are palpated distinctly from the testis, which differentiates them from hydroceles.
- Sudden onset of scrotal/testicular pain should always be considered a testicular torsion until proved otherwise.
- A possible testicular mass in a male with a history of undescended testicle requires immediate scrotal ultrasound examination with urological referral.
- Use lubricant under the foreskin while performing the manual reduction. Make sure no lubricant adheres to the glove itself to be able to apply firm traction while pulling down on the foreskin.

RESOURCES FOR THE CLINICIAN AND PATIENT

Mayo Clinic patient education: www.mayoclinic.org/diseases-conditions/hydrocele/basics/definition/CON-20024139; www.mayoclinic.org/diseases-conditions/varicocele/basics/definition/con-20024164

Urology Health: www.urologyhealth.org/urologic-conditions/spermatoceles; www.urologyhealth.org/urologic-conditions/hydroceles-and-inguinal-hernia; www.urologyhealth.org/urologic-conditions/varicoceles

REFERENCES

Boisen, K. A., Kaleva, M., Main, K. M., Virtanen, H. E., Haavisto, A. M., Schmidt, I. M., ... Skakkebaek, N. E. (2004). Difference in prevalence of congenital cryptorchidism in infants between two Nordic countries. *The Lancet*, *363*(9417), 1264–1269. doi:10.1016/S0140-6736(04)15998-9

Borgmann, H. (2014). Hydrocele. In A. S. Merseburger, M. A. Kuczyk, & J. W. Moul (Eds.), *Urology at a glance* (pp. 279–281). Berlin Heidelberg: Springer Verlag.

Buckley, S. R. (2017). Penile and scrotal disorders. In D. Newman-Kaschak, J. F. Wyman, & V. W. Welsh (Eds.), *Core curriculum for urologic nursing* (pp. 585–604). Pitman, NJ: Anthony J. Jannetti.

Crawford, P., & Crop, J. A. (2014). Evaluation of scrotal masses. American Family Physician, 89, 723–727.

Gomella, L. G. (2015). *The 5-minute urology consult* (3rd ed.). Philadelphia, PA: Wolters Kluwer.

Hirsh, I. H., & Gomella, L. G. (2015). Spermatocele. In L. G. Gomella (Ed.), *The 5-minute urology consult* (3rd ed., pp. 472–473). Philadelphia, PA: Wolters Kulwer Health.

Lallas, C. D., & Gomella, L. G. (2015). Hydrocele. Adult & pediatric. In L. G. Gomella (Ed.), *The 5 minute urology consult* (3rd ed., pp. 190–191). Philadelphia, PA: Wolters Kulwer Health.

Lip, S. Z. L., Murchison, L. E. D., Cullis, P. S., Govan, L., & Carachi, R. (2013). A meta-analysis of the risk of boys with isolated cryptorchidism developing testicular cancer in later life. *Archives of Disease in Childhood*, *98*(1), 20–26. doi:10.1136/archdischild-2012-302051

Newman, D. K., Wyman, J. F., & Welch, V. W. (2017). *Core curriculum for urological nursing*. Pittman, NJ: Jannetti.

Ohlander, S., & Niederberger, C. S. (2015). Varicocele, adult. In L. G. Gomella (Ed.), *The 5-minute urology consult* (pp. 624–625). Philadelphia, PA: Wolters Kluwer Health.

Simon, A. (2014). Varicocele. In A. S. Merseburger, M. A. Kuczyk, & J. W. Moul (Eds.), *Urology at a glance* (pp. 275–277). Verlag Berlin Heidelberg: Springer.

van Brakel, J., Kranse, R., de Muinck Keizer-Schrama, S. M., Hendriks, A. E. J., de Jong, F. H., Hack, W. W., ... Dohle, G. R. (2014). Fertility potential in a cohort of 65 men with previously acquired undescended testes. *Journal of Pediatric Surgery*, *49*(4), 599–605. doi:10.1016/j.jpedsurg.2013.09.020

Wood, H. M., & Elder, J. S. (2009). Cryptorchidism and testicular cancer: Separating fact from fiction. Journal of Urology, 181, 452–461. doi:10.1016/j.juro.2008.10.074

CHAPTER 24

Erectile Dysfunction: Introduction to Diagnosis and Management

Susanne A. Quallich and Michelle Lajiness

INTRODUCTION

Direct-to-consumer advertising for erectile dysfunction (ED) medications has raised awareness of ED as a medical issue affecting millions of men. While historically ED may have been managed by urologists and sometimes mental health providers, contemporary management can happen across healthcare disciplines that include primary care, cardiology, and urology. The association of ED with vascular disease risk factors places primary care providers and those with a men's health focus in a unique position for evaluation and management: Many men who may consider themselves "otherwise healthy" will self-refer for sexual function issues. It is well established that diabetes, hypertension, dyslipidemia, tobacco use, obesity, and coronary artery disease are contributors to a decline in erectile function, and these may all be newly diagnosed in the setting of the ED concern.

The classic Massachusetts Male Aging Study (MMAS) included investigation of ED, demonstrating that age and prevalence were closely correlated. Up to 52% of men between the ages of 40 and 70 in this study had some degree of ED, with a frequency that was linearly correlated with age: At 40 the prevalence was roughly 40%, while at age 70 the prevalence was as high as 67% (Feldman, Goldstein, Hatzichristou, Krane, & McKinlay, 1994). Primary care providers will note that up to half of the men in their practices will report some degree of erectile difficulty, and this percentage will rise with increased numbers of men aging, as the number of comorbid risk factors increases. Worldwide, the United Nations estimates that by 2025 there will be more than 356 million people over the age of 65 by 2025, with parallel increases in the percentages of men who have ED risk factors (Shabsigh, 2006).

ETIOLOGY OF ERECTILE DYSFUNCTION

Erections occur with mental or physical stimulation that progresses from the frontal lobes, down the spinal cord to the sacral area (S2-4), and peripherally out to the parasympathetic system, resulting in smooth muscle relaxation and the inflow of blood into the paired corporal bodies of the penis. The primary chemical mediators, nitric oxide and cyclic guanosine monophosphate (cGMP), further promote relaxation of cavernosal smooth muscle and promote inward blood flow into these paired corpora cavernosa as well as the corpus spongiosum. When filled, these cylinders press against the superficial veins, thereby trapping blood in the penis, resulting in an erection. This rigidity is due to the tunica albuginea, one of the strongest connective tissue layers in the body. The corpus spongiosum is a separate vascular system, which surrounds the urethra and distally enlarges to become the glans penis. It is also engorged during the process of erection, but does not contain tough fascial covering and does not become rigid.

Testosterone aids in the maturation and the maintenance of penile tissue architecture. Its major role is with libido; but testosterone does have a role in penile sensation, ejaculatory function, and erectile function (Chapter 29).

Historically, most ED cases were treated as psychogenic, in part owing to the limited medical treatment options. Presently, the origin of erectile issues can be psychogenic, organic, or most commonly with contributions from both. It is well established that ED in a majority of men can be attributed to vascular diseases (Table 24.1). In fact, ED may be considered an indicator of early systemic vascular endothelial cell and smooth muscle dysfunction (Jones et al., 2002). Psychogenic contributors to erectile issues include anxiety, stress, tension, fatigue, and depression, all of which can result in decreased libido and/or impaired nitric oxide release. These psychogenic contributors also result in decreased self-esteem and result in perceived sexual failure, creating feelings of shame, inadequacy, or embarrassment that can enter other aspects of a man's life.

TABLE 24.1 Contributing Factors to the Development of Erectile Dysfunction

Factor	Comments
Anatomic	Contributing factor with spina bifida and other neural tube defects, depending on severity of congenital defect
	Seen with Peyronie's disease, in which fibrosis and structural changes within the penis cause decreased flexibility of penile tissue
	May result after penile fracture, severe pelvic injuries
	Also seen after untreated (or recurrent) priapism, with significant scarring of the corporal tissue
Arteriogenic	Arterial and/or venous vascular compromise
	Unable to increase blood flow the 20–40-fold necessary to fill the penis for rigid erection
	Due to atherosclerotic disease, diabetic small vessel disease, trauma
	Factor in two thirds of patients with ED
	Penile vascular bed may be a sensitive indicator of early systemic endothelial cell and/or smooth muscle dysfunction
	Increase in the risk of future cardiac events when ED presents in younger men; up to 80% risk of subsequent CAD
Drug-induced	Illicit drugs (cocaine, ecstasy, marijuana)
	Antihypertensives
	SSRIs
	TCAs
	Antihistamines
	Antiandrogens
	Antianxiety medications
	Antipsychotics
	Opioids

(continued)

TABLE 24.1 Contributing Factors to the Development of Erectile Dysfunction (*continued*)

Factor	Comments
Hormonal	Typically a contributing factor rather than sole cause
	Low testosterone levels contribute to decreased nocturnal erections and libido
	Influences efficacy of PDE5 medications depending on other comorbid conditions
	Potential issue in men with kidney and liver disease, but reversible once primary condition treated, for example, testosterone returns to normal after kidney transplant
Neurogenic	Impaired neurological transmission
	Penile tissue does not receive signal that initiates vascular changes
	Can be seen with lumbar back issues, alcoholic neuropathy, medications, neurodegenerative conditions, after chemotherapy
	Pelvic or perineal surgeries can results in ED via incidental injury to nerves
Psychogenic	Anxiety about sexual function causes release of adrenaline, which counteracts the process of erection
	Differentiated by establishing presence/absence of morning erections; presence of morning erections indicates that physiology of erection itself is intact
Veno-occlusive dysfunction	Lack of smooth muscle relaxation in the cavernosal bodies: "venous leak"
	Result of tissue degeneration from ischemia, trauma, damage; peripheral nerve damage; lack of blood flow
	Usually a progressive problem that worsens with time

CAD, coronary artery disease; ED, erectile dysfunction; PDE5, type 5 phosphodiesterase; SSRIs, serotonin reuptake inhibitors; TCAs, tricyclic antidepressants.

■ HISTORY

Men can be unwilling to bring up sexual issues of any kind (Eardley, 2013) even when referred directly for evaluation. As with any condition, it is vital to have the individual describe exactly what his concern is, and the provider should elicit a targeted sexual, medical, and psychosocial history (Shamloul & Ghanem, 2013) and list of medications and supplements. There can be misunderstanding about what ED truly is, and it can be confused with rapid ejaculation, retrograde ejaculation, or sexually transmitted infections. Establish the duration and onset of the ED, the circumstance in which the problem occurs (with partner, self-stimulation), the presence of nocturnal/early morning erections, the percentage of the time he is not able to have sexual relations, and the percentage of "normal erection" he feels able to attain. Spontaneous erections are an important clue to psychological causes; if present, they indicate that the neurological reflex and cavernosal blood flow are intact. Ask about previous treatments and how successful they were. A thorough sexual history will also include the degree to which this has affected personal relationships, if this information is not freely volunteered (Althof, Rosen, Perelman, & Rubio-Aurioles, 2013).

It is vital to include cardiac risk stratification because of the strong connection between ED and atherosclerotic disease (Nehra et al., 2012). Men should also have a thorough examination of their cardiac risk factors (Chapters 33, 34, 35), including blood pressure, body mass index (BMI), and waist circumference measurements (independent predictor of ED when waist ≥ 42 inches).

Use of standardized questionnaires is common practice. The Sexual Health Inventory for Men (SHIM; Cappelleri & Rosen, 2005) and International Index of Erectile Function ([IIEF]; Rosen, Cappelleri, Smith, Lipsky, & Pena, 1999) allow men to describe their concern in advance of meeting the provider. Additional questions should include investigation of life stressors (divorce, newborn child, relocation for job), energy level, libido, orgasm, ejaculation issues, and new medications that may have been added in the same time frame when he noticed the ED. Providers may choose to screen separately for depression, either by using a form or verbally during the interview.

The discussion of sexual function concerns can be heavily influenced by cultural and religious factors, causing men to seek same-gender providers (Burd, Nevadunsky, & Bachmann, 2006). Providers should acknowledge the cultural variations regarding discussion of sexual and reproductive health concerns, but a full discussion of this issue relative to sexual health concerns is beyond the scope of this chapter.

Risk Factors for Erectile Dysfunction

A healthy lifestyle promotes preservation of erectile function; this is clear from the comorbid conditions that are seen with a diagnosis of ED, such as obesity, smoking, and elevated cholesterol. Tight control of these contributors can slow progression of ED, but it cannot be fully reversed once there is some evidence of erectile difficulties. (The exception to this would be in a case of purely psychogenic ED, in which case identification and treatment of the underlying condition can reverse the ED complaint.)

Men are at risk for the development of ED with any diagnosis that compromises vascular function, neurological transmission, and to a lesser extent hormone balance. Disease processes that compromise nerve function will impact erectile function; the predominant basic neural tone of the male genitals is sympathetic, and during the process of erection, the parasympathetic tone must override the resting state to produce an erection. In many instances, there can be multiple contributors to ED (Tables 24.1 and 24.2).

TABLE 24.2 Specific Erectile Dysfunction Contributors

Cause	Description	Comments
Depression	Frequently comorbid with ED	ED can be the result of depression or a factor in depression development
Diabetes	Micro- and macrovascular damage	Poor glycemic control is cause for worse ED Improved glycemic control halts progression of ED Improved glycemic control contributes to better efficacy of PDE5i medications
LUTS	Results from age and enlarging prostate	Emerging epidemiological evidence for a link between ED and LUTS PDE5i has recently been identified as improving both ED and LUTS via effects of smooth muscle relaxation in prostate
Sleep apnea	May be due to decreased REM sleep resulting in decreased nocturnal erections	Increasingly strong correlation between the severity of sleep apnea and ED severity Sleep apnea also associated with low testosterone Direct causative link elusive

ED, erectile dysfunction; LUTS, lower urinary tract symptoms; PDE5i, phosphodiesterase type 5 inhibitor; REM, rapid eye movement.

PHYSICAL EXAMINATION AND LABORATORY TESTING

Because men with erectile concerns may consider themselves "otherwise healthy" they may benefit from a complete physical examination and laboratory evaluation if they have not had contact with the healthcare system or do not have a primary care provider. Details for the focused male genitourinary examination can be found in Chapter 4, and should include note of secondary sexual characteristics as insight into the potential for a hormone contributor to the ED complaint. The physical examination is typically unrevealing, demonstrating age-appropriate virilization, penis, and testicle size, with the possible exception of identification of a Peyronie's plaque or absent/atrophic testis. Rarely are signs of profound hypogonadism noted.

In the man with recognized and treated comorbid conditions, the focus of the examination should be on the routine genital examination along with a cardiovascular examination and cardiovascular risk assessment. Even a brief cardiovascular assessment should include blood pressure, notation of BMI, heart sounds, and peripheral pulses in the lower extremities. Decreased pulses can suggest the presence of vascular disease, prompting additional cardiovascular assessment or referral to cardiology.

A general neurological assessment can be included as well, including assessment of anal sphincter and the bulbocavernous reflex.

Depending on the degree of past health maintenance, the laboratory evaluation can be quite extensive; if the provider is the first point of contact for the individual in many years, the initial evaluation for ED includes general health screening lab tests: fasting lipid profile, glycosylated hemoglobin, urinalysis, complete chemistry profile, complete blood count, testosterone and luteinizing hormone with possible prolactin, liver profile, and other tests deemed appropriate after history and examination (for instance, if fatigue is an issue, a thyroid evaluation might be considered).

If there is some question about psychogenic and organic contributors, a Rigiscan (GOTOP Medical, Inc.) test can help differentiate between the two. Additional options for evaluation include penile Doppler study (evaluates blood flow after injection of prostaglandin into the corporal tissue) and in some men an arteriogram to evaluate for issues with penile and pelvic vasculature. Imaging studies are rarely indicated in the evaluation of ED, unless there is a history of trauma or some suspicion of anatomical compromise to the vasculature (e.g., metastatic disease).

MANAGEMENT OF ERECTILE DYSFUNCTION

Referral to urology, endocrinology, cardiology, neurology, and/or psychiatry may be considered as testing and laboratory results are reviewed, depending on diagnostic findings. Ideally treatment should be one that is safe for the individual, and that is acceptable in term of possible side effects, cost, and efficacy. Although there are a variety of medical treatments available for men diagnosed with ED, the recent changes in insurance coverage over the past 5 to 10 years has resulted in a pattern of noncoverage for medical therapies for ED.

Once comorbid conditions have been identified, successful management of ED will always involve management of these contributing conditions through lifestyle changes such as weight loss, diet, and exercise.

It is also worth noting that no medical treatment for ED is covered by Medicare, making many of the following options cost-prohibitive for a large number of insured men. Commercial insurances may offer some coverage for medical management but are likely to limit monthly quantities. Vacuum erection devices (VEDs) are no longer a covered benefit under Medicare, and commercial coverage varies. As of publication, both Medicare and commercial insurances continue to cover penile implant surgery.

First-Line Therapies

Specialized sexual therapy can always be an adjunct for the treatment of ED. Many facilities may allow direct referral to a specialized sexual therapist and community providers may offer the service as well. It is important to emphasize to men that suggestion of specialized sexual therapy does not imply that they will need this treatment method for many years; many courses of sexual therapy last from a few months to a year or two at most. These appointments can involve basic sexuality education, and patients may choose to attend alone or with their partner. These appointments will also screen for other psychological contributors to sexual dysfunctions such as anxiety disorders and depression.

VEDs are a suitable method of improving erectile function in men who cannot tolerate medications. The device works by creating external negative pressure which then pulls venous blood directly into the penis, creating turgidity. The patient then places a constriction band at the base of the penis to prevent outflow of this blood; this band can remain in place for up to 30 minutes. Men may find this option very mechanical and awkward, as well as finding the constriction ring uncomfortable. This constriction ring can also interfere with ejaculation. However, once properly trained, most men will achieve a erection sufficient for sexual activity using the VED. There is a high dropout rates with use of this device, however, due to many factors including manual dexterity, a lack of spontaneity, the partner noting change in the erection, and the cumbersome nature of the device. Adverse effects with use of the VED may include hematoma, ecchymosis, petechiae, numbness of penis, pain, and pulling of scrotal tissue; men who were anticoagulated must be counseled that they are likely to bruise when using this device. The VED can be used safely in combination with other medical therapies.

Oral Agents

Type 5 phosphodiesterase (PDE5) inhibitors are considered first-line therapy in the treatment of ED, and require sexual stimulation to be effective, as they are promoters of nitric oxide production of the penis. There are four PDE5 inhibitors available (Table 24.3), with various restrictions based on specific insurance coverage. Although these agents are different, as a class they have a similar mechanism of action: they are a competitive and selective inhibitor of cyclic guanosine monophosphate (cGMP); PDE5 increases the level of intracellular cGMP, resulting in smooth muscle relaxation. These medications do not affect libido, climax, or ejaculation. All agents are equally effective and safe, and presently there are no data to suggest that any one is superior to another.

Prior to the prescription of these medications, it is important to stratify an individual's cardiovascular risk; men must be able to tolerate the "work" of sexual activity in order for these medications to truly be safe. The Princeton III Consensus Panel guidelines offer a structure for categorizing patients to one of three risk levels (high, intermediate, and low) based on their cardiovascular risk factors (Jackson, Rosen, Kloner, & Kostis, 2006). These guidelines recommend that patients at high risk should not receive treatment for sexual dysfunction until their cardiac condition has stabilized. Patients at low risk may be considered for oral agents.

These medications should always be started at the lowest effective dose, work best on an empty stomach, and offer no protection from sexually transmitted infections. Medications in this class may result in dyspepsia, nasal stuffiness, and flushing. They should be used cautiously in men who have hepatic impairment or renal impairment. Coadministration

TABLE 24.3 FDA-Approved Medications for Treatment of Erectile Dysfunction

Medication	Trade Name	Dose	Route	Comments
Avanafil	Stendra	50, 100, 200 mg	Oral	More rapid onset of action than other medications in this category: approved for 15-minute onset of action Possible muscle or back pain May be taken with or without food
Sildenafil	Viagra	25, 50, 100 mg	Oral	Possible color change disturbances, described as a "blue halo" effect No protection from sexually transmitted diseases Systemic vasodilator that can result in transient decreases in supine blood pressure Effective treatment for ED in men with Parkinson's disease Needs to be taken on an empty stomach
Tadalafil	Cialis	Daily: 2.5 or 5 mg On-demand: 5, 10, 20 mg	Oral or sublingual	Possible muscle or back pain May be taken with or without food May be more effective as daily dose in men with "difficult" ED due to sustained plasma levels Not recommended in combination with alpha-blockers for the treatment of BPH because efficacy of the combination has not been adequately studied Men with creatinine clearance <30 mL/min or on hemodialysis: Dose should not exceed 5 mg every 72 hours; daily use is not recommended
Vardenafil	Levitra	50, 100, 200 mg	Oral	Available as orally disintegrating tablet with more rapid onset of action May be taken with or without food, but high-fat meals may delay absorption Systemic vasodilator that can result in transient decreases in supine blood pressure Use 5 mg in patients with moderate hepatic impairment; maximum dose in patients with moderate hepatic impairment should not exceed 10 mg Effective in the context of diabetes, nerve-sparing prostatectomy

(*continued*)

TABLE 24.3 FDA-Approved Medications for Treatment of Erectile Dysfunction (*continued*)

Medication	Trade Name	Dose	Route	Comments
Alprostadil (prostaglandin E1)	EDEX (prefilled syringes)	10–40 mcg	Intracavernosal injection	May report pain in the penis, urethra, or testes with use Overdosage can cause priapism Do not use with men who have conditions that predispose them to priapism or with anatomical deformation of the penis
	Caverject (powder for mixing)	10–40 mcg	Intracavernosal injection	May report pain in the penis, urethra, or testes with use Overdosage can cause priapism Do not use with men who have conditions that predispose them to priapism or with anatomical deformation of the penis
	MUSE	125, 250, 500, 1,000 mcg	Interurethral suppository	Potential for symptomatic hypotension and syncope during in-clinic dosing May report pain in the penis, urethra, or testes with use Overdosage can potentially cause priapism Contraindicated in men with urethral stricture, balanitis, severe hypospadias and curvature, and acute or chronic urethritis

BPH, benign prostatic hyperplasia; ED, erectile dysfunction; FDA, Food and Drug Administration.

with strong CYP3A4 inhibitors is a direct contraindication. All PDE5 inhibitors potentiate the hypotensive effects of nitrates and should not be used in men who are prescribed organic nitrates on any dosing regimen. These medications should not be used in men within 6 months of a myocardial infarction, stroke, life-threatening arrhythmia, or unstable angina.

Men should be counseled to notify their provider of any changes in vision or hearing, and to stop the medication immediately and seek immediate medical treatment if such changes are noted. It is possible that vision changes while taking these medications may be a sign of nonarteritic anterior ischemic optic neuropathy (NAION), a cause of decreased vision that can progress to permanent loss of vision. Sudden hearing loss while on PDE5 medications has also been reported.

Daily tadalafil may be appropriate for men with ED who also have symptoms consistent with benign prostatic hyperplasia (BPH) and related lower urinary tract symptoms.

Treatment failures are often more a failure of education and men's understanding of how these medications work. Additional teaching may be all that is necessary to salvage the use of these very effective oral agents, but switching to another agent can be an option as well. As the severity of their underlying comorbid conditions increases, these agents may well no longer be sufficient in order to promote blood flow and a successful erection.

Second-Line Therapies

Both injection treatment and intraurethral treatment should be accompanied by in-office instruction and trial dosing. This is for patient safety, and there is a risk of priapism with use of these medications. It is also to ensure proper technique and that manual dexterity is sufficient to administer these products safely. Men should be provided with written information and verbal instruction; there are also company videos that provide demonstration. Whenever possible, partners should be included. These medications should always be started at the lowest effective dose and offer no protection from sexually transmitted infections.

Intracavernosal Injection Therapy

Self-administered intracavernosal injections (ICIs) revolutionized the diagnosis and treatment of ED in the mid-1980s, and they have a long history of efficacy and safety. Vasoactive drugs are injected directly into the corpora, resulting in an erection as the smooth muscles of the arterioles and the cavernous trabeculae relax. Intracavernosal injections may be effective in those patients who have failed oral or intraurethral therapies, and effective dosing can be established in up to 89% of men with ED regardless of cause (Coombs, Heck, Guhring, Narus, & Mulhall, 2012).

Three medications are used in injection therapy (papavarine hydrochloride, phentolamine, prostaglandin [PGE1]) in combinations as a bimix, trimix, or alone (prostaglandin). Only prostaglandin is approved by the Food and Drug Administration (FDA) for the ED indication (Edex or Caverject); the other injection options must be compounded.

Successful use of these medications requires extensive patient (or partner) education; injection sites must be rotated to prevent fibrosis or plaque. These injections can be prescribed to men who are anticoagulated, but they must understand the need to maintain pressure for 5 minutes after injection. These injections should not be prescribed if men have penile implants, a history of priapism or sickle cell disease, or their pannus prevents them from reaching their penis. Several adverse effects are possible, despite the overall safety of the product: hypotension, penile pain, priapism, fibrosis over time at injection sites, hematoma, or ecchymosis. Injection treatment can be used once in 24 hours, and up to three times a week; it is also an option for ED treatment that can safely be used in men who are starting or adding to their family.

Men should also have information regarding their present dosing to give to emergency room staff should their erection last longer than 4 to 6 hours. Prolonged erections lasting less than 4 hours after cessation of sexual activity can be treated initially at home, with trials of ice packs, cold showers, increased physical activity, or short-acting pseudoephedrine hydrochloride.

Intraurethral Therapy

Alprostadil (MUSE) is also formulated as an intraurethral suppository (Meda Pharmaceuticals Inc.) that will be absorbed into the surrounding corpora cavernosa. It is less invasive than injection therapy, has a longer onset, and has an overall lower efficacy. MUSE has a lower risk of priapism than injection therapy, but is contraindicated in men with any condition that would predispose them to priapism or an anatomical deformity of the penis (curvature, fibrosis, severe hypospadias). Men who are starting or adding to their family should not use MUSE, as its effects on sperm are not well described; it should not be used by men with their pregnant partners, as reports of vaginal irritation have been noted.

MUSE can be used once in 24 hours, and up to three times a week. Possible side effects include hypotension, pain in the penis or groin, burning from insertion, bleeding from scratching self with applicator, increase in heart rate, or fainting. Changes to insurance coverage have made this option cost-prohibitive under most plans.

Third-Line Therapies

Third-line treatment options are surgical; many men prefer to proceed step-wise from oral to injectable agents before considering surgery. Some men prefer to proceed directly to the implant as a definitive treatment. Regardless of their perspective, men should be supported as they consider options.

Penile Implants

Penile prostheses were first introduced in the 1970s and are available in two forms: malleable or inflatable devices. Inflatable devices are the most realistic option and most popular, and advances in surgical technique have made this a low-risk procedure. Malleable implants always have some degree of rigidity and can be difficult to conceal.

As it is surgery, it is essentially an irreversible option for treatment, and men should be advised to seek high-volume implanters (who will be urologists) to ensure the best outcome. Complications can be significant and include erosion of the device through the skin, infection, and mechanical failure (although this is rare). Although an implant makes use of VED unnecessary, men can use oral medication or MUSE to promote blood flow in the spongiosum (glans).

Vascular Surgery

It may seem intuitive that an option be available for penile revascularization. But historically, when this was attempted in men with vascular comorbid conditions, the outcomes were exceedingly poor, owing to the presence of some degree of venous leak. Presently this option is reserved for young men after genital/pelvic trauma, or those with demonstrated defects on angiogram. This option is only available in large medical centers by experienced surgeons.

Follow-up of Men Treated for ED

There is no standard recommendation for follow-up after starting medication for ED, but follow-up within the first 3 months after starting treatment is reasonable, as it will provide ample opportunity for a medication trial. A return visit also allows an opportunity for men to again complete any forms such as SHIM or IIEF for comparison with pretreatment values. Men should be encouraged to modify risk factors that can improve overall health such as diet and exercise. Oral medications, in particular, are safe and easy to use, but men may report failures or suboptimal results. A return visit allows for a reminder of how these medications work and dosage adjustment as needed.

Referral for ED Management

Men can be referred for management of ED if the provider is uncomfortable with the evaluation and management, or if this is a specific request of the patient or his partner. A common pattern is that men may also self-refer directly to urology practices for evaluation and management of their sexual function complaints.

If beginning treatment for ED, it is reasonable to start with oral medications, increasing the dose until the maximum dose is reached. If this is insufficient to produce satisfactory erections, then it is reasonable to refer men to a urology practice for consideration for penile injection therapy or possibly direct progression to penile implant.

If men have significant endocrine, cardiac, or psychological issues, they may benefit from referral to these specialties for additional evaluation and management. Treatment of ED may involve a multidisciplinary approach to manage these comorbid conditions, and as ED is successfully managed, and they are able to regain intimacy, men may be more likely to improve their adherence to other aspects of their medical management, such as diet and diabetic control.

THE CONTROVERSY SURROUNDING PENILE REHABILITATION

Penile rehabilitation programs are designed to improve, or preserve, erectile function after pelvic surgery, and in particular radical prostatectomy. The philosophy behind these rehabilitation programs centers on the fact that the presumed mechanism for the decline in erectile function is damage to the cavernous nerves, despite both the precision of a robotic approach and nerve-sparing approaches. This results in a period of neuropraxia after surgery contributing to smooth muscle fibrosis after a lowered oxygen supply.

Overall the literature on success rates in penile rehabilitation is sparse: this is particularly true of intracavernosal injection and MUSE as treatment options. This literature is also inconsistent in terms of sample sizes, dosing regimens, as well as suspected mechanism of injury (Fode, Ohl, Ralph, & Sønksen, 2013). A significant flaw in this literature also relates to the fact that there is a consistent definition of normal erectile function by which to gauge either damage or improvements. PDE5 inhibitors have never been compared head-to-head, resulting in a lack of consensus in the literature about which one might be best in this context. This has not stopped the increasing popularity of penile rehabilitation programs, and certainly their proposed methods of treatments have established records of success treating ED of many causes. This is further complicated by the fact that many of these men have existing comorbid conditions that also impact erectile function and blood flow.

Presently there is insufficient data to recommend one method of "penile rehabilitation" over another, and a better approach may simply be to find a regimen that works for an individual patient. Unfortunately, this will bring to mind the previous discussion regarding insurance covering and cost and that many men may not be able to maintain a consistent regimen of medication use due to cost.

CONCLUSION

ED is a common disorder, and its diagnosis may uncover risk factors for other diseases, especially diabetes and cardiovascular disease. Providers must be aware that issues with erectile function may drive men who have had a long absence from the healthcare system toward evaluation, and recognition of ED as a precursor of atherosclerotic disease represents an opportunity for early intervention and treatment. Treatment can be easily initiated by primary care providers, or referred to other specialty providers, but can create significant improvement in overall quality of life for successfully treated men.

CLINICAL PEARLS

- Difficulty attaining or sustaining erections should be referred to as "erectile dysfunction" and not "impotence," which is considered archaic and disparaging.
- Both American Urological Association (AUA) and the European Association of Urology (EAU) recommend oral PDE5 inhibitor (PDE5i) medications as first-line medical management for ED.
- The blood supply that results in penile erection originates in the cavernosal, or deep, penile arteries.

(continued)

CLINICAL PEARLS (*continued*)

- Underlying vascular disease is a contributor to ED in many men, and treatment of conditions such as smoking, obesity, hypertension, and dyslipidemia is a vital adjunct to ED treatment.
- ED that has an abrupt onset is usually due to psychosocial factors.
- Many classes of medications have side effects that include issues with erectile or ejaculatory function.
- All PDE5 inhibitors are contraindicated in men taking nitrates.
- Inflatable penile prostheses have consistently had the highest patient and partner satisfaction ratings of all ED treatments.
- Yohimbine blocks presynaptic alpha-2-adrenergic receptors, resulting in increased cholinergic and decreased adrenergic tone. It can be an ingredient in virility supplements and can mimic panic attacks and cause arrhythmias in large enough doses.
- Patients who have no spontaneous erectile function do not usually respond to oral or intraluminal medications.

RESOURCES FOR PROVIDERS

American Academy of Family Physicians. Curriculum for Men's Health: www.aafp.org/dam/AAFP/documents/medical_education_residency/program_directors/Reprint257_Men.pdf

American Urological Association (AUA) Guideline (2014). AUA Men's Health Checklist. AUA Board of Directors: www.auanet.org/Documents/education/clinical-guidance/Mens-Health-Checklist.pdf

American Urological Association. Sexual activity and cardiovascular risk: www.circ.ahajournals.org/content/125/8/1058

Centers for Disease Control and Prevention. Statistics on Men's Health: www.cdc.gov/nchs/fastats/mens-health.htm

RESOURCES FOR PATIENTS

Men's Health Network (MHN): www.menshealthnetwork.org

Men's Health Month: www.menshealthmonth.org

The Urology Care Foundation: www.urologyhealth.org

REFERENCES

Althof, S. E., Rosen, R. C., Perelman, M. A., & Rubio-Aurioles, E. (2013). Standard operating procedures for taking a sexual history. *The Journal of Sexual Medicine, 10*(1), 26–35. doi:10.1111/j.1743-6109.2012.02823.x

Burd, I. D., Nevadunsky, N., & Bachmann, G. (2006). Impact of physician gender on sexual history taking and a multispecialty practice. *Journal of Sexual Medicine, 3*, 194–200. doi:10.1111/j.1743-6109.2005.00168.x

Cappelleri, J. C., & Rosen, R. C. (2005). The Sexual Health Inventory for Men (SHIM): A 5-year review of research and clinical experience. *International Journal of Impotence Research, 17*(4), 307–319. doi:10.1038/sj.ijir.3901327

Coombs, P. G., Heck, M., Guhring, P., Narus, J., & Mulhall, J. P. (2012). A review of outcomes of an intracavernosal injection therapy programme. *BJU International, 110*(11), 1787–1791. doi:10.1111/j.1464-410X.2012.11080.x

Eardley, I. (2013). The incidence, prevalence, and natural history of erectile dysfunction. *Sexual Medicine Reviews, 1*(1), 3–16. doi:10.1002/smrj.2

Feldman, H. A., Goldstein, I., Hatzichristou, D. G., Krane, R. J., & McKinlay, J. B. (1994). Impotence and its medical and psychosocial correlates: Results of the Massachusetts Male Aging Study. *Journal of Urology, 151*(1), 54–61. doi:10.1016/S0022-5347(17)34871-1

Fode, M., Ohl, D. A., Ralph, D., & Sønksen, J. (2013). Penile rehabilitation after radical prostatectomy: What the evidence really says. *BJU International, 112*(7), 998–1008. doi:10.1111/bju.12228

Jackson, G., Rosen, R. C., Kloner, R. A., & Kostis, J. B. (2006). The second Princeton consensus on sexual dysfunction and cardiac risk: New guidelines for sexual medicine. *Journal of Sexual Medicine, 3*(1), 28–36; discussion 36. doi:10.1111/j.1743-6109.2005.00196.x

Jones, R. W., Rees, R. W., Minhas, S., Ralph, D., Persad, R. A., & Jeremy, J. Y. (2002). Oxygen free radicals and the penis. *Expert Opinion Pharmacotherapy, 3*(7), 889–897. doi:10.1517/14656566.3.7.889

Nehra, A., Jackson, G., Miner, M., Billups, K. L., Burnett, A. L., Buvat, J., ... Guay, A. T. (2012, August). The Princeton III Consensus recommendations for the management of erectile dysfunction and cardiovascular disease. *Mayo Clinic Proceedings, 87*(8), 766–778. doi:10.1016/j.mayocp.2012.06.015

Rosen, R. C., Cappelleri, J. C., Smith, M. D., Lipsky, J., & Pena, B. M. (1999). Development and evaluation of an abridged, 5-item version of the International Index of Erectile Function (IIEF-5) as a diagnostic tool for erectile dysfunction. *International Journal of Impotence Research, 11*(6), 319–326. doi:10.1038/sj.ijir.3900472

Shabsigh, R. (2006). Epidemiology of erectile dysfunction. In J. J. Mulcahy (Ed.), *Male sexual function: A guide to clinical management* (2nd ed., pp. 47–59). Totowa, NJ: Humana Press.

Shamloul, R., & Ghanem, H. (2013). Erectile dysfunction. *Lancet, 381*(9861), 153–165. doi:10.1016/S0140-6736(12)60520-0

CHAPTER 25

Benign Prostatic Hyperplasia

Stanley Mukundi

INTRODUCTION

This chapter will review the anatomy of the prostate and the common clinical presentation of men with benign prostate hyperplasia (BPH), as well as diagnostic and management options. The prostate is the only solid organ in the male pelvis and it is located posterior to the pubic symphysis, inferior to the bladder, but superior to the perineal membrane and can be easily palpated across the anterior rectal wall especially when enlarged.

Historically, as life expectancy has gradually improved over centuries, chronic issues associated with aging, and in particular BPH, have increased. Urinary retention was the most ominous complication of prostatic obstruction leading to renal insufficiency, urinary tract infection (UTI), and sometimes death of the patient (Sosnowski, 2014). BPH is a histological diagnosis, referring to the proliferation of smooth muscles and epithelial cells within the transition zone of the prostate (Chughtai et al., 2016). It is the most common non-neoplastic condition that afflicts American men, affecting 3 out of every 4 men by their seventh decade in life (Miller, Saigal, & Litwin, 2009). The prevalence is strongly related to age, revealing a chronic, gradual, and often progressive incidence of presentation, from approximately 8% of the men in their 50s to 90% of men older than 80 (Briganti & Gandaglia, 2014). Interestingly, the clinical manifestation of BPH is represented by a presentation of lower urinary tract symptoms (LUTS), although the relationship between the two is complex—denoting not all men with BPH will develop LUTS and inversely not all men with LUTS have significant BPH (Buchman & De La Rosette, 2012). It is important therefore to understand that although BPH is a common cause of LUTS in men, it certainly is not the only cause, and therefore, other potential causes of LUTS must be ruled out.

ANATOMY AND PHYSIOLOGY

The adult prostate is a tubular-alveolar gland, with its embryological origin, development, and function capturing the keen interest of scientists for centuries. According to Chapple and Tubaro (Sosnowski, 2014) the *Anatomiae Liber Introductorius* by Nicola Massa (1504–1589) in 1536 and the *Tabulae Anatomicae* by the anatomist Andreas Vesalius (1514–1564) in 1538 both displayed the prostate gland for the first time. There are four distinct zones of the prostate, namely the peripheral, central, transition, and anterior zones (Figure 25.1). These zones can be distinguished as early as embryological week 12 and become increasingly distinct over time.

The embryological development of the prostate begins through an interaction of four critical units in genetically normal individuals, namely the wolffian duct, the müllerian duct, the urogenital sinus (UGS), and the fetal gonad (Aaron, Franco, & Hayward, 2016). The müllerian ducts develop at about 6 weeks of gestation and by the eighth week, they are between the wolffian ducts, proximal to the UGS, forming the müllerian tubercule, which distally forms

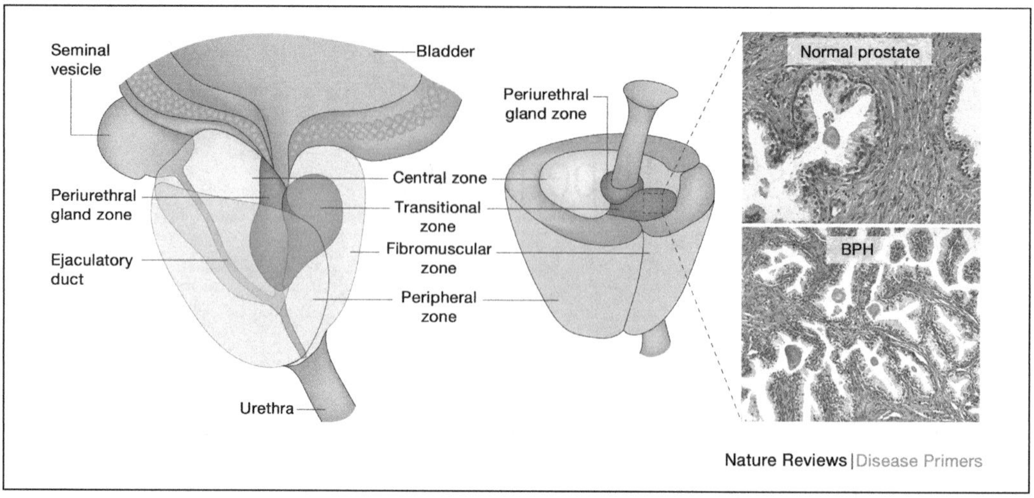

FIGURE 25.1 Benign prostatic hyperplasia.

Source: Chughtai, B., Forde, J., Thomas, D., Laaor, L., Hossack, T., Woo, H., ... Kaplan, S. (2016). Benign prostatic hyperplasia. *Nature Reviews Disease Primers, 2*, 16031. doi:10.1038/nrdp.2016.31

the penile urethra while the UGS forms the urethra (Aaron et al., 2016). The wolffian ducts develop into the seminal veiscles, epididymis, vas deferens, ampula, and ejaculatory duct through an androgen-mediated process. The prostate and seminal vesicles are responsible for production of seminal fluid, whereas the testicular Sertoli cells are responsible for spermatogenesis. The peripheral zone of the prostate is the largest of the four zones and is most common site of carcinomas. The anterior zone is mostly composed of smooth muscles, whereas the central zone surrounds the ejaculatory ducts.

On average, the adult prostate is a walnut-sized organ measuring 20 g in volume: 3 cm wide, 4 cm in length and 2 cm in depth (Khanna, Bratslavsky, & Stein, 2015). The hallmark of BPH is the proliferation of both stromal and epithelial cells within the transitional zone of the prostate surrounding the urethra (Chughtai et al., 2016) resulting in bladder outlet obstruction (BOO) due to a narrow/compressed prostatic urethra, which in turn causes a decreased urine flow. There is a cylindrical sleeve of smooth muscle that stretches from the base of the bladder to the verumontanum, the periprostatic sphincter, which is adjacent to the peripheral zone and plays an important role in maintaining urine continence.

The prostate has both parasympathetic and sympathetic innervation, the former arising from the S2 to S4 levels of the pelvic plexus and the latter from the L1 to L2 levels enabling contraction of the smooth muscles. With this in mind, it is easy to see how prostate surgery (in particular prostatectomy) can impact sexual and urinary continence. The pudendal nerve is the major nerve supply of the striated sphincter and levator ani. The most common adrenoceptor subtype present in prostate tissue is alpha-1A which mediates active tension in human prostatic smooth muscle, with stimulation of these receptors leading to dynamic increase in prostatic urethral resistance and inhibition resulting in a decrease in prostatic urethral resistance (Roehrborn, et al., 2011). Clinically, understanding this mechanism is important because it explains the mechanism of action of alpha antagonists and their potential side effects discussed later.

BPH results in compression of the urethra, causing resistance to urine flow known as BOO. This resistance can also result in obstruction-induced changes of bladder function, such as overactivity of the detrusor muscle or reduced contractility of the detrusor muscle (Roehrborn et al., 2017). BOO can present as LUTS, infections, or retention, as well as other conditions. BPH and BOO impose considerable burden on the health of older men and on healthcare costs.

The pathophysiology of BPH is incompletely understood, although there is clear understanding of the histological features within the prostate that are dependent of testosterone and its active metabolite dihydrotestosterone (Sarma & Wei, 2012). This is why exogenous testosterone supplementation leads to glandular hypertrophy, whereas castration leads to atrophy and regression of LUTS.

HISTORY

Examination begins with a complete medical history. This step includes detailing the patient's prior medical conditions, because LUTS can be due to multifactorial causes including cardiovascular, renal dysfunction, pulmonary/respiratory such as obstructive sleep apnea (OSA), or even neurological (central versus peripheral). A detailed history will allow the clinician to screen for potential ominous causes including infections, stones, and malignancy while understanding the severity, degree of bother, and impact on the patient's quality of life (QOL) (Woodard, Manigault, McBurrows, Wray, & Woodard, 2016). Asking appropriate and detailed questions will help the clinician understand the patient's most bothersome symptoms, but also will help in predicting the appropriate therapy, and once instituted, an accurate response or lack thereof. It is important to understand the onset (acute versus gradual), quantify frequency (day versus night), rate the urgency, and quantify episodes of urge incontinence and pad usage as well as query the severity of subjective symptoms including sensation of incomplete voiding, straining, hesitancy, and intermittency. Finally, burning and blood in the urine can point to a potential ominous urological cause of LUTS, aside from BPH, such as infection, stones, or malignancy.

Having a patient keep a voiding diary for 2 to 3 days while adhering to the normal routine might reveal behavioral causes of symptoms, such as excessive fluid and caffeine consumption. It is also helpful in distinguishing polyuria (defined as greater than 3 L output in 24 hours) from nocturnal polyuria (diagnosed when greater than 1/3 of urine output occurs at night). The voiding diary is also helpful in evaluating the patient's functional bladder capacity.

Reviewing an updated medication list is important because various medications affect LUTS differently. For instance, diuretics can lead to increased urine output, whereas anticholinergics can slow the bladder and colon, potentially causing urinary retention and constipation, respectively. Atypical antipsychotic medications can affect urinary symptoms in various ways including weight gain, which has been associated with OSA, and in turn nocturnal polyuria, whereas antihistamines weaken the detrusor and can precipitate urinary retention.

Attention must be given to the patient's family history and surgical/procedure history. It is key to specifically ask about any neurological symptoms and any past urological surgeries and procedures such as genitourinary reconstruction, urethral instrumentation, or recent biopsies.

Normal micturation normally depends on the ability of the detrusor muscle to generate a contraction that is able to overcome the resistance from the prostate and bladder neck (Sarma & Wei, 2012). Therefore, it is important to assess the severity and impact of LUTS on the patient's quality of life.

The American Urological Association (AUA) Symptom Index (AUASI) and the International Prostate Symptom Score (IPSS) are validated questionnaires that the patients can complete that quantify the severity of LUTS. Specifically, it addresses three storage symptoms (frequency, urgency, and nocturia) and four voiding symptoms (sensation of incomplete voiding, intermittency, straining, and a weak urinary stream). Scores range between 0 indicating no symptoms to 35 indicating severe symptoms, and the IPSS additionally assesses the degree of bother, specifically on the patient's QOL. This questionnaire is also extremely useful in assessing the potential response to therapy, whereby a minimum 3-point change in either direction is considered clinically significant (Sarma & Wei, 2012). Specifically, taking a good medical history, performing a thorough physical examination in conjunction with obtaining the appropriate laboratory testing will ensure exclusion of other potential causes of LUTS prior to attributing them to BPH.

Common Presentation

To better understand the common presentation, signs and symptoms of BPH, and associated LUTS, it is important to understand the pathogenesis. The main mechanisms in which an enlarged prostate contributes to LUTS involve a static component, whereby the enlarged prostate causes direct BOO, and a second dynamic component marked by increase in tone of the smooth muscles and resistance within the enlarged prostate—the alpha-adrenergic axis (Sarma & Wei, 2012). Therefore, symptoms of BPH can be viewed in two broad categories—obstructive symptoms secondary to BOO due to prostate enlargement versus irritative voiding symptoms due to bladder overactivity secondary to an enlarged prostate.

Signs and Symptoms

The resulting urethral constriction from an enlarged prostate results in mostly obstructive voiding symptoms including a weak force of stream, urinary hesitancy and intermittency, as well as sensation of incomplete voiding. Bladder detrusor hyperactivity, mediated by M2 and M3 muscarinic receptors, contributes of LUTS in approximately 15% of men (Sarma & Wei, 2012) and presenting symptoms might include urinary frequency, nocturia, and urinary urgency with or without incontinence. It is noteworthy that newer studies are showing significant expression of nonmuscarinic targets such as phosphodiesterase-5 in bladder and prostate smooth muscles, subsequently expanding the array of pharmacotherapy available for patient reprieve from LUTS.

As discussed previously, BPH is often progressive, meaning the prostate gradually increases in size over a man's lifetime. Similarly, over time, LUTS can be progressive and the rates of progression necessitating either pharmacological or surgical intervention can be predicted by the baseline prostate volume, age, PSA level, and severity of presenting symptoms (McConnell et al., 2003). These factors individually predict the risk of symptom progression, whereby in severe cases men can present with urinary retention, renal insufficiency, or UTIs. This means that an advanced age at presentation, large prostate volume, severe baseline LUTS, high PSA values, and a decreased urine flow rate are all individually associated with the risk of symptom progression.

Risk Factors

Recently, the role of chronic inflammation of the prostate (prostatitis) is emerging as the pathogenesis of BPH continues to be researched. This is hypothesized to be cytokine mediated, whereby upregulation of inflammatory cytokines has been widely reported in the prostate tissue of patients with BPH (Popovics, Schally, Salgueiro, Kovacs, & Rick, 2017; Sosnowski, 2014). Other associated risk factors that include smoking, race (African American > Caucasian), alcohol intake, and sexual activity have all been hypothesized (Sosnowski, 2014).

Additional risk factors include genetics, obesity, metabolic syndrome, diabetes, hypertension, body mass index (BMI), and waist circumference (Sosnowski, 2014; Sarma & Wei, 2012). Therefore, from a clinical standpoint, it is imperative to counsel patients on lifestyle modification aimed at not only lowering their risk factors for coronary artery disease (CAD) and the morbidity and mortality associated with it, but also at potentially improving or preventing progression of LUTS.

Morbidity and mortality from the prostate arise from either malignancy, inflammation/prostatitis, or severe outlet obstruction resulting in renal impairment or infections. Screening is the most common and effective method of early cancer detection; however, there is a clear lack of consensus among medical groups on who and how to screen. The current AUA guidelines (2013) recommend shared decision making and screening men at a high risk of cancer—African American men and those with a family history of prostate cancer as well as men age 55 to 69 years—after weighing the benefits of preventing prostate cancer death (1 man for every 1,000 screened over a decade) against known harms associated with screening and treatment. The risk of BPH disease progression has been shown to be greater in African American men compared to Caucasians (Figure 25.2; Collon & Payne, 2008).

Cultural Considerations

When it comes to BPH and LUTS, it is important to remember there are well-established socioeconomic factors that lead to healthcare disparities in management and progression of LUTS, such as men with lower incomes being associated with higher IPSS scores and an increased risk of moderate/severe LUTS (Fowke, Munro, Signorello, Blot, & Penson, 2011). It is therefore important to consider this when recommending or initiating treatment by balancing the cost/affordability versus efficacy of the proposed treatment. There are several cultural factors to be considered, including knowledge, health beliefs, barriers, and relationships with primary healthcare providers (Woods et al., 2004).

Patient reporting of LUTS can be affected by multiple factors including sociocultural factors and patient education/literacy (Fowke et al., 2011), and therefore, it is important to consider patient comprehension, especially when it comes to the use of validated questionnaires, patient education materials, and clinic communication.

Finally, it is important to understand men and their cultural background given the potential implications on the patient care and potential outcomes. For instance, some immigrant communities/religions do not allow any physical contact whatsoever (for instance, handshake or even a physical examination) from a person of the opposite sex. Such limitations, combined with the intrusive nature of a prostate examination and any potential procedures on the prostate or bladder, have been shown in other similar fields to be associated with negative outcomes including inadequate screening, delayed diagnosis, and presentation with advanced disease (Vahabi & Lofters, 2016).

PHYSICAL EXAMINATION

A thorough physical examination for assessment and planning of management for BPH should include the following:

- **Vital signs**: Blood pressure and temperature can point to the severity of a potential infection, and height, weight, and BMI calculations are important because obese patients are at a risk of OSA and consequently nocturnal polyuria (Unnikrishnan, Almassi, & Fareed, 2017).
- **Neurological and musculoskeletal:** Observing the patient walk, transition between positions, and even checking their reflexes are important. Diminished reflexes especially in the lower extremities, muscle weakness, and altered gait might point to an underlying cause such as multiple sclerosis, Parkinson's disease, or neurological deficits from a central or peripheral process. Additional neurological examination can be done by assessing the tone of the rectal sphincter.
- **Abdomen**: Palpating the suprapubic region might reveal a distended bladder, and additional dullness to percussion.

- **Genitourinary**: Examine the urethral meatus to ensure it is patent, normally positioned with no narrowing, and has no palpable mass or stone. Any abnormality here should prompt a referral to a urologist.
- **Digital rectal examination (DRE):** Although modestly accurate for checking prostate volume (Stone et al., 2017), DRE is also useful in checking for any palpable nodules, induration, or significantly enlarged prostate, which should similarly prompt a referral to a urologist (see Chapter 4 for details of how to perform).
- **Lower extremities:** Assess for pedal edema, which could be secondary to venous insufficiency or heart failure.

According to the current AUA guidelines on BPH management (2013) if the initial evaluation demonstrates an abnormal prostate on DRE, such as nodules or induration, or if the patient is presenting with hematuria, a palpably distended bladder, a history or risk of urethral strictures such as trauma or a history of UTIs or urethral instrumentation, or any neurological diseases that might raise the possibility of a primary bladder disorder, then an immediate referral to a urologist is appropriate before advising on treatment focused on medical management.

Diagnostic Tests

As recommended by the AUA 2013 guidelines, upon shared decision making, a PSA test should be obtained and the patient should be referred to the urologist for any abnormal results. A urinalysis is helpful to screen for UTI, but also to look for hematuria, which might signal a stone or cancer involving the kidneys, ureter, bladder, prostate, or urethra. In this context, referral to a urologist is similarly warranted. Glucosuria is an abnormal finding that should prompt further evaluation of the patient's fasting blood sugar. Routine serum creatinine is not indicated in the initial evaluation of men with LUTS secondary to BPH (AUA guidelines, 2014).

Patients with a palpable bladder on examination and those complaining of isolated, significant obstructive voiding symptoms can be evaluated with an ultrasound scan to rule out urinary retention (Sarma & Wei, 2012). An enlarged prostate can be assessed by transrectal ultrasound or cross-sectional imaging, although it is not necessary prior to a referral to a urologist or prior to instituting initial medical management. A transrectal ultrasound examination is appropriate, however, to assess for the size of the prostate by the urologist to determine the appropriate surgery based on prostate size, whereas a transrectal or transperineal ultrasound-guided prostate biopsy might be indicated for men with a high PSA upon consultation with a urologist.

MANAGEMENT

The AUA has developed the AUASI, a validated, self-administered questionnaire that is diagnostic and predictive of the severity of LUTS due to BPH and extremely useful in reliably capturing changes in symptoms over time (Barry et al., 2017). It differs from the standard AUA Symptoms Score (AUASS) in that the AUASI is one question shorter, and validation testing of the instrument showed it measures symptoms that more closely represent the clinical presentation of BPH. Men with mild or no symptoms (assessed on AUASI score of <8), or those not bothered by their symptoms, despite the symptoms being moderate or severe (assessed by AUASI >8), can be managed by watchful waiting according to the AUA 2014 guidelines. At each subsequent visit, patients should be asked if their symptoms are sufficiently bothersome to necessitate medical therapy (Sarma & Wei, 2012; Woodard et al., 2016). Previous testing of medication efficacy has been with the AUASS as the primary assessment instrument.

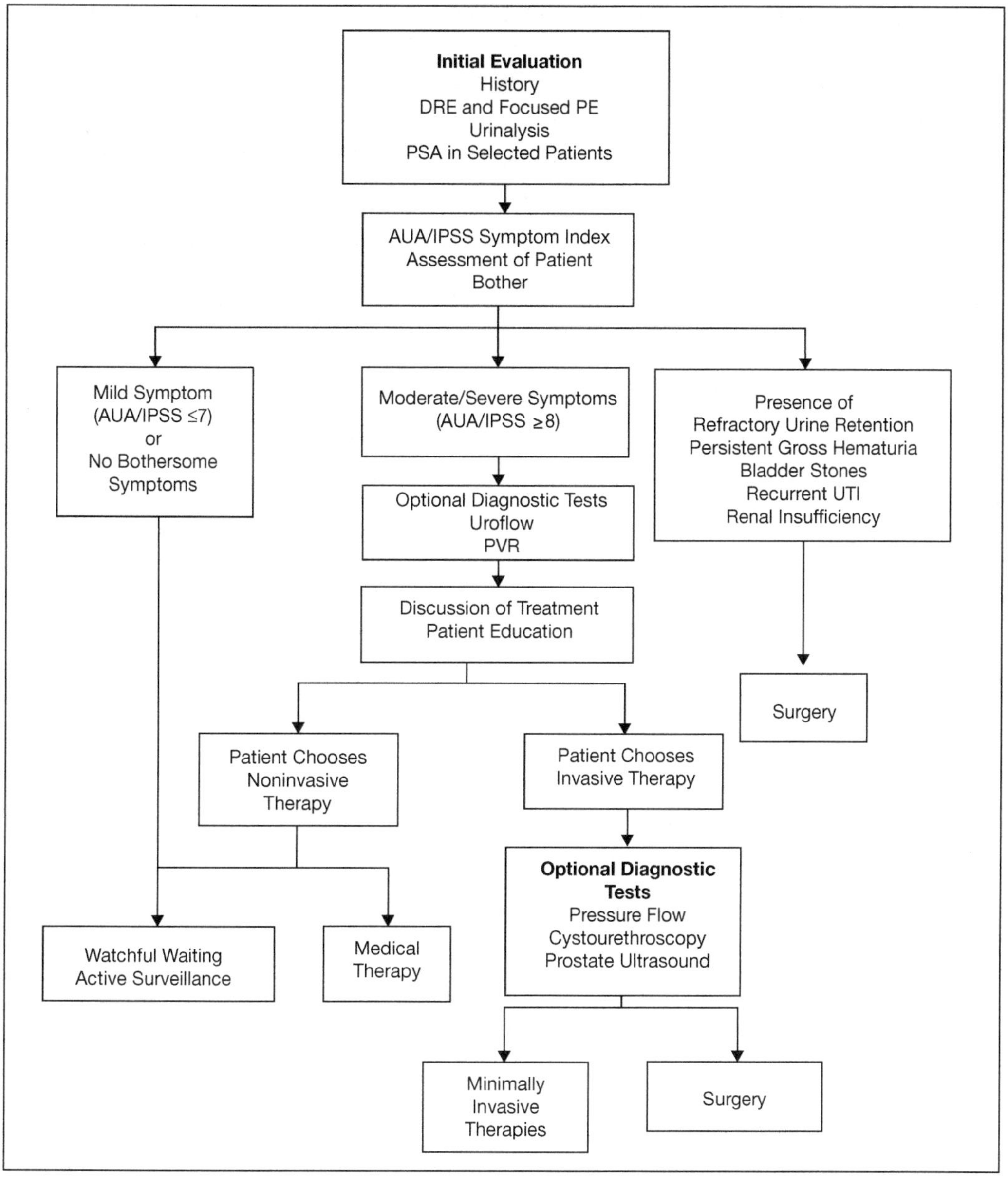

FIGURE 25.2 Benign prostatic hyperplasia diagnosis and treatment algorithm.

AUA, American Urological Association; DRE, digital rectal examination; IPSS, International Prostate Symptom Score; PE, physical examination; PSA, prostate-specific antigen; PVR, postvoid residual urine; UTI, urinary tract infection.

Source: Reprinted with permission from Collon, I., & Payne, E. (2008). Benign prostatic hyperplasia and lower urinary tract symptoms in African Americans and Latinos: Treatment in the context of common comorbidities. The American Journal of Medicine, 121, S18–S26. doi:10.1016/j.amjmed.2008.05.023.

Medical Management

Medical management is centered around four classes of medications: Alpha antagonists, 5-alpha-reductase inhibitors (5-ARI), antimuscarinic agents, and phosphodiesterase-5 inhibitors (PDE5i; Table 25.1). Patients with moderate or severe symptoms, or those bothered

TABLE 25.1 Approved Medication Classes in the Treatment of Benign Prostatic Hyperplasia (BPH)

Medication Class	Name (Trade Name)	Daily Dose	Common Side Effects
Alpha antagonists	Alfuzosin	10 mg	Headache, nasal congestion, hypotension, dizziness, malaise, fatigue, retrograde ejaculation, and erectile dysfunction **Caution:** Floppy intraoperative iris syndrome
	Doxazosin	1–8 mg	
	Terazosin	1–20 mg	
	Tamsulosin	0.4–0.8 mg	
	Silodosin	4–8 mg	
5-Alpha-reductase inhibitors (5-ARI)	Dutasteride	0.5 mg	Ejaculatory disorder, impotence, gynecomastia **Caution:** • Women and pediatric patients should avoid contact • Decreases prostate-specific antigen (PSA) • Increased risk of high-grade prostate cancer
	Finasteride (Proscar)	5 mg	
Phosphodiesterase type 5 inhibitor (PDE5i)	Tadalafil (Cialis)	2.5–5 mg	Flushing, headache, nasal congestion, blood pressure changes, and chest pain **Caution:** Concomitant use with nitrates or even alpha blockers could lead to fatal hypotension
Beta 3 agonist	Mirabegron	25–50 mg	Hypertension, tachycardia, dizziness
Anticholinergics	Oxybutynin	2.5–20 mg	Dizziness, drowsiness, confusion, dry mouth, dry eyes, constipation, urinary retention **Caution:** Contraindicated for narrow angle glaucoma
	Tolerodine	2–4 mg	
	Fesoterodine	4–8 mg	
	Trospium	40 mg	
	Darifenacin	7.5–15 mg	
	Solifenacin	5–10 mg	

Patients who do not wish to take any medication and prefer surgical intervention.
Patients intolerant to oral LUTS medications or in whom such medications are contraindicated.
Patients who have failed maximum medical therapy such as combination alpha blocker and 5-ARI and/or anticholinergics.
Patients with severe symptoms such as urinary retention.
Patients with gross hematuria or persistent/progressive LUTS.
Patients with recurrent urinary tract infections, kidney stones, or prior genitourinary reconstructive surgeries.

by their symptoms, can be offered medical management upon discussion of risks and benefits. Alpha-antagonists are the first-line therapy for LUTS when symptoms are predominantly BOO due to BPH (AUA guidelines, 2014). Alfuzosin, doxazosin, and terazosin, as well as more selective alpha blockers silodosin and tamsulosin, are approved by the Food and Drug Administration (FDA) for treatment of BPH symptoms. Doxazosin and terazosin require dose titration, usually over several weeks for optimal efficacy. They all appear to be equally effective clinically, excreting their effect on the prostatic smooth muscles and bladder neck by blocking the sympathetic adrenergic receptor mediated contraction (Sarma & Wei, 2012). These medications work by relaxing the smooth muscle tone around the prostate and bladder neck (Woodard et al., 2016). This leads to improved voiding. Owing to their effects on smooth muscles however, they can lead to a decrease in blood pressure, especially with the nonspecific alpha-blockers, which can lead to dizziness and, especially for geriatric patients, increase their risk of falls.

Other important side effects include nasal congestion, blurry vision, and retrograde ejaculation in which semen is redirected into the bladder instead of the normal forward propulsion outward upon reaching an orgasm. It is important as well for patients potentially undergoing cataract surgery to inform their eye surgeon that they are taking alpha blockers owing to their association with intraoperative floppy iris syndrome (IFIS), a condition in which the iris becomes flaccid, billowing, and prolapses and additionally associated with pupil constriction (Woodard et al., 2016).

There are two 5-ARIs (dutasteride 0.5 mg and finasteride 5 mg), which lead to significantly decreased serum dihydrotestosterone levels by blocking the 5-alpha-reductase isoenzyme. If the patient has an enlarged prostate on either DRE or imaging or if he has a PSA > 1.5 ng/mL (after ruling out malignancy), 5-ARIs have been shown to be effective alone or in combination with alpha antagonists than with alpha blockers alone. The randomized, double-blind study looking at the combination of Avodart (dutasteride) and tamsulosin (combAT) trial by Roehrborn et al. (2011) demonstrated a reduced relative risk of acute urinary retention, clinical symptom progression, and deterioration as well as BPH-related surgery on combo therapy (dutasteride and Flomax) or dutasteride monotherapy when compared with tamsulosin monotherapy. According to Toren et al. (2013), 5-ARIs have a demonstrated prophylactic benefit in mildy symptomatic and perhaps even asymptomatic men to prevent symptom progression, lower need for future BPH-related surgery, and also to improve bladder emptying, decrease the effects of bladder outlet obstruction, and prevent future incidents such as hematuria and urinary retention. 5-ARIs reduce prostate volume by as much as 25% and the PSA by 50% (Emberton et al., 2008), and decrease the AUASS by as much as 4 to 5 points in patients with prostates >30 g over a period of 2 to 6 months (Sarma & Wei, 2012). Potential side effects of these medications include gynecomastia, decrease in libido, hair growth, and depression.

When storage symptoms predominate without indication of BOO, lifestyle modification including timed voiding and fluid intake regulation as well as anticholinergics are effective. It is important to understand, however, that there are no FDA-approved antimuscarinics for BPH symptoms, although the AUA recognizes their potential role in symptom management (Woodard et al., 2016). These medications work by blocking the neurotransmitter acetylcholine in the central and peripheral nervous system, and there are five muscarinic subgroups described in the bladder muscles (M1–M5), with M2 and M3 comprising the majority. The broad distribution of acetylcholine receptors explains the side effect profile of these medications, with dose-dependent side effects that increase with less selective antimuscarinic agents. Caution should be used in patients with postvoid residual urine volumes greater than 250 mL because of the risk of urinary retention, and it is advised to initiate an alpha blocker beforehand (Woodard et al., 2016).

PDE5i have been studied with some promise in improvement of LUTS, although their exact mechanism of reducing these symptoms remains unclear. However, theories are converging toward the understanding that phosphodiesterase-5 is present in prostatic tissue, especially within the transition zone, detrusor, and vascular smooth muscle cells within the urinary tract and therefore its inhibition results in increases in cyclic adenosine monophosphate (AMP) and cyclic guanosine monophosphate, leading to smooth muscle relaxation, and perhaps antiproliferative effects in prostatic and bladder smooth muscle cells (Sarma & Wei, 2012; Woodard et al., 2016). Tadalafil is the only FDA-approved medication within this category. It might take 2 to 4 weeks to notice a positive impact on symptoms. Common side effects include flushing, nasal congestion, headache, and significant hypotension when combined with alpha blockers. Although tadalafil daily has the dual indication to relieve LUTS and erectile dysfunction symptoms, it is expensive and not covered by most insurance plans.

The list below, although not comprehensive, offers a guide as to when it is most appropriate to refer patients to a urology clinic, although clinicians should feel free to reach out to a local urologist if there are any questions.

- Patients who do not wish to take any medication and prefer surgical intervention
- Patients intolerant to oral LUTS medications or in whom such medications are contraindicated
- Patients who have failed maximum medical therapy such as combination alpha blocker and 5-ARI and/or anticholinergics
- Patients with severe symptoms such as urinary retention
- Patients with gross hematuria or persistent/progressive LUTS
- Patients with recurrent urinary tract infections, kidney stones, or prior genitourinary reconstructive surgeries

Brief Overview of Surgical Procedures and Their Indications; Basic Postoperative Considerations

According to the AUA 2014 guidelines, transurethral resection of the prostate (TURP) is the gold standard of interventional treatment of LUTS and it is indicated for patients with moderate to severe symptoms, patients with urinary retention due to prostatic outlet obstruction, patients intolerant to or who have failed medications but also patients with recurrent urinary tract infections, bladder calculi, renal insufficiency, or even persistent hematuria due to prostatic hyperplasia. It is the most definitive prostate procedure; however, it also carries the most significant potential risks including bleeding, infection, persistence of irritative bladder symptoms such as frequency and incontinence in addition to the known anesthesia risks. The different modalities of performing the transurethral resection include monopolar versus bipolar TURP, transurethral vaporization of the prostate (TUVP), and transurethral holmium laser enucleation of the prostate (HoLEP) among others.

There are minimally invasive procedures, which are meant to be performed in the office minimizing the risks that can be associated with a TURP. These procedures are appropriate and mostly effective on bothersome moderate and severe symptoms, although the long-term need for re-treatment limits their adoption and use. There are several modalities of treatment such as TUNA (transurethral needle ablation of the prostate), which is heat-induced coagulation necrosis using interstitial radiofrequency delivered to the prostate through transurethral needles; TUMT (transurethral microwave therapy), which heats the prostate using microwave antennae; and most recently Rezūm, which uses water vapor.

CONCLUSION

Presently there are a variety of modalities (transurethral electrovaporization, holmium laser resection, transurethral incision, photoselective vaporization) available for the treatment of benign enlarged prostate, with the development of additional targeted procedures likely for the future. As the population ages, the burden of BPH to the healthcare system will increase, creating the need for providers to maintain working knowledge of a variety of approaches that are useful for treating BPH and its symptoms, and inclusion of a sociodemographic perspective. This will include lifestyle management (such as diet) and management of comorbid conditions seen with an enlarged prostate, such as obesity.

CLINICAL PEARLS

- LUTS can be divided into two categories based on pathogenesis—outlet (weak force of stream, urinary hesitancy, intermittency and sensation of incomplete voiding) versus storage symptoms (urinary frequency, nocturia, urgency with or without incontinence).
- LUTS occur in more than half the men in their sixth decade of life.
- The AUASI is a validated, self-administered, questionnaire that can assess the severity of symptom and provide a reliable and objective measure of response to therapy.
- Risk of LUTS progression necessitating either pharmacological or surgical intervention has been individually linked to baseline larger prostate volumes, high PSA levels, severe LUTS, decreased urine flow rate, and advanced age at presentation.
- Men with mild symptoms or those not bothered by moderate and severe symptoms can be offered watchful waiting, deferring any pharmacological intervention after a comprehensive evaluation.
- Alpha blockers are a good initial option for patients with significant LUTS, since they can be combined with either 5-ARIs or anticholinergics for synergy.

RESOURCES FOR THE CLINICIAN

The American Urological Association (AUA; www.auanet.org) offers an excellent resource for clinicians, with up-to-date evidence-based clinical practice guidelines in addition to patient care resources such as handouts, and video tutorials. Clinical Guidelines Benign Prostatic Hyperplasia (2010; Reviewed and Validity Confirmed 2014): www.auanet.org/guidelines/benign-prostatic-hyperplasia-(2010-reviewed-and-validity-confirmed-2014)

European Association of Urology (EAU) Guidelines: www.uroweb.org/wp-content/uploads/EAU-Guidelines-Non-Neurogenic-Male-LUTS-Guidelines-2015-v2.pdf

The National Institute of Diabetes and Digestive and Kidney Diseases is another excellent resource: www.niddk.nih.gov

UpToDate: www.uptodate.com/contents/benign-prostatic-hyperplasia-bph-beyond-the-basics

RESOURCES FOR THE PATIENT

The AUA publishes a quarterly magazine (UrologyHealth Extra) which is an excellent resource for patients to get information that is concise, accurate and up-to-date. www.urologyhealth.org/educational-materials/magazine-subscription

The National Institute of Diabetes and Digestive and Kidney Diseases-Prostate Enlargement (Benign Prostatic Hyperplasia): www.niddk.nih.gov/health-information/urologic-diseases/prostate-problems/prostate-enlargement-benign-prostatic-hyperplasia

Urology Care Foundation: www.urologyhealth.org; www.urologyhealth.org/urologic-conditions/benign-prostatic-hyperplasia-(bph)

REFERENCES

American Urological Association. (2013). *Early detection of prostate cancer*. Linthicum, MD: Author.

American Urological Association. (2014). Management of benign prostatic hyperplasia. Retrieved from http://www.auanet.org/benign-prostatic-hyperplasia-(2010-reviewed-and-validity-confirmed-2014)

Aaron, L., Franco, O. E., & Hayward, S. W. (2016). Review of prostate anatomy and embryology and the etiology of benign prostatic hyperplasia. *Urologic Clinics, 43*(3), 279–288. doi:10.1016/j.ucl.2016.04.012

Barry, M., Fowler, F., O'leary, M., Bruskewitz, R., Holtgrewe, H., Mebust, W., & Cockett, A.; Measurement Committee of the American Urological Association. (2017, February). The American Urological Association Symptom index for benign prostatic hyperplasia. *Journal of Urology, 197*(2S), 189–197. doi:10.1016/j.juro.2016.10.071

Briganti, A., & Gandaglia, G. (2014). Epidemiology and pathophysiology of LUTS/BPO. In: C. Chapple, & A. Tubaro (Eds.), *Male LUTS/BPH made easy*. London, UK: Springer.

Buchman, A., & De La Rosette, J. (Eds.). (2012). *Benign prostatic hyperplasia and lower urinary tract symptoms in men* (pp. 1–5). New York, NY: Oxford University Press.

Chughtai, B., Forde, J., Thomas, D., Laaor, L., Hossack, T., Woo, H., ... Kaplan, S. (2016). Benign prostatic hyperplasia. *Nature Reviews Disease Primers, 2*, 16031. doi:10.1038/nrdp.2016.31

Collon, I., & Payne, E. (2008). Benign prostatic hyperplasia and lower urinary tract symptoms in African Americans and Latinos: Treatment in the context of common comorbidities. *The American Journal of Medicine, 121*, S18–S26. doi:10.1016/j.amjmed.2008.05.023

Emberton, M., Cornel, E., Bassi, P., Fourcade, R., Gomez, J., & Castro, R. (2008). Benign Prostatic hyperplasia as a progressive disease: A guide to the risk factors and options for medical management. *International Journal of Clinical Practice, 62*(7), 1076–1086. doi:10.1111/j.1742-1241.2008.01785.x

Fowke, J. H., Munro, H., Signorello, L. B., Blot, W. J., & Penson, D. F. (2011, November). Association between socioeconomic status (SES) and lower urinary tract symptom (LUTS) severity among black and white men. *Journal of General Internal Medicine, 26*(11), 1305–1310. doi:10.1007/s11606-011-1776-8

Khanna, R. V., Bratslavsky, G., & Stein, R. J. (Eds.). (2015). *Surgical techniques for prostate cancer*. New York, NY: Springer Publishing Company.

McConnell, J. D., Roehrborn, C. G., Bautista, O. M., Andriole Jr, G. L., Dixon, C. M., Kusek, J. W., ... Crawford, E. D. (2003). The long-term effect of doxazosin, finasteride, and combination therapy on the clinical progression of benign prostatic hyperplasia. *New England Journal of Medicine, 349*(25), 2387–2398. doi:10.1056/NEJMoa030656

Miller, D. C., Saigal, C. S., & Litwin, M. S. (2009). The demographic burden of urologic diseases in America. *Urologic Clinics, 36*(1), 11–27. doi:10.1016/j.ucl.2008.08.004

Popovics, P., Schally, A., Salgueiro, L., Kovacs, K., & Rick, F. (2017). Antagonists of growth hormone -releasing hormone inhibit proliferation induced by inflammation in prostate epithelial cells. *Proceedings of the National Academy of Sciences of the United States of America, 114*(6), 1359–1364. doi:10.1073/pnas.1620884114

Roehrborn, C. G., Barkin, J., Siami, P., Tubaro, A., Wilson, T. H., Morrill, B. B., & Gagnier, R. P. (2011). Clinical outcomes after combined therapy with dutasteride plus tamsulosin or either monotherapy in men with benign prostatic hyperplasia (BPH) by baseline characteristics: 4-year results from the randomized, double-blind Combination of Avodart and Tamsulosin (CombAT) trial. *BJU International, 107*, 946–954. doi:10.1111/j.1464-410X.2011.10124.x

Sarma, A. V., & Wei, J. T. (2012). Benign prostatic hyperplasia and lower urinary tract symptoms. New England Journal of Medicine, 367, 248–257. doi:10.1056/NEJMcp1106637

Sosnowski, R. (2014). History of LUTS/BPO and evolution of concepts and terminology. In C. Chaple & A. Tubaro (Eds.), *Male LUTS/BPH made easy* (pp. 1–5). New York, NY: Springer.

Stone, B. V., Shoag, J., Halpern, J. A., Mittal, S., Lewicki, P., Golombos, D. M., ... Lee, R. K. (2017). Prostate size, nocturia and the digital rectal examination: a cohort study of 30 500 men. *BJU International, 119*(2), 298–304. doi:10.1111/bju.13613

Toren, P., Margel, D., Kulkarni, G., Finelli, A., Zlotta, A., & Fleshner, N. (2013). Effect of dutasteride on clinical progression of benign prostatic hyperplasia in asymptomatic men with enlarged prostate: A post hoc analysis of the REDUCE study. *BMJ, 346*, f2109. doi:10.1136/bmj.f2109

Unnikrishnan, R., Almassi, N., & Fareed, K. (2017). Benign prostatic hyperplasia: Evaluation and medical management in primary care. *Cleveland Clinic Journal of Medicine, 84*(1), 53–64. doi:10.3949/ccjm.84a.16008

Vahabi, M., & Lofters, A. (2016). Muslim immigrant women's views on cervical cancer screening and HPV self-sampling in Ontario, *Canada. BMC Public Health, 16,* 868. doi:10.1186/s12889-016-3564-1

Woodard, T. J., Manigault, K. R., McBurrows, N. N., Wray, T. L., & Woodard, L. M. (2016). Management of benign prostatic hyperplasia in older adults. *The Consultant Pharmacist®, 31*(8), 412–424. doi:10.4140/TCP.n.2016.412

Woods, V. D., Montgomery, S. B., Belliard, J. C., Ramírez-Johnson, J., & Wilson, C. M. (2004). Culture, black men, and prostate cancer: What is reality? *Cancer Control, 11*(6), 388–396. doi:10.1177/107327480401100606

CHAPTER 26

Controversies in PSA Screening

Michelle Lajiness and Susanne A. Quallich

■ INTRODUCTION

Prostate cancer is the number one cancer diagnosis in in North American men, and accounts for up to 28% of all cancers diagnosed in a given year. In 1980, risk of diagnosis of prostate cancer was 1 in 11. At present it is the most common noncutaneous cancer in U.S. men, and the risk of diagnosis is 1 in 6 men, with invasive prostate cancer cases representing 21% of all new cancers in men for 2016 (Siegel, Miller, & Jemal, 2016). Prostate cancer remains the leading cause of cancer death in men. Death rates have decreased over 40% in the last 20 years, and this decline has been closely associated with the use of the prostate-specific antigen (PSA) test for screening, and not just for monitoring treatment, as it was originally approved by the Food and Drug Administration (FDA). In the United States, more than 50% of men were screened annually (Draisma et al., 2003).

Owing to the aging population, society can anticipate a 45% increase in cancer detection by 2030 in the United States alone. Prostate cancer is affecting a larger proportion of the male population, and with increasing public awareness and improving detection methods, more men are seeking screening. Furthermore, prostate cancer is common comorbidity among men who are dying of other causes.

Early-stage prostate cancer is largely asymptomatic and found as a result of screening by digital rectal examination (DRE) and PSA testing. Specimens obtained during transrectal ultrasound-guided biopsy of the prostate provides a tissue diagnosis Gleason score, or a rating for the degree of differentiation of the prostate gland cells that describes the aggressiveness of the prostate tumor. An increased risk for prostate cancer is associated with more than two first-order relatives diagnosed with prostate cancer; and the finding of family members, such as grandfathers, with prostate cancer should raise the index of suspicion for that individual patient.

The true issue with prostate cancer is applying treatment selectively, allowing the timing and aggressiveness of treatment to reflect both disease and patient characteristics. It is promoting selective therapy that allows for early identification of men with higher grade cancer that may have been identified on the original diagnostic biopsy and avoiding overtreatment of those men whose cancer might never become clinically significant. Only a small proportion of prostate cancer patients die within 10 to 15 years of diagnosis. Ideally, life expectancy should guide treatment options, but estimation of life expectancy based on clinical impression is difficult and creates problems for assessment of prostate cancer treatment options.

■ SCREENING ISSUES

When widespread PSA screening began in the late 1980s, there was a ~70% increase in prostate cancer incidence (Siegel et al., 2016). PSA screening has all but doubled the chance that an individual man will be diagnosed with prostate cancer. There is an estimated 87% to 94%

overdiagnosis rate for prostate cancer due to the high prevalence of microfocal disease in otherwise healthy men, which has been reported from 30% to 70% (Carter et al., 2013). This wide range for prostate cancer prevalence is secondary to a number of factors:

- High incidence of latent prostate cancer in aging men
- Widespread availability of PSA test
- Screening results in identification of potentially lethal prostate cancer any curable stage
- Long-term effects of therapy

Debate continues to rage regarding the sensitivity and specificity for PSA, which is still under debate owing to this overall low specificity. Comorbid conditions can influence PSA accuracy for an individual; a higher body mass index (BMI) can lead to a lower PSA, and other physiological factors (e.g., insulin resistance, carbohydrate intake) can influence the PSA value as well. Furthermore, PSA alone cannot differentiate between indolent and lethal prostate cancer.

But screening probably misses the most aggressive cancers; the basic assumption with the use of PSA for screening that screening for early-stage disease prevents late-stage/metastatic disease may not be true. Screening may not be done frequently enough to detect lethal tumors and prevent death. Frequent screening also increases the risk that men will be overtreated, because the PSA and rectal examination combination cannot distinguish between minimal risk tumors and those posing risk, or those that may develop into more aggressive tumors. Up to 7% to 56% might never cause clinical symptoms (Heinsdijk et al., 2009) because of the low likelihood of "true" microfocal low-grade disease progressing to metastatic disease.

The three most common prostatic diseases—prostatitis, benign prostatic hyperplasia (BPH), and prostate cancer—can all be associated with elevations of serum PSA levels. But other factors can artificially elevate the PSA as well (Carter et al., 2013), making it vital to carefully assess the medical history before testing the PSA:

- Recent ejaculation
- DRE
- Physical activity, such as cycling or jogging
- Infection
- Medications

Medications can also suppress PSA levels, resulting in false-negative results on tests. Instrumentation (such as catheterization or minimally invasive prostate procedures) will increase PSA and therefore, such testing should be delayed 3 to 4 weeks. The PSA should always be repeated and treatment is rarely decided on one value.

Screening has increased local disease detection without a corresponding increase in regional disease detection. This has created increased costs related to the morbidity associated with any treatment for prostate cancer and contributed to overdetection and overtreatment of non-life-threatening disease, as well as quality of life issues after treatment. Screening can be proposed with some greater accuracy for individual men (Box 26.1) by investigating specific aspects of their medical and family histories. Social Security data for 2017 suggests that the average 65-year-old male lived to be 84 years old, but the life expectancy drops below 10 years by age 78. This highlights the importance of shared decision making regarding PSA screening for men who are 75 years or older.

Improved screening involves appropriate patient selection, shared decision making, risk stratification for individual patients, improved biopsy safety, and improved surveillance for men with low-risk disease. Risk stratification will improve the use of biomarkers specific to prostate cancer and newer technologies such as the MRI diffusion biopsy to

BOX 26.1 FACTORS CONTRIBUTING TO INCREASED RISK OF PROSTATE CANCER

- Increasing age
- Obesity
- African American (later stage at diagnosis)
- High dietary fat intake: increased risk with regular consumption of deep-fried foods (>1×/week)
- Cadimum exposure (cigarette smoke, batteries, welding)
- # First-degree relatives and age at onset
- More than two first-order relatives diagnosed with prostate cancer: Family members, such as grandfathers, with prostate cancer, should raise index of suspicion
- Gene for familial cancer is on chromosome 1
- Increased prevalence in farmers, commercial pesticide applicators
- Whole milk: increased risk of progression/death
- Increased mortality rate in areas with low ultraviolet light

improve both sensitivity and specificity of significant disease, while improving on the random biopsy.

BIG DATA STUDIES THAT EVALUATED PROSTATE CANCER SCREENING

There have been studies evaluating the utility of prostate cancer screening. Some of these studies enroll large numbers of men and immediately attempt to randomize the participants to an arm for screening or an arm for no screening. However, to date, none have provided definitive data on the utility of screening or recommended a conclusively productive screening interval.

- The U.S. PLCO (prostate, lung, colon, ovarian) study randomized 76,000 men from the ages of 55 to 74 for an annual PSA over 6 years and a rectal exam for 4 years, or an arm with no screening. This study was limited by the fact that 45% of enrolled men had had a baseline PSA and 52% of the control group had also undergone PSA screening. This study demonstrated more diagnoses of prostate cancer but no decrease in deaths over the 13-year follow-up of the study (Andriole et al., 2009; 2012; Crawford et al., 2010), suggesting that annual screening is not superior to episodic screening based on personal history.
- The European Screening Study (ERSPC) screened to 182,000 men every 4 years, and most men were followed over 11 years. This study reported a relative decrease in risk of prostate cancer death of 21% but the number of men who had to be screened to prevent one prostate cancer death was 1,055, and the number of that group who needed to be treated to prevent one death was 37 (Schröder et al., 2012). Screening above age 63 years was less cost effective because of loss of quality-adjusted life-years (QALY) due to overdiagnosis; most favorable results for screening cessation occurred below age 60 years. This study also reported only an incremental cost effectiveness of these strategies.
- Most recently, data from a Swedish study that began in 1994 that randomized 20,000 men to PSA testing every 2 years or men without PSA testing reported

a median follow-up over 18 years. This study also defined a threshold for PSA biopsy of 2.5–3.0 ng/mL. This study included a control group that did not get PSA screening, has the longest follow-up to date, and has the lowest PSA threshold for biopsy. A youth rate of death from prostate cancer was 1.5% in the control group and 1% in the group that was screened; men who are screened had a 42% lower risk of death from prostate cancer, and most choose surveillance rather than surgery or radiation therapy. This study reported that 139 men were needed to screen and only 1,380 to be diagnosed to prevent one death (Arnsrud, Holmberg, Lilja, Stranne, & Hugosson, 2015; Godtman et al., 2016).

The results of the population-based survey from National Health Interview Survey (NHIS) reviewed data from 2005, 2010, and 2013 and reported a trend toward increased PSA screening in elderly men and those with limited life expectancies. It also reported underscreening with PSA in younger men (Drazer, Huo, & Eggener, 2015). Recent abstracts (Aragon-Ching et al., 2016) have demonstrated a decline in PSA screening rates that has contributed to decline in diagnosis in older men and that the attitude of primary care providers suffers from confusion and disconnect about the value of any of the available guidelines (Rosenberg, Crawford, Newmark, & Steiner, 2016).

Population level data cannot establish causality of elevated PSA and eventual metastatic disease. However, the benefits of screening may extend to other quality-of-life and cost issues including a reduced morbidity rate from other symptoms such as bone pain, bladder outlet obstruction, and chronic hematuria. It may be that younger men might be more apt to proceed with screening (and possible eventual treatment), in light of their anticipated longer life expectancy. Older men may be more skeptical of screening, feeling that the trade-off with the potential side effects after treatment are not worth the potential changes to their quality of life.

DISCUSSING SCREENING WITH YOUR PATIENTS

Because of the PSA controversy, overall rates of PSA screening have been declining, in part because of the lack of consensus among professional societies (Table 26.1) and because of the unclear benefits for widespread population screening. This is not unreasonable, as prostate cancer is not a homogeneous disease that presents the same way in each patient. However, this controversy has left many men, their families, and their providers unclear about how best to proceed and when to proceed with screening. Life expectancy remains one of the key metrics when approaching the value of PSA screening for an individual. One of the key limitations to the existing evidence base is the benefit to screening in younger men (ages below 55); present data are limited in part due to sparse literature that extends follow-up in prostate cancer screening trials beyond 10 years. Despite the controversy the randomized studies that have evaluated the utility of PSA in screening have noted that screening allows men to be identified with a lower grade of cancer at diagnosis. Patients with less than 10-year life expectancy should not be screened, although all agencies acknowledge the difficulty in predicting this in otherwise healthy men.

Several potential adverse events and issues are associated with PSA screening (assuming elevation of PSA and eventual biopsy):

- False-positive tests, creating anxiety and uncertainty in men screened
- A positive test that suggests the president prostate cancer, leading to anxiety about choosing a treatment path
- Overdiagnosis of low-grade cancer that is unlikely to progress
- *Lead time,* or the average time by which screening promotes diagnosis among men who would otherwise have been diagnosed without screening

- Hematuria and/or hematospermia after biopsy
- Complications after biopsy such as infection or urinary difficulties
- Possible hospitalization after biopsy for significant infection

It is also important to note that data regarding the benefits of PSA screening include PSA both with and without DRE. A DRE is not useful as a primary screening test alone; however, it is useful in the context of an elevated PSA.

Shared Decision Making

The American Urological Association (AUA) supports shared decision making between clinician and individual patients when deciding to move forward with prostate cancer screening via a PSA test. This process allows for discussion in the valuation of not only the choice to proceed with the PSA test, but investigation of the potential outcomes of both positive and negative PSA tests. This process helps the patient to understand his choices, and potential outcomes of those choices, while providing the clinician with insight into the value system

TABLE 26.1 Clinical Management Guide With PSA Screening

Routine or urgent referral to a urologist	Degree of PSA elevation and/or Degree to which it has risen since previous PSA value (PSA velocity) Obstructive symptoms (BUN/Cr)
Signs	Early stages asymptomatic Symptoms suggest locally advanced or metastatic disease Obstructive or irritative voiding complaints Bone pain Disease to the vertebral column can result in spinal cord-related symptoms • Paresthesias • Lower extremity weakness • Urinary/fecal incontinence DRE mandatory • Induration • Bulky regional lymphadenopathy • Lower extremity lymphedema • Signs of cord compression
Possible laboratory findings (advanced disease)	Azotemia, if bilateral ureteral obstruction Anemia Alkaline phosphatase elevations Serum acid phosphatase elevations
Definitive diagnosis is made via prostate biopsy	Does not have the specification to rule out clinically important disease, regardless of definition Product of a biopsy gives minimum amount of disease that might be present, not the maximum Risk of morbidity and mortality due to infection after biopsy remains an issue, even with pre procedure antibiotics

BUN, blood urea nitrogen; Cr, creatinine; DRE, digital rectal examination; PSA, prostate-specific antigen.

of the individual. This process can be facilitated with patient decision aids, such as the one offered by the AUA on its website. Shared decision making promotes individual participation in screening and treatment choices and avoids the traditional paternalistic approach that can be seen in healthcare arenas. In this context the AUA (Carter et al., 2013) anticipates that shared decision making encourages discussions relative to

- Acknowledgment that no screening test is perfect
- The mortality benefit of PSA screening
- Description of options after an abnormal PSA test
- Likelihood of both false-positive and false-negative results
- Conclusion of the discussion of other tests that may be needed after an elevated PSA
- Potential harms of screening, such as infection after biopsy
- Providing information about the prostate gland itself
- Providing information about the incidence of prostate cancer and associated mortality risk
- Treatment options for both early and advanced prostate cancer
- Discussion of the complications of these treatment options
- Acknowledgment that the risk of dying from prostate cancer is approximately 3% over an individual man's life, and only a small subset will progress toward significant disease

CONCLUSION

The decision to screen a patient for prostate cancer is controversial, and even in the best of circumstances the perception of the need for screening and the impression of material are likely to be different between provider and patient (Talcott, Aharonoff, Bezuhly, & Osborne, 2016). Documentation of the discussion is paramount. Keep two things in mind when determining screening: (1) the patient's life expectancy should be greater than 10 years and (2) the provider should work toward ensuring that the patient (and any family member who may be present) understands the risks and benefits of screening and is making an informed choice.

CLINICAL PEARLS

- Always repeat a newly elevated PSA level.
- Don't automatically treat an elevated PSA with antibiotics in the absence of other symptoms.
- Stratify in individual man's risk based on his baseline PSA.
- Do not refer for prostate biopsy based only on an individual's PSA velocity in the absence of other indications, such as established risk factors (Box 26.1).
- When starting a job that may involve counseling and screening men with PSA testing, survey the facility and the community standards to determine which guidelines are being followed (Table 26.2). Because of the lack of consensus globally regarding PSA screening, the best policy from a medical-legal standpoint is to follow the guidelines that are prevalent within your place of work or community. For example, if working in a urology environment, the AUA guidelines would be the standard.
- Know when to *stop* screening.

TABLE 26.2 Summary of PSA Screening Guidelines by Organization

Organization	Baseline Testing (Age)	Invitation to Screening[a] (Age)	High-Risk Groups[b] (Age)	Screening Interval	PSA Threshold for Biopsy (ng/mL): Referral to Urology
American Cancer Society (2010)	None	Beginning at 50 years as long as life expectancy ≥ 10 years	Beginning at 40 years as long as expectancy ≥ 10 years	• Annually if PSA ≥ 2.5 ng/mL • Every 2 years if PSA < 2.5 ng/mL	• 2.5 ng/mL in select high-risk patients • 4.0 ng/mL in most patients
U.S. Preventive Services Task Force (2012)	None	None	None	None	None
American Urological Association (2013)	None	55–69 years	40–69 years	Every 2 years	None specified
European Association of Urology (2013)	40–45 years	Any age while life expectancy ≥ 10 years	Any age while life expectancy ≥ 10 years	• Every 2–4 years if baseline PSA > 1 ng/mL • Every 8 years if baseline PSA ≤ 1 ng/mL	None specified
American College of Physicians (2013)	None	50–69 years	40–69 years	Annually if PSA ≥ 2.5 ng/mL	None specified
National Comprehensive Cancer Network (2014)	45–49 years	50–70 years	Consider change in biopsy threshold; lower threshold to biospy to reflect risk stratification	• For 40–49 years: Every 1–2 years if PSA > 1 ng/mL	3.0 ng/mL *or*
		70–75 years as long as life expectancy ≥ 10 years		• Repeat at age 50 if PSA ≤ 1 ng/mL • For 50–70 years: Every 1–2 years	<3.0 ng/mL with excess risk based on established risk factors for prostate cancer

[a] For men who are well informed on the risks and benefits of PSA screening.

[b] African American race and first-degree relatives diagnosed with prostate cancer.

RESOURCES FOR PROVIDERS

American Urological Association Prostate Cancer Screening Decision Tool: www.urologyhealth.org/Documents/Product%20Store/Prostate-Cancer-Screening-Decision-tool-english.pdf
American Urological Association Guidelines: www.auanet.org/education/aua-guidelines.cfm
Centers for Disease Control and Prevention-Men's Health: www.cdc.gov/men/
National Institutes of Health—Men's Health: health.nih.gov/search_results.aspx?terms=Men%27s+Health; www.nlm.nih.gov/medlineplus/menshealth.html
Society of Urologic Nurses and Associates: www.SUNA.org

RESOURCE FOR PATIENTS

Is prostate screening right for me? Urology Care Foundation, www.urologyhealth.org/knowyourstats/take-the-test

REFERENCES

Andriole, G. L., Crawford, E. D., Grubb III, R. L., Buys, S. S., Chia, D., Church, T. R., ... Weissfeld, J. L. (2009). Mortality results from a randomized prostate-cancer screening trial. *New England Journal of Medicine, 360*(13), 1310–1319. doi:10.1056/NEJMoa0810696

Andriole, G. L., Crawford, E. D., Grubb III, R. L., Buys, S. S., Chia, D., Church, T. R., ... Weissfeld, J. L. (2012). Prostate cancer screening in the randomized Prostate, Lung, Colorectal, and Ovarian Cancer Screening Trial: Mortality results after 13 years of follow-up. *Journal of the National Cancer Institute, 104*(2), 125–132. doi:10.1093/jnci/djr500

Aragon-Ching, J. B., Hussey, H. M., Chen, D., Nguyen, H., Henson, D., & Simmens, S. (2016). Effects of PSA screening guidelines on trends of diagnosis and treatment for prostate cancer: Analysis from the National Cancer Data Base (NCDB). *Journal of Clinical Oncology, 34*(2 Suppl.), 74. doi:10.1200/jco.2016.34.2_suppl.74

Arnsrud, G. R., Holmberg, E., Lilja, H., Stranne, J., & Hugosson, J. (2015). Opportunistic testing versus organized prostate-specific antigen screening: outcome after 18 years in the Goteborg randomized population-based prostate cancer screening trial. *European Urology, 68*(3), 354–360. doi:10.1016/j.eururo.2014.12.006

Carter, H. B., Albertsen, P. C., Barry, M. J., Etzioni, R., Freedland, S. J., Greene, K. L., ... Zeitmen, A. L. (2013). *Early detection of prostate cancer: AUA Guideline*. Linthicum, MD: American Urological Association Education and Research.

Crawford, E. D., Grubb III, R., Black, A., Andriole Jr, G. L., Chen, M. H., Izmirlian, G., ... D'Amico, A. V. (2010). Comorbidity and mortality results from a randomized prostate cancer screening trial. *Journal of Clinical Oncology, 29*(4), 355–361. doi:10.1200/JCO.2010.30.5979

Draisma, G., Boer, R., Otto, S. J., van der Cruijsen, I. W., Damhuis, R. A., Schröder, F. H., & de Koning, H. J. (2003). Lead times and overdetection due to prostate-specific antigen screening: Estimates from the European Randomized Study of Screening for Prostate Cancer. *Journal of the National Cancer Institute, 95*(12), 868–878. doi:10.1093/jnci/95.12.868

Drazer, M. W., Huo, D., & Eggener, S. E. (2015). National prostate cancer screening rates following the 2012 United States Preventive Services Task Force recommendation discouraging prostate-specific antigen (PSA)-based screening. *Journal of Clinical Oncology, 33*(22), 2416–2423. doi:10.1200/JCO.2015.61.6532

Godtman, R. A., Holmberg, E., Khatami, A., Pihl, C. G., Stranne, J., & Hugosson, J. (2016). Long-term results of active surveillance in the Göteborg randomized, population-based prostate cancer screening trial. *European Urology, 70*(5), 760–766. doi:10.1016/j.eururo.2016.03.048

Heijnsdijk, E. A. M., der Kinderen, A., Wever, E. M., Draisma, G., Roobol, M. J., & De Koning, H. J. (2009). Overdetection, overtreatment and costs in prostate-specific antigen screening for prostate cancer. *British journal of cancer, 101*(11), 1833. doi:10.1038/sj.bjc.6605422

Rosenberg, M., Crawford, D., Newmark, J., & Steiner, M. (2016). MP39-01 use of PSA screening guidelines among primary care physicians. *The Journal of Urology*, *195*(4), e541. doi:10.1016/j.juro.2016.02.126

Schröder, F. H., Hugosson, J., Roobol, M. J., Tammela, T. L., Ciatto, S., Nelen, V., … Denis, L. J. (2012). Prostate-cancer mortality at 11 years of follow-up. *New England Journal of Medicine*, *366*(11), 981–990. doi:10.1056/NEJMoa1113135

Siegel, R. L., Miller, K. D., & Jemal, A. (2016). Cancer statistics, 2016. *CA: A Cancer Journal for Clinicians*, *66*(1), 7–30. doi:10.3322/caac.21332

Talcott, J. A., Aharonoff, G., Bezuhly, M., & Osborne, M. P. (2016). Do patients and physicians perceive PSA screening discussions the same? *Journal of Clinical Oncology*, *34*(2suppl), 160. doi:10.1200/jco.2016.34.2_suppl.160

CHAPTER 27

Male Infertility and Cryopreservation

Puneet Sindhwani, Zane Giffen, Ashwin Raghavan, and Tariq Shah

INTRODUCTION: EPIDEMIOLOGY AND ACCESS TO REPRODUCTIVE CARE

Infertility is generally defined as the inability of a couple to achieve pregnancy after 1 year of regular unprotected intercourse. According to the World Health Organization (WHO), 15% of couples are affected by infertility. In the United States, the prevalence of infertility is approximately 12% for men and 16% for women; however, the true prevalence of male infertility is unknown (Louis et al., 2013). Male factor infertility is present in 50% of couples affected by infertility, with men being the sole infertile partner in 20% of couples and a combined male and female factor present in 30% of couples (American Urological Association, 2010). Failure to obtain pregnancy has to be viewed as couples' disease. Unlike other health issues in which there is focus only on the evaluation and treatment of a patient presenting with a problem, an infertile couple requires evaluation of both partners.

Male infertility is often underrepresented epidemiologically and socially, even though it contributes to half of all infertile couples. This may be due to several reasons including cultural views toward male infertility as well as access to male reproductive care. It is the female partner who typically first seeks the infertility evaluation, which puts the onus of triaging these couples on the gynecologists. Most of these initial referrals are then directed to the reproductive endocrinologists. This may lead to primary evaluation of the female partner first, with male partner being evaluated only secondarily. In the United States, there is no national registry that systematically collects and organizes information regarding male reproductive health and access to reproductive care; therefore, information on the prevalence of infertility is based on limited sampling and the true prevalence of male fertility issues is not known. There is limited access to assisted reproductive technology (ART) centers for both men and women in underserved areas. Men of reproductive age are 2 to 2.5 times less likely to visit a medical professional for medical care in general and subsequently reproductive evaluation. This is compounded by the fact that men usually pay higher out-of-pocket costs due to limited insurance coverage or limited public funding for infertility treatment. Additionally, many medical practitioners in primary care practice and even in urological practice have limited training to recognize or evaluate male infertility; therefore, information about the prevalence of infertility is based on limited sampling and cannot be accurately reported.

In addition, there are some unique challenges that are faced by infertility patients (Pasch & Sullivan, 2017). There may be unrecognized socioeconomic, religious, or philosophical barriers that may need to be addressed in these couples. In many states insurances provide no or minimal coverage for diagnosis or treatment of male infertility. The financial burden on a younger couple who has not yet maximized their earning potential can be significant and can play a critical role in their decision making. Some of the assisted reproductive techniques can cost $12,000 to $25,000 per cycle. This does not include financial losses due to clinic visits, medical treatments, and lost wages. The repeated treatment cycles can accrue a large cumulative financial burden (Mottla, Richter, Kaplan, Hayward, & Mahony, 2017).

Unique social pressures due to expectations of fertility from the extended family such as parents and grandparents can exert external stressors on the relational dynamics of the couple. This may manifest as depression, anxiety, and interrelational strife. The social stigma attached with male infertility can prevent these patients from being seen in the infertility clinics (Fisher & Hammarberg, 2017). Some religious-philosophical barriers against in vitro manipulation of gametes may prevent some couples from seeking treatment. These beliefs may be personal, social, or sectarian. Some denominations may consider reproductive technologies unacceptable means to treat infertility (Mehta, Nangia, Dupree, & Smith, 2016). In some societies (sub-Saharan, Northern African) there is often greater cultural aversions to evaluation for male infertility as this is may be perceived as a diminution of male virility (Agarwal, Mulgund, Hamada, & Chyatte, 2015). In these cultures, women have developed religious coping mechanisms to deal with evaluation in these high stress situations (Oti-Boadi & Asante, 2017), as men may not undergo infertility testing readily. Polygamy or polyandry is common in some of these societies to bypass infertility or subfertility issues.

It is important to ask a patient about beliefs and/reservations toward masturbation, which might be needed for acquisition of semen samples (Pottinger, Carroll, & Mason, 2016). This discussion becomes very sensitive when the patient is a young pubescent male who may not be sexually active and is referred for cryopreservation prior to spermatotoxic treatments (Ramstein, Halpern, Gadzinski, Brannigan, & Smith, 2017). And, lastly, in many cultures and countries, there is no definite classification of male infertility as a disease, which presents difficulties in both quantifying, evaluating, and treating infertile men.

CLASSIFICATION OF MALE INFERTILITY

There are four different ways to classify male infertility (Wieder, 2014). The first category separates infertility based on a man having never been fertile (primary infertility) or previously having been fertile and presently having difficulty with impregnation (secondary infertility).

The second categorization is based on the site of a specific abnormality in the process of sperm production or transportation leading to infertility. These causes are broadly divided into:

1. Pretesticular causes of infertility (e.g., hypogonadotropic hypogonadism)
2. Testicular causes (e.g., Klinefelter syndrome)
3. Post-testicular causes (e.g., impaired delivery of sperms from testis to the female genital tract due to problems with obstruction, ejaculatory disorders, and abnormal penile anatomy)

Infertility can also be categorized by specific sperm parameters based on semen analysis. These include no sperm found in the ejaculate (azoospermia), impaired sperm concentration (oligospermia), impaired sperm motility (asthenospermia), abnormal sperm morphology (teratospermia), normal sperm parameters on semen analysis (normospermia), and no ejaculate (aspermia) (Kumar & Singh, 2015).

Another way to classify infertility is based on whether or not there is partial or complete obstruction of the genitourinary tract (obstructive) as opposed to a completely patent tract (nonobstructive) as evidenced by seminal volume. In the clinical setting, these classifications are commonly intermixed to give a complete picture of patient's infertility.

EMBRYOLOGY, ANATOMY, AND PHYSIOLOGY OF MALE FERTILITY

Development of the male genital tract is closely related to development of the urological tract. The ureteric bud gives rise to the ureter, renal pelvis and calyces, and distal collecting ducts. The Wolffian ducts develop into critical reproductive structures, which include the epididymis, vas deferens, seminal vesicles, and ejaculatory ducts. This development is mediated by testosterone, produced by Leydig cells in the testes. The portion of the bladder adjacent to the vas deferens later becomes the posterior urethra and moves the implantation site of the vas deferens to the verumontanum.

Testicular volume provides an estimation of sperm production, as the majority of the testis is constituted by seminiferous tubules, where spermatogenesis occurs. **Spermatogenesis** is the process by which spermatozoa are produced from spermatogonial stem cells present in the seminiferous tubules. This process takes approximately 74 to 80 days to complete. The first step is the division of the spermatogonia to make spermatocytes. This is followed by the meiotic division of spermatocytes to spermatids, which are haploid (contain half the genetic material). The third step that occurs, a process called **spermiogenesis,** involves conversion of spermatids to spermatozoa. Once formed, spermatozoa, or sperm, are transported to the epididymis through the rete testis and efferent ducts. Sperm maturation (acquisition of motility and capacity to fertilize) takes place in the epididymis. Sperm are then stored in the tail of the epididymis until ejaculation occurs.

The process of ejaculation consists of two phases: **emission and expulsion**. The first phase, emission, consists of the deposition of seminal fluid into the posterior urethra and closure of the bladder neck. This process is under sympathetic nervous system control (T12-L2). The process of emission can be impaired by injury to the sympathetic pathways, for example, iatrogenic injury during retroperitoneal lymph node dissection for testicular cancer. Expulsion is the second phase of ejaculation and is constituted by rhythmic contractions of the urethral muscular complex: the bulbospongiosus, ischiocavernosus, perineal, and levator muscles. This complex is supplied by sacral spinal cord (S2-S4) via the pudendal nerve.

In addition to the exocrine function of spermatogenesis, testes are also involved in the endocrine function due to steroidal hormonal excretion. The Leydig cells are responsible for testosterone production and do so under the influence of luteinizing hormone (LH). Pulsatile secretion of LH is in turn controlled by gonadotropin-releasing hormone (GnRH) from the hypothalamus. Sertoli cells, also called supporting or nursing cells, aid in the process of maturation of spermatogonia. This cell type is also critical in maintaining the blood-testis barrier. Sertoli cells are responsive to follicle-stimulating hormone (FSH) excretion and secrete inhibin, which exerts negative feedback on FSH production in males.

Testosterone, LH, and FSH are a few of the key hormones responsible for proper spermatogenesis. Secretion of these hormones can be affected by input from higher centers in the neurohormonal axis, medications like opioids, estrogen and its derivatives as well as by anabolic and sex steroids.

RISK FACTORS AND ETIOLOGY OF MALE INFERTILITY

Spermatogenesis is a finely tuned process. Production of healthy sperm in the ejaculate requires a functional neuroendocrine axis and the absence of significant chromosomal abnormalities, as well as functional urogenital anatomy. Any disruption of these elements may cause infertility and these disruptions can be categorized into four main classes (Punab et al., 2017):

1. Endocrine and systemic disorders
2. Primary testicular impairment of spermatogenesis

3. Sperm transportation and deposition disorders
4. Idiopathic infertility

A healthy hypothalamic-pituitary-gonadal (HPG) axis is required not only for proper development of male urogenital tract, but also for proper spermatogenesis and ultimately male fertility. Any disruption at this level, whether congenital or acquired, can present with male infertility in association with hormonal deficiency syndromes. These include multi-organ congenital disorders such as prune belly syndrome and congenital GnRH deficiency (Kallmann syndrome), acquired infertility from trauma/surgery, pituitary tumors, exogenous androgens/psychotropic drugs, and systemic disease such as diabetes mellitus and morbid obesity.

Primary testicular failure and impairment of sperm formation can also occur from both congenital and acquired causes. Congenital causes include genetic conditions such as Klinefelter syndrome (the most common genetic disorder associated with male infertility), androgen insensitivity syndrome, and myotonic dystrophy. Other congenital causes include failure of testicular descent (cryptorchidism) and deletions/mutations causing impairment of sperm morphology. Acquired disorders may be due to varicocele (the most common overall cause of male infertility), infections such as viral orchitis (e.g., postpuberty mumps) and epididymo-orchitis due to sexually transmitted diseases (STDs), and occupational exposure (Punab et al., 2017). Additionally, systemic illness such as hepatic cirrhosis, sickle cell disease, and celiac disease are known to be associated with testicular sperm impairment. Rarely, primary testicular malignancies can present with infertility (Chowdhary & Tiwari, 2016).

Sperm transport disorders can result from systemic disease that cause impairment of ciliary motion and sperm motility such as cystic fibrosis or Kartagener syndrome, or abnormalities in the urogenital tract (e.g., Young syndrome). Abnormalities in genitourinary anatomy causing obstruction (e.g., urethral strictures) can impair sperm translocation into the female genital tract. Additionally, abnormal physiology, present in ejaculatory disorders such as retrograde ejaculation, can reduce the amount of viable sperm available for fertilization to occur.

Exposure to chemicals (e.g., agricultural, volatile hydrocarbons, organic solvents, biphenyls), radiation (direct radiation to the testes or indirect scatter radiation during radiotherapy to surrounding organs, including the pituitary-hypothalamic area), hyperthermia (certain occupations with high temperature environments such as factory workers, varicocele), certain chronic infections or inflammatory states (e.g., epididymitis, orchitis, urethritis, or prostatitis), trauma (e.g., testicular rupture, testicle torsion, pelvic disruption), exposure to heavy metals (e.g., lead, mercury, cobalt, chromium, cadmium), and recreational agents (e.g., anabolic steroids, narcotic opioids, exogenous testosterone and supplements, tobacco, marijuana) have all been linked to male infertility (Chowdhary & Tiwari, 2016).

Certain iatrogenic risk factors for infertility can be easily overlooked. Previous surgical history in the area of pelvis, genitourinary tract, or testicles can predispose to infertility. A history of hernia repair, especially with the use of mesh, can induce intense scarring, which can lead to obstruction of the vas deferens. Vasectomy can cause obstruction not only at the site of surgery but also by causing proximal "blow-outs" in the epididymal tubules due to back pressure. Testicular torsion can cause ischemic damage and scarring of the involved testicle. Torsion or other testicular injuries can also affect sperm production in the contralateral testicle owing to breakdown of the blood-testis barrier and subsequent formation of antisperm antibodies.

Exposure to chemotherapeutic agents, particularly alkylating agents, can cause damage to DNA. Commonly used cytotoxic agents typically lead to transient oligospermia, teratospermia, or even azoospermia in a small percentage of patients. The damage can be long lasting and potentially permanent. Infertility has been reported in up to 46% of cancer survivors in a study done by Wasilewski-Masker et al. (2014). Certain pharmacological agents such as sulfasalazine, cyclosporine, ketoconazole, tetracyclines, and nitrofurantoin can also cause impaired spermatogenesis.

In some cases of male infertility, patients can have normal sperm parameters, normal ejaculatory volume, and no identifiable cause of extrinsic damage. These patients are labeled as having idiopathic infertility (American Urological Association, 2010). Defects in sperm DNA integrity and morphology are thought to be the cause of many of such cases, and genetic testing, ultrastructural studies, and chromatin assays may shed further light on the true cause.

EVALUATION OF THE INFERTILE MALE

The goal of the infertility evaluation is threefold. The primary objective is to identify, categorize, and if possible, treat any reversible causes of male infertility. In doing so, this can help with maximizing outcomes of assisted reproductive techniques from the male partner's standpoint. And finally, proper evaluation can identify conditions that can be detrimental to the patient's overall health, such as hypogonadism, unrecognized testicular cancer, or hypothalamic-pituitary issues. It is important to remember that men with infertility are at a higher risk of testicular cancer (2 to 20 times increased risk as compared to general population) and also at a higher risk of developing some other malignancies. Moreover, evaluation of male infertility may unmask underlying transmissible genetic abnormalities, such as cystic fibrosis. These can then help in deciding the need of doing preimplantation genetic diagnosis on the embryos and to use only the nonaffected embryos for implantation.

HISTORY

A detailed reproductive history and physical examination is the key to unmasking underlying causes of male infertility. Initial screening evaluation for infertility in a man should begin after pregnancy has not been achieved after a year of unprotected sexual intercourse. Evaluation can be started earlier if there are known male or female risk factors or if a patient questions his fertility status. Reproductive history and two properly performed semen analyses should be included within an initial evaluation. A full workup is warranted if there are any abnormalities. Additionally, further evaluation of a man is necessary if a couple presents with unexplained infertility after thorough workup of the female partner or if a female partner is treated and there is still persistent infertility (American Urological Association, 2010). These patients usually present independently, but often are referred by the gynecologist of the female partner.

A comprehensive infertility evaluation begins with a detailed history to elucidate potential factors contributing to the patient's infertility (Wieder, 2014). A clinician should first determine the duration of infertility (i.e., how long the couple has been trying to achieve pregnancy). It is important to establish if there has been prior evaluation or treatment for infertility. A male patient should be asked about past pregnancies with other partners. Sexual history should include couple's frequency of intercourse and coital timing to ensure that sperms are present in the female genital tract 2 days prior, on the day of, and 2 days after the ovulation. The use and type of lubricants are important to know as some commercial lubricants such as Vaseline, Surgilube, and K-Y Jelly can be spermatotoxic.

A brief reproductive history of the current partner is important to document. It is necessary to know the age of the female partner, any previous pregnancies with the same or different partner, and the outcome of those pregnancies. One should briefly inquire about any history of irregular menstrual cycles or pelvic inflammatory disease, use of ovulation kits, previous contraceptive methods, family history of early menopause, previous gynecological surgeries, and any prior gynecological workup.

Detailed sexual history including libido and quality of erections and orgasm should be discussed, as these can indicate any underlying endocrine issues. Any problems with ejaculation such as pain may indicate infection or inflammation. Absence of ejaculation after orgasm may be due to lack of emission, retrograde flow of semen into the bladder due to nonclosure of bladder neck, or ejaculatory duct obstruction. A change in the force of ejaculation, such as dripping ejaculation, may indicate obstruction due to a urethra stricture. Decreased libido, erectile dysfunction and loss of nocturnal erection can indicate hypogonadal state. The patient should be asked about any history of genitourinary infections, including STDs, urinary tract infections, postpuberty mumps, orchitis, epididymitis, or prostatitis.

Male patients may present with hormone-related symptoms that would require further workup for specific hormonal imbalances or underlying genetic disorders. These include morbid obesity, signs and symptoms of hypo- or hyperthyroidism, depression, gynecomastia, galactorrhea, hot flashes, sudden or progressive loss of libido, and loss of facial/body hair. Additionally, patients may present with chronic headaches or visual changes, which could indicate a pituitary tumor, or anosmia, which is associated with Kallmann syndrome. These patients may also have previous history of cleft lip/palate surgery. A broad review of systems should be collected, with specific attention to sexual and urinary symptoms, including hematospermia, as well as genital/abdominal pain or noted scrotal swelling. Scrotal swelling or a lump/mass should alert a clinician to the possible likelihood of malignancy, which should be appropriately evaluated.

A patient's past medical and surgical history can also provide key information as to the cause(s) of infertility. A clinician should determine if the patient has any current medical illness such as diabetes mellitus or other chronic systemic disease. A history of recurrent sinopulmonary infection may indicate cystic fibrosis, Kartagener syndrome, or Young syndrome, which are associated with infertility.

Additionally, a detailed surgical history should be obtained, with particular attention to surgery involving the inguinal and scrotal areas. This would include prior vasectomy or vasectomy reversal, inguinal hernia repair, orchiectomy, prostate surgery, as well as previous history of breast reduction for gynecomastia. The patient should be asked about any prior head trauma or trauma to the genitals, pelvis, or perineum. The patient's sexual developmental history should be documented, specifically the age of puberty, testicular descent, and facial/body hair development. Delayed puberty could indicate hypogonadism or Klinefelter syndrome. Any history of cryptorchidism or testicular torsion is important to note as well. Cryptorchidism in particular has been associated with decreased sperm production later in life; this is more detrimental in men with a history of bilateral undescended testicles.

A family history of infertility, genetic conditions associated with infertility/subfertility, or systemic diseases such as cystic fibrosis may provide further diagnostic information to the clinician. A recent history of febrile illness, surgical procedures under anesthesia especially within 1 to 3 months, or recent emotional stressor(s) can contribute to transient subfertility. The clinician should also inquire about conditions contributing to hyperthermia of the genitals, including sauna, hot tub, or frequent warm baths. The patient should be asked about tobacco, alcohol, and drug use/abuse (e.g., marijuana, opioids) as well as occupational exposures to pesticides and heavy metals. The clinician should review a complete list of the patient's current medications, both prescription and nonprescription, including herbal supplements and vitamins. The patient should also be questioned about current or prior radiation or cytotoxic chemotherapy treatment, exogenous testosterone or steroid use (e.g., anabolic steroids, corticosteroids), and drugs such as antipsychotics that may cause hyperprolactinemia.

PHYSICAL EXAMINATION

A general physical examination with emphasis on the male genitalia is an essential part of the evaluation of the infertile male. Key components of the exam include (American Urological Association, 2010):

1. Examination of the penis including the location of the urethral meatus
2. Assessment of the size and consistency of the testes
3. Presence and consistency of the vas deferens and epididymides
4. Presence of a varicocele
5. Digital rectal examination

The examiner should also take note of secondary sex characteristics including body habitus, hair distribution, and breast development (Practice committee of the American Society for Reproductive Medicine, 2015).

Examination of the scrotum is best performed in a warm room to allow for relaxation of scrotal skin. Cold temperatures or patient anxiety may lead to tightening of the scrotal skin, making examination and detection of varicoceles more difficult (Belay, Huang, Shen, & Ko, 2016). Assessment of suspected varicocele should include examination of the patient while both standing and supine. Examination in the supine position allows for the evaluation of the emptying of the dilated veins. A varicocele that does not empty with the patient supine raises concern for intra-abdominal obstruction of venous outflow. Similarly an isolated right-sided varicocele is unusual and may be a sign of retroperitoneal obstruction. These patients should be evaluated with cross-sectional abdominal imaging (Mittal et al., 2017). Palpation during Valsalva maneuver should also be performed, as the grading of varicoceles is based on the physical examination and early stages of varicocele may only be detected during Valsalva maneuvers. This maneuver can be performed by asking the patient to bear down and complete a forceful expiration against a closed airway. Care should be taken if the patient has an overactive vasovagal reflex or is prone to syncope with such maneuvers.

Assessing testicular volume is a key component of the physical exam. Normal testicular volume is greater than 15 to 20 mL (Mittal et al., 2017), and can be assessed clinically using an orchidometer or calipers. Testicular atrophy suggests hypogonadism or testicular damage. This can be due to environmental exposures or, more commonly, to varicocele. Testicular enlargement or the presence of a testicular mass should always be ruled out, as infertility may be the presenting symptom in a subset of patients with underlying testicular cancer. Testicular tenderness on palpation suggests an infectious process. Likewise, the epididymides should be palpated for tenderness suggestive of epididymitis. Epididymal cysts, or spermatoceles may be felt; these are usually benign and are seldom of any significance in terms of causing infertility.

A proper physical examination will also include palpation of the vas deferens bilaterally. Each testicle is placed on gentle downward traction with one hand while the other rolls the spermatic cord structures between the first and third fingers until a thin, rubbery, firm cord structure is palpated. One to 2% of men evaluated for infertility will have an absent vas deferens. Unilateral agenesis of the vas deferens (UAVD) can be associated with ipsilateral renal agenesis (Miller et al., 2016). Follow-up imaging with renal ultrasound may be considered to rule out renal abnormalities. Congenital bilateral absence of the vas deferens (CBAVD) is associated with cystic fibrosis and mutations of the cystic fibrosis transmembrane conductance regulator (CFTR) gene.

Digital rectal examination should be performed in all men. Palpation of a midline cystic structure on digital rectal examination may suggest the presence of a midline prostatic cyst, which may be a cause of ejaculatory duct obstruction (Cheng et al., 2015). Tenderness on exam indicates prostatitis which may result in pyospermia, and can impair sperm parameters. Symptomatic patients should be treated with antibiotics. Genitourinary tuberculosis is a major problem in Asia, and may account for 10% to 14% of presentations of extrapulmonary tuberculosis (Dikshit, Singh, Jadhav, & Nongmaithem, 2016). Involved organs may include the prostate, seminal vesicles, epididymis, or testes. Palpable, indurated seminal vesicles or beaded, firm vas deferens may suggest genitourinary tuberculosis infection.

Further scrotal imaging in the form of ultrasound testing may be beneficial in cases of limited physical examination due to obesity, tight scrotum, or scrotal scarring from prior surgeries. Ultrasound is noninvasive, safe, and offers views of testicular structures in multiple planes. Scrotal ultrasound imaging provides accurate testicular volumes, evaluates for testicular masses, and can identify varicoceles with high sensitivity and sensitivity in patients who have unfavorable scrotal anatomy or do not tolerate physical examination (Belay et al., 2016). The clinical significance of varicoceles that are not palpable (subclinical), however, has not been demonstrated (Practice committee of the American Society for Reproductive Medicine, 2015). Imaging with ultrasound identifies nonpalpable testicular masses in 0.8% to 7.4% of patients (Rocher et al., 2016). This may be especially important in patients with a history of an undescended testis or prior malignancy in the contralateral testis, both of which are associated with a higher risk of testicular malignancy.

DIAGNOSTIC TESTS

Initial laboratory evaluation of the infertile male should include semen analysis. Proper semen collection should involve sexual abstinence 48 to 72 hours prior to collection. Samples may be collected by masturbation or by intercourse using specially designed condoms that are not detrimental to sperm (American Urological Association, 2010). The sample should be kept at room temperature and be analyzed within 1 hour of collection. Two separate samples are required for proper analysis and diagnostics. Postejaculation urinalysis is recommended for patients with ejaculatory volume less than 1 mL to rule out retrograde ejaculation. Other causes of low ejaculate volume include ejaculatory duct obstruction, incomplete semen collection, or androgen deficiency. Complete absence of sperm, or azoospermia, should not be diagnosed until the patient's specimen is centrifuged for 15 minutes (American Urological Association, 2010). In additional to semen volume, semen analysis provides diagnostic information on sperm concentration, motility, and morphology.

Other important aspects of evaluation are serum studies, including FSH and testosterone levels, to unmask only hypothalamic-pituitary-testicular axis abnormalities. If testosterone levels are low, testing should be repeated, and prolactin and LH should be checked (American Urological Association, 2010). The sample ideally should collected after 6 to 8 hours of restful sleep, preferably between 8 a.m. and 11 a.m., as testosterone levels may vary significantly throughout the day. In patients with high prolactin levels or very low LH and FSH levels in presence of hypogonadism, it may be necessary to perform cross-sectional imaging of the brain with CT or MRI to rule out hypothalamic or pituitary lesions.

Genetic abnormalities may contribute to up to 20% of cases of azoospermia (Flannigan & Schlegel, 2017). Therefore, a chromosomal analysis or karyotype can be a useful adjunct to the infertility workup, especially in men with atrophic testes or elevated FSH levels. Testing for cystic fibrosis mutations should be conducted in patients with CBAVD. Moreover, up to 15% of men with azoospermia or severe oligospermia have small deletions in the long arm of the Y chromosome called Y chromosome microdeletions. These deletions are labeled *AZF* (azoospermia factor region) a, b, and c. *AZFc* microdeletions are the most common form, and are favorable to surgical sperm retrieval techniques; 50% to 60% of men with *AZFc* deletions ultimately have successful sperm retrieval (Flannigan & Schlegel, 2017). In contrast, sperm retrieval is not feasible in men with *AZFa* or *AZFb* deletions.

A number of procedures are available to retrieve semen from patients who are anejaculatory due to neurological injury. Penile vibratory stimulation (PVS) involves applying personal vibratory devices to the glans penis to induce ejaculation. It requires an intact ejaculatory reflex (T10-S4). PVS is the recommended first-line treatment for anejaculatory men with spinal cord injury (SCI) and achieves high ejaculatory rates (Chong, Ibrahim, Aballa, Lynne, & Brackett, 2017). In contrast to PVS, electroejaculation (EEJ) can be used at all spinal cord injury levels. For EEJ, a probe containing electrodes is placed in the rectum and directed toward the prostate, and direct current (DC) is delivered until ejaculation occurs. Some degree of retrograde ejaculation typically occurs, and a postprocedure catheterized urine specimen may be the only source of available semen (Ibrahim, Lynne, & Brackett, 2015). In all procedures involving SCI patients, those at risk for autonomic dysreflexia should be pretreated with nifedipine (Ibrahim et al., 2015).

In patients suspected to have ejaculatory duct obstruction as evidenced by low volume ejaculate with acidic pH and semen negative for fructose, transrectal ultrasound imaging may be required to evaluate for midline prostatic cysts, dilated seminal vesicles, or ejaculatory ducts.

MANAGEMENT

Management of infertility depends upon the underlying cause. A discussion with patients about lifestyle modification and diet should be the starting point regardless of specific cause. Behavioral modifications include cessation of tobacco, exogenous androgenic supplements, opioid narcotics, and marijuana use. Additionally, adopting an active lifestyle and maintaining a healthy body mass index (BMI) (ideally 20–25 kg/m^2) promote sperm health and viability (Kahn & Brannigan, 2017). Approximately 4 to 6 hours per week of aerobic exercise has also been associated with improved semen parameters.

Diet and Fertility

It is difficult to recommend a specific diet for improving fertility as there are no large randomized controlled trials that evaluate/compare specific diets. Anecdotal studies have shown some benefits with certain supplements. These should be recommended to patients with caution, as most supplements are not standardized or regulated, and the potential for harm may exist if there are contaminants such as heavy metals or androgenic steroids.

Dairy intake and semen quality has been controversial and conflicting. In a recent study published by Afeiche, Bridges et al. (2014), 155 men were prospectively evaluated to look at dietary intake of dairy products and semen parameters (2014). The authors of this study concluded that a low-fat dairy intake was positively related to sperm concentration and progressive motility, whereas cheese intake was related to lower sperm concentration among past or current smokers. Another study by Vujkovic et al. (2009), however, failed to show this correlation. In another study by Afeiche, Gaskins, et al. (2014) correlating meat, poultry, and fish intake to semen analysis parameters, various forms of processed red meat had a weak negative effect on sperm morphology, whereas fish intake was positively correlated to improved sperm density and morphology.

In a comprehensive review published in 2017 by Salas-Hueto, Bulló, M., and Salas-Salvadó (2017), the authors concluded that in general diets rich in omega-3 fatty acids and antioxidants (e.g., beta carotene, vitamin E, vitamin C, lycopene, and folate) and low in saturated fatty acids and transfatty acids were inversely associated with low semen quality parameters.

Diets rich in processed meats, potatoes, coffee, alcohol, sweetened beverages, and sweets had a negative impact on semen quality. High intake of alcohol, caffeine, and red meat by males had a negative influence on fertilization rates in their partners.

Ahmadi et al. performed a literature review evaluating antioxidant supplementation and its effect on male infertility (Ahmadi, Bashiri, Ghadiri-Anari, & Nadjarzadeh, 2016). They concluded that the combination of antioxidants including vitamin C, vitamin E, and CoQ10 intake improved semen parameters. However, in other studies, the impact of these antioxidants was minimal, especially when taken individually. In general, a heart-healthy diet is a fertility-friendly diet.

TREATMENT OPTIONS

As mentioned previously, the most common reversible cause of infertility found is varicocele. Varicocele is the dilation of the pampiniform plexus of veins in the scrotum. It can be found in up to 40% to 60% of men with subfertility or infertility. It can present with dull aching pain, which is worse after prolonged standing/strenuous activity, or in many patients it can be totally asymptomatic. It is most commonly seen on the left side and can be associated with the ipsilateral loss of volume of the testicle. Varicoceles can be graded as grades 1 to 3, or mild, moderate, and severe. Grade 1 varicocele is usually palpated with Valsalva maneuver, grade 2 is palpable without Valsalva maneuver, and grade 3 is a visible varicocele. Subclinical varicoceles (grade 0) are found incidentally on scrotal ultrasound imaging only. These are usually not of clinical significance and repair is not indicated. Varicoceles can affect parameters of sperm function and quality. Patients may present with oligospermia, asthenospermia, teratospermia, or a combination of all these abnormalities. Some of these patients may have low testosterone levels as well. Treatment for this condition is surgical correction via open, laparoscopic, or microscopic approach. Intervention radiological coiling has been done in some European countries but may have higher failure rates. Varicocelectomy involves ligation of dilated veins in the spermatic cord, sparing the testicular artery and typically three to five lymphatics. Common complications are recurrence, bleeding, and formation of hydrocele after the surgery. Procedure is typically performed in an outpatient setting. By using magnification intraoperatively, using micro-Doppler probe and a subinguinal approach, the recurrence rates and hydrocele formation can be minimized (less than 1% chance). This approach avoids muscle cutting and is associated with less pain than muscle-splitting approaches. Postoperatively using ice pack to the scrotum, use of scrotal support, and avoiding heavy lifting more than 10 pounds and straining can further decrease the convalescence. Improvement in sperm parameters can be seen in as early as 3 months. Serial semen analyses are recommended every 3 months at intervals at 3, 6, and 9 months postoperatively (American Urological Association, 2010).

In patients with specific hormonal abnormalities, treatment can be targeted medically toward the underlying defect. Patients with hypogonadotropic hypogonadism may benefit from treatment with human chorionic gonadotropin (hCG) with or without human menopausal gonadotropin (hMG). Nonspecific antiestrogenic agents such as clomiphene in select patients can increase testosterone and transiently improve sperm concentrations. However, a clinician should be aware that this is an off-label use of clomiphene, and should be used with informed patient consent and under close physician supervision. In patients who have low testosterone and high estradiol levels, treatment with anastrozole may also restore hormonal balance temporarily. This medication inhibits peripheral conversion of testosterone into estrogen at the level of adipocytes.

If men present with high levels of prolactin, other causes of hyperprolactinemia should be investigated. These include hepatic, iatrogenic (due to medication), or chronic stress.

If this elevation persistents on repeat laboratory evaluation, cross-sectional imaging of the pituitary hypothalamic area should be done (see *Evaluation of the Infertile Male*). In patients with pituitary microadenoma and mild hyperprolactinemia, dopamine agonists such as cabergoline can be used. Patients with larger tumors of the pituitary need referral for transnasal ablation.

In select patients with retrograde ejaculation, medications that cause contraction of the bladder neck (e.g., pseudoephedrine or imipramine) can help some patients to reestablish antegrade ejaculation. In other patients, penile vibratory stimulus or electroejaculation with bladder wash can be used to retrieve sperm (see *Diagnostic Tests*). Transurethral resection of ejaculatory duct may be required in select patients who have midline cysts or obstruction, but this can create issues with retrograde ejaculation.

Testicular biopsy in isolation is usually not performed. A diagnostic biopsy may be needed in patients who have nonobstructive azoospermia with normal hormones and normal testicular examination. In azoospermic patients with ejaculatory duct obstruction, biopsy may be used to confirm spermatogenesis. It is advisable to combine biopsy with simultaneous sperm cryopreservation if possible.

Sperm retrieval from the testicle can be performed either percutaneously using fine-needle aspiration, or by incising the testicle to create a window through which the seminiferous tubules are excised. In patients with Klinefelter syndrome, microscopic testicular sperm extraction may be required.

In patients with previous history of vasectomy, a reversal can be offered, especially if the patient is within 8 years of the original procedure. During the reversal, freshened ends of both vasa can be anastomosed together (vasovasostomy), or the vas can be anastomosed to the smaller tubules in the epididymis, which is known as vasoepididymovasostomy. These procedures can be done in conjunction with sperm retrieval and cryopreservation.

In male patients when there are no options of fathering a biological child, there are still other options available to become a parent. One should discuss options of artificial insemination using donor sperm, child adoption, or embryo adoption.

SEMEN CRYOPRESERVATION

Current and evolving therapeutic regimens of chemotherapy and radiation therapy have improved survival for a majority of young adults diagnosed with a wide variety of cancers. In these patients, spermatogenesis can be adversely affected as a result of both the disease and the treatment (Shah & Keye, 2005). Because these patients are now surviving and leading healthy and productive lives, sperm preservation should be considered prior to cancer treatment, if possible (Wasilewski-Masker et al., 2014).

With recent advances in assisted reproductive technologies (including cryopreservation technology), it has become possible for male cancer survivors to have children after using sperm derived from their ejaculated samples or from testicular tissues cryopreserved before the onset of anticancer treatments. It has been recommended that all male patients of reproductive age who are at risk for loss of testicular function and who may desire children in the future should cryopreserve sperm prior to initiation of therapy (Loren et al., 2013). Sperms lack cytoplasm and hence are less susceptible than normal cells by freezing. Healthy sperms can successfully withstand freezing and thawing without incurring damage to their function in the future.

Only a few spermatozoa are needed for successful in vitro fertilization with the intracytoplasmic sperm injection (ICSI) procedure, from fresh or frozen samples. Male patients between the ages of 14 to 50 are usually eligible for cryopreservation. Fertility preservation is not just available for oncology patients receiving anticancer therapies, patients with some rheumatic diseases such as lupus, rheumatoid arthritis, or Crohn's disease can also have their sperm sample cryopreserved. In addition, patients facing bone marrow or stem cell transplantation for hematological diseases or those seeking gender reassignment can also access and benefit from these technologies.

Fertility preservation laws are state specific and closely regulated. Patients must be counseled properly in common aspects of cryopreservation, especially regarding the descendant's ownership of the sample; and in the event of death, policies regarding disposition of the sample if they lose contact with the clinic or fail to pay for the storage of the sample.

This requires close cooperation and coordination among caregivers across multiple specialties including social workers, counselors, and financial coordinators. Historically, a major barrier in implementation of cryopreservation technology has been lack of awareness about the emerging trends in fertility preservation among oncologists, pathologists, and oncology nurses. Recently, however, there is a growing awareness among specialists about the importance of counseling patients regarding the effects of cancer treatments on fertility and the available options for the fertility preservation. In addition, there is an increasing recognition of role of oncology social workers. They typically are the primary source of psychosocial services and often develop long-term relationships with patients through prolonged recovery periods (King et al., 2008).

It is of paramount importance that specialists discuss fertility preservation with all patients of reproductive age as well as with those who have not yet attained reproductive maturity. Conversations about fertility preservation can be particularly difficult with prepubertal boys. Under these circumstances, specialists should have candid conversations with the parents or guardians. Clinicians should also be mindful of religious and cultural nuances in these matters, since a great diversity exits across cultures on how to deal with matters of life and death, paternity, and posthumous procreation.

CONCLUSION

Male infertility is a topic to which few providers may be exposed in the course of their healthcare training. Problems of male infertility can seem minor within the larger realm of urology and men's health; but infertility is a disease of the reproductive system that can be presenting symptoms of a serious underlying health problem, and treating it is not addressing an inconvenience or an indulgence. Providers should feel comfortable addressing basic male and female reproductive health questions, and referring men to a male infertility specialist or an andrologist for additional evaluation. Failure to establish paternity can impact mental well-being and social standing in some communities, highlighting that a full evaluation and treatment is vital to an individual's overall quality of life.

CLINICAL PEARLS

- Male infertility is a hidden issue within the context of overall fertility care, and evaluation can be initiated if the male or couple is concerned about their fertility status.
- Research from disciplines such as social work, psychology, and anthropology reports that the overall infertility experience marginalizes the experience and role of men.
- Fertility evaluation may be the first time men have contact with the healthcare system as adults.

(continued)

CLINICAL PEARLS (*continued*)

- The goal of the male fertility evaluation is to identify any potentially reversible, treatable causes.
- Most medical therapies for men are empiric, but medical management can be successful if a specific contributing factor is identified.
- Because sperms take approximately 90 days to grow and mature, follow-up for male fertility treatment occurs every 3 months.
- The precise mechanism by which obesity influences male fertility is unknown.

RESOURCES FOR THE CLINICIANS

American Urological Association Best Practice Statement: Optimal Evaluation of the Infertile Male: www.auanet.org/guidelines/male-infertility-optimal-evaluation-(reviewed-and-validity-confirmed-2011)
American Society for Reproductive Medicine: www.reproductivefacts.org
Diagnostic Evaluation of the Infertile Male: A Committee Opinion. American Society for Reproductive Medicine: www.asrm.org/globalassets/asrm/asrm-content/news-and-publications/practice-guidelines/for-non-members/diagnostic_evaluation_of_the_infertile_male_a_committee_opinion-noprint.pdf
Fertility Preservation for Patients with Cancer: American Society of Clinical Oncology Clinical Practice Guideline Update. (2013). *Journal of Clinical Oncology. 31*(19), 2500–2510.
Neiderberger, C. S. (2016). Male infertility. In: A. J. Wein (Ed.). *Campbell-Walsh Urology* (pp. 556–579). (11th ed.). Philadelphia, PA: Elsevier.

RESOURCES FOR THE PATIENTS

American Society for Reproductive Medicine: www.reproductivefacts.org
Anawalt, B. D., Page, S. T. (2017). Patient information: Treatment of male infertility (Beyond the basics). In: Snyder, P. J., (ed.). *UpToDate*. Waltham, MA: UpToDate. www.uptodate.com/contents/treatment-of-male-infertility-beyond-the-basics
RESOLVE: The National Infertility Association: www.resolve.org
Urology Care Foundation. Male Infertility: www.urologyhealth.org/urologic-conditions/male-infertility

REFERENCES

Afeiche, M. C., Bridges, N. D., Williams, P. L., Gaskins, A. J., Tanrikut, C., Petrozza, J. C., … Chavarro, J. E. (2014). Dairy intake and semen quality among men attending a fertility clinic. *Fertility and Sterility, 101*(5), 1280–1287. doi:10.1016/j.fertnstert.2014.02.003
Afeiche, M. C., Gaskins, A. J., Williams, P. L., Toth, T. L., Wright, D. L., Tanrikut, C., … Chavarro, J. E. (2014). Processed meat intake is unfavorably and fish intake favorably associated with semen quality indicators among men attending a fertility clinic. *The Journal of Nutrition, 144*(7), 1091–1098. doi:10.3945/jn.113.190173
Agarwal, A., Mulgund, A., Hamada, A., & Chyatte, M. R. (2015). A unique view on male infertility around the globe. *Reproductive Biology and Endocrinology, 13*(37), 1–9. doi:10.1186/s12958-015-0032-1
Ahmadi, S., Bashiri, R., Ghadiri-Anari, A., & Nadjarzadeh, A. (2016). Antioxidant supplements and semen parameters: An evidence based review. *International Journal of Reproductive Biomedicine, 14*(12), 729–736. doi:10.29252/ijrm.14.12.729

American Urological Association. (2010). *The optimal evaluation of the infertile male: AUA Best Practice Statement*. Retrieved from http://www.auanet.org/guidelines/male-infertility-optimal-evaluation-(reviewed-and-validity-confirmed-2011)

Belay, R. E., Huang, G. O., Shen, J. K., & Ko, E. Y. K. (2016). Diagnosis of clinical and subclinical varicocele: How has it evolved? *Asian Journal of Andrology, 18*, 182–185. doi:10.4103/1008-682X.169991

Cheng, G., Bianjiang, L., Song, Z., Xu, A., Song, N., & Wang, Z. (2015). A novel surgical management for male infertility secondary to midline prostatic cyst. *BMC Urology, 15*, 18. doi:10.1186/s12894-015-0015-8

Chong, W., Ibrahim, E., Aballa, T. C., Lynne, C. M., & Brackett, N. L. (2017). Comparison of three methods of penile vibratory stimulation for semen retrieval in men with spinal cord injury. *Spinal Cord, 55*, 921–925. doi:10.1038/sc.2017.60

Chowdhary, R., & Tiwari, B. (2016). Understanding male infertility and its causes: A review. *International Journal of Biomedicine Research, 7*(10), 702–707. doi:10.7439/ijbr

Dikshit, V., Singh, G., Jadhav, D., & Nongmaithem, M. (2016). Tuberculosis epididymitis masquerading as acute scrotal abscess. *International Surgery Journal, 3*(3), 1674–1676. doi:10.18203/2349-2902.isj20162774

Fisher, J., & Hammarberg, K. (2017). Psychological aspects of infertility among men. *Endocrinology of the Testis and Male Reproduction, 1*, 1287. doi:10.1007/978-3-319-44441-3_46

Flannigan, R., & Schlegel, P. (2017). Genetic diagnostics of male infertility in clinical practice. *Best Practice and Research Clinical Obstetrics and Gynecology, 44*, 26–37. doi:10.1016/j.bpobgyn.2017.05.002

Ibrahim, E., Lynne, C. M., & Brackett, N. L. (2015). Male fertility following spinal cord injury: An update. *Andrology, 4*(1), 13–26. doi:10.1111/andr.12119

Kahn, B. E., & Brannigan, R. E. (2017). Obesity and male infertility. *Current Opinion in Urology, 27*(5), 441–445. doi:10.1097/MOU.0000000000000417

King, L., Quinn, G. P., Vadaparampil, S. T., Miree, C. A., Wilson, C., Clayton, H., & Zebrack, B. (2008). Oncology social workers' perceptions of barriers to discussing fertility preservation with cancer patients. *Social Work in Health Care, 47*(4), 479–501. doi:10.1080/00981380802255215

Kumar, N., & Singh, A. K. (2015). Trends of male factor infertility, an important cause of infertility: A review of literature. *Journal of Human Reproductive Sciences, 8*(4), 191–196. doi:10.4103/0974-1208.170370

Loren, A. W., Mangu, P. M., Beck, L. N., Brennan, L., Magdalinski, A. J., Partridge, A. H., Quinn, G., … Oktay, K. (2013). Fertility preservation for patients with cancer: American Society of Clinical Oncology clinical practice guideline update. *Journal of Clinical Oncology, 31*(19), 2500–2510. doi:10.1200/JCO.2013.49.2678

Louis, J. F., Thoma, M. E., Sørensen, D. N., McLain, A. C., King, R. B., Sundaram, R., … Buck Louis, G. M. (2013). The prevalence of couple infertility in the United States from a male perspective: Evidence from a nationally representative sample. *Andrology, 1*(5), 741–748. doi:10.1111/j.2047-2927.2013.00110.x

Mehta, A., Nangia, A. K., Dupree, J. M., & Smith, J. F. (2016). Limitations and barriers in access to care for male factor infertility. *Fertility and Sterility, 105*(5), 1128–1137. doi:10.1016/j.fertnstert.2016.03.023

Miller, S., Couture, S., James, G., Plourde, S., Rioux, J., & Labrecque, M. (2016). Unilateral absence of vas deferens: Prevalence among 23,013 men seeking vasectomy. *International Brazilian Journal of Urology, 42*(5), 1010–1017. doi:10.1590/S1677-5538.IBJU.2015.0717

Mittal, P. K., Little, B., Harri, P. A., Miller, F. H., Alexander, L. F., Kalb, B., … Moreno, C. C. (2017). Role of imaging in the evaluation of male infertility. *RadioGraphics, 37*, 837–854. doi:10.1148/rg.2017160125

Mottla, G. L., Richter, K. S., Kaplan, B., Hayward, B., & Mahony, M. C. (2017). Treatment decision trends in the infertility patient journey from 78,958 cycles in a real-world database: Impact of age, diagnosis, and year of treatment. *Fertility and Sterility, 107*(3), e41. doi:10.1016/j.fertnstert.2017.02.078

Oti-Boadi, M., & Asante, K. O. (2017). Psychological health and religious coping of Ghanaian women with infertility. *BioPsychoSocial Medicine, 11*(1), 20. doi:10.1186/s13030-017-0105-9

Pasch, L. A., & Sullivan, K. T. (2017). Stress and coping in couples facing infertility. *Current Opinion in Psychology, 13*, 131–135. doi:10.1016/j.copsyc.2016.07.004

Pottinger, A. M., Carroll, K., & Mason, G. (2016). Male attitude towards masturbating: An impediment to infertility evaluation and sperm parameters. *Andrologia, 48*, 774–778. doi:10.1111/and.12511

Practice committee of the American Society for Reproductive Medicine. (2015). Diagnostic evaluation of the infertile male: A committee opinion. *Fertility and Sterility, 103*(3), 18–25. doi:10.1016/j.fertnstert.2014.12.103

Punab, M., Poolamets, O., Paju, P., Vihljajev, V., Pomm, K., Ladva, R., … Laan, M. (2017). Causes of male infertility: A 9-year prospective monocentre study on 1737 patients with reduced total sperm counts. *Human Reproduction, 32*(1), 18–31. doi:10.1093/humrep/dew284

Ramstein, J. J., Halpern, J., Gadzinski, A. J., Brannigan, R. E., & Smith, J. F. (2017). Ethical, moral, and theological insights into advances in male pediatric and adolescent fertility preservation. *Andrology, 5*(4), 631–639. doi:10.1111/andr.12371

Rocher, L., Ramchandani, P., Belfield, J., Bertolotto, M., Derchi, L. E., Correas, J. M., … Richenberg, J. (2016). Incidentally detected non-palpable testicular tumors in adults at scrotal ultrasound: Impact of radiological findings on management. Radiologic review and recommendations of the ESUR scrotal imaging subcommittee. *European Radiology, 26*, 2268–2278. doi:10.1007/s00330-015-4059-7

Salas-Huetos, A., Bulló, M., & Salas-Salvadó, J. (2017). Dietary patterns, foods and nutrients in male fertility parameters and fecundability: A systematic review of observational studies. *Human Reproduction Update, 23*(4), 371–389. doi:10.1093/humupd/dmx006

Shah, T. A., & Keye, W. R. (2005). Fertility: Tissue and cell banking overview. *Clinics in Laboratory Medicine, 25*(3), 557–569. doi:10.1016/j.cll.2005.06.007

Vujkovic, M., de Vries, J. H., Dohle, G. R., Bonsel, G. J., Lindemans, J., Macklon, N. S., … Steegers-Theunissen, R. P. (2009). Associations between dietary patterns and semen quality in men undergoing IVF/ICSI treatment. *Human Reproduction, 24*(6), 1304–1312. doi:10.1093/humrep/dep024

Wasilewski-Masker, K., Seidel, K. D., Leisenring, W., Mertens, A. C., Shnorhavorian, M., Ritenour, C. W., … Robison, L. L. (2014). Male infertility in long-term survivors of pediatric cancer: A report from the childhood cancer survivor study. *Journal of Cancer Survivorship, 8*(3), 437–447. doi:10.1007/s11764-014-0354-6

Wieder, J. A. (2014). *Pocket guide to urology* (5th ed., pp. 419–450). Berkeley, CA: Author.

CHAPTER 28

Male UCPPS and Orchialgia

Susanne A. Quallich

INTRODUCTION

Historically, the term "prostatitis" has been used nonspecifically to describe genital or pelvic discomfort in men. There may or may not be lower urinary tract symptoms or sexual complaints present. Management of men with prostatic-urethral and/or pelvic pain and/or pain on voiding (dysuria) is a problematic and frustrating clinical entity. The clinician must identify potential specific causes, excluding an infectious or malignant cause. But the majority of men with prostatic pain (approximately 90%) do not have an identifiable infective etiology, resulting in classification as chronic pelvic pain syndrome (CPPS) (Clemens et al., 2015).

Prostatitis (inflammation of the prostate gland) and urological chronic pelvic pain syndrome (UCPPS) represent a complex problem ranging from an acute and possibly life-threatening bacterial infection to a challenging set of chronic and debilitating symptoms that can defy effective treatment and degrade quality of life. Prostatitis is a common genitourinary infection affecting 10% to 15% of all men (Pontari, 2015), although this incidence is wholly dependent on how prostatitis is defined. Younger and middle-aged men present for evaluation more commonly, and it is the presenting complaint responsible for up to 25% of all urology office visits (Nguyen, 2014; Wagenlehner, Weidner, Pilatz, & Naber, 2014). Prostatitis was classified into four categories by the National Institutes of Health (NIH) in 1999 (Krieger, Nyberg, & Nickel, 1999; Table 28.1).

(UCPPS until recently was evaluated from only a urology perspective. This resulted in a record of unpredictable results and poor treatment success (Clemens, 2014). But a contemporary shift in focus, due to large epidemiological studies (Multidisciplinary Approach to the Study of Chronic Pelvic Pain [MAPP]), pointed toward the possibility of an underlying chronic pain syndrome in patients with UCPPS (Krieger et al., 2014). Treating UCPPS from only the urology perspective did not take into account the multifactorial nature of what eventually would be identified as a chronic pain, not urologic, condition. A shift in focus from a strictly urology component of UCPPS included related disciplines (basic scientists, epidemiologists, pain specialists, neuroimaging, translational animal models) and refocused the investigation into the etiology of UCPPS in men and women, allowing for potential systemic syndromes that may have a relationship with UCPPS. Exploration of UCPPS through application of the principles of chronic pain resulted in progress toward identification of characteristics that UCPPS patients shared with other chronic pain populations. Two phenotypes of UCPPS patients have been identified, one with bladder-focused symptoms and one with more systemic, centralized pain (Clemens, 2014; Krieger et al., 2014). Clemens et al. (2015) reported that perineal pain appears to be a defining characteristic in male UCPPS.

TABLE 28.1 National Institutes of Health (NIH) Classification of Prostatitis

Description	NIH Designation	Clinical Presentation
Acute bacterial prostatitis	Type I	Acute symptoms + bacterial infection
Chronic bacterial prostatitis (CP)	Type II	Recurrent symptoms + documented bacterial infection with same organism
Chronic prostatis/chronic pelvic pain syndrome (CPPS)	Type III	Chronic, intermittent, or recurrent urogenital symptoms > 3 months No evidence of bacterial infection
Chronic prostatis/chronic pelvic pain syndrome (CPPS)	Type IIIa: inflammatory	Semen and prostate secretion leukocytes Inflammation, but no infection
	Type IIIb: noninflammatory (previous term: prostatodynia)	No semen and prostate secretion leukocytes No inflammation or infection
Asymptomatic	Type IV	No symptoms Incidental finding (e.g., with prostate biopsy) No treatment necessary

Source: Krieger, J. N., Nyberg, L., & Nickel, J. C. (1999). NIH consensus definition and classification of prostatitis. *JAMA, 282*(3), 236–237. doi:10-1001/pubs.JAMA-ISSN-0098-7484-282-3-jac90006

ACUTE PROSTATITIS

Clinical Presentation

Acute prostatitis affects all age groups, tends to occur more frequently in young and middle-aged men, and has a rapid and severe onset. It is easily recognized, but less common than chronic bacterial prostatitis (CP) or UCPPS. Etiological features include ascending urethral infection or intraprostatic reflux, or as a complication of sexually transmitted infection. Men will be acutely ill, and may present because they are unable to void. They can report fever and chills, dysuria, urinary frequency, urgency, perineal/flank/low back pain, possible generalized malaise, and an exquisitely tender, swollen prostate on rectal examination. Prompt diagnosis and treatment are critical to prevent complications of sepsis. Prostate abscess is rare; it should be part of any differential diagnosis if there is no improvement or if symptoms worsen on initial antibiotic therapy and in men with decreased sensation to the pelvic region, such as men with spinal cord injuries.

Risk factors for acute prostatitis are multifactorial (Table 28.2), influenced by the overall health of the patient and his comorbid conditions, existing dysfunctional voiding, constipation, and pelvic floor dysfunction. Anatomical issues that affect voiding, such as phimosis, enlarged prostate, or urethral stricture disease increase the risk for prostate infection.

Physical Examination

Vital signs may demonstrate fever and possible blood pressure changes. The patient's appearance overall may be toxic, especially if there has been a problem with voiding. On digital rectal examination (DRE), the prostate may be firm, edematous, and exquisitely tender; avoid vigorous DRE to reduce the risk of urosepsis. The bladder may be palpable, and there may be costovertebral angle (CVA) tenderness on examination. Genital examination may be inconclusive, with any complaints of pain not reproduced on examination.

TABLE 28.2 Acute and Chronic Bacterial Prostatitis: Representative Symptoms and Risk Factors

Most Common Symptoms	Risk Factors
Dysuria	Bladder dysfunction
Elevated prostate-specific antigen (PSA)	Chronic pain syndromes
Erectile dysfunction	Dehydration
Fever, chills	HIV
Hematospermia	Indwelling catheter or intermittent catheterization
Hematuria	Marathon runners
Malaise or flu-like symptoms	Benign prostate hyperplasia (BPH)
New-onset urinary hesitancy or dribbling	Recent prostate biopsy or other genitourinary instrumentation/procedure
Nonspecific back pain	Recurrent urinary tract infection
Painful ejaculation	Sexually transmitted diseases
Perineal, rectal, pelvic, groin, or penis pain	Trauma
Prostate tenderness on digital rectal examination (DRE)	Urethral stricture
Urge incontinence	
Urinary urgency or frequency	

Diagnosis/Evaluation

Obtain urinalysis, Gram stain, urine culture, and complete blood count. Depending in the presentation, a basic metabolic panel, erythrocyte sedimentation rate (ESR), and C-reactive protein can be added. Prostate-specific antigen (PSA) elevation is common during acute infection. Blood cultures are needed only if sepsis is suspected. Imaging is not usually indicated; however, if prostatic abscess is suspected, obtain transrectal ultrasound (TRUS) or CT imaging. Ultrasound postvoid residual test can aid in treatment decisions if retention is suspected.

Results will show elevated white blood cells (WBCs), likely pyuria/bacteriuria, and positive urine culture. Cultured organisms are primarily gram-negative (*Escherichia coli* [~80%], *Klebsiella* [3%–11%], *Proteus* [3%–6%], *Pseudomonas* [3%–7%]) (Wagenlehner et al., 2013). Instrumentation (prostate biopsy or resection) may be a factor in acute prostatitis with resistant pathogens, possibly secondary to periprocedure antibiotics (Meyrier & Fekete, 2015a; Nguyen, 2014; Sharp, Takacs, & Powell, 2010).

Treatment

Men who are in acute retention may need a suprapubic tube placed to avoid unnecessary manipulation of the prostate with catheter placement. Treatment requires antibiotics, but the recommendation may vary by facility and society recommendations (Table 28.3). Some men require hospitalization for hydration and IV antibiotics, while others will improve with outpatient antibiotics. While the most common causative organism is *E. coli*, monitor culture/sensitivity results to be certain the patient is on appropriate antibiotic regimen. Treat for 4 to 6 weeks to avoid chronic prostatitis, emphasizing increased fluid intake and avoidance of pressure to the prostate. Men may benefit from a probiotic such as Align, which can help prevent gastrointestinal (GI) distress due to the lengthy course of antibiotics. Symptomatic management with nonsteroidal anti-inflammatory drugs (NSAIDs) or

TABLE 28.3 Treatment of Prostatitis by Type

<table>
<tr><th>Description</th><th colspan="2">Treatment Guide</th></tr>
<tr><td>Acute bacterial prostatitis*</td><td colspan="2">Severe symptoms
Sulfamethoxazole and trimethoprim 800–160 mg orally
Fluoroquinolones orally
Trimethoprim 300 mg orally
Cephalexin 500 mg
Amoxicillin and clavulanic acid 500 mg + 125 mg orally
Appears septic, unable to urinate or unable to tolerate oral therapy
Admit to hospital, offer parenteral therapy according to facility guidelines</td></tr>
<tr><td>Chronic bacterial prostatitis* (CP)</td><td colspan="2">Norfloxacin 400 mg orally every 12 h for 4 wk, or
Trimethoprim 300 mg orally daily for 4 wk
If Chlamydia or Ureaplasma noted
• Doxycycline 100 mg orally every 12 h for 2–4 wk</td></tr>
<tr><td rowspan="3">Chronic prostatis/ chronic pelvic pain syndrome (CPPS)</td><td>Type III</td><td rowspan="3">Treatment aimed at both symptom relief and improving quality of life
Pelvic floor physical therapy
Alpha-1-adrenergic receptor antagonist (α blockers)
NSAIDs
5α-Reductase inhibitors
Pregabalin or other anticonvulsants
PDE5i
Trigger point injections
Cognitive-based therapy/stress management
Sitz baths
Phytotherapy: pollen extracts, saw palmetto, quercetin
Yin yoga</td></tr>
<tr><td>Type IIIa: inflammatory</td></tr>
<tr><td>Type IIIb: noninflammatory</td></tr>
<tr><td>Asymptomatic</td><td colspan="2">None required</td></tr>
</table>

*Specific choice of antibiotic may be guided by facility guidelines, culture results, society guidelines.

NSAIDs, nonsteroidal anti-inflammatory drugs; PDE5i, phosphodiesterase type 5 inhibitor.

acetaminophen, stool softeners, and alpha blockers may help with overall comfort levels. At the beginning of treatment, men should be advised that they may notice only modest improvement of symptoms over the first few weeks of treatment.

At a return clinic visit, after men have been treated for the acute manifestations, the provider can consider referral to a urology provider. This will enable assessment of voiding function and bladder emptying, along with consideration for repeat urinalysis/culture after treatment (Meyrier & Fekete, 2015a; Nguyen, 2014). If the patient is not improving, he should be referred urgently to urology, as an ultrasound-guided perineal puncture of any abscess may be needed to better tailor any antibiotic regimen. Assessment of bladder function may reveal voiding dysfunction that can respond to management and prevent future acute infections.

■ CHRONIC BACTERIAL PROSTATITIS

Clinical Presentation

Chronic bacterial prostatitis (CBP) almost always involves recurrent documented bacterial infections with the same pathogens as previous episode of acute prostatitis, and can be due to inadequate treatment of acute prostatitis. CBP is accompanied by urogenital symptoms similar to those in acute prostatitis, with similar risk factors (Table 28.2), but may not demonstrate the fever and acute symptoms, or urinary retention. Men with prostate or bladder calculi, diabetes, and tobacco abuse are at higher risk for chronic prostatitis. History may include waxing and waning of symptoms, especially if they had been treated with short courses of antibiotics; this can include a history of "chronic epididymitis" when the cause is recurrent bacterial migration from the prostate to the epididymis after inadequate treatment for acute prostatitis or CBP. There may also be a history of repeated urinary tract infections, and left untreated, CBP can contribute to male factor infertility as the ejaculatory ducts can become obstructed, and chronic WBCs in the semen may be a contributor to decreased rates of fertilization.

Physical Examination

Overall presentation will be nontoxic, general examination is benign, and vital signs will be normal. DRE may reveal hypertrophy, tenderness, irregularity, or edema (soft to palpation), but the prostate may not be tender to examination.

Diagnosis/Evaluation

The historical gold standard of bacterial localization for CBP is the Meares-Stamey four-glass test: first-voided urine, midstream urine, expressed prostatic secretions, and postprostatic massage urine are sampled. Although this test is classic for diagnosis purposes, it is infrequently used in clinical practice (Nickel et al., 2006; Nickel et al., 2015).

Semen culture can be ordered, but it may identify pathogens in only about 50% of specimens. The laboratory evaluation for CBP is usually normal, with negative results for the urinalysis and dipstick evaluation. But the most likely causative bacteria is *E. coli*. Postvoid residual test, either via bladder scan or bladder ultrasound, can be performed to confirm retention is not an issue. In the absence of proven bacterial infection, providers can find it difficult to distinguish CBP from UCPPS (Meyrier & Fekete, 2015b; Wagenlehner et al., 2013).

Treatment

Table 28.1 discusses treatment; the length of treatment should be a minimum of 4 weeks, but can range between 4 and 12 weeks depending on past episodes of treatment. Symptomatic management with NSAIDs or acetaminophen, stool softeners, probiotics, and alpha blockers may help with overall comfort levels and improve associated symptoms. If CBP is refractory to treatment, refer to urology or infectious disease for additional evaluation.

Follow-up

Some men may benefit from assessment of voiding function, stricture disease, or pelvic floor dysfunction as a way to prevent future episodes. Men should be advised to avoid constipation and focus on proper hydration. At the beginning of treatment, men should be advised that they may notice only modest improvement of symptoms over the first few weeks of treatment.

CHRONIC PROSTATITIS/UROLOGICAL CHRONIC PELVIC PAIN SYNDROME

Chronic prostatitis/urological chronic pelvic pain syndrome (CP/UCPPS) is a clinical syndrome defined as pelvic pain associated with urinary symptoms and/or sexual dysfunction, lasting for at least 3 of the past 6 months in the absence of other identified causes (NIH standardized definition). It remains a diagnosis of exclusion, and occurs in 2% to 10% of all adult men, but there is no precise incidence for this condition (Nickel, Shoskes, & Wagenlehner, 2013). The symptoms and clinical presentation are similar to prostate infection, yet with no evident source of infection.

In CP/UCPPS, the term "prostatitis" may not be indicative that the source of symptoms is the prostate, but some initiation of symptoms may have been the result of urine reflux into prostatic ducts. Recent research indicates an association between nonurological somatic syndromes and symptom severity of CP/UCPPS (Krieger et al., 2014). Breaking research by the MAPP network has identified overrepresentation of *Burkholderia cenocepacia* (gram-negative bacteria) in the initial urine stream of men with chronic pelvic pain syndrome (Krieger et al., 2014; Nickel et al., 2015), and suggests there may be two types of patients: those with pelvic and urinary symptoms and those with both urological symptoms and nonurological syndromes, suggesting a more systemic condition (Table 28.4) that may be influenced by other chronic pain conditions. Table 28.2 also distinguishes between inflammatory (IIIa) and noninflammatory (IIIb) subtypes.

Clinical Presentation

Men will provide a history of urological and pelvic symptoms for greater than 3 months without a positive culture. A detailed history is essential: present urinary symptoms; pain sites and description of the pain; sexual history and current sexual activity; mental health history; attempt to elicit history of physical, emotional, or sexual trauma; and nonurological somatic disorders (Table 28.4). There may be reports of waxing and waning symptoms, including pelvic pain, low back pain, painful erections or ejaculation, irritative and/or obstructive voiding symptoms, and hematuria or hematospermia. Sexual dysfunction complaints may be present, but pelvic floor tenderness, depression, and catastrophizing are more clinically significant. For perspective, catastrophizing is defined as an exaggerated negative mental

TABLE 28.4 Conditions Associated With UCPPS

Associated Nonurological Somatic Syndromes
Chronic fatigue syndrome
Irritable bowel syndrome or Crohn's disease
Fibromyalgia/chronic fatigue syndrome
TMJ disorder
Anxiety disorder
Widespread chronic pain
Interstitial cystitis/painful bladder syndrome (IC/PBS)

TMJ, temporomandibular joint; UCPPS, urological chronic pelvic pain syndrome.

Sources: Krieger, J. N., Stephens, A. J., Landis, J. R., Clemens, J. Q., Kreder, K., Lai, H. H., ... Williams DA; MAPP Research Network. (2014). Relationship between chronic nonurological associated somatic syndromes and symptom severity in urological chronic pelvic pain syndromes: Baseline evaluation of the MAPP study. *The Journal of Urology, 193*(4), 1254–1262. doi:10.1016/j.juro.2014; Pontari, M. (2015). Chronic prostatitis/chronic pelvic pain syndrome. *UpToDate*. Retrieved from http://www.uptodate.com/contents/chronic-prostatitis-chronic-pelvic-pain-syndrome?topic; Wagenlehner, F., van Till, J., Magri, V., Perletti, G., Houbiers, J., Weidner, W., & Nickel, J. C. (2013). National Institutes of Health Chronic Prostatitis Symptom Index (NIH-CPSI) symptom evaluation in multinational cohorts of patients with chronic prostatitis/chronic pelvic pain syndrome. *European Urology, 63*(5), 953–959. doi:10.1016/j.eururo.2012.10.042

set brought to bear during actual or anticipated painful experience (Sullivan et al. 2001; Sullivan, 2009) that consists of three distinct components: rumination, magnification, and helplessness, and it has been implicated as predictor of treatment success.

Physical Examination

General physical examination is typically unrevealing. Examination of the pelvic floor may demonstrate point tenderness and suggest trigger points. Rectal examination may show tenderness or be benign. Examination may reproduce complaints of pain (including genital pain) or fail to reproduce pain; men may demonstrate hyperesthesia (increased sensitivity to stimulation) and allodynia (pain from a stimulus that does not normally provoke pain) as well.

Diagnosis/Evaluation

All other causes of pelvic pain should be eliminated; this can include imaging studies such as pelvic CT or MRI, depending on the individual presentation (Pontari, 2015; Sharp et al., 2010; Stein, May, & Dekel, 2015). Initial laboratory evaluation should include urinalysis and culture, urine cytological test if hematuria noted, PSA, and inflammatory markers. If undergoing evaluation with a urology provider, additional tests may include cystoscopy and/or prostate ultrasound or biopsy, bladder ultrasound and/or catheterization for post-void residual may be indicated. There are short, validated instruments that help assess symptoms and guide treatment, including the NIH Chronic Prostatitis Symptom Index (NIH-CPSI), American Urological Association/International Prostate Symptom Score (AUA/IPSS) questionnaire, and UPOINTS classification system (Table 28.5; Kartha, Kerr & Shokes, 2013; Nickel & Shoskes, 2010; Shoskes & Nickel, 2013).

Treatment

At present there is no universally accepted treatment regimen for UCPPS, and no therapy that will be effective in all cases, which is an important concept to emphasize to men undergoing treatment. But the UPOINTS screening tool can suggest domains (urinary, psychosocial, orgain-specific, infection, neurological, tenderness, sexual) in which to initially focus

TABLE 28.5 UPOINTS Classification for UCPPS

Domain	Evaluation
Urinary	Postvoid residual test measured by ultrasound
Psychosocial	Evaluate depression and catastrophizing
Organ-specific	Pain improvement with bladder emptying, prostate tenderness
Infection	Culture for *Mycoplasma* and *Ureaplasma*, urine culture Consider expressed prostatic secretions or a post-prostate massage urine
Neurological/systemic	Pain beyond the pelvis Investigate history of other chronic pain syndromes
Tenderness	Palpate the abdominal and pelvic skeletal muscles (via rectum) Check for spasm and trigger points
Sexual	Sexual dysfunction, pain with sexual activity

UCPPS, urological chronic pelvic pain syndrome.

treatment or multimodal therapies (Herati & Moldwin, 2013). Management goals should improve functional status, quality of life, and sexual function. Cognitive-based therapy or psychological/psychiatric evaluation may assist with identification and management of conditions such as anxiety and depression and provide direction for stress reduction. Successful management of UCPPS involves introducing the concept that this condition has to be managed, like any other chronic condition; some men may benefit from referral to a multidisciplinary pain management program.

ASYMPTOMATIC INFLAMMATORY PROSTATITIS

Clinical Presentation/Diagnosis

Asymptomatic inflammatory prostatitis is an incidental finding in men who undergo urological procedures, such as prostate biopsy, infertility assessment, or cancer workup. Leukocytospermia (elevated WBCs in the semen) without infection may be noted on fertility evaluation. Men do not present with symptoms.

Treatment

No treatment is required unless symptoms develop. Antibiotics may be prescribed if a couple is planning for in vitro fertilization cycles. There is little evidence to support either the natural history or treatment for asymptomatic inflammatory prostatitis (Krieger et al., 1999; Sharp et al., 2010).

CHRONIC UNEXPLAINED ORCHIALGIA

Chronic unexplained orchialgia (CUO) is "a subjective negative experience of adult men, perceived as intermittent or continuous pain of variable intensity, present at least three months, localizing to the testis(es) in the absence of objective organic findings, that interferes with quality of life" (p. 8, Quallich & Arslanian-Engoren, 2014). It is a difficult clinical entity, as men may seek care episodically over its course. This is a male genital pain condition without a contemporary evidence-based treatment algorithm, and a lack of research into the condition (Quallich & Arslanian-Engoren, 2013). Men with CUO will seek repeated evaluation and treatment, as seen with many other chronic pain populations. Initial evaluation includes elimination of causes of acute scrotal and testicular pain (Chapter 23).

Background and Risk Factors

No specific ethnic or genetic risk factors have been identified, and onset of CUO may be spontaneous or pain may linger after an infection or injury. Some men report constant pain, while the pattern may be intermittent for others, often without specific aggravating or alleviating factors. Previous guidelines have suggested that CUO is a regional extension of male chronic pelvic pain syndrome (Engeler et al., 2013) but actual evidence for this is sparse, as despite the sparse representation the literature, reported symptoms in CUO do not typically involve voiding symptoms or pelvic floor complaints.

Clinical Presentation and History

Clinical presentation and history are the same as for UCPPS. Individuals should be asked specifically about a history of vasectomy, as complaints of CUO can be improperly diagnosed as postvasectomy pain syndrome.

Physical Examination and Diagnostic Testing

A thorough examination of the male genitals must be performed, with attempts to precisely locate the source of pain. Similar to UCCPS, examination may reproduce complaints of pain or fail to reproduce pain; men may demonstrate hyperesthesia and allodynia as well.

A scrotal ultrasound scan is mandatory to rule out intrascrotal pathology that could be causing pain, if the patient has not undergone this imaging in more than 6 months. Depending on the specific history, screening for sexually transmitted infections can be added, along with cultures for *Ureaplasma*. In men with symptoms consistent with possible radiculopathy (e.g., testicular pain at the same time pain shoots down the leg) imaging of the low back may be helpful.

Management

As men with CUO present like many other chronic pain populations, and similar to UCPPS, proceed from a noninvasive perspective, which may involve referral to a multidisciplinary pain management program. Clinical management of symptoms can proceed as detailed for UCPPS (Table 28.3). Men can be referred to a urology provider for more focused evaluation, including a spermatic cord block.

■ CONCLUSION

Both UCPPS and chronic orchialgia can significantly affect quality of life. Presently the evidence-based guidance for treating these conditions is in its infancy, meaning that providers can best proceed with an evaluation that screens for significant causes (such as testicular cancer) and symptomatic management based on the individual's presentation at the time, although this lack of defined process and diagnosis can be a source of frustration for men. There is also value in treating these conditions in a multidisciplinary fashion by including a psychology evaluation to help identify stress and other psychosocial factors that may act as triggers that can provoke and sustain pain complaints.

■ CLINICAL PEARLS

- If acute prostatitis is suspected, avoid vigorous DRE, which may cause bacteremia.
- Imaging studies are not usually needed to diagnose acute prostatitis unless prostate abscess is suspected.
- Recurrence of chronic bacterial prostatitis is common. Consider antibiotic resistance, impaired absorption, and failure to complete prior treatment when planning for a longer course of antibiotics.
- Most CP/UCPPS is a diagnosis of exclusion.
- There is NO universally accepted treatment regimen for CP/UCPPS. Individual presentation should guide treatment regimen.
- Only emerging, low-level evidence guides "best practice" for treating chronic orchialgia.

RESOURCES FOR THE PROVIDER

The Multidisciplinary Approach to the Study of Chronic Pelvic Pain (MAPP) is a research network conducting collaborative research on urological chronic pelvic pain disorders—specifically, interstitial cystitis/painful bladder syndrome (IC/PBS) and chronic prostatitis/chronic pelvic pain syndrome (CP/CPPS): www.mappnetwork.org

National Guideline Clearinghouse: Chronic Pelvic Pain: www.guideline.gov/content.aspx?id=38626#Section424

The National Institutes of Health Chronic Prostatitis Symptom Index (NIH-CPSI): www.prostatitis.org/symptomindex.html

UPOINT clinical phenotyping system for CP/CPPS to guide multimodal treatment: www.upointmd.com/index.php

RESOURCES FOR THE PATIENT

AUA: Urology Care Foundation (2015). "Prostatitis (Infection of the Prostate)": www.urologyhealth.org/urologic-conditions/prostatitis-(infection-of-the-prostate)/symptoms

British Medical Journal (BMJ) "Prostatitis" (patient handout—note that some of the information refers to European medication names, but overall topic coverage is solid): www.bestpractice.bmj.com/best-practice/pdf/patient-summaries/532707.pdf

NIH: "What I need to know about prostate problems" (English and Spanish): www.niddk.nih.gov/health-information/health-topics/urologic-disease/prostatitis-disorders-of-the-prostate/Pages/ez.aspx

SUNA: "Prostatitis—Patient Fact Sheet" (English and Spanish): www.suna.org/download/members/prostatitis.pdf

Up to Date—"Patient Information: Prostatitis (The Basics)": www.uptodate.com

REFERENCES

Clemens, J. Q. (2014). *Update on the MAPP Project* (plenary session May 19). American Urologic Association Annual Conference, Orlando, FL.

Clemens, J. Q., Clauw, D. J., Kreder, K., Krieger, J. N., Kusek, J. W., Lai, H. H., … Landis, J. R. (2015). Comparison of baseline urological symptoms in men and women in the MAPP research cohort. *The Journal of Urology, 193*(5), 1554–1558. doi:10.1016/j.juro.2014.11.016

Engeler, D. S., Baranowski, A. P., Dinis-Oliveira, P., Elneil, S., Hughes, J., Messelink, E. J., … Williams, A. C. (2013). The 2013 EAU guidelines on chronic pelvic pain: is management of chronic pelvic pain a habit, a philosophy, or a science? 10 years of development. *European Urology, 64*(3), 431–439. doi:10.1016/j.eururo.2013.04.035

Herati, A., & Moldwin, R. (2013). Alternative therapies in the management of chronic prostatitis/chronic pelvic pain syndrome. *World Journal of Urology, 31*, 761–766. doi:10.007/s00345-011097-0

Kartha, G. K., Kerr, H., & Shoskes, D. A. (2013). Clinical phenotyping of urologic pain patients. *Current Opinion in Urology, 23*(6), 560–564. doi:10.1097/MOU.0b013e3283652a9d

Krieger, J. N., Nyberg, L., & Nickel, J. C. (1999). NIH consensus definition and classification of prostatitis. *JAMA, 282*(3), 236–237. doi:10-1001/pubs.JAMA-ISSN-0098-7484-282-3-jac90006

Krieger, J. N., Stephens, A. J., Landis, J. R., Clemens, J. Q., Kreder, K., Lai, H. H., … Williams DA; MAPP Research Network. (2014). Relationship between chronic nonurological associated somatic syndromes and symptom severity in urological chronic pelvic pain syndromes: Baseline evaluation of the MAPP study. *The Journal of Urology, 193*(4), 1254–1262. doi:10.1016/j.juro.2014

Meyrier, A., & Fekete, T. (2015a). Chronic bacterial prostatitis. In S. B. Calderwood (Ed.), *UpToDate*. Retrieved from http://www.uptodate.com/contents/chronic-bacterial-prostatitis?topicKey=ID%2F86802&el

Meyrier, A., & Fekete, T. (2015b). Acute bacterial prostatitis. In S. B. Calderwood (Ed.), *UpToDate*. Retrieved from http://www.uptodate.com/contents/acute-bacterial-prostatitis?topicKey=ID%2F8062&elaps

Nguyen, N. (2014). Treating prostatitis effectively: A challenge for clinicians. *US Pharmacist, 39*(4), 35–41.
Nickel, J. C., & Shoskes, D. A. (2010). Phenotypic approach to the management of the chronic prostatitis/chronic pelvic pain syndrome. *BJU International, 106*(9), 1252–1263. doi:10.1111/j.1464-410X.2010.09701.x
Nickel, J. C., Shoskes, D. A., & Wagenlehner, F. M. (2013). Management of chronic prostatitis/chronic pelvic pain syndrome (CP/CPPS): the studies, the evidence, and the impact. *World Journal of Urology, 31*(4), 747–753. doi:10.1007/s00345-013-1062-y
Nickel, J. C., Shoskes, D. A., Wang, Y., Alexander, R. B., Fowler, J. E., Zeitlin, S., ... Propert, K. J. (2006). How does the pre-massage and post-massage 2-glass test compare to the Meares-Stamey 4-glass test in men with chronic prostatitis/chronic pelvic pain syndrome? *The Journal of Urology, 176*(1), 119–124. doi:10.1016/j.juro.2008.06.061
Nickel, J. C., Stephens, A., Landis, J. R., Chen, J., Mullins, C., van Bokhoven, A., ... Ehrlich, G. D.; The MAPP Research Network. (2015). Search for Microorganisms in men with Urologic Chronic Pelvic Pain Syndrome: A culture-independent analysis in the MAPP Research Network. *The Journal of Urology, 194*(1), 127–135. doi:10.1016/j.juro.2015.01.037
Pontari, M. (2015). Chronic prostatitis/chronic pelvic pain syndrome. *UpToDate*. Retrieved from http://www.uptodate.com/contents/chronic-prostatitis-chronic-pelvic-pain-syndrome?topic
Quallich, S. A., & Arslanian-Engoren, C. (2013). Chronic testicular pain in adult men: An integrative literature review. *American Journal of Men's Health. 7*(5), 402–413. doi:10.1177/1557988313476732
Riegel, B., Bruenahl, C. A., Ahyai, S., Bingel, U., Fisch, M., & Löwe, B. (2014). Assessing psychological factors, social aspects and psychiatric co-morbidity associated with Chronic Prostatitis/Chronic Pelvic Pain Syndrome (CP/CPPS) in men – A systematic review. *Journal of Psychosomatic Research, 77*(5), 333–350. doi:10.1016/j.jpsychores.2014.09.012
Sharp, V., Takacs, E., & Powell, C. (2010). Prostatitis: diagnosis and treatment. *American Family Physician, 82*(4), 397–406. Retrieved from http://www.aafp.org/afp/2010/0815/p397.html
Shoskes, D., & Nickel, J. C. (2013). Classification and treatment of men with chronic prostatitis/chronic pelvic pain syndrome using the UPOINT system. *World Journal of Urology, 31*(4), 755–760. doi:10.1007/s00345-013-1075-6
Stein, A., May, T., & Dekel, Y. (2015). Chronic pelvic pain syndrome: A clinical enigma. *Postgraduate Medicine, 126*(4), 115–122. doi:10.3810/pgm.2014.07.2789
Sullivan, M. J. (2009). *The Pain Catastrophizing Scale user manual.* Montréal: McGill University.
Sullivan, M. J., Thorn, B., Haythornthwaite, J., Keefe, F., Martin, M., Bradley, L., & Lefebvre, J. (2001). Theoretical perspectives on the relation between catastrophizing and pain. *The Clinical Journal of Pain, 17*(1), 52–64. doi:10.1097/00002508-200103000-00008
Wagenlehner, F., Pilatz, A., Bschleipfer, T., Diemer, T., Linn, T., Meihardt, A., ... Weidner, W. (2013). Bacterial prostatitis. *World Journal of Urology, 21*, 711–716. doi:10.1007/s00345-013-1055-x
Wagenlehner, F. M., Weidner, W., Pilatz, A., & Naber, K. G. (2014). Urinary tract infections and bacterial prostatitis in men. *Current Opinion Infectious Diseases, 27*(1), 97–101. doi:10.1097/QCO.0000000000000024

CHAPTER 29

Hypogonadism and Testosterone Replacement Issues

Kenneth A. Mitchell

INTRODUCTION

Hypogonadism is a medical term for decreased functional activity of the gonads. The gonads (ovaries or testes) produce hormones (testosterone, estradiol, antimüllerian hormone, progesterone, inhibin B, activin) and gametes (eggs or sperm) (Yialamas & Hayes, 2003). Generally, testosterone deficiency (TD) is defined as a decrease in the concentration of serum total testosterone (TT; <300 ng/dL) and/or a decrease in sperm production (Bhasin et al., 2010). Signs and symptoms include decreased libido, fatigue, erectile dysfunction, loss of body and facial hair, decreased bone mineral density (BMD), increased body fat, decreased lean muscle mass, weakness, depressed mood, sleep disturbance, and anemia. Prevalence of hypogonadism in men aged ≥45 years visiting primary care practices in the United States is estimated to be approximately 38.7%. Further evidence indicates that there is a higher prevalence of hypogonadism in men with obesity, diabetes, hypertension, rheumatoid arthritis, hyperlipidemia, and osteopenia/osteoporosis (Mulligan, Frick, Zuraw, Stemhagen, & McWhirter, 2006).

Testosterone has been available to clinicians as a medical therapy since the 1930s; however, its use was limited until the last 10 to 15 years, at which point prescription rates began to increase at a rapid rate. The increase in testosterone therapy (TTh) is attributed to a combination of factors, including consumer marketing increasing awareness of TD (also known as low testosterone, or low T) as a treatable condition, the publication of numerous studies documenting benefits of TTh, and decreased concern regarding safety risks, particularly prostate cancer (Morgentaler, Khera, Maggi, & Zitzmann, 2014).

EVALUATION OF HYPOGONADISM

Initial evaluation of men with hypogonadism should include a comprehensive medical history to assess the presenting symptoms and identify any associated comorbid conditions. Patients with one or more objective symptoms of hypogonadism (Table 29.1) should undergo a thorough physical examination to identify the presence of gynecomastia and the presence of secondary sex characteristics (decreased body hair (pubic/axillary), decreased beard growth), a testicular examination paying close attention to the size and consistency of the testicles (adult testes are usually between 20 and 30 mL in volume and from 4.5 to 6.5 cm long by 2.8 to 3.3 cm wide), prostate examination, and body mass index (BMI) (Bhasin et al., 2010; Petak et al., 2002). Laboratory testing parameters vary between the published guidelines; however, all agree that measurement of a morning TT level by a reliable assay confirmed by repeat measurement should be obtained to confirm the diagnosis.

Men with TT near the lower limit of normal or men whom sex hormone binding globulin (SHBG) abnormality is suspected (e.g., older men, men with obesity, diabetes mellitus,

TABLE 29.1 Clinical Presentation of Hypogonadism

Physical	Psychological	Sexual
Decreased BMD Decrease muscle mass and strength Gynecomastia Anemia Frailty Increased BMI Fatigue Insulin resistance Enlarged liver/elevated LFTs	Diminished energy, sense of vitality, or well-being Impaired cognition and memory Decreased mood	Decreased spontaneous erections Erectile dysfunction Difficulty achieving orgasm Diminished libido

BMD, bone mineral density; BMI, body mass index; LFTs, liver function tests.

chronic illness, liver disease, or thyroid disease) should have additional laboratory testing performed. Further lab testing should include serum luteinizing hormone (LH) and follicle-stimulating hormone (FSH) levels to distinguish between primary (testicular) and secondary (pituitary-hypothalamic) hypogonadism. Measurement of LH and FSH concentrations can help distinguish between primary and secondary hypogonadism. In addition, usage of the quantitative Androgen Deficiency in the Aging Male (qADAM) questionnaire can be helpful to initiate a conversation about the symptoms they may be having, identify patients with a high probability of having low testosterone, and quantify the severity of androgen deficiency in older men (Mohamed et al., 2010).

Primary Hypogonadism

Primary hypogonadism is caused by testicular failure of various causes. Testicular failure is characterized by low serum testosterone and elevated LH and FSH concentrations. Primary hypogonadism, also known as hypergonadotropic hypogonadism, is commonly attributed to testicular injury, tumor, infection (e.g., mumps orchitis), genetic defects (e.g., Klinefelter's syndrome), chemotherapy, radiation therapy, and alcohol abuse (Petak et al., 2002; Seftel, 2006).

Secondary Hypogonadism

Secondary hypogonadism is characterized by low testosterone with low or normal LH concentrations. Serum LH levels in men with secondary hypogonadism may be below the normal range or in low-normal range, but clearly inappropriate in relation to the low testosterone concentrations. In patients in whom secondary hypogonadism is suspected, further evaluation should include measurements of serum prolactin, pituitary function testing, and MRI of the pituitary gland. In men with primary testicular failure of unknown cause and a physical examination yielding low testicular volume, obtaining a karyotype to exclude Klinefelter's syndrome (XXY male) is recommended. Men with Klinefelter's syndrome can benefit from genetic counseling and need surveillance for certain disorders for which they are at increased risk (Dean et al., 2015).

Infertility

Many experts believe that all infertile males should undergo an endocrine evaluation; however, no consensus regarding this has been reached. In the context of a male infertility evaluation, providers may consider an endocrine evaluation if there is (a) an abnormal semen analysis (sperm concentration less than 10 million/mL); (b) impaired sexual function; or (c) other clinical findings suggestive of a specific endocrinopathy. In men being evaluated for infertility and/or suspected TD, the Endocrine Society Guidelines and the American Urological Association (AUA) publication, *The Optimal Evaluation of the Infertile Male: AUA Best Practice Statement* both recommend performing an endocrine evaluation on all infertile males. This evaluation is detailed further in Chapter 27.

HYPOGONADISM-ASSOCIATED COMORBID CONDITIONS

Higher incidence of hypogonadism has been associated with several common diseases or conditions. The Hypogonadism in Males study noted the calculated odds ratios for conditions associated with hypogonadism (Table 29.2). Interestingly, there is also an observable correlation with known causes of erectile dysfunction, hypogonadism, and the top 10 leading causes of death in men (Table 29.3). The current state of the science for hypogonadism does not suggest whether low testosterone levels are a consequence of the disease, connected with the disease's cause, or have a proven causal relationship identified. Experts concluded that randomized controlled trials will be needed to determine if treating the hypogonadism is likely to improve the patient's disease symptoms.

Hypogonadism and Cardiometabolic Syndrome

TD has been shown to be associated with the following increased cardiovascular events and risk factors: dyslipidemia (including low high-density lipoprotein [HDL] and triglycerides), hypertension, obesity, diabetes mellitus, and insulin resistance. In addition, testosterone has an inverse relationship with BMI, waist circumference, low-density lipoprotein, and triglycerides (Ebeling, 2008; Nettleship, Jones, & Channer, & Jones, 2009; Shabsigh, Katz, Yan, & Makhsida, 2005). However, it is not known whether hypogonadism is the cause of, or the consequence of, these conditions. Physiologically, it is understood that an increase in adiposity in adult males followed by aromatization of adipose tissue results in an increase in estradiol and adipokine production leading to suppression of the hypothalamic pituitary secretion of LH resulting in

TABLE 29.2 Prevalence Rates and Odds Ratios for Selected Risk Factors in Enrolled Untreated Hypogonadal Patients

Risk Factor/Condition	Hypogonadism Prevalence Rate (95% CI)	Odds Ratio (95% CI)
Obesity	52.4 (47.9–56.9)	2.38 (1.93–2.93)
Diabetes	50.0 (45.5–54.5)	2.09 (1.70–2.58)
Hypertension	42.4 (39.6–45.2)	1.84 (1.53–2.22)
Rheumatoid arthritis	47.3 (34.1–60.5)	1.59 (0.92–2.72)
Hyperlipidemia	40.4 (37.6–43.3)	1.47 (1.23–1.76)
Osteoporosis	44.4 (25.5–64.7)	1.41 (0.64–3.01)
Asthma/COPD	43.5 (36.8–50.3)	1.40 (1.04–1.86)
Prostatic disease/disorder	41.3 (36.4–46.2)	1.29 (1.03–1.62)
Chronic pain	38.8 (33.7–44.0)	1.13 (0.89–1.44)
Headaches (within last 2 weeks)	32.1 (25.3–38.8)	0.81 (0.58–1.11)

CI, confidence interval; COPD, chronic obstructive pulmonary disease.

TABLE 29.3 Male Sexual Health Correlates

Causes of Erectile Dysfunction	Top 10 Leading Causes of Death	Hypogonadism
Coronary artery disease (CAD)	Heart disease (CAD)	Obesity (52.4)
Hormonal problems	Cancer	Diabetes (50.0)
Injuries	Stroke	Hypertension (42.4)
Nerve damage (RRP, MS, Parkinson's disease)	Accidents	Hyperlipidemia (40.4)
Infections	Lung disease (COPD)	Osteoporosis (44.4)
Diabetes	Pneumonia	Asthma/COPD (43.5)
Stress, depression, and anxiety	Diabetes	Prostate disease (41.3)
Alcohol and drug abuse	Suicide	
Hypertension	Liver disease (cirrhosis)	
	Homicides	

COPD, chronic obstructive pulmonary disease; MS, multiple sclerosis; RRP, radical retropubic prostatectomy.

decreased testosterone production by Leydig cells in the testicles. Additionally, an increase in insulin resistance also occurs which further inhibits Leydig cell production of testosterone (Aso, 2008; Kapoor, Malkin, Channer, & Jones, 2005).

Hypogonadism and Diabetes

According to the National Diabetes Statistics Report 2017 (Centers for Disease Control and Prevention [CDC], 2017), reported estimates showed 15.3 million men (95% confidence interval [CI]: 13.8–17.0) or 12.7% (95% CI: 11.5–14.1) had either diagnosed or undiagnosed diabetes in the United States. The estimated number of adult males ≥18 years of age reported as prediabetic was 44.5 million (95% CI: 40.5–48.7), or 36.9% (95% CI: 33.6–40.4). Meanwhile, the percentage of men aware of prediabetes was a mere 9.4% (95% CI: 6.6–13.3). Low testosterone concentrations are known to occur in association with type 2 diabetes requiring clinicians to be aware of the relationship between low testosterone concentrations and diabetes. Dhindsa et al. (2004) were the first to measure free testosterone and establish hypogonadism as a feature of male type 2 diabetes.

In the HIM study, a diabetic man was approximately twice as likely to be hypogonadal compared with a nondiabetic man (Mulligan et al., 2006). The prevalence in diabetic men has been estimated at 33% to 50% suggesting that hypogonadism must be considered a common complication of type 2 diabetes in adult males. Measurement of gonadotropin levels indicates that the hypogonadism in type 2 diabetes is predominately secondary hypogonadism and that there is no demonstrable relation between the degree of hyperglycemia and testosterone concentration (Tomar et al., 2006).

However, markers of systemic inflammation, specifically C-reactive protein, have been found to be markedly elevated in patients with secondary hypogonadism and type 2 diabetes. Concentrations of C-reactive protein in these patients are noted to be twice as high as those in eugonadal type 2 diabetics whose C-reactive protein levels are already elevated compared with nondiabetics. Furthermore, these patients have also been shown to be mildly anemic, are osteopenic in the arms and ribs, and have increased adiposity compared with eugonadal type 2 diabetics (Bhatia et al., 2006; Dhindsa et al., 2007; Mascarenhas et al., 2017). These findings are markedly similar to findings in hypogonadal patients without diabetes; low testosterone concentrations have been shown to predict the development of type 2 diabetes. According to data from the National Health and Nutrition Examination Survey (NHANES III), men in the lowest free testosterone tertile were four times as likely to have diabetes as those in the highest free testosterone tertile (Selvin et al., 2007). However, these studies have not demonstrated an association with type 1 diabetes and hypogonadism, suggesting that hypogonadism is specifically related to pathophysiological features of type 2 diabetes and not specifically to hyperglycemia (Tomar et al., 2006).

Hypogonadism, Obesity, and Metabolic Syndrome

According to the 2011–2014 NHANES review, obesity among adult men had a prevalence of 34.3% (Ogden, Carroll, Fryar, & Flegal, 2015). Adults who have a BMI between 25 and 29.9 kg/m^2 are classified overweight, whereas adults with a BMI of 30 kg/m^2 or higher are considered obese. However, BMI does not directly measure body fat, so athletes, for example, may have high BMIs even though they are not overweight. The increased health risks associated with obesity are well known: type 2 diabetes, hypertension, atherosclerotic diseases, and coronary heart disease. It is reported that nearly 83% of diabetic patients are overweight or obese (Ogden et al., 2015). Moreover, there is a known association with obesity, low TT, reduced SHBG levels, and an inverse linear relationship between TT, BMI, and free testosterone concentrations, decreasing with increasing BMI. There also exists an inverse relationship between serum total and free testosterone concentrations and central obesity. Studies have confirmed that the degree of hypogonadism is positively correlated with the degree of obesity in obese men.

The metabolic syndrome is a constellation of interrelated risk factors of metabolic origin—*metabolic risk factors*—that appear to directly promote the development of atherosclerotic cardiovascular disease (ASCVD). Experts specifically define a person with metabolic syndrome as having any three of the following five factors: elevated waist circumference (≥102 cm [≥40 inches]), hypertension (≥130/80 mmHg) or on antihypertensive drug treatment in a patient with a history of hypertension, reduced HDL (<40 mg/dL in males) or on drug treatment for reduced HDL, raised triglycerides (≥150 mg/dL) or on drug treatment for elevated triglycerides, and raised fasting plasma glucose (≥100 mg/dL) or on drug treatment for elevated glucose (Grundy et al., 2005). Men with metabolic syndrome are considered at increased risk for developing type 2 diabetes mellitus and are at high risk for developing coronary heart disease. Individuals with these characteristics commonly manifest a prothrombotic state and a proinflammatory state as well.

As noted previously, the constituent elements of metabolic syndrome themselves are correlated with testosterone concentrations; therefore, it would be accurate to conclude that hypogonadism is also associated with the metabolic syndrome, as has been shown in several epidemiological studies (Morgentaler et al., 2015; Traish, Guay, Feeley, & Saad, 2009).

The hypogonadal-obesity cycle describes the pathophysiological process correlating testosterone concentrations and obesity in obese men. During the hypogonadal state, there is an increase in the deposition of abdominal adipose tissue containing high concentrations of aromatase. Increased aromatase activity leads to a greater formation of estradiol from testosterone. This results in further reduction in serum and tissue testosterone concentrations, increased deposition of abdominal fat, and progressive hypogonadism. One significant factor may be leptin, the adipocyte-secreted protein product of the *ob* gene. Leptin is strongly linked to obesity and regulates weight and adipose tissue mass. Serum leptin levels correlate positively with age, BMI, serum insulin, and fat mass, and inversely with testosterone. Additional findings indicated that leptin levels are higher in aging males with lower testosterone and testosterone replacement therapy (TRT) corrects this. The mechanism

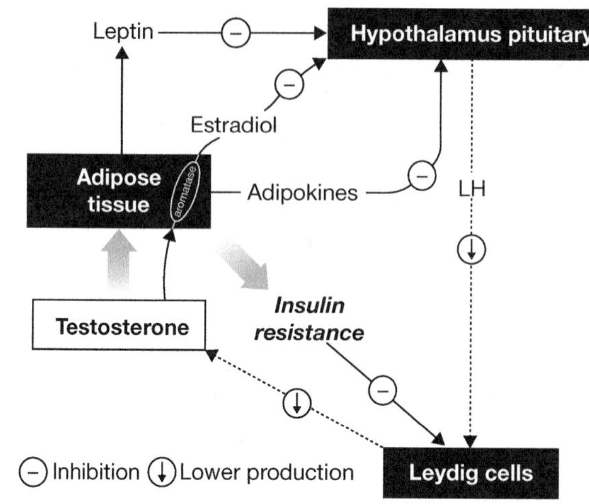

FIGURE 29.1 The interrelationship between hypogonadism and insulin resistance. Leptin, released in response to increased adiposity, also inhibits the release of LH via its effect on the release of gonadotropin-releasing hormone (Dhindsa et al., 2010).

LH, luteinizing hormone.17, 18, 19.

Source: Dandona, P., & Rosenberg, M. T. (2010). A practical guide to male hypogonadism in the primary care setting. *International Journal of Clinical Practice*. doi:10.1111/j.1742-1241.2010.02355.x?

is unclear but is likely to be related to a combination of reduction in adipose tissue mass and a direct suppressive effect on *ob* gene expression (Cohen, 2001). The estradiol negatively feeds back on the hypothalamic pituitary gonadotropin (HPG) system, reducing testosterone production in the Leydig cells. Increasing adipose tissue also increases insulin resistance, which negatively impacts the Leydig cells as well as inhibiting the release of LH via the release of adipokines (inflammatory cytokines) such as tumor necrosis factor-alpha (TNF-alpha). Leptin, released in response to increased adiposity, also inhibits the release of LH via its effect on the release of gonadotropin-releasing hormone (GnRH) (Figure 29.1).

Consequently, hypogonadal, obese patients with diabetes mellitus are at further risk of poor glycemic control resulting in an increased risk of development of complications of diabetes and an increase in overall mortality risk. Recent studies have shown that TTh can ameliorate cardiometabolic risk. In a study conducted by the Veterans Administration, researchers conducted an observational study to determine if TRT improved overall mortality rate. The data showed that over a 4-year period, overall mortality rate decreased by 10.3% in the treated group and 20.7% in the untreated group (Luukkaa et al., 1998). In men with type 2 diabetes, researchers showed that over a 6-year period, all-cause mortality rate was 19.2% in untreated men and 8.4% in men treated with TRT (Muraleedharan, Marsh, Kapoor, Channer, & Jones, 2013).

Hypogonadism and Opiates

The opioid crisis in the United States is attributed to increased use of prescription and illegal long-acting opioids such as heroin, methadone, morphine, fentanyl, and oxycodone for both recreational use and for the treatment of chronic pain. This surge in opiate use has led to an increased prevalence of opioid-induced androgen deficiency (OPIAD). The mechanism for OPIAD is thought to involve the suppression of GnRH by the hypothalamus, resulting in a secondary hypogonadism. Findings from a case–control study of 40 cancer survivors found that 90% of those on opioid treatment were hypogonadal compared with only 40% of the control group. When identifying men who present with symptoms of hypogonadism they must be screened for current, past, or potential use of opiates (Daniell, Lentz, & Mazer, 2006; Howell, Radford, Ryder, & Shalet, 1999).

Hypogonadism and Cancer Treatment

Men undergoing cancer treatment, independent of testicular cancer, are at risk for developing hypogonadism. Radiation treatments, chemotherapy, corticosteroid, or opiates for pain may impair Leydig cell function or germinal epithelial failure and result in a secondary hypogonadism. The HPG axis may also be affected by androgen- or ectopic adrenocorticotropic hormone (ACTH)–producing tumors, leading to secondary hypogonadism (Kalyani, Gavini, & Dobs, 2007).

HUMAN IMMUNODEFICIENCY VIRUS

Approximately 20% to 50% of HIV-infected men receiving highly active antiretroviral therapy are hypogonadal. TD in this patient population is strongly associated with AIDS wasting syndrome. The cause of hypogonadism in this patient population is multifactorial, for example, testicular atrophy caused by opportunistic infection; disruption of the HPG axis resulting from malnutrition; and the effects of antimitotic medications which inhibit steroid biosynthesis. TRT, given to HIV-positive hypogonadal men, has been shown to increase lean muscle mass, improve mood, and improve perceived well-being (Gennari & Bilezikian, 2007; Grinspoon et al., 1998; 2000).

Osteoporosis

Osteoporosis remains largely underdiagnosed in males. The number of males with osteoporosis is not currently known, mainly due to the infrequency of screening and controversies in BMD testing standards in men. Using the World Health Organization (WHO) diagnostic criteria, it is estimated that 1 to 2 million men in the United States have osteoporosis and an additional 8 to 13 million have osteopenia (Gennari & Bilezikian, 2007). Using data from 2002, researchers estimated that about 25% of the male Medicare population had osteoporosis (Blume & Curtis, 2011). Because testosterone stimulates bone formation and inhibits bone resorption that involve both androgen and estrogen receptor–mediated processes, older men are at greater risk of low trauma fracture (Ebeling, 2008; Jackson, Riggs, & Spiekerman, 1992; Mascarenhas et al., 2017). In men with severe androgen deficiency with or without low trauma fracture, measurement of BMD by dual-energy x-ray absorptiometry (DEXA) scanning is also recommended (Bhasin et al., 2010; Mascarenhas et al., 2017).

■ DIAGNOSIS

The increased prevalence of hypogonadism and subsequent surge in treatment has forced experts to establish effective guidelines for the evaluation and treatment of hypogonadism. The Endocrine Society recommends that the diagnosis of testosterone be made in men who have consistent signs and symptoms and low TT levels. Serum TT is the easiest and most common initial laboratory measurement to lead to a diagnosis of hypogonadism. However, many experts suggest an initial evaluation of a total and free testosterone for the initial measurement followed by a second confirmatory laboratory measurement. Most clinic and hospital laboratories can provide TT measurements of good accuracy and reliability.

Testosterone is secreted in a pulsatile manner and is subject to circadian and circannual rhythms; therefore, it is recommended to draw the blood sample in the morning. There is ongoing debate regarding the lower threshold of serum testosterone; consequently, no consensus exists among experts establishing an absolute testosterone level below which a man can unequivocally be stated to be hypogonadal. The Endocrine Society recommends 300 ng/dL as a reliable level to consider as the lower threshold for normal TT, and the American Association of Clinical Endocrinologists (AACE) (Petak et al., 2002) suggests 200 ng/dL. TT represents the total of free, SHBG-bound, and albumin-bound testosterone. Some experts feel that free testosterone may be more reliable to correlate with symptoms of hypogonadism owing to the variability in SHBG. SHBG levels are easily affected by many conditions such as diabetes, obesity, and the normal consequence of aging.

TT measurements may be misleading indicators of hypogonadism due to elevated or depressed levels of SHBG (Table 29.4). Obese or elderly men are not uncommonly seen in routine clinical practice; therefore, it is prudent not to rely on TT concentrations for diagnosing hypogonadism for these patients. There are mixed opinions regarding free testosterone or bioavailable testosterone (BAT) measurements in all men other than healthy lean young men whose SHBG levels are presumably normal and whose measured TT concentration is expected to be unaffected in this manner. It is important that clinicians use reliable laboratories and are aware of the laboratory reference ranges for testosterone. One can calculate free testosterone reliably by using TT, albumin, and SHBG concentrations and using an online calculator (www.issam.ch/freetesto.htm) or smartphone app (T Calc, ViralMD). Some laboratories can accurately perform a free testosterone measurement by equilibrium dialysis.

As with TT measurements, there is no general agreement as to what constitutes the lower limit of normal free testosterone levels; however, the Endocrine Society recommends 50 pg/mL for free testosterone measured by equilibrium dialysis and most organizations recommend 65 pg/mL for calculated free testosterone. The International Society of Andrology (ISA)/International Society for the Study of the Aging Male (ISSAM)/European Association of Urology (EAU)/European Association of Andrology (EAA)/American Society of Andrology (ASA) guidelines recommend that subjects with TT levels falling between 230 and 350 ng/dL (8–12 nmol/L) could benefit from having a repeat measurement of TT together with a measurement of SHBG concentrations so as to calculate free testosterone levels, or free testosterone levels can be measured directly via equilibrium analysis in these cases (Wang et al., 2009a; 2009b). Whether a patient has primary or secondary hypogonadism can be determined by measuring the serum LH and FSH. Elevated LH and FSH levels (Table 29.5) suggest primary hypogonadism, whereas low or low-normal LH and FSH levels suggest secondary

TABLE 29.4 Conditions That Affect SHBG Levels

Increased SHBG	Decreased SHBG
HIV	Opioids
Liver disease	Androgens
Hyperthyroidism	Hypothyroidism
Estrogens	Nephrotic syndrome
Anticonvulsants	Glucocorticoids
Low testosterone	Acromegaly
Age (1%/year)	Obesity (IR)

IR, insulin resistant; SHBG, sex hormone binding globulin.

TABLE 29.5 The Relationship of Testosterone, LH, FSH, and Prolactin with Clinical Condition

Clinical Condition	FSH	LH	Testosterone	Prolactin
Normal spermatogenesis	Normal	Normal	Normal	Normal
Hypogonadotropic hypogonadism	Low	Low	Low	Normal
Abnormal spermatogenesis	High/normal	Normal	Normal	Normal
Complete testicular failure/ hypergonadotropic hypogonadism	High	High	Normal/low	Normal
Prolactin-secreting pituitary tumor	Normal/low	Normal/low	Low	High

FSH, follicle-stimulating hormone; LH, luteinizing hormone.

hypogonadism. Normal LH or FSH levels with low testosterone suggest primary defects in the hypothalamus and/or the pituitary (secondary hypogonadism). As mentioned previously, in cases in which fertility is an issue, it is recommended to measure FSH and LH levels. In patients in whom secondary hypogonadism is suspected, further evaluation should include measurements of serum prolactin, pituitary function testing, and MRI of the pituitary gland. In men with primary testicular failure of unknown cause and a physical examination yielding low testicular volume, obtaining a karyotype to exclude Klinefelter's syndrome (XXY male) is recommended. Men with Klinefelter's syndrome can benefit from genetic counseling and need surveillance for certain disorders for which they are at increased risk (Dean et al., 2015).

■ TREATMENT

TRT is indicated in men with primary or secondary hypogonadism. The goal of TRT is to treat the signs and symptoms of hypogonadism and achieve and maintain eugonadal serum testosterone levels. Food and Drug Administration (FDA)-approved testosterone replacement treatments are numerous and varied in their routes of administration and duration of action (Table 29.6). The eugonadal range for adult men has been considered in most studies to be in the range of 300 to 1,000 ng/dL (the AACE recommends 280–800 ng/dL), and it is usually considered best to aim for a testosterone level in the mid-normal range, avoiding excessive supraphysiological peaks (Dean et al., 2015; Petak et al., 2002).

Many issues presently surround testosterone replacement for men, especially in the era of insurance prior authorizations. This prior authorization aspect is unregulated, and many insurance companies have created their own independent definition of hypogonadism, which may be in conflict with the definitions established by medical societies. This can cause treatment delays for men and can require additional documentation and lab work before the testosterone replacement is approved.

Intramuscular Injections

Testosterone injections have been available for at least 50 years and are usually the cheapest choice for treatment. The testosterone esters, testosterone enanthate or cypionate, are either administered in the office or self-administered at home by the patient or a caregiver. Injected testosterone esters reach peak concentration within 2 to 5 days after the injection, causing the serum testosterone levels to rise to supraphysiological levels followed by a gradual decline in the hypogonadal range by the end of the dosing interval (Shoskes, Wilson, & Spinner, 2016). The usual frequency of injections is once every 2 weeks. Peak serum testosterone levels can be reduced by decreasing the dose and/or frequency of injections to once a week.

TABLE 29.6 Testosterone Preparations Available in the United States

Formulation	Dosage	Adverse Effects	Benefits
Topical/Transdermal			
Formulation	**Dosage**	**Adverse Effects**	**Benefits**
Androgel 1%, Androgel 1.62%, Testim, Fortesta 2%	5–10 g qd	Skin irritation, transference	Maintain T level concentration over a 24-hour period. High patient adherence
Transdermal patch, Androderm	2–4 mg patch qd	Skin irritation, transference	T levels mimic circadian rhythm Low incidence of polycythemia
Topical solution, Axiron	60–120 mg applied to axilla qd	Skin irritation, transference	Maintain T levels over a 24-hour period Unique administration presumed to minimize risk of transference
Buccal/Oral			
Formulation	**Dosage**	**Adverse Effects**	**Benefits**
Buccal system, Striant	30 mg q12h	Alterations in taste and irritation of gums and oral mucosa	Testosterone levels within physiological range
Fluoxymesterone, Halotestin	5–40 mg daily	Hepatotoxicity	Pill form
Injectable			
Formulation	**Dosage**	**Adverse Effects**	**Benefits**
Testosterone cypionate, Depo-Testosterone	50–400 mg IM q 10–14 days	Mood fluctuations or changes in libido, pain at injection site, excessive erythrocytosis	Effective in relieving symptoms, inexpensive
Testosterone enanthate, Delatestryl	50–400 mg IM q 1 week	Mood fluctuations or changes in libido, pain at injection site, excessive erythrocytosis	Effective in relieving symptoms, inexpensive
Testosterone undecanoate, Nebido, Aveed	1,000 mg IM q 6 weeks during first 12 weeks, then 1,000 mg q 3 months 750 mg IM Initial followed by 2nd injection 4 weeks later, then q 10 weeks (REMS Certification required)	Mood fluctuations or changes in libido, pain at injection site, excessive erythrocytosis, pulmonary oil microembolism (POME)	Effective in relieving symptoms, inexpensive, long-acting

(continued)

TABLE 29.6 Testosterone Preparations Available in the United States (*continued*)

Implantable			
Formulation	**Dosage**	**Adverse Effects**	**Benefits**
Testopel 75 mg pellets	6 pellets implanted q 3–4 months	Pain at insertion site, infection, expulsion, expensive, requires Office Visit	Long-acting, convenient, consistent delivery for a prolonged period of time (3–6 months)

REMS, Risk Evaluation and Mitigation Strategy; T, testosterone.

TABLE 29.7 Endocrine Society Guidelines for the Monitoring of Testosterone Therapy

	Start of Treatment (Baseline)	Each Visit	3 Months	Annually	1–2 Years
Symptom response		√	√	√	
Adverse events (AEs)		√	√	√	
Formulation-specific AEs		√			
Testosterone levels	√		√		
Hematocrit	√		√	√	
BMD of Lumbar spine Femoral neck					√
DRE	√		√		
PSA test	√		√		

BMD, bone mineral density; DRE, digital rectal examination; PSA, prostate-specific antigen.

Common side effects seen are variable breast tenderness, increase or decrease in sexual activity, emotional lability (anger or depression), and general well-being (fatigue) as the testosterone levels change over time. Patients who are sensitive to injectable testosterone and have fluctuating responses (e.g., mood and sexual function) in relation to time of dosing and duration of action may benefit from lower doses given more frequently and slowly titrated upward in dose with a reduction in frequency (Table 29.7). Testosterone undecanoate (Aveed, Nebido) is a long-acting depot preparation that carries some similar side effect profile as shorter acting injectable preparations. However, owing to a reported increased risk of pulmonary oil microembolism (POME), clinicians in the United States are required to undergo Risk Evaluation and Mitigation Strategy (REMS) training prior to obtaining authorization to prescribe testosterone undecanoate.

Transdermal Patches

Transdermal testosterone patches are applied to the skin, typically at night. These preparations are known for approximating normal circadian plasma testosterone concentrations. The first available testosterone patches were applied to the scrotum due to the 40-fold higher rate of absorption than the forearm. Scrotal patches are rarely prescribed as compliance is noted to be low due mostly to the need to keep the scrotum clean shaven to better ensure adherence of the patch to the skin. More commonly used transdermal patches are applied once daily to the back, abdomen, thighs, or upper arms, preferably in the evening. Skin irritation is a common side effect of these delivery systems. In cases of significant skin irritation, a preapplication of a corticosteroid cream to the skin can help reduce the skin irritation but may also decrease absorption.

Transdermal Gels and Solutions

Transdermal gels and solutions are most commonly prescribed after injections. Gel preparations are currently available in 1%, 1.62%, and 2% concentrations, whereas topical solutions are available in a standardized 30 mg of testosterone per pump actuation. Testosterone gels are typically applied in the morning. Application sites for gels include the upper arms and shoulders, front and/or upper inner thigh, or the abdomen, and topical solutions are applied to the axilla. Reported advantages of topical gels and solutions are their relative ease of use, lower incidence of skin irritation, consistent delivery, and dosing flexibility. Several reported issues with gels and solutions are related to transference from patient to partner or family member, particularly a child. Patients should be instructed to take necessary precautions to minimize the risk of transference by washing their hands with soap and water after applying the gel or solution, covering the application site with clothing after the gel or solution has dried, and washing the application site when skin-to-skin contact is anticipated. Men should be given further instruction regarding proper and secure storage of the gel or solution to avoid accidental application of the gel or solution to a woman or child.

Buccal Tablets

These adhesive tablets containing testosterone are applied to the gum just above the incisor teeth. They release testosterone slowly, allowing for absorption through the gum and cheek surfaces. In this manner, they bypass first-pass hepatic metabolism. The tablet must remain in the mouth for a full 12 hours and two are needed for the 24-hour dosing period. The incidence of adverse effects is low, although gum and buccal irritation and alterations in taste have been reported (Dhindsa et al., 2010).

Subcutaneous Pellets

These are among the earliest effective formulations for administering testosterone, dating back to the 1940s. Although not frequently used, they remain available. The testosterone pellets are usually implanted under the skin of the lower abdomen using a trocar and cannula or are inserted into the gluteus muscle. Six to ten pellets are implanted at one time and they last 4 to 6 months, when a new procedure is required to implant more. Testosterone pellets currently are the only long-acting testosterone treatment approved for use in the United States. As a result of their long-lasting effect and the inconvenience of removing them, it is best to use pellets in men for whom the beneficial effects and tolerance for TRT have already been established.

Oral Testosterone Tablets or Capsules

There are no FDA-approved orally ingested testosterone preparations currently available in the United States. There are concerns with hepatotoxic side effects and the development of liver tumors seen with previously available orally ingested testosterone preparations. However, a new orally ingested formulation of testosterone undecanoate has competed phase III Safety Oversight, Adjudication and Reporting (SOAR) Trials and is expected

TABLE 29.8 Testosterone Undecanoate Dosing Schedule and Monitoring

Testosterone Undecanoate—Initial Series				
Week	**Injection**	**Lab**	**Office Visit**	**Rationale**
1	X			
4	X			
6		X		Monitor that loading dose was sufficient at 6 weeks (day 42)
14	X			
16		X		Check if reached steady state after 14 weeks (day 70) Based on the pharmacokinetics statement: ***Steady state serum testosterone concentration was achieved with the 3rd injection at 14 weeks.***
18			X	Review labs and assess symptoms
24	X			
34	X			
44	X			
54	X	X		
56			X	Review labs and assess symptoms. If stable, order continued series of testosterone undecanoate injections.
Testosterone Undecanoate—Continued Series				
Week	**Injection**	**Lab**	**Office Visit**	**Rationale**
Initial	X			
10	X			
20	X	X		Routine monitoring
30	X			
40	X	X		
42			X	Review labs and assess symptoms. If stable, order continued series of testosterone undecanoate injections.

to be available in the near future pending FDA approval. The advantage of this new oral preparation versus previous available preparations is that it bypasses first-pass metabolism in the liver and is preferentially absorbed through the lymphatic system, thus avoiding the previously seen hepatotoxic side effects.

Contraindications and Precautions with Testosterone Replacement

The most important contraindications related to TRT are for prostate and male breast cancer (Table 29.8). There is a fair amount of controversy surrounding the role of testosterone in prostate cancer disease development, progression, and recurrence; details regarding this controversy will be discussed later in this chapter. However, because the suspicion of "feeding a hungry tumor" with androgens is widely accepted, and no evidence to completely support or refute this claim has been elucidated, it is recommended that clinicians proceed with caution in these populations. The evidence is much clearer regarding male breast cancer and the role testosterone plays in its development and progression. Men with breast cancer should never take testosterone because it causes breast cancer cells to grow (Osterberg, Bernie, & Ramasamy, 2014). Further recommendations include performing a baseline digital rectal examination (DRE) and a baseline prostate-specific antigen (PSA) level measurement before starting TTh for any man, regardless of age.

Testosterone is also contraindicated in pregnant or breastfeeding women and children. Clinicians must inform and instruct men using topical preparations to follow the previously mentioned precautions to minimize transference to pregnant or breastfeeding women or children.

MONITORING TREATMENT

Once TRT has started, patients need to be carefully monitored. The Endocrine Society recommends a PSA test and DRE be performed initially and repeated during the course of treatment (Table 29.9). The clinical response to TTh typically occurs as early as 1 month up to 3 months. It is recommended that serum testosterone levels and hematocrit be measured at baseline and at 1 and 3 months after initiating therapy. The clinical response of testosterone should be evaluated by assessing the serum testosterone levels, PSA levels, performing a DRE, and correlating the testosterone levels with symptom relief. PSA levels and DREs can be performed thereafter at the recommended intervals based on age and clinical history. Any elevations in PSA should prompt discontinuing testosterone replacement and either refer or conduct the recommended urological evaluation for elevated PSA. From then on, PSA levels need to be checked according to the usual guidelines for prostate cancer screening.

Testosterone is a known stimulant of erythropoiesis and carries a 3% to 18% risk of elevated red blood cells or hemoglobin values; elevated hematocrit values above 54% should prompt reduction or discontinuing TRT until the hematocrit decreases to the normal range. Persistent elevations in hematocrit should prompt a referral to a hematologist/oncologist for further evaluation.

BMD measurement should also be carried out at baseline; hypogonadism is an important cause of male osteoporosis. BMD measurement in a male with osteopenia/osteoporosis or history of low trauma fracture can be repeated 1 to 2 years after TRT is initiated (Bhasin et al., 2010; Mascarenhas et al., 2017).

Men with benign prostatic hyperplasia (BPH) with or without lower urinary tract symptoms (LUTS) treated with androgens are at an increased risk for worsening of signs and symptoms of BPH and/or LUTS. Interestingly, it is widely accepted that development of

TABLE 29.9 Contraindications and Precautions with TRT

Contraindications	Precautions
Male breast cancer	BPH
Prostate cancer (known or suspected)	LUTS
Known or suspected sensitivity to ingredients used in the preparation.	Edema in patients with preexisting cardiac, renal, or hepatic disease
	Gynecomastia
	Precipitation or worsening of sleep apnea
	Azoospermia
	Testicular atrophy

BPH, benign prostatic hyperplasia; LUTS, lower urinary tract symptoms, TRT, testosterone replacement therapy.

BPH requires androgens; however, studies have failed to show an association with testosterone treatment. Prostate volume has been shown to increase during TRT, however this is usually similar to the normal volume seen in eugonadal men. Nevertheless, patients may experience irritative voiding symptoms and should be counseled regarding the possible development of and/or worsening voiding symptoms.

HYPOGONADISM AND PROSTATE CANCER

Use of TRT in men with prostate cancer remains controversial. Numerous studies have shown that TRT can decrease the overall mortality risk in hypogonadal men with or without prostate cancer (Kaplan, Lenis, Shah, Rajfer, & Hu, 2015; Khera et al., 2009). Historically it had been widely accepted that testosterone may potentiate the growth of prostate cancer cells, resulting in the recommendation that TRT not be utilized or be used with extreme caution in men with a known diagnosis of prostate cancer regardless of treatment. However, recent data provided evidence supporting that there is no increased risk of progression or recurrence of prostate cancer in men treated or untreated with a confirmed diagnosis of prostate cancer (Kaplan et al., 2015; Khera et al. 2009).

More recent data suggest that TRT may be safe in men with a known history of prostate cancer; however, researchers concluded that more studies are needed. Further evidence has shown low serum testosterone levels to be associated with a greater risk of prostate cancer and higher grade of disease (Khera, 2015). Furthermore, the rate of prostate cancer progression and recurrence in men treated for prostate cancer tends to be lower in hypogonadal men treated with TRT than in those men not treated with TRT. Recent data now suggest that TRT may be protective against the development and recurrence of prostate cancer. The prostate saturation model explains the changes in PSA in response to TRT and androgen deprivation therapy (ADT) to treat prostate cancer (Lackner, Koller, Schatzl, Marberger, & Kratzik, 2009).

SOCIETAL ISSUES

Societal pressure and widespread advertising have contributed in large part to men inappropriately seeking treatment for hypogonadism. In cities across the nation, "Low T" centers have been established to treat men with presumed hypogonadism. Many of these establishments provide suboptimal evaluations and often initiate inappropriate treatment, which often leads to adverse reactions. Clear communication between the clinician and the patient is paramount to dispelling inaccurate information or advertised promises that lead patients to have unrealistic expectations about the benefits of TRT. Further clarification is important for both the clinician and the patient to understand the difference between testosterone *supplementation* and TRT. Testosterone supplementation involves the addition of testosterone where the levels of testosterone are already in the normal range. This practice is typically done by bodybuilders or athletes to increase muscle mass or recover from injuries quickly, whereas testosterone replacement is the act of restoring abnormally low or deficient testosterone levels back to the normal range. Patient counseling defining these terms and the expected treatment outcomes is essential to help the patient understand the true benefits of TRT while setting realistic expectations for the patient. Clinicians should counsel patients with hypogonadism to make appropriate lifestyle modifications that support normal androgen production and/or improve response to therapy. Improving nutrition, increasing exercise, and decreasing or discontinuing medications contributing to the patient's hypogonadism will also support improvement in endogenous testosterone production and symptom relief.

LACK OF CONSENSUS

Despite the long history of TRT, there has been little standardization regarding the evaluation and management of hypogonadism. This lack of consensus causes confusion among clinicians and represents a significant hurdle and contributes greatly to inappropriate use of TRT. Morgentaler et al. (2014) report that the confusion stems from a number of factors: availability of multiple assays to determine androgen status, such as total, free, and bioavailable testosterone, with proponents for each; widely differing laboratory reference ranges; limited clinical correlation between serum testosterone concentrations and symptoms; and clinical experiences that differ from published guidelines.

Published guidelines from several expert specialty societies have attempted to address these issues. As mentioned previously, the Endocrine Society in the United States (Bhasin et al., 2010), joint guidelines from various international andrological societies (Wang et al., 2009), recommendations from the International Consultation on Sexual Medicine (Buvat et al., 2010), and the International Society for Sexual Medicine (ISSM) guidelines (Dean et al., 2015), with minor variations, suggest that the diagnosis of TD should only be made in men with characteristic symptoms or signs of TD in combination with a documented serum testosterone that is low. Variations of the Endocrine Society occurred over a narrow period of 4 years. In the 2006 version of the Endocrine Society guidelines, a serum testosterone below 300 ng/dL (10.4 nmol/L) was set as the diagnostic threshold; however, in the 2010 updated version, clinicians were referred to their own laboratory's reference ranges. The joint international societies recommended a threshold of 350 ng/dL (12 nmol/L) asserting that men with serum testosterone concentrations above this level generally do not benefit from treatment (Wang et al., 2009a; 2009b). The International Consultation on Sexual Medicine repeats this threshold, but notes that treatment may be reasonably offered to symptomatic men with higher concentrations based on clinical judgment (Buvat et al., 2010). All groups recommend obtaining a second confirmatory TT test prior to initiating treatment. There is a lack of consensus regarding the use of free or bioavailable testosterone with these groups recommending that these tests be utilized as secondary measures of when serum testosterone provides unclear results. Experts agree that guidelines provide a valuable guide for clinicians new to the field; however, it is important to understand that guidelines have significant limitations in more advanced clinical practice (Powers, 2011). Morgentaler et al. (2014) report that the quality of supporting evidence regarding evaluation and treatment of TD is poor and no studies to date have provided sufficient evidence that reveals evidence to help predict which men will respond. Furthermore, it must be understood that guidelines represent the consensus opinions of experts of various practice styles and methodologies which lends to a tendency to regard guidelines as reflecting "ideal" practices, which may not exist.

CONCLUSION

Advanced practice providers caring for men with hypogonadism must be able to accurately diagnose, treat, and manage these patients effectively. The increased prevalence of hypogonadism and subsequent surge in treatment has forced experts to establish effective guidelines for the evaluation and treatment of hypogonadism. The ISSM guidelines provide the most comprehensive and current data pertinent to patients who are more likely to present to a urology practice (Morgentaler et al., 2015). The ISSM guidelines contain information and guidance regarding patients with urological disease including recommendations for patients with prostate cancer and BPH. The ISSM guidelines also address the controversy surrounding cardiovascular risk associated with TRT. Experts reviewing the literature in search of evidence to support the claim that TRT increased cardiovascular risk published their findings indicating that there were no studies conducted that produced evidence to support the claim that TRT increased cardiovascular risk. The data discovered by the researchers indicated that TRT in hypogonadal men decreased the risk of cardiovascular disease. The researchers further concluded that randomized controlled trials will be critical to accurately determine the efficacy and safety of TRT with or without significant comorbid conditions.

CLINICAL PEARLS

- The goal of TRT is to treat the signs and symptoms of hypogonadism and achieve and maintain eugonadal serum testosterone levels.
- Screen for hypogonadism in men who participate in pain management programs or in any man on long-term (>3 months) opioid therapy.
- Diminished libido and sexual function complaints are sensitive for the indication of hypogonadism.
- No thromboembolic events have been reported with men on TRT.
- There is no increased risk for prostate cancer for men on TRT.

RESOURCES FOR CLINICIANS

American Academy of Family Physicians curriculum for Men's Health: www.aafp.org/dam/AAFP/documents/medical_education_residency/program_directors/Reprint257_Men.pdf
Men's Health Month: www.menshealthmonth.org
Smartphone apps: T Calc, ViralMD

RESOURCES FOR PATIENTS

Men's Health Month: www.menshealthmonth.org
Men's Health Network (MHN): www.menshealthnetwork.org
The Urology Care Foundation: www.urologyhealth.org

REFERENCES

Aso, Y. (2008). Cardiovascular disease in patients with diabetic nephropathy. *Current Molecular Medicine, 8*(6), 533–543. doi:10.2174/156652408785747960

Bhasin, S., Cunningham, G. R., Hayes, F. J., Matsumoto, A. M., Snyder, P. J., Swerdloff, R. S., & Montori, V. M. (2010). Testosterone therapy in men with androgen deficiency syndromes: An endocrine society clinical practice guideline. *The Journal of Clinical Endocrinology & Metabolism, 95*(6), 2536–2559. doi:10.1210/jc.2009-2354

Bhatia, V., Chaudhuri, A., Tomar, R., Dhindsa, S., Ghanim, H., & Dandona, P. (2006). Low testosterone and high C-reactive protein concentrations predict low hematocrit in type 2 diabetes. *Diabetes Care, 29*(10), 2289–2294. doi:10.2337/dc06-0637

Blume, S. W., & Curtis, J. R. (2011). Medical costs of osteoporosis in the elderly Medicare population. *Osteoporosis International, 22*(6), 1835–1844. doi:10.1007/s00198-010-1419-7

Buvat, J., Maggi, M., Gooren, L., Guay, A. T., Kaufman, J., Morgentaler, A., … Zitzmann, M. (2010). Endocrine aspects of male sexual dysfunctions. *The Journal of Sexual Medicine, 7*(4), 1627–1656. doi:10.1111/j.1743-6109.2010.01780.x

Centers for Disease Control and Prevention. (2017). *National Diabetes Statistics Report, 2017*. Atlanta, GA: Centers for Disease Control and Prevention, U.S. Department of Health and Human Services.

Cohen, P. G. (2001). Aromatase, adiposity, aging and disease. The hypogonadal-metabolic-atherogenic -disease and aging connection. *Medical hypotheses, 56*(6), 702–708. doi:10.1054/mehy.2000.1169

Daniell, H. W., Lentz, R., & Mazer, N. A. (2006). Open-label pilot study of testosterone patch therapy in men with opioid-induced androgen deficiency. *The Journal of Pain, 7*(3), 200–210. doi:10.1016/j.jpain.2005.10.009

Dean, J. D., McMahon, C. G., Guay, A. T., Morgentaler, A., Althof, S. E., Becher, E. F., … Hellstrom, W. J. (2015). The International Society for Sexual Medicine's process of care for the assessment and management of testosterone deficiency in adult men. *The Journal of Sexual Medicine, 12*(8), 1660–1686. doi:10.1111/jsm.12952

Dhindsa, S., Bhatia, V., Dhindsa, G., Chaudhuri, A., Gollapudi, G. M., & Dandona, P. (2007). The effects of hypogonadism on body composition and bone mineral density in type 2 diabetic patients. *Diabetes Care, 30*(7), 1860–1861. doi:10.2337/dc07-0337

Dhindsa, S., Miller, M. G., McWhirter, C. L., Mager, D. E., Ghanim, H., Chaudhuri, A., & Dandona, P. (2010). Testosterone concentrations in diabetic and nondiabetic obese men. *Diabetes Care, 33*(6), 1186-1192. doi:10.2337/dc09-1649

Dhindsa, S., Prabhakar, S., Sethi, M., Bandyopadhyay, A., Chaudhuri, A., & Dandona, P. (2004). Frequent occurrence of hypogonadotropic hypogonadism in type 2 diabetes. *The Journal of Clinical Endocrinology & Metabolism, 89*(11), 5462–5468. doi:10.1210/jc.2004-0804

Ebeling, P. R. (2008). Osteoporosis in men. *New England Journal of Medicine, 358*(14), 1474–1482. doi:10.1056/nejmcp0707217

Gennari, L., & Bilezikian, J. P. (2007). Osteoporosis in men. *Endocrinology and Metabolism Clinics of North America, 36*(2), 399–419. doi:10.1016/j.ecl.2007.03.008

Grinspoon, S., Corcoran, C., Askari, H., Schoenfeld, D., Wolf, L., Burrows, B., … & Basgoz, N. (1998). Effects of androgen administration in men with the AIDS wasting syndrome: A randomized, double-blind, placebo-controlled trial. *Annals of Internal Medicine, 129*(1), 18–26. doi:10.7326/0003-4819-129-1-199807010-00005

Grinspoon, S., Corcoran, C., Lee, K., Burrows, B., Hubbard, J., Katznelson, L., … Klibanski, A. (1996). Loss of lean body and muscle mass correlates with androgen levels in hypogonadal men with acquired immunodeficiency syndrome and wasting. *The Journal of Clinical Endocrinology & Metabolism, 81*(11), 4051–4058. doi:10.1210/jcem.81.11.8923860

Grinspoon, S., Corcoran, C., Stanley, T., Baaj, A., Basgoz, N., & Klibanski, A. (2000). Effects of hypogonadism and testosterone administration on depression indices in HIV-infected men. *The Journal of Clinical Endocrinology & Metabolism, 85*(1), 60–65. doi:10.1210/jcem.85.1.6224

Grundy, S. M., Cleeman, J. I., Daniels, S. R., Donato, K. A., Eckel, R. H., Franklin, B. A., … Spertus, J. A. (2005). Diagnosis and management of the metabolic syndrome: An American Heart Association/National Heart, Lung, and Blood Institute scientific statement. *Circulation, 112*(17), 2735–2752. doi:10.1161/CIRCULATIONAHA.105.169404

Howell, S. J., Radford, J. A., Ryder, W. D. J., & Shalet, S. M. (1999). Testicular function after cytotoxic chemotherapy: Evidence of Leydig cell insufficiency. *Journal of Clinical Oncology, 17*(5), 1493–1498. doi:10.1200/jco.1999.17.5.1493

Jackson, J. A., Riggs, M. W., & Spiekerman, A. M. (1992). Testosterone deficiency as a risk factor for hip fractures in men: A case-control study. *The American Journal of the Medical Sciences, 304*(1), 4–8. doi:10.1097/00000441-199207000-00003

Kalyani, R. R., Gavini, S., & Dobs, A. S. (2007). Male hypogonadism in systemic disease. *Endocrinology and Metabolism Clinics, 36*(2), 333–348. doi:10.1016/j.ecl.2007.03.014

Kaplan, A. L., Lenis, A. T., Shah, A., Rajfer, J., & Hu, J. C. (2015). Testosterone replacement therapy in men with prostate cancer: A time-varying analysis. *The Journal of Sexual Medicine, 12*(2), 374–380. doi:10.1111/jsm.12768

Kapoor, D., Malkin, C. J., Channer, K. S., & Jones, T. H. (2005). Androgens, insulin resistance and vascular disease in men. *Clinical Endocrinology, 63*(3), 239–250. doi:10.1111/j.1365-2265.2005.02299.x

Khera, M. (2015). *Testosterone replacement therapy: Controversies versus reality*. Grand Rounds in Urology. Retrieved from http://www.grandroundsinurology.com/TRT-Mohit-Khera-testosterone-replacement-therapy-controversies-versus-reality

Khera, M., Grober, E. D., Najari, B., Colen, J. S., Mohamed, O., Lamb, D. J., & Lipshultz, L. I. (2009). Testosterone replacement therapy following radical prostatectomy. *The Journal of Sexual Medicine, 6*(4), 1165–1170. doi:10.1111/j.1743-6109.2009.01161.x

Lackner, J. E., Koller, A., Schatzl, G., Marberger, M., & Kratzik, C. (2009). Androgen deficiency symptoms in testicular cancer survivors are associated with sexual problems but not with serum testosterone or therapy. *Urology, 74*(4), 825–829. doi:10.1016/j.urology.2009.03.051

Luukkaa, V., Pesonen, U., Huhtaniemi, I., Lehtonen, A., Tilvis, R., Tuomilehto, J., ... Huupponen, R. (1998). Inverse correlation between serum testosterone and Leptin in men. *The Journal of Clinical Endocrinology & Metabolism, 83*(9), 3243–3246. doi:10.1210/jcem.83.9.5134

Mascarenhas, M. R., Barbosa, A. P., Gomes, A. R. C., Silvestre, C., Barbosa, D., Paixao, R., ... Bugalho, M. J. (2017). Effects of male hypogonadism treatment on the bone mineral density. *Endocrine Abstracts, 49*, EP1083. doi:10.1530/endoabs.49.ep1083

Mohamed, O., Freundlich, R. E., Dakik, H. K., Grober, E. D., Najari, B., Lipshultz, L. I., & Khera, M. (2010). The quantitative ADAM questionnaire: A new tool in quantifying the severity of hypogonadism. *International Journal of Impotence Research, 22*(1), 20–24. doi:10.1038/ijir.2009.35

Morgentaler, A., Khera, M., Maggi, M., & Zitzmann, M. (2014). Commentary: Who is a candidate for testosterone therapy? A synthesis of international expert opinions. *The Journal of Sexual Medicine, 11*(7), 1636–1645. doi:10.1111/jsm.12546

Morgentaler, A., Miner, M. M., Caliber, M., Guay, A. T., Khera, M., & Traish, A. M. (2015). Testosterone therapy and cardiovascular risk: Advances and controversies. *Mayo Clinic Proceedings, 90*(2), 224–251. doi:10.1016/j.mayocp.2014.10.011

Mulligan, T., Frick, M., Zuraw, Q., Stemhagen, A., & McWhirter, C. (2006). Prevalence of hypogonadism in males aged at least 45 years: The HIM study. *International Journal of Clinical Practice, 60*(7), 762–769. doi:10.1111/j.1742-1241.2006.00992.x

Muraleedharan, V., Marsh, H., Kapoor, D., Channer, K. S., & Jones, T. H. (2013). Testosterone deficiency is associated with increased risk of mortality and testosterone replacement improves survival in men with type 2 diabetes. *European Journal of Endocrinology, 169*(6), 725–733. doi:10.1530/EJE-13-0321

Nettleship, J., Jones, R. D., & Channer, K. S., & Jones, T. H. (2009) Testosterone and coronary artery disease. In T. H. Jones (Ed.), *Advances in the management of testosterone deficiency* (Vol. 37, pp. 91–107). Basel, Switzerland: Karger.

Ogden, C. L., Carroll, M. D., Fryar, C. D., & Flegal, K. M. (2015). *Prevalence of obesity among adults and youth: United States, 2011–2014*. NCHS data brief, no 219. Hyattsville, MD: National Center for Health Statistics.

Osterberg, E. C., Bernie, A. M., & Ramasamy, R. (2014). Risks of testosterone replacement therapy in men. *Indian Journal of Urology 30*(1), 2–7. doi:10.4103/0970-1591.124197

Petak, S. M., Nankin, H. R., Spark, R. F., Swerdloff, R. S., & Rodriguez-Rigau, L. J.; American Association of Clinical Endocrinologists. (2002). American Association of Clinical Endocrinologists Medical Guidelines for clinical practice for the evaluation and treatment of hypogonadism in adult male patients—2002 update. *Endocrine Practice, 8*, 440–456.

Powers, J. H. (2011). Practice guidelines. *Archives of Internal Medicine, 171*(1), 15–17. doi:10.1001/archinternmed.2010.453

Seftel, A. (2006). Male hypogonadism. Part II: Etiology, pathophysiology, and diagnosis. *International journal of Impotence Research, 18*(3), 223–228. doi:10.1038/sj.ijir.3901365

Selvin, E., Feinleib, M., Zhang, L., Rohrmann, S., Rifai, N., Nelson, W. G., ... Platz, E. A. (2007). Androgens and diabetes in men: Results from the Third National Health and Nutrition Examination Survey (NHANES III). *Diabetes Care, 30*(2), 234–238. doi:10.2337/dc06-1579

Shabsigh, R., Katz, M., Yan, G., & Makhsida, N. (2005). Cardiovascular issues in hypogonadism and testosterone therapy. *The American Journal of Cardiology, 96*(12), 67–72. doi:10.1016/j.amjcard.2005.10.009

Shoskes, J. J., Wilson, M. K., & Spinner, M. L. (2016). Pharmacology of testosterone replacement therapy preparations. *Translational Andrology and Urology, 5*(6), 834–843. doi:10.21037/tau.2016.07.10

Tomar, R., Dhindsa, S., Chaudhuri, A., Mohanty, P., Garg, R., & Dandona, P. (2006). Contrasting testosterone concentrations in type 1 and type 2 diabetes. *Diabetes Care, 29*(5), 1120–1122. doi:10.2337/diacare.2951120

Traish, A. M., Guay, A., Feeley, R., & Saad, F. (2009). The dark side of testosterone deficiency: I. Metabolic syndrome and erectile dysfunction. *Journal of Andrology, 30*(1), 10–22. doi:10.2164/jandrol.108.005215

Wang, C., Nieschlag, E., Swerdloff, R., Behre, H. M., Hellstrom, W. J., Gooren, L. J., ... Wu, F. C. W. (2009). Investigation, treatment, and monitoring of late-onset hypogonadism in males: ISA, ISSAM, EAU, EAA, and ASA recommendations. *European Urology, 55*(1), 121–130. doi:10.1016/j.eururo.2008.08.033

Yialamas, M. A., & Hayes, F. J. (2003). Androgens and the ageing male and female. *Best Practice & Research Clinical Endocrinology & Metabolism, 17*(2), 223–236. doi:10.1016/S1521-690X(03)00018-6

CHAPTER 30

Brief Guide to Penile and Testicular Cancer

Anne E. Calvaresi

PENILE CANCER IN THE UNITED STATES

Introduction and Incidence

In 2017, there were an estimated 2,120 new cases of penile cancer in the United States. Cases are more prevalent among rural, underdeveloped countries, especially in Africa, Asia, Latin America, and South America. It is predicted that 10% to 20% of male cancers in certain parts of South America and Africa are penile cancer. The median age at presentation is 58 years, and age at presentation is nearly always greater than 40 years old (American Cancer Society, 2017a). With the risk being much higher in uncircumcised patients, the risk of developing the disease in the United States and having been circumcised at birth is less than 1 in 1,800. In the Jewish population, for example, penile cancer is rare owing to circumcision at birth (Pow-Sang, Ferreira, Pow-Sang, Nardi, & Destefano, 2010). Caucasians are much less likely to be diagnosed than African Americans (Cookson & Whittam, 2010).

Pathophysiology

Nearly all penile cancers are squamous cell carcinomas (95%; Cookson & Whittam, 2010, pp. 252–253). In 80% of cases, cure can be attained; however, metastatic penile cancer has a poor prognosis. It is still unknown, whether squamous cell carcinoma is precluded by nonmalignant lesions (Hakenberg et al., 2014). Other malignant presentations include sarcoma, melanoma, basal cell carcinoma, and lymphomas. Buschke-Lowenstein tumor is benign, but because of its aggressive local extension, it may destroy the penis if not treated. Spread of disease by squamous cell carcinomas typically spread first to superficial inguinal lymph nodes, then to deep inguinal lymph nodes, and third to the pelvic nodes. Either one or both sides of the groin may be involved (Cookson & Whittam, 2010).

Pertinent Anatomy and Physiology

Providers should be familiar with the penile glans (foreskin, if applicable), prepuce, coronal sulcus, shaft, and urethra as well as the tunica albuginea, corpus spongiosum, and corpus cavernosum. Lymph nodes associated with penile cancer should also be reviewed, including deep and superficial inguinal lymph nodes and, in some cases, the pelvic lymph nodes. Thorough knowledge of the urethra and perineum should be established, as surgical treatments for penile cancer may require reconstruction or redirecting the urethra (Held-Warmkessel, 2017).

Risk Factors and Causes

Risk factors include human papillomavirus (HPV) infection, especially HPV16, HPV6, and HPV18 (Hakenberg et al., 2014). Chronic inflammation such as balanitis, not being circumcised as an infant or child, phimosis (inability to retract the foreskin), smegma (thick accumulation of secretions underneath the foreskin), smoking, history of ultraviolet (UV) light treatment for psoriasis (with exposure of genitals), increasing age, history of condylomata acuminata (American Cancer Society, 2017d), prior injury to the patient, and cigarette smoking, especially in patients who smoke more than 10 cigarettes daily for at least 5 years, or with a greater than 30 pack-year history (Pow-Sang et al., 2010). No data support a link between AIDS/HIV diagnosis and penile cancer (Hakenberg et al., 2014). The direct causes of penile cancer are unknown; however, evidence shows that more high-risk HPV types inhibit tumor gene suppression, linking directly, high-risk HPV with proteins including E6 and E7 to the cause of penile cancer (Held-Warmkessel, 2017). Additionally, the carcinogens that are released with smoking can cause DNA structural changes that result in the development of certain cancers, including penile cancer (American Cancer Society, 2017a).

CULTURAL CONSIDERATIONS

Treatment is often delayed for fear of loss of the penis, disfigurement of the penis, or loss of sexual function. Reminding patients of improved outcomes following early intervention should be utilized in this patient population. Treatment can be devastating, owing to genital mutilation, and detrimental to the psychological state of the patient (Hakenberg et al., 2014). It is estimated that up to 50% of patients have had a penile lesion for at least 1 year prior to seeking medical intervention (Pow-Sang et al., 2010).

Physical Examination

Physical examination requires palpation of the shaft to assess for corporal involvement and rectal examination for urethral/prostatic involvement. Retraction of the foreskin should be performed (if possible). Palpate bilateral groins for identification of lymphadenopathy (Cookson & Whittam, 2010, pp. 252–253).

Typical presenting symptoms of penile cancer include an uncircumcised male, often with long duration of phimosis (unretractable foreskin). Also be sure to question patient for history of balanitis or other chronic inflammation, herpes simplex virus, tobacco use, poor hygiene, or any past treatment for lichen sclerosis. Patients may report a history of itching or burning with progression to ulceration. Men do not typically report pain; however, there may be a secondary infection or other inflammatory conditions. They may or may not report a visible or palpable lesion. In advanced stages, there may be changes in voiding, or difficulty with elimination (Held-Warmkessel, 2017).

On physical examination, there may be changes in the penile skin, especially at the glans or foreskin, prepuce, coronal sulcus, and along the shaft of the penis. Lesions may not always be visible without retraction of the foreskin. Skin changes that are commonly seen include a change in color; a lump on the penis; an ulcer that may or may not bleed; a reddish rash, with or without velvety appearance or with or without white lesions; crust-covered bumps; blue/brown growths; discharge, especially from the foreskin; and swelling of the penis, especially at the glans. Other symptoms that might be representative of more advanced disease include changes in voiding or urinary retention and lymph node enlargement, especially within the groin region and identified on palpation (American Cancer Society, 2017b).

Diagnostic Tests

Biopsy of the lesion with normal adjacent penile skin for pathologic testing is required, and this may be done in a clinic procedure room or the operating room. Establishing the depth of invasion will be important for treatment planning. Further workup includes CT of the abdomen and pelvis (MRI and, in some cases, ultrasound can also be used). Biopsy of questionably involved lymph nodes may also be required (Cookson & Whittam, 2010).

Staging and Management

The tumor-node-metastasis staging system is utilized for staging purposes. The involvement of nodal metastasis is the most negative predictive factor in predicting outcomes and prognosis (American Cancer Society, 2017b). Referral to urology with undiagnosed/unknown penile lesion should occur if the provider is concerned or the lesion(s) have not responded to initial management. In Tis cases, topical treatment may be indicated, however most penile cancers will require treatment with surgery, chemotherapy, and/or radiation treatment. Early treatment of penile cancer will result in improved outcomes and cure; therefore, encourage patients to follow up for immediate care (Cookson & Whittam, 2010).

Treatment

Treatment will be based upon staging and may include topical treatment, chemotherapy, radiotherapy, or surgical intervention. Topical treatment of Tis lesions include fluorouracil 5% to the area for 12 hours every 3 days for 28 days and may be repeated. Topical imiquimod 5% is used as a second-line therapy. Follow-up is necessary because of the risk of recurrence. Side effects of topical treatments include a local inflammatory response, crusting, erythema, dermatitis, pigment changes, pain, and itching (Held-Warmkessel, 2017). Systemic chemotherapy of a cisplatin-based regimen, usually four cycles, may be used in the neoadjuvant (before surgery) setting, especially for patients with nodal and distant metastases.

Surgery is used in the majority of presentations. The aims of treatment are radical tumor excision with maximum organ preservation (Hakenberg et al., 2014). Surgery can range from a circumcision to a complete penectomy. Circumcision is the removal of the foreskin and can treat the lesion, prepare for radiation, or treat phimosis depending on the presentation. Nodal metastases may be evaluated through fine needle aspiration, sentinel lymph node biopsy, or frozen section during lymph node dissection. Nodal involvement is treated through lymph node dissection, based upon the extent of involvement (Held-Warmkessel, 2017). Radiation therapy may be used with the goal of penile preservation, to treat inguinal lymph node metastases, as a radiosensitizer, or for recurrent disease that cannot be managed surgically.

Follow-Up

Recurrences may occur, either locally, nodally, or distantly. Close and long-term follow-up is required in this patient population. Follow-up includes imaging of chest, abdomen, and pelvis along with laboratory tests and physical examination every 3 months for the first 1 to 2 years and then at increasing intervals. Resection of residual mass, radiation treatment, and/or chemotherapy may be indicated for recurrent disease, dependent upon extent (Cookson & Whittam, 2010).

Side effects and results of treatment may include urethral obstruction or difficulty urinating, radiation burns or radiation cystitis, ureteral obstruction, lymphedema, alteration in appearance and length of penis, alteration in urethra, and changes in mood, especially depressed mood and effect on relationships. These all need to be managed based upon presentation and may require referral to specialists. Be especially concerned for depression and suicidal ideation following radical penectomy.

Education and counseling is key in this patient population. Posttraumatic stress disorder or depressive mood may occur. Sex therapy is strongly encouraged; support and involvement of family in the healing process should be encouraged. Patients must adapt to both sexual and urinary physiologic changes during the posttreatment stages. Include social work and psychology when needed (Held-Warmkessel, 2017).

Encourage patients to practice good hygiene, to routinely retract the foreskin, and to practice safe sex. The most important factor in decreasing the incidence of penile cancer may be circumcision in the infant (see discussion in Chapter 9). Elimination of cigarette smoking is also key. Finally, refer to urology at the first indication of a suspicious lesion or presentation.

TESTICULAR CANCER IN THE UNITED STATES

Introduction and Incidence

There were 8,850 new cases of testicular cancer predicted in 2017, and approximately 440 deaths occur yearly as a result of the disease. Testicular cancer is the most common solid tumor among males ages 15 to 35, but accounts for only 1% of all cancers. Incidence has increased worldwide, nearly 50% over the past 40 years, without a known cause for the increase (Stackhouse & Moul, 2010). The average age at diagnosis is 33 years, with the majority of cases presenting in young and middle-aged men (Stackhouse & Moul, 2010). Chances of cure are quite high, with a risk of dying of testicular cancer being only 1 in 5,000 (American Cancer Society, 2017c). Even in cases of recurrent disease, cure can often be achieved with second- and potentially third-line chemotherapy regimens. This is especially true in cases of germ cell tumor (Hanna & Einhora, 2014). In a 25-year follow-up study, young men diagnosed with testicular cancer had an increased mortality rate in the 2 years following diagnosis, but reached annual survival probabilities of 99.9% following that 2-year interval (Capocaccia, Gatta, & Dal Maso, 2015). Follow-up for long-term health side effects is important in this population because of early age at presentation and treatment and likely chance of cure (Hashibe et al., 2016).

PERTINENT ANATOMY AND PHYSIOLOGY

Thorough knowledge of the scrotal structures should be understood: skin and tunica dartos, the spermatic cord containing the vas deferens, blood vessels, nerves, cremasteric muscle, epididymis, testicle, and tunica albuginea. Additionally, because of the concern for spread to the retroperitoneal lymph nodes, providers should be familiar with the retroperitoneal lymph nodes and the corresponding vascular and arterial blood supply (Flick & Russell, 2017).

History

It is important to evaluate for the history of a noted testicular mass either by the patient or their partner, including when the mass was initially identified and length of time to seeking consultation. Longer delay increases risk of metastatic disease. Family and personal history of testicular cancer or personal history of an undescended testicle should also be assessed. With personal history of undescended testicle, it is important to note the location of the testicle and age the patient underwent orchiopexy, if possible.

COMMON PRESENTATION

Patients typically present with a solitary painless lump, swelling, or hardened testicle identified by either the patient or partner. Some report a change in the size of the testicle, or discomfort, increased awareness, or heaviness in the scrotum (Stackhouse & Moul, 2010, pp. 440–441). The most common presenting symptom is painless swelling or enlargement of the testicle. Additionally, evaluation may show pain in the scrotum, gynecomastia, feminization, early puberty, or history of dysplastic syndromes (Stackhouse & Moul, 2010).

SIGNS AND SYMPTOMS

In addition to a solitary, painless lump in or on the testicle, and feelings of dullness or heaviness in the scrotum, patients often report increased sensation or heightened awareness of their scrotum. Pain is rarely reported in the scrotum; however, some patients do report a dull ache in the abdomen or groin. Additionally, change in appearance of the breasts, breast growth or tenderness, and nipple tenderness may be present. Symptoms of advanced disease include abdominal pain, supraclavicular or mediastinal masses, or cough (Stackhouse & Moul, 2010).

RISK FACTORS

The most common risk factors include a family history of testicular cancer, especially in first-degree relatives, a history of undescended testicle(s), infertility, and testicular atrophy (Stackhouse & Moul, 2010).

CULTURAL FACTORS

The private nature of the genitals and sexual function requires an added complexity of consideration for patients with the diagnosis. This factor can lead to added delay in treatment and hesitancy for treatment. Concern for providers of the opposite gender may need to be considered. Survivorship and sperm banking are key to this population, as the disease is most often curable (Flick & Russell, 2017, pp. 373–381). Fertile patients who wish to father a child following radical orchiectomy may delay further treatment prior to completion, when pathologic diagnosis is favorable (Albers et al., 2015).

Physical Examination

Providers should assess the supraclavicular region for evidence of mass or palpable adenopathy. Next, a thorough breast examination should occur to assess for evidence of gynecomastia, tenderness, nipple pain, or swelling. The abdomen should be examined for evidence of masses, lymphadenopathy, or mass. The testicular exam includes palpation of all areas of the testicle, bimanually, including all scrotal contents, beginning with the normal side (Flick & Russell, 2017). Abnormal findings include lymphadenopathy, gynecomastia or tender breasts or nipples, hepatomegaly, and any firm, painless mass on or connected to the testicle.

Diagnosis

LABORATORY EVALUATION

Laboratory tests should include routine complete blood count (CBC) and comprehensive metabolic panel (CMP). Serum tumor markers are key elements in the workup, diagnosis, and treatment of testicular cancer. Serum tumor markers include AFP (alpha-fetoprotein), beta-hCG (beta-human chorionic gonadotropin), and LDH (lactate dehydrogenase). AFP and beta-hCG are typically elevated in nonseminomatous germ cell tumors. Pure seminomas do not typically cause a rise in AFP, rarely in beta-hCG. Elevated LDH is concerning for metastatic disease (Gomella, 2010). Contralateral biopsy has been advocated in some cases, especially with testicular intraepithelial neoplasia. Because of the low incidence of contralateral malignancy, however, this practice is not currently recommended (Albers et al., 2015).

IMAGING STUDIES

Scrotal ultrasound scan should be ordered for prompt diagnosis of involvement of the testicle, looking for a hypoechoic mass to determine whether the mass is intra- or extratesticular. Initially, men will have a chest x-ray study, followed by a CT scan of the chest, abdomen, pelvis, and brain (with neurologic symptoms) to rule out metastatic disease and to evaluate efficacy following neoadjuvant chemotherapy. Following chemotherapy, seminomas may have residual masses that will likely resolve within the first 18 months following treatment.

Management

Germ cell tumors are the most common types of testicular cancers and cell type will determine treatment. Seminomas are typically well demarcated with sheets of relatively uniform cells, usually presenting later in life. They are typically considered low to intermediate risk depending upon the primary tumor, lymph node status, metastasis status, and serum tumor marker levels. Patients with seminoma diagnosis and no metastatic disease are considered low risk. The presence of any nonpulmonary visceral metastases are considered intermediate risk (Flick & Russell, 2017).

Nonseminomas include embryonal carcinomas, choriocarcinomas, yolk sac tumors, and teratomas. Embryonal carcinomas tend to present in the earlier decades of life and are less differentiated, making them more aggressive and concerning for metastases. Choriocarcinomas tend to present with metastases. Yolk sac tumors typically present along with another component of germ cell tumors, as mixed germ cell tumors, and are similar to the embryonic yolk sac in appearance. Teratomas are rare and can occur at any age (Flick & Russell, 2017).

Nonseminomatous germ cell tumors presenting with primary tumors in the testis or retroperitoneal lymph nodes without nonpulmonary visceral metastases are considered low to intermediate risk dependent upon tumor markers. AFP less than 1,000 ng/mL, beta-hCG less than 5,000 U/L, and LDH less than 1.5 times the upper limit of normal range are low risk. Intermediate-risk markers include an AFP between 1,000 and 10,000 ng/mL, beta-hCG between 5,000 and 50,000 U/L, and LDH between 1.5 and 10 times the upper limits of normal. High-risk disease includes levels above those listed here, or involvement of mediastinal lymph nodes or other visceral metastases (Flick & Russell, 2017).

Treatment and Follow-Up

Prior to initiating treatment, ensure that patients are offered the ability to bank their sperm for purposes of future conception.

A radical orchiectomy with high ligation of the spermatic cord is indicated in most cases of suspected testicular cancer. Following a radical orchiectomy with stage 1 seminoma and normal tumor markers, follow-up with surveillance tumor markers and chest/abdominal/pelvic imaging is utilized. More advanced disease has varying follow-up depending on pathology of the tumor and stage. Retroperitoneal lymph node dissection (RPLND) is less commonly used in cases of lower risk disease; however, in cases of concern for relapse, this procedure may be an option. Patients should seek an experienced surgeon, able to perform a nerve-sparing RPLND via a laparoscopic or robotic approach (Albers et al., 2015).

Follow-up is dependent upon the risk of disease and adjuvant treatment following an orchiectomy. Regardless of the stage and grade of disease, some close schedule of imaging including chest, abdominal, and pelvic, with either CT or PET, will be utilized along with serum tumor markers. Physical examination with close attention to the breasts and solitary testicle at close follow-up schedules and patient monthly testicular self-exams are required (Gomella, 2010). For exact follow-up schedules, providers should consult guidelines via the

National Comprehensive Cancer Network (NCCN), American Joint Committee on Cancer (AJCC), or the American Urological Association (AUA).

Close follow-up with primary care physicians and routine health maintenance following treatment for testicular cancer is very important. Testicular cancer survivors tend to experience a 24% increase in long-term health effects in the greater than 5 years following treatment. Obesity prior to treatment for testicular cancer appears to be the strongest risk factor; however, treatment with chemotherapy and retroperitoneal lymph node dissection also increased the risk of long-term health effects. Hypercholesterolemia, orchitis, and infertility were among the highest rates of late effects (Hashibe et al., 2016). Additional concern for secondary malignancies, especially after frequent exposure to diagnostic radiation, chemotherapy, and surgery should also be considered. Secondary leukemia after etoposide is also a consideration. Further health effects in this population include metabolic syndrome, cardiovascular disease, neurotoxicity, nephrotoxicity, pulmonary toxicity, hypogonadism, and psychosocial effects.

CLINICAL PEARLS

- Encourage use of the HPV vaccination series in both males and females.
- Emphasize safe sex practices with all patients.
- Explain retraction of foreskin and proper hygiene.
- A scrotal ultrasound examination must be ordered and obtained quickly when a testicular mass is noted.
- All testicular masses should be treated urgently, as long as there is no history of acute onset of pain, and considered to be testicular cancer until proved otherwise.
- Staging is very important for this disease.
- Men undergoing treatment require fertility counseling, option for sperm banking, and psychosocial support options.

RESOURCES FOR THE CLINICIAN

American Cancer Society: www.cancer.org/cancer/penile-cancer.html
American Society for Reproductive Medicine: www.reproductivefacts.org
American Urological Association Guidelines
National Comprehensive Cancer Network Guidelines: www.nccn.org
RESOLVE: The National Infertility Association: www.resolve.org
Spiess, P.E. (2017). *Penile Cancer*. New York, NY: Humana Press.
The Urology Care Foundation: www.urologyhealth.org

RESOURCES FOR THE PATIENT

American Society for Reproductive Medicine: www.reproductivefacts.org
American Cancer Society: www.cancer.org/cancer/penile-cancer.html
Cancer Survivors Network, American Cancer Society: www./csn.cancer.org/node/152457
Cancer Support Community: www.cancersupportcommunity.org/learn-about-cancer-types/penile-cancer/more-about-understanding-penile-cancer
RESOLVE: The National Infertility Association: www.resolve.org
Testicular Cancer Foundation: www.testicularcancer.org
Testicular Cancer Society: www.testicularcancersociety.org

REFERENCES

Albers, P., Albrecht, W., Algaba, F., Bokenmeyer, C., Cohn-Cedermark, G., Fizazi, K., ... Oldenburg, J. (2015). Guidelines on testicular cancer: 2015 update. *European Urology, 68*, 1054–1068. doi:10.1016/j.eururo.2015.07.044

American Cancer Society. (2017a). *Do We Know What Causes Penile Cancer?* Pitman, NJ: Society of Urologic Nurses and Associates.

American Cancer Society. (2017b). Penile cancer. Signs and symptoms of penile cancer. Retrieved from https://www.cancer.org/cancer/penile-cancer/detection-diagnosis-staging/signs-symptoms.html

American Cancer Society. (2017c) Testicular cancer. What are the key statistics about testicular cancer? Retrieved from https://www.cancer.org/cancer/testicular-cancer/about/key-statistics.html

American Cancer Society. (2017d). What are the risk factors for penile cancer? Retrieved from https://www.cancer.org/cancer/penile-cancer/causes-risks-prevention/risk-factors.html

Capocaccia, R., Gatta, G., & Dal Maso, L. (2015). Life expectancy of colon, breast, and testicular cancer patients: An analysis of US-SEER population-based data. *Annals of Oncology, 26*, 1263–1268. doi:10.1093/annonc/mcv131

Cookson, M. S., & Whittam, B. M. (2010). Penis, squamous cell carcinoma. In L. G. Gomella (Ed.), *The 5-minute urology consult* (2nd ed, pp. 252–253). Philadelphia, PA: Lippincott Williams & Wilkins.

Flick, S. M., & Russell, S. S. (2017). Testicular cancer. In D. K. Newman, J. F. Wyman, & V. W. Welch (Eds.), *Core curriculum for urologic nursing* (pp. 373–381). Pitman, NJ: Society of Urologic Nurses and Associates.

Gomella, L.G. (2010). The 5-Minute Urology Consult (2nd ed.). Philadelphia, PA: Lippincott Williams & Wilkins.

Hakenberg, O. W., Compérat, E. M., Minhas, S., Necchi, A., Protzel, C., & Watkin, N. (2015). EAU guidelines on penile cancer: 2014 update. *European Urology, 67*(1), 142–150. doi:10.1016/j.eururo.2014.10.017

Hanna, N., & Einhorn, L. H. (2014). Testicular cancer: A reflection on 50 years of discovery. *Journal of Clinical Oncology, 32*(28), 3085–3092. doi:10.1200/JCO.2014.56.0896

Hashibe, M., Abdelaziz, S., Al-Temimi, M., Fraser, A., Boucher, K. M., Smith, K., ... Holton, A. E. (2016). Long-term health effects among testicular cancer survivors. *Journal of Cancer Survivorship, 10*(6), 1051-1057. doi:10.1007/s11764-016-0548-1

Held-Warmkessel, J. (2017). Penile cancer. In D. K. Newman, J. F. Wyman, & V. W. Welch (Eds.), *Core curriculum for urologic nursing* (1st ed., pp. 363–371). Pitman, NJ: Society of Urologic Nurses and Associates.

Pow-Sang, M. R., Ferreira, U., Pow-Sang, J. M., Nardi, A. C., & Destefano, V. (2010). Epidemiology and natural history of penile cancer. *Urology, 76*(2), S2–S6. doi:10.1016/j.urology.2010.03.003

Stackhouse, D. A., & Moul, J. W. (2010). Testis, seminoma. In L. G. Gomella (Ed.), *The 5-minute urology consult* (2nd ed., pp. 440–441). Philadelphia, PA: Lippincott Williams & Wilkins.

CHAPTER 31

Survivorship Basics and the Male Urological Cancer Survivor

Hilary Shreves and Amy Leatherwood

INTRODUCTION

Late in the 20th century there was a flurry of scientific discoveries and innovations in the area of cancer diagnostics, prevention, and treatment that led to earlier detection of cancer and more effective therapies to treat it. This in turn has led to an increase in the number of cancer survivors. The increase in cancer survivors is also due in part to a growing and aging population that is living longer and is more likely to encounter a cancer diagnosis, if not more than one, in their lifetime (DeSantis et al., 2015). In the United States alone there were an estimated 15.5 million cancer survivors as of January 2016 and that number is continually growing (Miller et al., 2016). Future projections estimate the United States will have nearly 20 million cancer survivors by the year 2026 (Miller et al., 2016). The care of cancer survivors, or survivorship, has become an area of pressing national concern, as the number of cancer survivors continues to increase along with our understanding of the magnitude of impact that their cancer diagnosis and treatment bring to their health and overall quality of life.

Cancer survivorship is a concept that focuses on the comprehensive care of a patient with cancer from the time of diagnosis until death. This includes thorough medical as well as holistic care. An individual is considered a cancer survivor from the time of diagnosis through the balance of his or her life. Family members, friends, and caregivers are also impacted by the survivorship experience and are therefore included in this definition (The National Coalition for Cancer Survivorship, 2017). Many cancer survivors experience physical, psychosocial, and long-term effects of cancer and its treatment; these effects can be severe and debilitating, and at times permanent. At a certain point the patient is usually discharged from the care of their oncologist and is often left feeling isolated and scared. Primary care providers (PCPs), who may now be assuming responsibility for their care, often do not know how best to meet the specific needs of the cancer survivor (Nekhlyudov, Aziz, Lerro, & Virgo 2014).

This chapter aims to assist the PCP in assuming the care of the male cancer survivor following active cancer treatment, by reviewing the general concepts of survivorship care with special attention on issues confronted by men with a history of urological cancer. Prostate, bladder, kidney, and testis cancers account for approximately 57% of all male cancer survivors (DeSantis et al., 2014). The male urological cancer survivor suffers from challenges common to all cancer survivors but also experiences unique medical and psychosocial challenges that require proactive assessment and management.

A BRIEF HISTORY OF CANCER SURVIVORSHIP

In 1971 the National Cancer Act was signed into law by President Richard Nixon establishing the National Cancer Institute. This represented the U.S. commitment to what President Nixon described as the "war on cancer," which had become the nation's second leading cause of death by 1970. As cancer treatments continued to advance, the long-held recognition of the burden of cancer treatment on the quantity and quality of life of cancer survivors was only reinforced. In 1986 the NCCS (National Coalition for Cancer Survivorship) was founded with the goal of replacing the term cancer "victim" with the term "survivor" and of improving the care of the cancer survivor through advocacy (The National Coalition for Cancer Survivorship, 2017; Selph & Peterson, 2017).

In 2004, almost 20 years after the NCCS was formed, The President's Cancer Panel, in observance of the National Cancer Act of 1971, published a report entitled Living Beyond Cancer: Finding a New Balance (Reuben, 2004). The panel exposed the unmet and growing needs of the community of cancer survivors and made recommendations on how to help alleviate the severe burden experienced by cancer survivors and their families (Reuben, 2004). Shortly thereafter, in 2006, the Institute of Medicine (IOM) published a seminal report entitled *From Cancer Patient to Cancer Survivor: Lost in Transition* (Hewitt, Greenfield, & Stoval, 2006). This report was a comprehensive assessment of the status of cancer survivors in the United States that revealed a significant number of cancer survivors suffered from chronic, long-term physical, social, and emotional distress. The study found that a pressing concern for most patients was a lack of access to healthcare and poor coordination of care, once the cancer treatment and intermediate surveillance was concluded. The report made 10 recommendations to improve the care of survivors; the first 5 were for healthcare providers and last 5 were for policymakers and governmental bodies (Box 31.1). The aim of their recommendation was specifically to increase access to care for cancer survivors, facilitate cancer survivors' transition to community providers, and to increase research funding (Hewitt et al., 2006). These IOM recommendations have laid the framework on which current progress in survivorship care has been built upon and for which future developments are spurred on.

BOX 31.1 INSTITUTE OF MEDICINE 10 RECOMMENDATIONS FOR IMPROVING SURVIVORSHIP CARE

1. Increase awareness and delivery of survivorship care.
2. Provide a survivorship care plan upon completion of treatment (i.e., a detailed treatment summary and follow-up plan).
3. Practice evidence-based medicine.
4. Develop and monitor quality-of-care measures.
5. Design educational programs for healthcare providers to address the healthcare care needs of survivors.
6. Eliminate employment discrimination against cancer survivors.
7. Ensure that cancer survivors have access to affordable and adequate insurance.
8. Support the Centers for Disease Control and Prevention comprehensive cancer control plans for survivors.
9. Support demonstration projects for survivorship care.
10. Increase funding for survivorship research.

THE EFFECTS OF CANCER AND CANCER TREATMENT

The physical problems in cancer survivors are varied. Common symptoms include pain, musculoskeletal issues, fatigue, urinary issues, bowel issues, lack of stamina, lymphedema, infertility, cognitive deficits, osteoporosis, cardiac issues, increased risk of second primary cancers, and sexual dysfunction. The symptoms a particular cancer survivor will experience depend mainly on the type of treatment utilized. For example, radiation to the pelvis can result in bowel, urinary, and sexual dysfunction as well as increased risk of second primary malignancies (Adams et al., 2014).

Second primary cancers occur at an overall higher incidence among cancer survivors than a first primary cancer occurs in the general population because of genetic susceptibilities, causative factors (smoking, obesity, environmental exposure), and the potential for mutagenic effects of cancer treatments (Chen et al., 2015; Wood et al., 2012). Screening for second primary cancers is an important aspect of survivorship care. The PCP providing survivorship care for a cancer survivor should follow routine cancer screening recommendations, and in addition should pursue any additional cancer screening that is recommended by the primary oncology team or from a clinical guideline for the particular type of cancer involved. One example of this is the recommendation for an annual urinalysis to screen for secondary bladder cancer in prostate cancer survivors who have undergone radiation treatments. Prostate radiation has been associated with an increased risk for developing a secondary bladder cancer (Keehn, A., Ludmir, Taylor, & Rabbani, 2017).

For some cancer survivors, the impact of cancer treatment is minimal, and they return to a normal life after the completion of treatment. In fact, studies have shown that most cancer survivors report being in good general health and claim an excellent quality of life following completion of cancer treatments (Bloom, Petersen, & Kang, 2007; Stein, Syrjala, & Andrykowski, 2008). A 2011 survey of colorectal, breast, and prostate cancer survivors found that the majority did not suffer from psychological morbidity or have a significant number of unmet supportive care needs (Harrison et al., 2011). Other studies have uncovered similar findings with cancer survivors reporting a high quality of life with minimal cancer-related symptoms (Hsu, Ennis, Hood, Graham, & Goodwin, 2013).

However, there are still many other cancer survivors who do experience adverse physical as well as psychosocial effects of cancer and its treatment. Some sequelae become evident during cancer treatments (long-term effects), whereas others may not manifest for months or even years after (late effects). These issues can range in severity and in some circumstances can even be life threatening. Some are temporary and treatable; others are progressive or permanent. One review suggests that 50% of all cancer survivors experience at least one late effect of cancer treatment (Valdivieso, Kujawa, Jones, & Baker, 2012). The Livestrong Foundation performed a survey of cancer survivors in 2006 and again in 2010 to understand the gap between what cancer survivors desire in their care and what they actually receive (Rechis & Boerner, 2010; Rechis & Reynolds, 2011). Of the approximately 2,300 respondents in 2006, 91% had at least one physical concern following their cancer treatment. The three most common concerns related to energy level in 59%, concentration in 55%, and sexual function in 46%. Furthermore, 22% of patients reported incontinence and 3% reported fertility concerns. What was particularly noteworthy was the lack of treatment offered by providers for these conditions with 50%, 69%, and 71% of patients responding that they did not receive treatment for incontinence, infertility, and sexual dysfunction, respectively (Rechis & Boerner, 2010). The survey was repeated in 2010 and the results revealed the same deficiencies. The care that was being received was coming primarily from oncologists and PCPs and the survey revealed a significant opportunity to improve the care provided to this patient population (Rechis & Reynolds, 2011; Selph & Peterson, 2017).

PHASES OF SURVIVORSHIP

In his 1975 essay, Seasons of Survival, Dr. Fitzhugh Mullan describes three distinct phases of survivorship both from the perspective of a patient's experience as well as from a clinical perspective: the acute phase, the intermediate phase, and the long-term phase (Mullan, 1985). The acute phase begins with the diagnosis of cancer and includes all the testing for cancer and all of the treatment of the malignancy. Clinical care during this phase is primarily delivered by surgical, radiation, and medical oncologists as well as advance practice providers. The focus of care is on eradication of the malignancy and on the management of any complications suffered from the treatment. From the perspective of the patient the experience is often one of illness, anxiety, fear of the cancer, as well as hope of a successful treatment or remission (Foxhall & Rodriguez, 2015).

The intermediate phase of survivorship begins when the patient has reached remission or upon concluding the primary treatment (Mullan, 1985). Depending on the type of malignancy and the treatment required, this phase could also include maintenance treatment or consolidation therapies for some patients. For example, some urothelial carcinomas of the bladder are treated with an initial course of immunotherapy instilled within the bladder, followed by 3 years of maintenance instillations. The primary focus of the intermediate phase of survivorship is watchful monitoring with physical examinations, cystoscopy, and studies to determine if an early relapse will occur. Clinical care during this phase continues to be primarily delivered by surgical, radiation, and medical oncologists as well as advance practice providers. Patients often experience anxiety and fear of recurrence during this phase, and the recovery from the acute phase of treatment may be prolonged and extend into this intermediate phase as well (Foxhall & Rodriguez, 2015).

The long-term phase of survivorship begins when the highest risk period for recurrence has passed and the patient is considered well from that episode of cancer (Foxhall & Rodriguez, 2015; Mullan, 1985). The focus of clinical care in long-term survivorship should turn to maintenance of health, management of latent complications of cancer treatment, reduction of risks of second malignancies, and cancer screening as appropriate for the type of cancer. This phase of survivorship care is often transitioned from the oncologist to the PCP. In 1985 a new category of long-term survivor began to emerge which included patients with chronic active cancer in a smoldering phase or with periodic remissions interrupted by expected relapses that require treatment (Foxhall & Rodriguez, 2015). The goals of clinical care for these patients are the same as for the cancer-free survivors, but they require more intense surveillance for recurrence and undergo intermittent treatments for their primary cancer as needed, repeating their trajectory through the earlier phases of survivorship (Foxhall & Rodriguez, 2015).

Models of Care

One of the ongoing challenges of survivorship care is finding the ideal model for delivering survivorship care that adequately addresses the comprehensive needs of the survivor. Multiple models of survivorship care exist, and have evolved over the years based on who is providing the care, the survivorship population, the site of care, and the capacity for delivery of certain services (Halpern, McCabe, & Burg, 2016). Three commonly proposed models include community-based shared care models, dedicated disease-specific clinics, and comprehensive survivor programs (Table 31.1). Regardless of the model of survivorship, the goal is the same: providing comprehensive care that is able to respond to the needs of a cancer survivor and is familiar enough with their unique concerns to anticipate those concerns, screen for them, and help to prevent them.

TABLE 31.1 Models of Survivorship Care

Community-Based Shared Care	Disease-Specific Clinics	Comprehensive Survivor Programs
• Oncologist provides cancer care. • Patient is then referred back to PCP for long-term survivorship care. • Oncologist and PCPs are encouraged to communicate via SCP.	• Group of providers who focus on one particular type of cancer and provide multidisciplinary survivorship care	• Varied structures • Typically a multidisciplinary program made up of oncologist, advance practice providers, social workers, psychologists, and consulting specialists

PCP, primary care provider; SCP, survivorship care plan.

Coordination of Care for Survivors

Cancer survivors are cared for by their primary oncology team and allied specialist throughout active treatment (acute phase of survivorship), and then transitioned to their PCP at some point after the conclusion of active treatment. In some cases, the patient is transitioned to the PCP for both the intermediate phase and the long-term phase of survivorship, and in other cases he is transitioned for long-term phase of survivorship only. During active cancer treatment it is in the best interest of the cancer survivor to continue to see the PCP on a regular basis in addition to the cancer specialist. This ensures that the routine healthcare is not overlooked, which is essential because many cancer treatments will impact comorbid conditions such as hypertension and diabetes. One example of this for the male urological cancer survivor is in the case of prostate cancer when androgen deprivation therapy (ADT) is utilized. ADT promotes metabolic changes that are associated with cardiovascular risk and the patient requires vigilant monitoring of his blood pressure, blood glucose, and lipids with his PCP or local urologist during active cancer treatment (Greiman & Keane, 2017; NCCN Clinical Practice Guidelines in Oncology: Survivorship, 2017).

The ideal time to transition a cancer survivor back to the PCP for ongoing survivorship care has not been well established, because the role of the specialist versus the PCP in providing survivorship care continues to be a matter of discussion (Nekhlyudov, O'Malley, & Hudson, 2017). Some authors report cancer survivors are reluctant to be discharged from their primary oncology team following active cancer treatment (Brennan, Butow, Spillane, & Boyle, 2010), while others have found that patients welcome transitioning survivorship care to their PCP (Brennan, M. E., Butow, P., Spillane, A. J., & Boyle et al., 2016). Importantly, there have been only two randomized trials comparing survivorship care administered by an oncologist versus a PCP (who had been provided guidelines outlining appropriate follow-up care) and no difference in disease-related outcomes was found, including survival (Grunfeldet al., 2006; Wattchow et al., 2006).

The concept of a survivorship care plan (SCP) has been developed as a tool that the primary oncology team prepares that provides a concise summary of the type of cancer and treatment utilized, and a plan for follow-up, including surveillance and preventive measures (Table 31.2). This is an important recommendation from the IOM survivorship report (Hewitt et al., 2006). A SCP can be of particular value as the patient transitions oncology follow-up from an oncology specialist to the PCP (Foxhall & Rodriguez, 2015), but SCPs have been slow to integrate into actual practice. One reason is that they are time consuming to prepare and not yet a reimbursable service, but research is lacking that demonstrates any benefit in long-term outcomes (Grunfeld et al., 2011). However, multiple studies have highlighted the perceived value to PCPs of SCPs in providing better care and coordination, and SCPs continue to be a IOM recommended part of a cancer survivor's care (Baravelli et al., 2009; Salz, Oeffinger, McCabe, Layne, & Bach, 2012). There are e-learning modules that exist to

TABLE 31.2 Example of a Survivorship Care Plan (SCP)

Treatment Summary	Follow-up Care Plan
• Contact information of treating institution/providers • Specific diagnosis/histological subtype • Disease stage at diagnosis • Surgery type, location, date • Chemotherapy agents given and end date • Radiotherapy performed, location, end date • Ongoing toxicity or adverse events of any treatment received • Likely course of recovery from toxicity • Any genetic testing results	• Contact information for oncology provider • Any need for ongoing adjuvant therapy, including duration and expected adverse effects • Schedule of follow-up visits • Surveillance testing for recurrence: what lab tests to order, when and by whom • Screening for new primary cancers • A general statement to continue all standard noncancer-related healthcare • Symptoms of disease recurrence to watch for • A list of potential late or long-term effects of treatment • A list of emotional, mental, work, financial, or insurance issues the survivor has experienced • A general statement emphasizing healthy diet, smoking cessation, exercise, and alcohol use reduction

Prostate Cancer Survivorship Care Plan		
General Information		
Patient Name:	DOB:	Age:
MRN:	Phone:	Email:
Healthcare Providers		
Primary Care Provider:		
Urological Surgeon:		
Radiation Surgeon:		
Medical Oncologist:		
Other Providers:		

Treatment Summary		
Diagnosis		
Cancer Type: Prostate Cancer	Diagnosis Date:	
Stage: ☐ I ☐ II ☐ III ☐ IV ☐ Not applicable		
Gleason Grade:	Pre-Treatment PSA:	
Clinical Trial Enrollment: ☐ Yes ☐ No Study Details:		
Treatment Completed		
Surgery: ☐ Yes ☐ No	Surgery Date:	Surgeon/Institution:
Surgical Procedure:	Surgical Pathology:	
Radiation: ☐ Yes ☐ No	Provider/Facility:	End Date:
	Treatment Site/Dose:	
Systemic Therapy (chemotherapy, hormonal therapy, other): ☐Yes ☐ No		
Details:		
Other Therapy (Cryotherapy/HIFU): ☐ Yes ☐ No		
Details		

(continued)

TABLE 31.2 Example of a Survivorship Care Plan (SCP) (*continued*)

Names of Agents Used	End Dates (year) or ongoing
☐ Casodex	
☐ Lupron (or similar LHRH agonist)	
☐ Other	

Persistent symptoms, toxicities, or side effects at completion of above treatment: ☐ Yes ☐ No

Details:

Expected resolution:

Treatment Ongoing

Need for ongoing (adjuvant) treatment for cancer ☐ Yes ☐ No

Additional treatment name	Planned duration	Possible side effects

Follow-up Care Plan

Schedule of Clinic Follow-Up Visits

Coordinating Provider	When/How Often

Cancer Surveillance or Other Recommended Tests

Coordinating Provider	Test	How Often
	PSA (Prostate-Specific Antigen) Blood Test	

Prostate Cancer Survivorship Care Plan

Please continue to see your primary care provider for all general health care recommended for a man your age, including screening tests for other primary cancers. Any symptoms should be brought to the attention of your provider:

1. Anything that represents a brand new symptom;
2. Anything that represents a persistent symptom;
3. Anything you are worried about that might be related to the cancer coming back.

Possible late and long-term effects that someone with this type of cancer and treatment may experience:

- Incontinence
- Erectile dysfunction
- Decreased sex drive
- Fatigue
- Hair loss
- Hot flashes
- Shortening of the penis
- Mood swings
- Osteoporosis
- Painful urination
- Rectal pain
- Enlarging breast tissue
- Skin irritation or darkening
- Sterility

(*continued*)

TABLE 31.2 Example of a Survivorship Care Plan (SCP) (*continued*)

• Increased body fat • Loss of muscle mass • Metabolic syndrome (increased blood pressure, blood sugar, cholesterol)		• Tiredness • Trouble emptying your bladder • Urinary frequency • Other:
Cancer survivors may experience issues with a variety of life circumstances. If you have any concerns in these or other areas, please speak with your providers to find out how you can get help with them.		
☐ Anxiety or depression	☐ Insurance	☐ Sexual functioning
☐ Emotional and mental health	☐ Memory or concentration loss	☐ Stopping smoking
☐ Fatigue/energy	☐ Parenting	☐ Weight changes
☐ Fertility	☐ Physical functioning	☐ Relationship concerns
☐ Financial advice or assistance	☐ School/employment	☐ Other
A number of lifestyle/behaviors can affect your ongoing health, including the risk of cancer coming back or developing a different cancer. Discuss these issues with your primary care provider:		
☐ Alcohol use	☐ Exercise	☐ Other
☐ Diet	☐ Sun screen use	
☐ Management of medications	☐ Tobacco cessation	
☐ Management of other illnesses	☐ Weight management	
Resources for prostate cancer survivors: • www.cancer.net • Other:		
Other comments:		
Prepared by:		Delivered on:

help educate and train PCPs on survivor's issues, as well as clinical practice guidelines that can assist the PCP in screening for late effects and long-term problems. Appendix 31.1 lists some of these resources.

COMPONENTS OF SURVIVORSHIP CARE

The comprehensive care of the cancer survivor includes four components: physical/medical, psychological, practical/social, and existential/spiritual components. The physical/medical component of cancer care focuses as first priority on the prevention, where possible, and then identification and treatment of recurrent cancers and secondary cancers. It addresses treatment side effects as pain, erectile dysfunction, incontinence, lymphedema, and cardiac dysfunction. Some of the physical impacts of cancer and the treatment of cancer are universal and some are unique to the type of cancer or treatment utilized (Figure 31.1).

The psychological domain focuses on the depression, anxiety, isolation, and uncertainty that can accompany cancer treatment (Andersen, Rowland, & Somerfield, 2015). Many cancer survivors experience a combination of positive and negative psychological effects. The positive effects include strengthened relationships, a sense of gratitude, and an increased appreciation for life (Bellizzi, Miller, Arora, & Rowland, 2007). Even if a patient is expressing positive psychological effects from their diagnosis, it is still important to screen for psychological distress as they often coexist.

The practical or social component of survivorship care focuses on identifying relationship changes, loss of job, insurance issues, and financial burden from medical expenses.

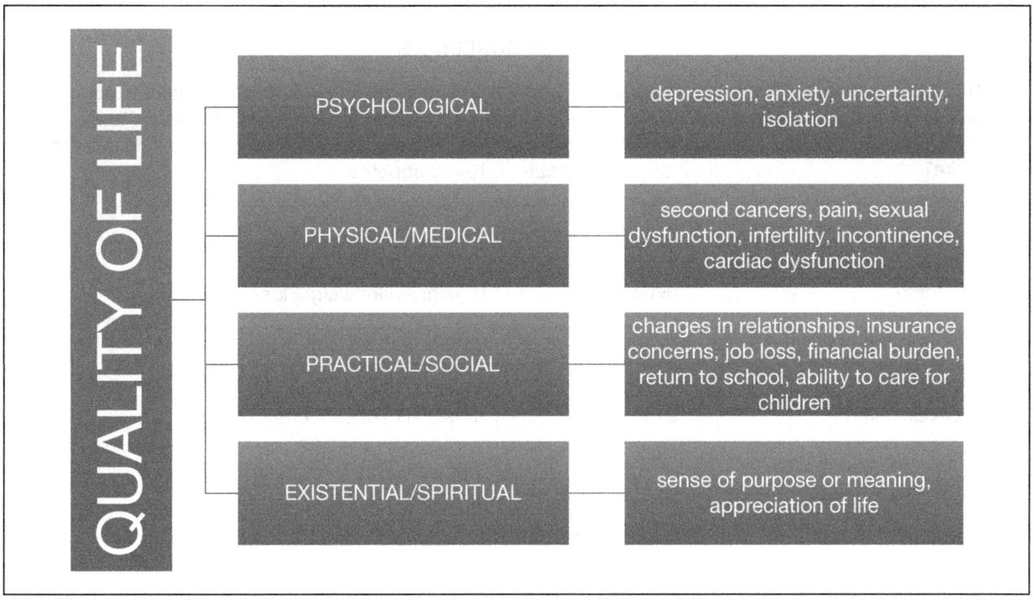

FIGURE 31.1 Realms of quality of life.

The assistance of social workers and counselors becomes very important in this realm of survivorship care. Research has shown that cancer treatment can have catastrophic consequence on the social aspect of a patient's life, with more than 55% of cancer survivors reporting going into financial debt to pay for medical treatments and with unpaid medical bills continuing to be the number one cause of bankruptcy in the United States (Banegas et al., 2016). Appendix 31.1 provides a list of resources available to patients which can help them navigate many of the practical and social issues they will confront.

Lastly, the spiritual realm has to do with faith, religion, purpose, peace, and meaning. Research has consistently shown that patients who consider themselves spiritual have less distress and a better reported quality of life then those who do not (Canada, Murphy, Fitchett, & Stein, 2016). Men with prostate cancer specifically who have low spirituality have worse health-related quality of life (Krupski et al., 2006).

Screening Tools for Comprehensive Care

Screening tools have been developed to assess for general areas of concern in these four realms of a cancer survivor's life, commonly referred to as distress screening tools. They are an important measure of a cancer survivor's overall quality of life and can lead to further, more focused assessments or referrals for support once areas of specific concern have been identified. One commonly used tool is the National Comprehensive Care Network (NCCN) distress thermometer, which can be found on the NCCN.org website, but distress screening tools can easily be created for a particular patient population, such as the one shown in Figure 31.2 for survivors of genitourinary cancers (NCCN Clinical Practice Guidelines in Oncology: Survivorship, 2017). Cancer survivors should be screened early after diagnosis and continue to be screened regularly thereafter (NCCN Clinical Practice Guidelines in Oncology: Survivorship, 2017). If areas of concern are uncovered, such as depression, the provider implementing the screening can assess this finding in more detail with a specific depression screening tool or can refer to a mental health specialist.

DISTRESS SCREENING

Here in the department of urology we are concerned not only with treating your cancer, but also with helping you cope with it. We want to help you with your emotional, social, and financial needs. Please tell us how you are doing today by circling the appropriate number on the number line for the following questions.

Appetite? 0=good appetite 10=no appetite

0	1	2	3	4	5	6	7	8	9	10

Weight loss? 0=no weight loss 10=significant weight loss

0	1	2	3	4	5	6	7	8	9	10

Fertility/Sexuality? 0=no concern 10=significant concern

0	1	2	3	4	5	6	7	8	9	10

Depression? 0=no depression 10=severe depression

0	1	2	3	4	5	6	7	8	9	10

Anxiety? 0=no anxiety 10=severe anxiety

0	1	2	3	4	5	6	7	8	9	10

Concerns about your children? 0=no concern 10=significant concern

0	1	2	3	4	5	6	7	8	9	10

Insurance or financial issues? 0=no issues 10=significant issues

0	1	2	3	4	5	6	7	8	9	10

Spouse or family concern? 0=no concern 10=significant concern

0	1	2	3	4	5	6	7	8	9	10

Strength issues? 0=average strength 10=significant low/weak strength issues

0	1	2	3	4	5	6	7	8	9	10

Memory issues? 0=no memory issues 10=significant memory issues

0	1	2	3	4	5	6	7	8	9	10

Other problems/Concerns?

If you would like to be contacted by one of our professionals, please indicate:

Cancer Social Worker	Cancer Nutritionist	Rehabilitation Specialist

FIGURE 31.2 Example of a Distress Screening Tool.

■ COMMON SURVIVORSHIP CONCERNS FOR MALE GENITOURINARY CANCER SURVIVORS

Sexual Function

Erectile dysfunction (ED) is defined as the inability of a man to achieve and maintain an erection of sufficient strength for satisfactory sexual activity (Philippou et al., 2016). Following treatment for prostate cancer, sexual function is an area of concern. Both surgery (if nerve-sparing) and radiation therapy may take a toll on erectile function, ability for pleasurable sensation, and orgasm. During radical prostatectomy (RP), the cavernosal nerves controlling erections are spared (if it is at all possible to do so without increasing risk of cancer recurrence). However, even after the nerves are dissected from the prostate gland before its removal, the trauma incurred to the nerve bundles during the surgery may affect their function after the surgery.

The International Index of Erectile Function (IIEF), a 15-question, self-administered questionnaire, asks the patient to answer by selecting a score from 1 to 5 on various qualities of erectile function, as pertaining to themselves. A commonly used, abbreviated version of this tool is a 5-question form, the IIEF-5, which is also referred to as the Sexual Health Inventory for Men (SHIM). This form is readily available on the Internet. Scoring results of the SHIM have been shown to reliably correlate with severity of ED. Generally, a score >21 is considered to represent normal erectile function.

Men who have undergone radiation, chemotherapy, and surgical dissection for testicular cancer also present with posttreatment ED. As testicular cancer typically strikes in younger men who are sexually active, the early identification and treatment of ED become even more paramount. In a recent study of 77 men treated for testicular cancer, it was noted that most (88%) had successful response to first-line treatment for ED (Tal, Stember, Logmanieh, Narus, & Mulhall, 2014). Younger age likely has a positive effect on the preservation of erectile function.

Treatment with type 5 phosphodiesterase inhibitors (PDE5i) such as sildenafil or tadalafil is typically started within 1 month after prostatectomy (as long as it is financially feasible for the patient). The goal of this early intervention is to encourage healing and improve circulation to the nerve bundles controlling erectile function, although the data on "penile rehabilitation" is inconclusive. In general, PDE5i are used as first-line therapy for treatment-induced ED from either prostatectomy or radiation therapy, due to oral route of administration, and subtlety of use for the patient (Chapter 24). Other forms of treatment for ED caused by prostate cancer treatment are the vacuum erection device (VED), penile injections, and penile implant. Providers should open a discussion with their patients about sexual health and not wait on the patient to raise concerns as many patients find this difficult to do. Additional information on evaluating and treating ED can be found in Chapter 24. All options for treating erectile dysfunction have copious literature describing their efficacy and safety, but can remain cost prohibitive for many men, owing to limited insurance coverage. However, men should be presented with multiple options to address their ED until they find the option that enables them to best maintain intimacy with their partner.

Fertility

Men who are diagnosed with cancer will find it important to preserve their fertility if they have not yet created or completed their families. Between 2008 and 2011, nearly 1 in 29 men under 50 years of age developed invasive cancer (Grover, Deal, Wood, & Mersereau, 2016). Many of these survivors are at increased risk for infertility, owing to removal of crucial sexual organs, radiation damage to the organs, or disruption of spermatogenesis by chemotherapy or radiation treatment (Krupski & Litwin, 2007). The testicular cancer survivor population is particularly susceptible to issues with fertility, as these patients typically require orchiectomy, radiotherapy, and chemotherapy, all of which are damaging to sperm count and viability. A large multicenter study of 446 patients reported a decrease of 30% in fertility after treatment in testicular cancer patients (Huyghe et al., 2004). Within this study, radiotherapy appeared to have the most negative effect on fertility. Prostate cancer is typically diagnosed in an older population, but treatments can also affect fertility afterward. The plan for expected future fertility should be discussed with patients prior to treatment and referral to sperm banking should be done at this time, if desired.

But referral rates to sperm banking and fertility counseling are low in men who have been diagnosed with cancer. In a recent study of 201 young men diagnosed with cancer requiring chemotherapy, only 29% received fertility counseling, and only 11% sperm banked (Grover et al., 2016). More work is needed to create opportunities for clinicians and patients to discuss the importance of fertility counseling and sperm banking early in the cancer treatment planning process.

Urinary Incontinence

One side effect that can occur after treatment in prostate cancer patients, in particular, is incontinence of urine. This issue persists, despite vast improvements in surgical technique and precise accuracy of location and dose of radiation. The magnitude of the issue varies from patient to patient, and typical time to full expected recovery of continence extends to 2 years after treatment. Variables that can affect outcomes include surgical skill and volume, pretreatment continence, age, and other pre-existing urinary conditions.

In postprostatectomy patients, the most common type of urinary leakage is stress incontinence, leakage that occurs with coughing, laughing, sneezing, or bearing down while increasing intra-abdominal pressure. The leakage is due to insufficient sphincter function, related to damage of the internal urinary sphincter during surgical removal of the adjacent prostate gland. Men who undergo radical prostatectomy are encouraged to begin strengthening the external (voluntary) urinary sphincter through Kegel exercises. These exercises require the patient to identify the muscles used to stop the flow of urine during evacuation and learn to squeeze these muscles to improve sphincter strength and continence. By approximately 2 years after prostatectomy, most men are unable to regain additional continence.

Approximately 2% of men undergoing surgery will have enough leakage to necessitate the use of incontinence pads for the rest of their lives (Krupski, Saigal, & Litwin, 2003). Stress incontinence is difficult to remedy; men will choose to wear an incontinence pad or diaper. Other options include the use of a Cunningham clamp—a device that is placed over the penis and clamps, or provides pressure, over the urethra to prevent leakage.

Surgical placement of an artificial urinary sphincter (AUS) by a urology specialist offers a definitive option for incontinence treatment, but demands additional surgical intervention. AUS has generally produced good long-term outcomes; patient satisfaction rates are usually between 80% and 90%, and the success rate of the AUS in recent longitudinal studies following patients out to 5 and 7 years after placement is around 70% (Llorens & Pottek, 2017). About 25% of men will require revision surgery, with the rate of revision increasing with time (Llorens & Pottek, 2017). Some of the complications that can arise from AUS placement include infection, urethral atrophy, erosion, and mechanical failure (Singla, Cordon, & Singla, 2016).

Urge incontinence can affect men who have been treated for prostate cancers, especially those who have undergone pelvic radiation treatment. This uncontrollable outflow of urine is related to bladder dysfunction following treatment, and symptoms are similar to overactive bladder disease (OAB). Men will describe urgency, frequency, and the inability to hold urine (even on the way to the toilet) due to the overwhelming activity of the bladder's detrusor muscle. Typical treatment for urge incontinence includes both behavioral and lifestyle changes, as well as medication (Chapter 32).

Bowel Dysfunction

Bowel dysfunction (BD), including urgency, frequency, diarrhea, bloody or painful bowel movements, and fecal incontinence can occur after treatment in prostate cancer patients. These symptoms are most common in patients who have undergone radiation therapy, due to the proximity of the rectum to the prostate and treatment field. As patients do not always readily discuss bowel issues, it is important to inquire about bowel function and specifically ask whether the patient is experiencing any of these symptoms following radiation for prostate cancer.

First-line therapy for radiation-induced BD includes initiation of a bulking agent taken daily, such as psyllium fiber or methylcellulose. Although these supplements are typically taken to help with constipation, their bulking action has been shown to have a regulating action on bowel that has been affected by radiation treatments. If diarrhea is the main symptom, this can additionally be treated with over-the-counter antidiarrheal products. If diarrhea is severe or uncontrollable, prescription medication can be used. In rare cases, patients may have ongoing mild fecal incontinence, and require pads or diapers; providers should advise men to use a barrier cream to protect the skin around the anus from breakdown due to fecal leakage.

Providers should also warn men of the possibility of significant blood after radiation treatment (rectal bleeding and hematochezia), a less common side effect related to close proximity of the radiation treatment fields to the rectum. This may cause considerable alarm in patients, depending on the amount of bleeding seen. In a few individuals, the radiation effects may cause the rectal mucosa to thin and become friable. This induces rectal bleeding that can be seen after treatment. Patients should be reassured that this may be a side effect from treatment, but to be comprehensive, a history of colonoscopy screening should be reviewed, as well as any other abrupt changes in bowel habits, and family history of colon cancer; and referral to gastroenterology for further workup should be arranged as needed.

Issues Related to Androgen Deprivation Therapy

Androgen deprivation therapy, or ADT, is a form of treatment specifically for prostate cancer patients. Androgens encourage the growth of both normal and cancerous prostate cells by binding to and activating the androgen receptor. The androgen receptor is a protein that is expressed in prostate cells. Once triggered, the androgen receptor stimulates the expression of specific genes that cause prostate cells to grow (Massie et al., 2011). Early in development, some prostate cancers need fairly high levels of androgens to flourish and are referred to as "androgen sensitive" because treatments that lower androgen levels or block androgen activity can impede their growth. ADT reduces androgen production by the testicles, blocks the action of androgens in the body, and blocks the production of androgens throughout the body. The side effects of ADT vary by individual. Unfortunately, side effects are not a predictable variable. Common side effects include fatigue, hot flashes, night sweats, mood swings, central weight gain with muscle mass loss, loss of libido and erectile function, gynecomastia, loss of bone density, and occasionally cognitive deficits. An estimated 80% of patients on ADT will experience hot flashes and up to 27% describe them as the most bothersome side effect (Khan, Lewis, & Hughes, 2014). If symptoms are

TABLE 31.3 Treatment Options for Men Experiencing ADT Side Effects

Therapy	Proposed Effects
Oral megestrol acetate	Reduce hot flashes
Soy products containing phytoestrogens	Reduce hot flashes
Herbal supplements: red clover, evening primrose oil, and black cohosh	Reduce hot flashes
Acupuncture (Harrison et al., 2011)	Reduce hot flashes

severe or intolerable, there are some options for lessening the severity and frequency of hot flashes (Table 31.3).

Because of other health-related risks associated with weight gain and increased risk of bone density loss on ADT, men undergoing this therapy should be encouraged to maintain a healthy weight through weight-bearing exercise and low-fat diet. Men who will be undergoing at least 1 year of continuous ADT should have a baseline bone density test. Vitamin D and calcium supplements for bone density maintenance are recommended; however, if the patient is found to have osteopenia or osteoporosis at baseline, concurrent treatment with a bisphosphonate medication is needed. Patients with bone loss will also require ongoing monitoring by the PCP in the long-term.

Continued monitoring of the ADT patient for depressive symptoms related to dealing with cancer and its treatment is necessary. ADT has been known to increase the risk for depression. Mental health status should be assessed at each visit with the PCP, and appropriate treatment initiated as needed. Cognitive changes related to ADT are less common, but include language ability, short-term memory loss, mental flexibility, and some loss of inhibitory control (Gunlusoy et al., 2017). There is no current recommended screening in place for cognitive dysfunction related to ADT; however, clinicians should remain watchful for new complaints that may reflect cognitive change.

Cognitive behavioral therapy (CBT) and cognitive training are available for patients who have noticeable cognitive decline with ADT. These are available through referral to psychotherapy or within a speech-language pathology service. These interventions have been shown to have benefits by patient self-report, but there have been no significant improvements noted on objective measures of function (NCCN Clinical Practice Guidelines in Oncology: Survivorship, 2017).

Fatigue

Fatigue has been defined as "a distressing, persistent, subjective sense of physical, emotional, and/or cognitive tiredness, or exhaustion related to cancer or cancer treatment that is not proportional to recent activity and interferes with usual functioning" (NCCN Clinical Practice Guidelines in Oncology: Survivorship, 2017). This bothersome symptom is very common in patients who undergo cancer treatments and can continue for months and years after completion of therapy. The management of fatigue first requires an assessment of other contributing factors such as pain, distress, anemia, and sleep disturbances. A recent survey of cancer patients noted that fatigue is experienced by about 80% of patients who undergo chemotherapy or radiation therapy; most report that this fatigue continues to affect their quality of life after treatment has ended, and 17% to 29% continue to experience ongoing fatigue in the long term (NCCN Clinical Practice Guidelines in Oncology: Survivorship, 2017). Cancer survivors should be routinely screened for fatigue levels following treatment to ensure that moderate to severe fatigue (which can be quite disabling) is quickly addressed. This can be done with a simple severity scale numbered 0 to 10, where 0 is no fatigue noted, and 10 is fatigue that severely limits daily activities. A score that is higher than 4 should be addressed further, and fatigue levels rechecked at future visits.

Education about timing of activities and energy conservation are helpful in managing fatigue. This includes helping the patient identify more energetic times while awake, and congregating activities around those times. Guiding patients to better self-awareness can be helpful in allowing them to listen to their bodies at low energy times and allow a period of rest.

A number of trials have confirmed that increasing physical activity through a regular exercise program can combat fatigue, and also increase tolerance for activity, decrease anxiety and depression, and improve body image perception. A recent meta-analysis of eight randomized controlled trials noted that a 12- to 16-week exercise intervention significantly improved fatigue symptoms when assessed by the Functional Assessment of Cancer Therapy (FACT) Fatigue scale (Vashistha, Singh, Kaur, Prokop, & Kaushik, 2016). Additionally, fatigue remained improved at 6 months after the intervention, showing promise for longer-term stability (Vashistha et al., 2016). The care provider should encourage the survivor to maintain a healthy exercise schedule to combat fatigue, and a referral to physical therapy may be made if the patient has become deconditioned.

Anxiety, Depression, and Distress

Survivors of cancer are at an especially high risk for anxiety, depression, and other forms of psychosocial distress due to multiple stressors, vulnerability, and other challenges they are faced with during and after treatment. Mental health can also suffer in relation to new physical limitations, social isolation, and financial issues stemming from treatment. Cancer patients often experience distress in the form of fear of recurrence and feelings of lack of control, which can manifest as anxiety or depression. Anxiety and/or depression can affect up to 29% of cancer survivors (NCCN Clinical Practice Guidelines in Oncology: Survivorship, 2017), with PTSD (posttraumatic stress disorder) symptoms being a common finding this group. In a recent Swedish study, it was found that cancer survivors were afflicted with mental health disorders for up to 10 years after treatment (Lu et al., 2016). This is not surprising given the predictable decrease in routine provider care and support following treatment. Adding to this issue, there is a lack of sufficient psycho-oncology services available through barriers in the referral process during the survivorship phase, creating a significant deficiency in psychological care.

Routine psychosocial distress screening is recommended by the NCCN, especially in light of the strong correlation between elevated psychosocial distress and the formation of mental health issues. This may be accomplished at regular follow-up intervals by questioning the patient about whether he feeling more anxious or sad than usual, and whether or not this mood is impacting his quality of life. It is particularly important to repeat screening if the patient has had a change in clinical status or is noting numerous somatic complaints (NCCN Clinical Practice Guidelines in Oncology: Survivorship, 2017). Patients may be referred as needed to mental health service professionals including psychiatrists, psychologists, social workers, or online and phone-based community support.

For patients who present with suicidal ideation and impending plan to do harm to themselves or others, an emergency intervention may be required, such as securing weapons, calling 911, or securing the patient for emergency psychiatric evaluation and treatment. Individuals who have intermittent suicidal ideation but no specific plan to do harm are at lower risk but will still require the preparation of a safety plan. This plan may include regular monitoring, access to a suicide hotline, or plans to go to the emergency room if thoughts become increasingly urgent.

Once depression and anxiety have been identified and diagnosed, management may include nonpharmacological and pharmacological interventions.

Role of Exercise

Regular exercise has been noted to be effective in increasing quality of life in studies involving cancer survivors, and results in the treatment of depression and anxiety have followed this curve. A recent study involving breast cancer survivors noted significant improvement in depression scores after patients were involved in a 22-week cardiac rehabilitation-based program, which offered personalized aerobic and resistance exercises plus 12 group educational sessions to encourage behavioral adoption to a healthy lifestyle (Dolan et al., 2018).

Physical therapy and exercise may be effective for treatment of pain in survivors, with the added benefit and goal of increasing overall mobility. Randomized controlled trials in cancer survivors have demonstrated a significant reduction in joint pain, severity of pain, and interference of pain in daily life. Yoga, in particular, may be beneficial to cancer survivors as it encompasses both the physical and spiritual side of self-care.

The role of exercise in the cancer survivorship phase is further discussed later in the chapter as an important factor in the posttreatment development of healthy lifestyle choices. It is a topic that should be discussed regularly at follow-up appointments; this regular discourse allows patients to identify barriers to exercise and collaborate with the provider on ideas for creating a feasible and sustainable exercise regimen.

Sleep Disorders

Within the general management of sleep disorders, and insomnia in particular, education about sleep hygiene is of utmost importance. Key points to discuss with the survivor include regular physical activity, daytime exposure to bright light, a dark and quiet sleep environment, and avoiding heavy meals, alcohol, and nicotine near bedtime.

Sleep disorders are commonly seen in patients with cancer, owing to disease or treatment-related changes in the sleep cycle, stress and anxiety related to cancer diagnosis and treatment, and other side effects from treatment including pain and fatigue. These disturbances may extend into the survivorship phase related to chronic side effects from treatment, anxiety, depression, medication, and change in sleep habits related to fatigue. Sleep disorders can include insomnia—trouble falling or staying asleep—excessive daytime sleepiness, and sleep-related movement disorders or breathing disorders, such as sleep apnea.

Cancer survivors should be screened for sleep disorders at regular intervals, and also when there is an alteration in health status. Assessment of sleep disorders can be challenging but should begin with ruling out obstructive sleep apnea (OSA) as a cause of sleep disruption and excessive sleepiness. There are various validated screening tools for OSA, including the STOP tool (www.sleepmedicine.com/files/files/StopBang_Questionnaire.pdf), and OSA can be confirmed with a sleep study referral.

Restless leg syndrome (RLS) is another cause of sleep disturbance and is associated with uncomfortable sensations and an urge to continuously move the legs when in a resting position. The symptoms can sometimes be alleviated with walking or stretching. If the patient is found to have RLS symptoms, he should be evaluated for iron deficiency, and a physical examination should be performed. Iron replacement can improve symptoms, and dopamine agonists, benzodiazepines, gabapentin, and opioids have also been used. Referral to a sleep specialist is always a suitable option.

Psychosocial therapy can help improve sleep in the survivor population. Several randomized controlled trials and meta-analyses have found strong evidence that cognitive behavioral therapy (CBT) can have significant and positive effects on the severity of insomnia, and the positive effects that CBT produced were found to be durable over time (Johnson et al., 2016).

Pharmacological treatments are also available for insomnia, and should be used discontinuously as needed during the survivorship phase to help the patient achieve healthy sleep habits and avoid other complications of sleep loss. Providers should keep in mind that many of the benzodiazepine receptor agonists are associated with dependence, abuse, and withdrawal, and these patients should be carefully assessed on a regular basis, and made aware of these possible side effects.

Pain

More than a third of cancer survivors experience chronic pain after treatment; predictors of pain include tumor characteristics, course of therapy used in cancer treatment, time since the cancer treatment, and efficacy of any initial pain therapy (Paice, Lacchetti, & Bruera, 2016). Pain can lead to psychological distress, decreased activity, low motivation, reduced personal interaction with others, and poor quality of life. Pain in cancer survivors is often undermanaged, with obstacles that include a lack of healthcare provider training, patient fears of addiction or side effects from medication, and cost. Screening for pain should be done at regular intervals in cancer survivors. If pain exists, its intensity must be quantified by the patient and is best accomplished by a subjective, self-reporting statement from the patient. A useful way to quantify pain intensity is by using a 0 to 10 numeric rating scale, categorical scale, or pictoral scale. A commonly used scale that utilizes both numeric and pictoral measurements is the Wong-Baker FACES Pain Rating Scale. Men should also be asked to characterize their pain: aching, burning, stabbing, or otherwise. If the patient is found to be in severe and uncontrolled pain, it should be considered an emergency, and the pain promptly addressed, as an increased level of pain should also be reason to rule out an oncological emergency.

Pain management goals for survivors include increasing comfort, maximizing function, and improving quality of life. This can be accomplished by a multidisciplinary approach including the involvement of pharmacological treatment, psychosocial intervention, physical therapy, exercise, occupational therapy, complementary therapy, and other interventional procedures. Psychological support for survivors experiencing chronic pain is of utmost importance, and referral to psychosocial services should always be an option.

A large part of pain management in cancer survivors includes pharmacological treatments. This group of medications includes opioids, adjuvant analgesics, nonsteroidal anti-inflammatory drugs (NSAIDs), and muscle relaxants. Local therapies may also include topical anesthetics.

Opioid medications are typically used in the treatment of neuropathic pain, skeletal pain, and chronic pain. Providers should be aware of the potential for abuse and misuse of these medications, and monitor these patients at regular intervals.

Adjuvant analgesics are antidepressants and anticonvulsants that are used in the treatment of patients with neuropathic pain, postradiation pain, chronic pain syndrome, myalgias, or arthralgias. These medications include serotonin and norepinephrine reuptake inhibitors (SNRIs), tricyclic antidepressants, gabapentin, and pregabalin. A recent review found that the use of these medications concurrently with opioids may provide additional neuropathic pain relief in cancer patients (NCCN Clinical Practice Guidelines in Oncology: Survivorship, 2017).

NSAIDs are effective at blocking the biosynthesis of prostaglandins, inflammatory mediators of pain and, along with acetaminophen, are commonly used in the treatment of myofascial and skeletal pain. NSAIDs are most effective for mild to moderate pain. A recent systematic review found that data supporting the use of NSAIDs for pain control in patients with advanced cancer are limited, but their use may assist in reducing opioid dose requirement (NCCN Clinical Practice Guidelines in Oncology: Survivorship, 2017).

Finally, muscle relaxants are known to reduce muscle spasm and can aid in treatment of skeletal pain, myalgia, and arthralgia. There is limited evidence for their effectiveness in noncancer settings and no evidence is available in studies of cancer-related pain.

Acupuncture is another complementary therapy should be considered as an option for the treatment of both myofascial and neuropathic pain in cancer survivors. There is currently limited evidence supporting the effectiveness of this method, but it is becoming a more popular choice for pain management. A recent online survey of 15 licensed acupuncturists in the United States required responses from the care providers about patient-reported response of neuropathic pain on chemotherapy treatment. Reported results included ratings of moderately successful outcomes with moderate improvement seen in 60% of treated patients (Lu, Moody, Marx, & Hammerstrom, 2017). Other local therapies for pain can include heat and cold packs, massages, and medicated topical ointments and patches. Other interventional procedures may include the use of transcutaneous electrical nerve stimulation (TENS) units, nerve blocks, neurotomy with radiofrequency ablation, and dorsal nerve stimulation.

Role of Support Groups

Support groups for cancer survivors are available online (Appendix 31.1) and through many local hospitals and cancer treatment centers. These groups offer opportunities to discuss common challenges in recovery and opportunities to both receive and offer advice. Many cancer survivors find support groups helpful, simply knowing that they are not alone in their recovery and gleaning helpful recommendations while also finding meaning in their suffering by being in a position to offer helpful advice themselves (Coffey et al., 2016).

Engaging with adjustment-focused self-management interventions in the form of support groups has been shown to enable cancer survivors to gain emotional and informational support from peers and/or facilitators in an open and nonjudgmental environment (Coffey et al., 2016; Gottlied & Wachala, 2007). Support groups have been shown to improve quality of life, anxiety, depression, and even fatigue among cancer survivors (Willems et al., 2017). Cancer survivors describe a process of becoming empowered by support groups by enhancement of knowledge and skills, regaining confidence and control, and the encouragement to move beyond cancer by accepting their illness, reprioritizing their goals, and adopting a positive outlook (Coffey et al., 2016; Gottlied & Wachala, 2007).

However, the extent to which cancer survivors engaged in support groups and benefited from support groups was mitigated by very diverse preferences among survivors for how these peer interventions were designed, the content of the groups, and delivery method (Coffey et al., 2016; Gottlied & Wachala, 2007). Having a wide variety of options in design, content, and mode of delivery of peer support groups enables the diverse body of cancer survivors to overcome barriers to participation and to be more likely to engage in peer support groups that effectively meet their needs.

■ HEALTHY LIFESTYLE FOR THE MALE GENITOURINARY CANCER SURVIVOR

Nutrition

Nutrition and eating habits can become a "hot topic" after cancer treatment. Many patients are interested in adjusting their eating habits and other health-related habits to increase their longevity and quality of life. Some of these patients may already be doing well at maintaining a healthy weight through diet and exercise, and for others who were overweight prior to treatment, their cancer diagnosis may be an incentive to action.

Weight gain can be a common problem during and after cancer diagnosis and treatment; the prevalence of obesity in the survivor population is higher than in the general population. This holds especially true for prostate cancer survivors undergoing ADT. Owing to the hormonal changes stimulated by ADT, these men are at particular risk for decreased insulin sensitivity, central weight gain, and muscle mass loss—with fatigue from treatment only compounding the problem of inactivity. Additional adverse effects of ADT include increases in high-density lipoprotein cholesterol and triglycerides. These changes have some overlap with metabolic syndrome, bringing concerns that long-term ADT may put prostate cancer survivors at greater risk for diabetes and cardiovascular disease (Saylor & Smith, 2013).

There are also concerns that obesity may cause increased risk for prostate cancer progression in treated patients. In a recent study of 5,158 men diagnosed with localized prostate cancer who were followed over 26 years, there was a positive association found between long-term weight gain and risk of lethal prostate cancer (Dickerman et al., 2017). The findings suggest that metabolic changes may stimulate prostate cancer progression.

Cancer survivor nutrition and weight management should be evaluated, and body mass index (BMI) should be calculated and discussed with patients. Whether they are underweight or overweight, it is important to inform survivors of their current weight status, and decide upon interventions, as needed, to attain a normal body weight. Survivors with an overweight BMI should be educated by the PCP about portion control, identifying lower calorie foods, choosing nutrient-dense foods, and tracking their diet and calorie intake, as well as physical activity. Behavioral modification training may also be useful for weight loss in this population.

Discussions about nutrition should also be conducted with survivors who fall into the underweight range of BMI. Education addressed to this group should include increasing meal frequency, avoiding fluid intake with meals, assessment of dental health, and smoking status. Evaluation of swallowing ability, detection of taste and smell disorders, and determination of gastrointestinal motility may also be necessary. Referral to a registered dietitian for individual counseling and treatment planning can be helpful for all cancer survivors.

Cancer survivors also should be counseled to limit alcohol intake to one drink per day for women, and two drinks per day for men. Survivors of liver, esophageal, kidney, and head and neck cancers should refrain from alcohol entirely, owing to increased risk of death with alcohol consumption.

Exercise

During cancer treatment, many patients become deconditioned and can develop deficiencies in cardiovascular fitness due to the direct and indirect effects of therapy. Physical activity during and after cancer treatment is an important tool for health maintenance in cancer survivors. Exercise training is a safe, supportable, and effective intervention for survivors. Structured exercise programs have shown improvements in cardiovascular health, with additional positive changes in balance, body composition, emotional well-being, and quality of life. In a recent randomized control trial of testicular cancer survivors, who had an increased risk of treatment-related cardiovascular disease, a high-intensity aerobic interval training program was found to have significant benefits for improving cardiorespiratory fitness and markers of cardiovascular mortality risk for testicular cancer survivors (Adams et al., 2017).

Sedentary behavior is a risk factor for postcancer mortality and also impacts mood and quality of life. Barriers to physical activity should be discussed and addressed in each visit with cancer survivors. Common barriers to physical activity for cancer survivors include time constraints, lack of access to a satisfactory exercise environment, uncertainty about safety of exercise following cancer treatment, lack of knowledge about appropriate exercise patterns, and lingering physical limitations following cancer treatment. It is important to mitigate pain, fatigue, distress, and nutritional deficits prior to commencement of an exercise program, as removal of these barriers will help the patient to include exercise as part of his healthy lifestyle.

Survivors who have been treated with chemotherapy are increased risk for peripheral neuropathy; and prostate cancer survivors who have been treated with ADT are at additional risk for poor bone health and possibly musculoskeletal issues related to muscle wasting. These patients should be considered at a moderate risk for exercise-related accident and injury, and their stability, balance, and gait must be assessed prior to initiation of an exercise program. These moderate risk survivors can often practice general recommendations for physical activity, and if there are safety concerns referral to a physical or occupational therapist can be considered.

Supplements

As many as 79% to 85% of cancer survivors take some type of vitamin or mineral dietary supplement, often without disclosing this information to their treating providers (NCCN Clinical Practice Guidelines in Oncology: Survivorship, 2017). There have been numerous systematic reviews and meta-analyses to assess the role of various vitamins and other dietary supplements in primary cancer prevention, cancer control, or cancer recurrence. To date, no clear evidence supports an effective dietary supplementation (Mayne, Ferrucci, & Cartmel, 2012).

Because of the possibility of interactions between supplements and other medications or treatments survivors may be taking, it is not recommended that cancer patients take supplements unless they are noted to have a deficiency, an inadequate diet, or some other comorbid illness requiring supplementation.

Common supplements used by men who have undergone treatment for prostate cancer include antioxidants such as green tea extract, pomegranate, and vitamin C. Other supplements marketed as being supportive of prostate health include selenium, saw palmetto, and African cherry. There are few studies referencing "alternative non-hormonal treatments" and their effectiveness for prostate cancer survivors, but there are indications that these treatments may be useful alternatives if patients are not willing to take prescribed medication (Drewe, Bucher, & Zahner 2015).

■ COMPLEMENTARY AND ALTERNATIVE CARE

Many cancer survivors reassess their health and lifestyle following cancer diagnosis and treatment; as an attempt to exert some control over their health, more patients are choosing to incorporate integrative approaches during their recovery. "Alternative" or "complementary" therapies are currently utilized by approximately 50% of Americans to maintain optimal health (Yates et al., 2005). The use of these therapies, along with traditional medicine, is also known as "integrative medicine." Approximately 90% of cancer patients and survivors employ this type of treatment during rehabilitation (Yates et al., 2005).

These approaches include several types: healing touch, mind–body approaches, creative arts, nutrition, and fitness. Many of these methods are effective in helping the patient manage symptoms and side effects from cancer treatment, while providing a sense of self-control and efficacy. Integrative medicine addresses mind, body, and spirit and encourages patients to be proactive partners in their treatment. This embraces the idea of a "holistic" well-being. Integrative medicine can include therapy through support groups, massage, acupuncture, meditation, yoga, art therapy, and music therapy.

There is a paucity of studies on the involvement of integrative therapy in cancer. Although these therapies have been shown to be effective for symptom relief, to date there is no evidence that they will slow the progression of cancer. It should be noted that the modern integration of complementary therapies with conventional medical treatment has allowed healthcare providers to fully address physical emotional spiritual and quality of life needs of cancer patients.

CONCLUSION

The male genitourinary cancer survivor confronts potential long-term and late effects that can be devastating to their quality of life if not identified when present and treated effectively. The potential burden of genitourinary (GU) complications of cancer is significant for all cancer survivors, not just those with cancers of the GU tract. Studies such as the Livestrong Foundation survey highlight how common urological side effects are and how infrequently they may be addressed (Rechis & Boerner, 2010). It is essential that any provider of survivorship care be familiar with the potential impact of urological cancer treatments and be comfortable speaking frankly with their patients about these concerns.

With improved diagnostics and treatment options the number of cancer survivors continues to climb. Many cancer survivors will experience long-term or late effects of cancer and its treatment, which often include physical as well as psychosocial problems. It is important that these issues are addressed comprehensively and in a regular and methodical way by providers familiar with the challenges confronted by cancer survivors. This initially requires the effort of the primary oncology team, but increasingly, this responsibility is being transitioned to the PCP soon after the completion of primary treatment. With adequate communication at the time of transfer of care and with access to survivorship educational resources the PCP is well suited to provide this care.

CLINICAL PEARLS

- Useful forms for the screening of anxiety and depression symptoms with guidelines for referral are available at the National Comprehensive Cancer Network (NCCN) website.
- Survivorship should include management of comorbid symptoms such as fatigue, weight gain, depression, and social aspects of being labeled as a cancer survivor.
- Pretreatment fertility preservation and management should be offered to all men undergoing treatment, not solely those planning chemotherapy.
- American Society of Clinical Oncology forms provide a way for men to record information about their cancer, cancer treatment, and planned follow-up care.
- Erectile dysfunction is a common late effect from cancer treatments and men should be routinely screened for it and treatment options should be offered. The IIEF-5 or SHIM are two screening tools that are effective and easy to use.
- There are e-learning tools that exist to help educate and train PCPs on how to care for cancer survivors, some of these are listed in Appendix 31.1.
- Survivors should be given a distress screening tool on a regular basis to capture the areas of their life impacted by cancer treatment. Interventions for for these areas of concern should then be discussed on a recurring basis.

REFERENCES

Adams, E., Boulton, M. G., Horne, A., Rose, P. W., Durrant, L., Collingwood, M., ... Watson, E. K. (2014). The effects of pelvic radiotherapy on cancer survivors: Symptom profile, psychological morbidity and quality of life. *Clinical Oncology, 26*(1), 10–17. doi:10.1016/j.clon.2013.08.003

Adams, S. C., DeLorey, D. S., Davenport, M. H., Stickland, M. K., Fairey, A. S., North, S., ... Courneya, K. S. (2017). Effects of high-intensity aerobic interval training on cardiovascular disease risk in testicular cancer survivors: A phase 2 randomized controlled trial: Exercise and CVD Risk in Testicular Cancer. *Cancer, 123*(20), 4057–4065. doi:10.1002/cncr.30859

Andersen, B. L., Rowland, J. H., & Somerfield, M. R. (2015). Screening, assessment, and care of anxiety and depressive symptoms in adults with cancer: An American Society of Clinical Oncology Guideline Adaptation. *Journal of Oncology Practice, 11*(2), 133–134. doi:10.1200/JOP.2014.002311

Banegas, M. P., Guy, G. P., Jr., de Moor, J. S., Ekwueme, D. U., Virgo, K. S., Kent, E. E., ... Yabroff, K. R. (2016). For working-age cancer survivors, medical debt and bankruptcy create financial hardships. *Health Affairs, 35*(1), 54–61. doi:10.1377/hlthaff.2015.0830

Baravelli, C., Krishnasamy, M., Pezaro, C., Schofield, P., Lotfi-Jam, K., Rogers, M., ... Jefford, M. (2009). The views of bowel cancer survivors and health care professionals regarding survivorship care plans and post treatment follow up. *Journal of Cancer Survivorship, 3*(2), 99–108. doi:10.1007/s11764-009-0086-1

Bellizzi, K. M., Miller, M. F., Arora, N. K., & Rowland, J. H. (2007). Positive and negative life changes experienced by survivors of non-Hodgkin's lymphoma. *Annals of Behavioral Medicine, 34*(2), 188–199. doi:10.1007/BF02872673

Bloom, J. R., Petersen, D. M., & Kang, S. H. (2007). Multi-dimensional quality of life among long-term (5+ years) adult cancer survivors. *Psycho-Oncology, 16*(8), 691–706. doi:10.1002/pon.1208

Brennan, M. E., Butow, P., Spillane, A. J., & Boyle, F. M. (2010). Survivorship care after breast cancer: Follow-up practices of Australian health professionals and attitudes to a survivorship care plan. *Asia-Pacific Journal of Clinical Oncology, 6*(2), 116–125. doi:10.1111/j.1743-7563.2010.01286.x

Canada, A. L., Murphy, P. E., Fitchett, G., & Stein, K. (2016). Re-examining the contributions of faith, meaning, and peace to quality of life: A report from the American Cancer Society's Studies of Cancer Survivors-II (SCS-II). *Annals of Behavioral Medicine, 50*(1), 79–86. doi:10.1007/s12160-015-9735-y

Chen, T., Fallah, M., Jansen, L., Castro, F. A., Krilavicuite, A., Katalinic, A., ... Castro, F. (2015). Distribution and risk of the second discordant primary cancers combined after a specific first primary cancer in German and Swedish cancer registries. *Cancer Letters, 369*(1), 152–166. doi:10.1016/j.canlet.2015.08.014

Coffey, L., Mooney, O., Dunne, S., Sharp, L., Timmons, A., Desmond, D., ... Gallagher, P. (2016). Cancer survivors' perspectives on adjustment-focused self-management interventions: A qualitative meta -synthesis. *Journal of Cancer Survivorship, 10*(6), 1012–1034. doi:10.1007/s11764-016-0546-3

DeSantis, C. E., Lin, C. C., Mariotto, A. B., Siegel, R. L., Stein, K. D., Kramer, J. L., ... Jemal, A. (2014). Cancer treatment and survivorship statistics, 2014. *CA: A Cancer Journal for Clinicians, 64*(4), 252–271. doi:10.3322/caac.21235

Dickerman, B. A., Ahearn, T. U., Giovannucci, E., Stampfer, M. J., Nguyen, P. L., Mucci, L. A., & Wilson, K. M. (2017). Weight change, obesity and risk of prostate cancer progression among men with clinically localized prostate cancer: Weight change, obesity and prostate cancer risk. *International Journal of Cancer, 141*(5), 933–944. doi:10.1002/ijc.30803

Dolan, L. B., Barry, D., Petrella, T., Davey, L., Minnes, A., Yantzi, A., ... Oh, P. (2018). The cardiac rehabilitation model improves fitness, quality of life, and depression in breast cancer survivors. *Journal of Cardiopulmonary Rehabilitation and Prevention, 38*(4), 246–252. doi:10.1097/hcr.0000000000000256

Drewe, J., Bucher, K. A., & Zahner, C. (2015). A systematic review of non-hormonal treatments of vasomotor symptoms in climacteric and cancer patients. *SpringerPlus, 4*(1), 65. doi:10.1186/s40064-015-0808-y

Foxhall, L. E., & Rodriguez, M. A. (2015). *Advances in cancer survivorship management*. New York, NY: Springer Publishing Company.

Gottlied, B. H., & Wachala, E. D. (2007). Cancer support groups: A critical review of empirical studies. *Psycho-Oncology, 16*(5), 379–400. doi:10.1002/pon.1078

Greiman, A. K., & Keane, T. E. (2017). Approach to androgen deprivation in the prostate cancer patient with pre-existing cardiovascular disease. *Current Urology Reports, 18*(6), 41. doi:10.1007/s11934-017-0688-5

Grover, N. S., Deal, A. M., Wood, W. A., & Mersereau, J. E. (2016). Young men with cancer experience low referral rates for fertility counseling and sperm banking. *Journal of Oncology Practice, 12*(5), 465–471. doi:10.1200/JOP.2015.010579

Grunfeld, E., Julian, J. A., Pond, G., Maunsell, E., Coyle, D., Folkes, A., … Levine, M. N. (2011). Evaluating survivorship care plans: Results of a randomized, clinical trial of patients with breast cancer. *Journal of Clinical Oncology, 29*(36), 4755–4762. doi:10.1200/JCO.2011.36.8373

Grunfeld, E., Levine, M. N., Julian, J. A., Coyle, D., Szechtman, B., Mirsky, D., … Whelan, T. (2006). Randomized trial of long-term follow-up for early-stage breast cancer: A comparison of family physician versus specialist care. *Journal of Clinical Oncology, 24*(6), 848–855. doi:10.1200/JCO.2005.03.2235

Gunlusoy, B., Ceylan, Y., Koskderelioglu, A., Gedizlioglu, M., Degirmenci, T., Ortan, P., & Kozacioglu, Z. (2017). Cognitive Effects of Androgen Deprivation Therapy in Men With Advanced Prostate Cancer. *Urology, 103*, 167–172. doi:10.1016/j.urology.2016.12.060

Halpern, M. T., McCabe, M. S., & Burg, M. A. (2016). The cancer survivorship journey: Models of care, disparities, barriers, and future directions. *American Society of Clinical Oncology Educational Book, 35*, 231–239. doi:10.14694/EDBK_156039

Harrison, S. E., Watson, E. K., Ward, A. M., Khan, N. F., Turner, D., Adams, E., … Rose, P. W. (2011). Primary health and supportive care needs of long-term cancer survivors: A questionnaire survey. *Journal of Clinical Oncology, 29*(15), 2091–2098. doi:10.1200/JCO.2010.32.5167

Hewitt, M., Greenfield, S., & Stoval, E. (2006). *From cancer patient to cancer survivor: Lost in transition*. Washington, DC: National Academies Press.

Hsu, T., Ennis, M., Hood, N., Graham, M., & Goodwin, P. J. (2013). Quality of life in long-term breast cancer survivors. *Journal of Clinical Oncology, 31*(28), 3540–3548. doi:10.1200/jco.2012.48.1903

Huyghe, E., Matsuda, T., Daudin, M., Chevreau, C., Bachaud, J.-M., Plante, P., … Thonneau, P. (2004). Fertility after testicular cancer treatments: Results of a large multicenter study. *Cancer, 100*(4), 732–737. doi:10.1002/cncr.11950

Johnson, J. A., Rash, J. A., Campbell, T. S., Savard, J., Gehrman, P. R., Perlis, M., … Garland, S. N. (2016). A systematic review and meta-analysis of randomized controlled trials of cognitive behavior therapy for insomnia (CBT-I) in cancer survivors. *Sleep Medicine Reviews, 27*, 20–28. doi:10.1016/j.smrv.2015.07.001

Keehn, A., Ludmir, E., Taylor, J., & Rabbani, F. (2017). Incidence of bladder cancer after radiation for prostate cancer as a function of time and radiation modality. *World Journal of Urology, 35*(5), 713–720. doi:10.1007/s00345-016-1934-z

Khan, A., Lewis, R., & Hughes, S. (2014). Managing hot flushes in men receiving androgen deprivation therapy for prostate cancer: ADT TOXICITY. *Trends in Urology & Men's Health, 5*(1), 31–33. doi:10.1002/tre.377

Krupski, T. L., Kwan, L., Fink, A., Sonn, G. A., Maliski, S., & Litwin, M. S. (2006). Spirituality influences health related quality of life in men with prostate cancer. *Psycho-Oncology, 15*(2), 121–131. doi:10.1002/pon.929

Krupski, T. L., & Litwin, M. S. M. S. (2007). Medical and psychosocial issues in prostate cancer. In P. A. Ganz (Ed.), *Cancer survivorship: Today and tomorrow* (pp. 145–152). New York, NY: Springer Publishing Company.

Krupski, T. L., Saigal, C. S., & Litwin, M. S. (2003). Variation in continence and potency by definition. *The Journal of Urology, 170*(4), 1291–1294. doi:10.1097/01.ju.0000085341.63407.46

Llorens, C., & Pottek, T. (2017). Urinary artificial sphincter ZSI 375 for treatment of stress urinary incontinence in men: 5 and 7 years follow-up report. *Urologia Journal, 84*(4), 263–266. doi:10.5301/uj.5000243

Lu, D., Andersson, T. M. L., Fall, K., Hultman, C. M., Czene, K., Valdimarsdóttir, U., & Fang, F. (2016). Clinical diagnosis of mental disorders immediately before and after cancer diagnosis. *JAMA Oncology, 2*(9), 1188. doi:10.1001/jamaoncol.2016.0483

Lu, Z., Moody, J., Marx, B. L., & Hammerstrom, T. (2017). Treatment of chemotherapy-induced peripheral neuropathy in integrative oncology: A survey of acupuncture and oriental medicine practitioners. *The Journal of Alternative and Complementary Medicine, 23*(12), 964–970. doi:10.1089/acm.2017.0052

Massie, C. E., Lynch, A., Ramos-Montoya, A., Boren, J., Stark, R., Fazli, L., ... Mills, I. G. (2011). The androgen receptor fuels prostate cancer by regulating central metabolism and biosynthesis: AR coordinates anabolic program in prostate cancer. *The EMBO Journal, 30*(13), 2719–2733. doi:10.1038/emboj.2011.158

Mayne, S. T., Ferrucci, L. M., & Cartmel, B. (2012). Lessons learned from randomized clinical trials of micronutrient supplementation for cancer prevention. *Annual Review of Nutrition, 32*, 369–390. doi:10.1146/annurev-nutr-071811-150659

Miller, K. D., Siegel, R. L., Lin, C. C., Mariotto, A. B., Kramer, J. L., Rowland, J. H., ... Jemal, A. (2016). Cancer treatment and survivorship statistics, 2016. *CA: A Cancer Journal for Clinicians, 66*(4), 271–289. doi:10.3322/caac.21349

Mullan, F. (1985). Seasons of survival: Reflections of a physician with cancer. *New England Journal of Medicine, 313*(4), 270–273. doi:10.1056/NEJM198507253130421

The National Coalition for Cancer Survivorship. (2017). Retrieved from https://www.canceradvocacy.org

NCCN Clinical Practice Guidelines in Oncology: Survivorship. (2017). Retrieved from https://www.nccn.org/professionals/physician_gls/pdf/survivorship.pdf

Nekhlyudov, L., Aziz, N. M., Lerro, C., & Virgo, K. S. (2014). Oncologists' and primary care physicians' awareness of late and long-term effects of chemotherapy: Implications for care of the growing population of survivors. *Journal of Oncology Practice, 10*(2), e29–e36. doi:10.1200/JOP.2013.001121

Nekhlyudov, L., O'Malley, D. M., & Hudson, S. V. (2017). Integrating primary care providers in the care of cancer survivors: Gaps in evidence and future opportunities. *The Lancet Oncology, 18*(1), e30–e38. doi:10.1016/S1470-2045(16)30570-8

Paice, J. A., Lacchetti, C., & Bruera, E. (2016). Management of chronic pain in survivors of adult cancers: ASCO clinical practice guideline summary. *Journal of Oncology* Practice, *12*(8), 757–762. doi:10.1200/JOP.2016.014837

Philippou, Y. A., Steggall, M. J., Treacy, C. L., Hirani, S., O'Driscoll, S. T., Bakker, C. J., & Dahm, P. (2016). Penile rehabilitation for post-prostatectomy erectile dysfunction. *Cochrane Database of Systematic Reviews*, (11), CD012414. doi:10.1002/14651858.CD012414

Reuben, S. H. (2004). *The President's cancer panel: Living beyond cancer: Finding a new balance*. Bethesda, MD: National Cancer Institute, National Institutes of Health, U.S. Department of Health and Human Services

Rechis, P., & Boerner, L. (2010). How cancer has affected post-treatment survivors: A livestrong report. Retrieved from https://d1un1nybq8gi3x.cloudfront.net/sites/default/files/what-we-do/reports/LSSurvivorSurveyReport.pdf

Rechis, P., & Reynolds, K. A. (2011). "I Learned To Live With It" is not good enough: Challeges reported by post-treatment cancer survivors in the livestrong surveys. Retrieved from https://d1un1nybq8gi3x.cloudfront.net/sites/default/files/what-we-do/reports/LSSurvivorSurveyReport_final_0.pdf

Salz, T., Oeffinger, K. C., McCabe, M. S., Layne, T. M., & Bach, P. B. (2012). Survivorship care plans in research and practice. *CA: Cancer Journal for Clinicians, 62*(2), 101–117. doi:10.3322/caac.20142

Saylor, P. J., & Smith, M. R. (2013). Metabolic complications of androgen deprivation therapy for prostate cancer. *The Journal of Urology, 189*(1), S34–S44. doi:10.1016/j.juro.2012.11.017

Selph, J. P., & Peterson, A. C. (2017). Review article: Past, present and future of cancer survivorship and the importance of the urologist. *Urology Practice, 4*(1), 60–70. doi:10.1016/j.urpr.2016.01.001

Singla, A., Cordon, B., & Singla, N. (2016). Artificial urinary sphincters for male stress urinary incontinence: Current perspectives. *Medical Devices: Evidence and Research, 9*, 175–183. doi:10.2147/MDER.S93637

Stein, K. D., Syrjala, K. L., & Andrykowski, M. A. (2008). Physical and psychological long-term and late effects of cancer. *Cancer, 112*(11 suppl.), 2577–2592. doi:10.1002/cncr.23448

Tal, R., Stember, D. S., Logmanieh, N., Narus, J., & Mulhall, J. P. (2014). Erectile dysfunction in men treated for testicular cancer. *BJU International, 113*(6), 907–910. doi:10.1111/bju.12331

Valdivieso, M., Kujawa, A. M., Jones, T., & Baker, L. H. (2012). Cancer survivors in the united states: A review of the literature and a call to action. *International Journal of Medical Sciences, 9*(2), 163–173. doi:10.7150/ijms.3827

Vashistha, V., Singh, B., Kaur, S., Prokop, L. J., & Kaushik, D. (2016). The effects of exercise on fatigue, quality of life, and psychological function for men with prostate cancer: Systematic review and meta-analyses. *European Urology Focus, 2*(3), 284–295. doi:10.1016/j.euf.2016.02.011

Wattchow, D. A., Weller, D. P., Esterman, A., Pilotto, L. S., McGorm, K., Hammett, Z., … Silagy, C. (2006). General practice vs surgical-based follow-up for patients with colon cancer: Randomised controlled trial. *British Journal of Cancer, 94*(8), 1116–1121. doi:10.1038/sj.bjc.6603052

Willems, R. A., Bolman, C. A. W., Mesters, I., Kanera, I. M., Beaulen, A. A. J. M., & Lechner, L. (2017). Short-term effectiveness of a web-based tailored intervention for cancer survivors on quality of life, anxiety, depression, and fatigue: Randomized controlled trial. *Psycho-Oncology, 26*(2), 222–230. doi:10.1002/pon.4113

Wood, M. E., Vogel, V., Ng, A., Foxhall, L., Goodwin, P., & Travis, L. B. (2012). Second malignant neoplasms: Assessment and strategies for risk reduction. *Journal of Clinical Oncology, 30*(30), 3734–3745. doi:10.1200/JCO.2012.41.8681

Yates, J. S., Mustian, K. M., Morrow, G. R., Gillies, L. J., Padmanaban, D., Atkins, J. N., … Colman, L. K. (2005). Prevalence of complementary and alternative medicine use in cancer patients during treatment. *Supportive Care in Cancer, 13*(10), 806–811. doi:10.1007/s00520-004-0770-7

Zhou, E. S., Bober, S. L., Nekhlyudov, L., Hu, J. C., Kantoff, P. W., & Recklitis, C. J. (2016). Physical and emotional health information needs and preferences of long-term prostate cancer survivors. *Patient Education and Counseling, 99*(12), 2049–2054. doi:10.1016/j.pec.2016.07.017

Appendix 31.1 Survivorship Resources for Healthcare Providers and Patients: General Information	
National Coalition for Cancer Survivorship (NCCS)	www.canceradvocacy.org
American Association for Cancer Research (AACR). A six-part podcast series about survivorship in partnership with CR Magazine and The Wellness Community:	www.aacr.org/http://www.crmagazine.org/archive/Crpodcasts/Pages/SurvivingThriving.aspx
American Cancer Society (ACS) • Survivorship information • Cancer Survivors Network • National Cancer Survivorship Resource Center • Physical side effects information, including sexual function	www.cancer.org/index www.cancer.org/treatment/survivorshipduringandafter treatment/index www.csn.cancer.org www.cancer.org/SurvivorshipCenter www.cancer.org/treatment/treatmentsandside effects/physicalsideeffects/index
American Institute for Cancer Research (AICR): Survivorship information. Nutrition, physical activity, weight management	www.aicr.org/patients-survivors/staying-healthy-after-treatment/
American Society of Clinical Oncology (ASCO) Survivorship information for patients and tools and resources for oncology providers	www.cancer.net/survivorship www.asco.org/practice-guidelines/cancer-care-initiatives/prevention-survivorship/survivorship/survivorship-compendium
Cancer Care: Free, professional support services for anyone affected by cancer	www.cancercare.org
Centers for Disease Control and Prevention: survivorship information	www.cdc.gov/cancer/survivorship/index.htm
George Washington University Cancer Survivorship e-learning Series for PCP	smhs.gwu.edu/gwci/survivorship/ncsrc/elearning
Leukemia and Lymphoma Society: survivorship information	www.lls.org/diseaseinformation/managingyourcancer/survivorship
LIVESTRONG: Advocacy and support	www.livestrong.org
National Cancer Institute: Cancer Survivorship Research Facing Forward series, designed to educate cancer survivors, family members, and healthcare providers about the challenges associated with life after cancer treatment	www.survivorship.cancer.gov cancercontrol.cancer.gov/ocs/resources/ffseries.html
National Comprehensive Cancer Network (NCCN) Life After Cancer: Patient and caregiver Information	www.nccn.org/index.asp www.nccn.org/patients/resources/life_after_cancer
MedlinePlus: Up-to-date, accurate information by cancer site	www.nlm.nih.gov/medlineplus/cancers.html

(continued)

Survivorship Resources for Healthcare Providers and Patients: General Information (*continued*)	
Oncology Nursing Society: Putting Evidence Into Practice	www.ons.org/practice-resources/pep
HELP LINES	
American Cancer Society	1.800.227.2345; www.cancer.org
American Psychosocial Oncology Society	1.866.276.7443; apos-society.org
Cancer Support Community	1.888.793.9355 www.cancersupportcommunity.org
LIVESTRONG Survivor Care	1.855.220.7777
National Cancer Institute's Cancer Information Service	1.800.4.CANCER

CHAPTER 32

Overactive Bladder and Incontinence in the Male Patient

Mashrin Lira Chowdhury and Min Suk Jun

INTRODUCTION

Urinary tract symptoms are frequently seen and treated in a primary care physician's office. Many patients can be evaluated in the office with a history, physical examination, or laboratory testing. This chapter will address overactive bladder (OAB) and urinary incontinence in male patients. Even though urge urinary incontinence is a more common type, other causes for incontinence will also be addressed. Included in the discussion will be how to perform a general evaluation of a patient with OAB symptoms, diagnose OAB and incontinence, and management considerations in male patients. Relevant anatomic considerations and physical examination will also be reviewed.

OAB encompasses a host of symptoms defined by the International Continence Society (ICS) as "urinary urgency, usually accompanied by frequency and nocturia are not terms unique to urology. They are known descriptive terms of symptoms." In addition, the Society of Urodynamics and Female Pelvic Medicine and Urogenital Reconstruction (SUFU) and American Urological Association (AUA) have created care pathways in treating patients with OAB (Gormley et al., 2014). OAB with or without incontinence afflicts both men and women. In fact, the incidence of OAB in males is nearly equal to women at up to 50% of the population (Dmochowski & Gomelsky, 2009). However, the incidence of urgency incontinence associated with OAB in men is less than that of women (Buckley, Lapitan, & Epidemiology Committee of the Fourth International Consultation on Incontinence, 2010; Wieder, 2014). OAB is often overlooked in males and sometimes dismissed as a symptom of an enlarged prostate. The diagnosis and treatment of men with benign prostatic hypertrophy (BPH) and related symptoms are discussed in Chapter 25. OAB may be present with other common comorbid conditions such as depression or diabetes mellitus (see Box 32.1) (Palleschi et al., 2014; Shamliyan, Wyman, Ping, Wilt, & Kane, 2009; Solmaz et al., 2017). Newer studies are showing that patients who present with OAB and/or incontinence are at a higher risk of falls. This may be due to other confounding factors such as age, polypharmacy, and comorbid conditions (Chung, Noguchi, Chan, & Tse, 2016).

Urinary incontinence is defined as an involuntary loss of urine. The male patient can present with OAB with or without urgency incontinence designated as OAB wet and OAB dry, respectively. It is important to keep in mind that different causes of incontinence exist and should be differentiated noting these differences drive the treatment plan.

With an aging population, the prevalence of urgency incontinence is increasing and can place great economic burden on the healthcare system (Gorina, Schappert, Bercovitz, Elgaddal, & Kramarow, 2014; Shamliyan et al., 2009; Yehoshua et al., 2016). Higher rates of urinary incontinence are seen in aging patients and patients who live in nursing homes

BOX 32.1 COMORBID CONDITIONS ASSOCIATED WITH OVERACTIVE BLADDER AND INCONTINENCE

Diabetes mellitus
Depression
Falls
Fractures
Urinary tract infection
Polypharmacy
Neurological conditions such as Parkinson's disease and stroke

(Stothers, Thom, & Calhoun, 2005; Wu et al., 2014). Male patients are less likely to report incontinence episodes due to embarrassment or shame, and are also less likely to seek help than their female counterparts. Male patients can experience more psychological distress from this condition (Clemens, 2016). They might be incorrectly treated for years before proper evaluation. Clinicians must be mindful that the management of these symptoms in males and females differs owing to different causes.

MALE ANATOMY AND PHYSIOLOGY OF THE LOWER URINARY TRACT

Urethra

The urethra is composed of six segments. From distal to proximal, they include the urethral meatus, fossa navicularis, penile urethra, bulbar urethra, membranous urethra, and prostatic urethra. The narrowest portion of the urethra is the fossa navicularis. The average diameter of the male urethra is 8 to 9 mm. The urethra is invested by the corpus spongiosum from the urethral meatus to the bulbar urethra. Glands of Littre are found along this segment as well—these glands serve to provide urethral lubrication. The external urinary sphincter is composed of skeletal muscle and is found at the level of the membranous urethra. Basal muscular tone is present to promote continence but can be consciously relaxed in order to void. The bulbospongiosus muscle surrounds the bulbar urethra, and it functions to evacuate residual urine from the urethra in addition to contributing to erectile and ejaculatory function. Cowper's glands are within the pelvic floor musculature, and their ducts insert into the bulbar urethra. Their secretions provide lubrication during sexual arousal. The verumontanum is a prominence within the prostatic urethra. The ejacularory ducts and the utricle, a vestigial remnant of embryological development, are found on the verumontanum (Kavoussi, 2016).

Prostate

The prostate is an exocrine gland found in males and is about the size of a walnut that sits in the pelvis anterior to the rectum. It contributes a variety of products for semen critical in normal male reproductive function. There are four zones of the prostate: the peripheral zone, transition zone, central zone, and anterior fibromuscular stroma. Prostate cancer is mainly found in the peripheral zone, and BPH is enlargement of the transition zone (Chapter 25) (Kavoussi, 2016).

Bladder

The bladder plays a vital role in storage and emptying of urine. The bladder neck directly abuts the prostatic urethra and is considered a smooth muscle sphincter. The trigone lies

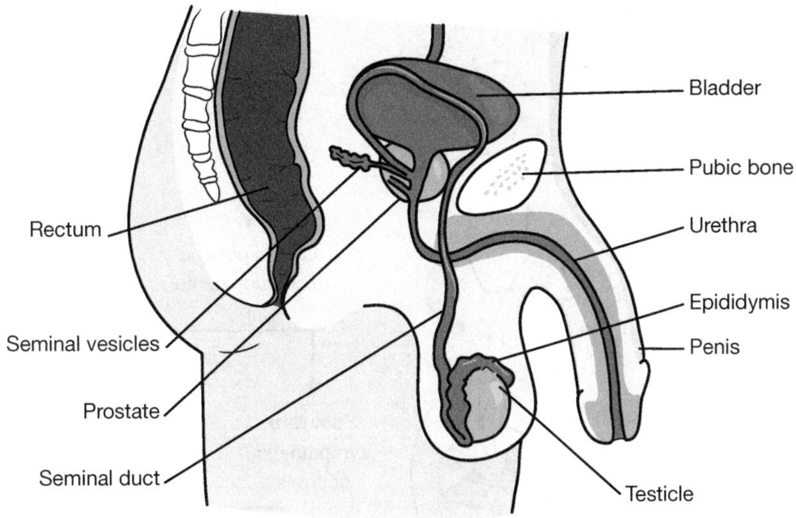

FIGURE 32.1 Diagram of male urethra, prostate, and bladder.

along posterior aspect of the bladder and contains the ureteric ridge where both ureters insert into the bladder. The bladder layers from inside to out include the urothelium, lamina propria, and two muscularis layers. Intact neurological pathways, functional detrusor muscle, and an open bladder outlet allow for the successful passage of urine.

Neurophysiology of the Bladder

Normal bladder function requires coordination among the sympathetic, parasympathetic, and somatic nervous systems. When the bladder senses it is full, voiding is initiated by the voluntary relaxation of the somatic muscle, the rhabdosphincter, which receives its innervation from the pudendal nerve (S2-S4). The sympathetic nervous system provides bladder neck relaxation by way of the hypogastric nerve (T10-L2). The detrusor muscle must then contract, which is under control of the pelvic nerve (S2-S4), which carries parasympathetic nerve fibers. Bladder storage requires inhibition of the parasympathetic system and activation of the sympathetic system. In short, the bladder outlet is actively closed while detrusor contraction is inhibited. This is collectively termed the guarding reflex for voiding control (Wieder, 2014; Wein, 2016). In summary, normally while the bladder is filing with urine, no bladder contractions exist while the sphincter remains closed to keep the patient continent. When the bladder senses a volume that reaches its capacity it stimulates the voiding cycle to evacuate the urine.

Pathophysiology of Overactive Bladder

Afferent nerve fibers carry bladder sensory information to various levels of the central nervous system (CNS). A-delta fibers are mechanoreceptors and sense the degree of stretch of the bladder—in short, they monitor bladder fullness. C fibers are nociceptors and detect bladder irritation (Juszczak, Ziomber, Wyczolkowski, & Thor, 2009). The brainstem, which is responsible for the body's primitive functions, is the integration center for most of the regulatory function of the bladder, including the voiding reflex. The cortex, however, integrates higher

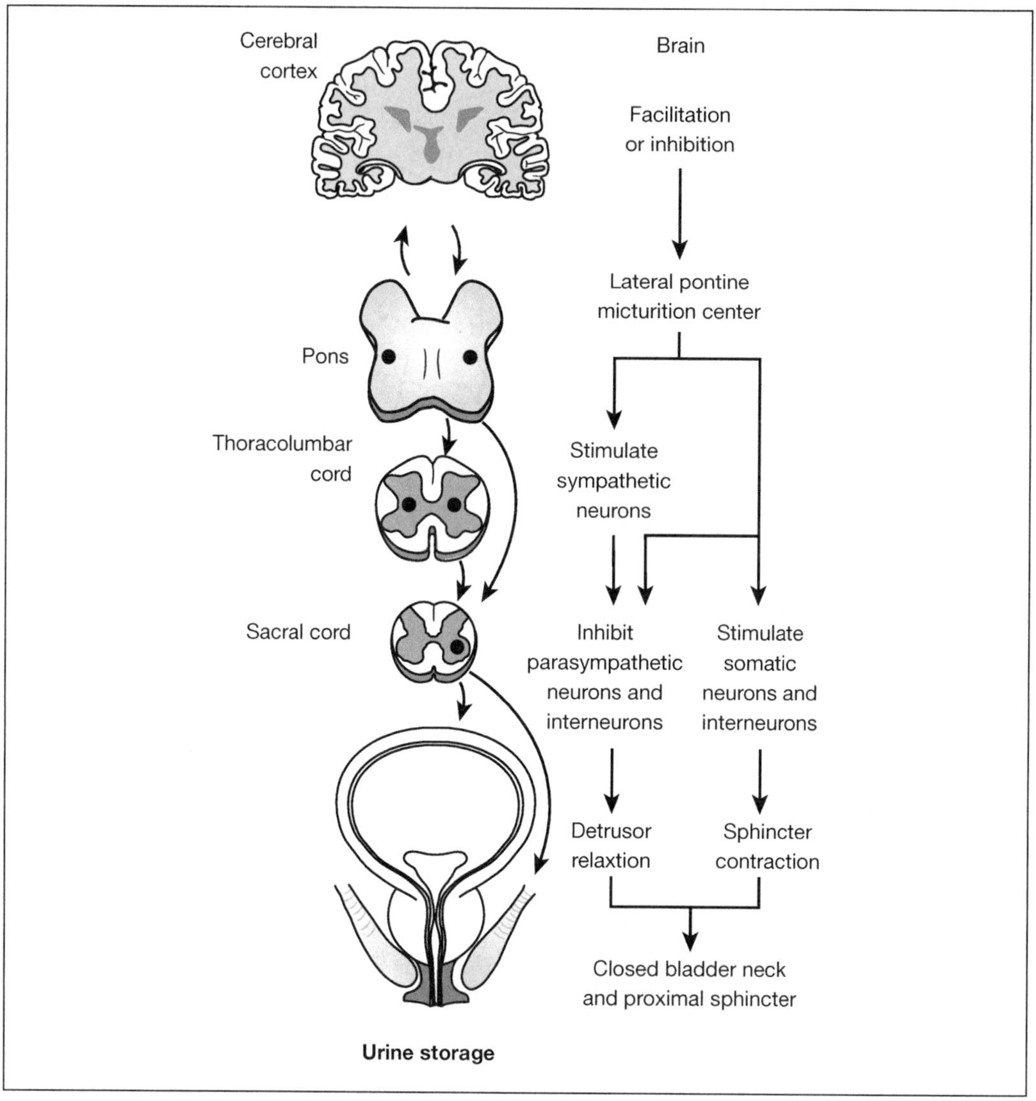

FIGURE 32.2 Physiology/pathophysiology of voiding. (*continued*)

level sensory information and "translates" these afferent inputs to subjective lower urinary tract sensations, such as bladder fullness and urgency. Overactive bladder begins with a state of dysfunction of the elements described above. For example, A-delta fibers may fire at inappropriately high rates for a given degree of bladder fullness while C fibers are firing in the absence of bladder irritants. It is also a reasonable theory that integration centers in the CNS can "misinterpret" otherwise normal afferent nerve activity from the bladder (Drake, 2007).

Bladder overactivity must also include activation of the detrusor muscle. The components that lead to detrusor contraction include afferent input, signal processing, efferent innervation, and smooth muscle contraction. Multiple hypotheses of the pathophysiology of OAB exist; some postulate that spontaneous excitation of smooth muscle cells leads to inappropriate nerve stimulation while others suggest that the primary defect is the nerve signaling to and/or from the bladder (Drake, Mills, & Gillespie, 2001).

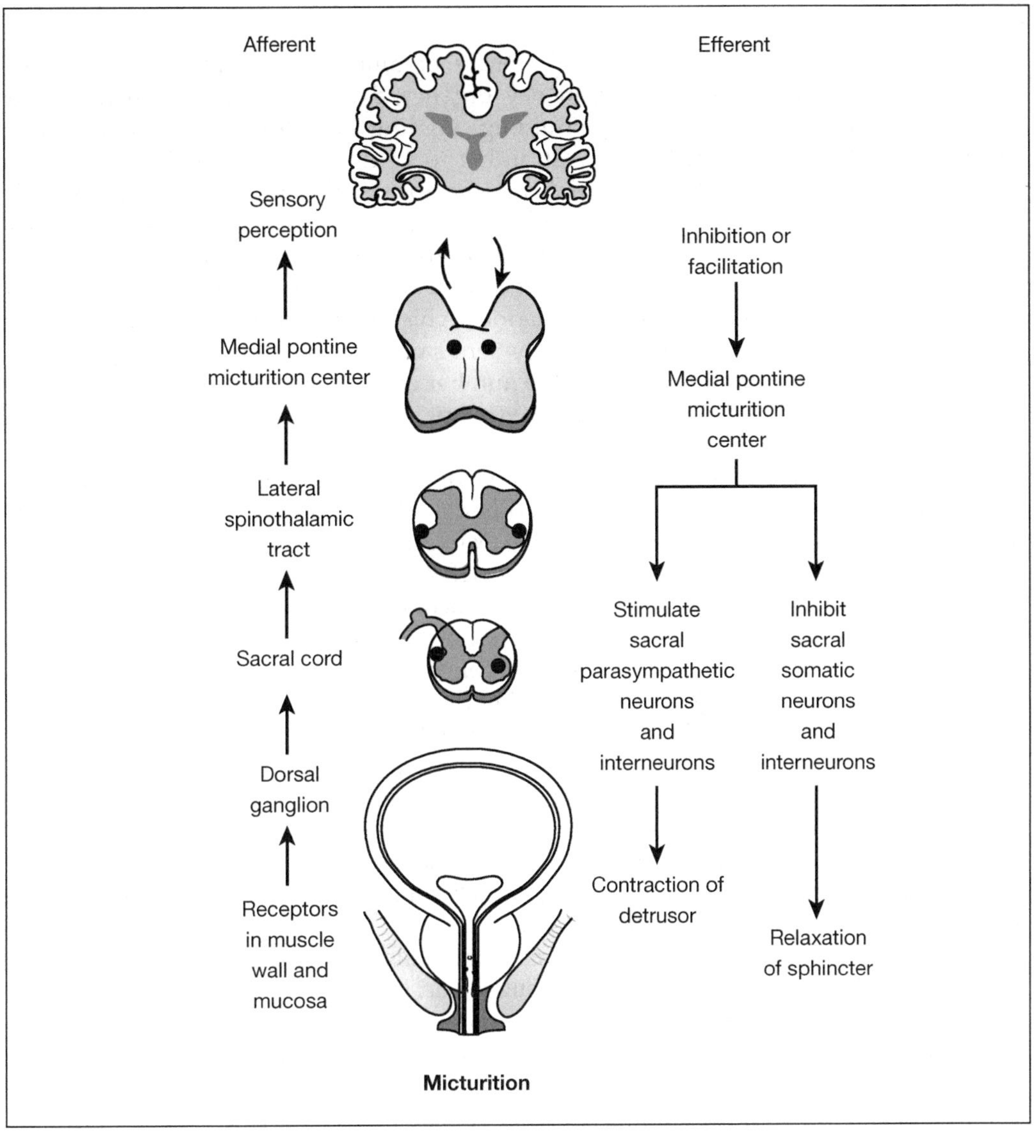

FIGURE 32.2 *(continued)*

Neurological disease is clearly linked with the development of bladder overactivity. The development of continence parallels the development of the cortex in children. It is believed that the cortex provides a continuous inhibitory signal with volitional suppression of this signal, thus enabling social continence. Injury, neurological disease, or aging is known to damage the cortex and may lead to the loss of this inhibitory signal. It is by this mechanism that strokes and aging lead to the development of detrusor overactivity (Drake, 2016).

EVALUATION OF THE MALE PATIENT WITH VOIDING SYMPTOMS

Before discussing the diagnosis and treatment of OAB and incontinence, it is imperative to discuss how to perform a directed history, physical examination, and any other diagnostic testing for these patients.

History

A focused history of present illness (HPI) must be obtained first and foremost. The clinician should differentiate irritative (frequency, urgency, dysuria) versus obstructive (slow stream, hesitancy, spraying of urine, straining) voiding symptoms. Decreased force of stream, hesitancy, intermittent stream, straining to void, and incomplete voiding may indicate underlying obstruction. Urethral stricture specific findings include genital pain, spraying of urinary stream, decreased force of stream, and dysuria. Men may have a history of previous urethritis, urethral instrumentation, or genital or perineal trauma. Gross hematuria in addition to lower urinary tract symptoms (LUTS) may indicate underlying bladder cancer or carcinoma in situ of the bladder. A history of culture-proven urinary tract infections (UTIs) may be the reason for the patient's urinary tract symptoms. In men with incontinence, it is important to quantify the number of pads or briefs used per day along with the weight of each change, as this may relate to quality-of-life issues (Mangera & Chapple, 2014).

Questionnaires provide objective measurement of a patient's symptoms and are an objective way to gauge how much the patient is bothered. The questionnaire can be distributed while the patient is waiting to be seen. Some examples include the AUA symptom score (AUASS), International Prostate Symptom Score (IPSS), and the International Consultation of Incontinence Modular Questionnaire Urinary Incontinence Short Form (ICIQ-UI-SF).

Another useful tool is a bladder diary, which should be provided to a patient at the time of the first visit. Simplified bladder diary components include the date and time of void, the volume of void, incontinence, pads per day (if symptoms include incontinence), and any habits (food, drink, volume of intake) that they find to exacerbate or improve symptoms. The International Consultation of Incontinence Modular Questionnaire (ICIQ-BD) is an example of a bladder diary that can be found online; however, simpler ones do exist. Easy-to-read formats should be provided to the patient; 3 days is usually adequate but the diary can be kept longer if desired by the clinician. The healthcare provider or staff member should educate the patient on how to appropriately fill this out. If done correctly, it can aid in a personalized treatment plan for the patient.

In addition to the HPI, the astute clinician must also perform a thorough review of comorbid conditions, surgical history, medications, social history, and family history. Disease states, such as poorly controlled diabetes or multiple sclerosis, can directly contribute to lower urinary tract dysfunction. Previous pelvic surgery can lead to LUTS masquerading as OAB. Many medications potentially contribute to the OAB, such as diuretics and stimulants. Chronic opioid use may cause chronic constipation, which is related to voiding dysfunction. Caffeine, tobacco, spicy foods, and polydipsia are all examples of habits or social factors that contribute to bladder pathology. Finally, it is important to obtain a urological family history, as bladder cancer and nephrolithiasis also contribute to OAB.

PHYSICAL EXAMINATION

A focused physical examination begins from the time the patient enters the exam room. The patient's functional status, body habitus, and gait can be immediately assessed. Is the patient ambulatory? Does he require a walker? Is he wheelchair bound? This may relate to functional status and how he may get to the bathroom.

An abdominal exam is performed in the supine position and includes palpation for masses such as hydronephrotic kidneys (albeit extremely difficult in an adult) or suprapubically, a distended bladder. Costovertebral angle (CVA) tenderness elicited by a gentle tap on the flank while the patient is sitting upright or suprapubic tenderness or fullness indicate obstruction or infection. The clinician should carefully inspect the meatus for size, location, or lesions. Phimosis can cause irritative voiding symptoms. Testicular and scrotal pathology rarely contribute to OAB or incontinence but should be included in a complete male genitourinary examination. Large hydroceles, testicular masses, or hernias may cause functional voiding issues. A digital rectal examination (DRE) should be performed in all men with voiding symptoms. This will give you information on rectal and pelvic muscle tone, stool impaction, prostate nodules, prostate size, prostatitis, or rectal masses. Keep in mind the normal prostate has the consistency of a thenar eminence (the group of muscles on the palm of the human hand at the base of the thumb). A proper DRE is performed with the patient either bent over the examination table or laying on the side with the knees to the chest (Gerber & Brendler, 2016).

DIAGNOSTIC TESTS

Diagnostic tests are a useful adjunct to the history and physical examination. Many tests such as a dipped urinalysis or postvoid residual (PVR) urine test can be done in the clinic.

A dipstick urinalysis (UA) is a chemical-based in-office test that provides valuable information. Nitrites are indicative of the presence of gram-negative bacteria, the most common bacteria responsible for UTIs. Leukocyte esterase indicates the presence of white blood cells, the sign of an immune response to pathogenic bacteria. If both of these components are positive in the setting of LUTS, the clinician should be highly suspicious of UTI. Inflammatory conditions like a UTI can thus be the cause of the patient's urinary symptoms. The presence of blood on dipstick UA is suggestive of but not diagnostic for hematuria; this must be fully evaluated with microscopy. Microscopic urinalysis in most settings is a "send-out" test. Microscopic hematuria, defined as more than 2 red blood cells per high-power field, in the absence of a UTI (negative nitrite, leukocyte esterase, and/or bacteria) may indicate underlying pathology and warrants further workup by a urology provider. White blood cells are directly reported in microscopy, obviating the need for leukocyte esterase. Bacteria are also reported with microscopy, which is obviously useful when suspicion is high for UTI and necessitating a urine culture as well.

Routine cases of OAB and incontinence do not warrant a complete blood count (CBC). Creatinine, an indicator of renal function, is not recommended in routine cases of LUTS. Prostate-specific antigen (PSA) testing is not performed for the diagnosis of LUTS, OAB, or urinary incontinence. The physical examination should suffice in the diagnosis of the enlarged prostate (Carter et al., 2013).

A renal and bladder ultrasound examination may be ordered in patients with suspected obstruction and/or abnormal renal function. A large distended bladder indicates urinary retention. Ultrasound may also detect bladder wall thickening, diverticulae, or hydronephrosis. Any of these findings prompt referral to a urologist for further evaluation. Further testing may include voiding cystourethrogram, uroflowmetry, and retrograde urethrogram to guide definitive treatment.

A bladder scanner uses ultrasound to determine bladder volume. A PVR test will show the amount of urine remaining after the patient voids. Elevated PVR urine amount indicates impaired emptying. After referral to a urologist the patient may undergo other procedures. Uroflowmetry plots urinary flow over time, and cystometry and electromyography measure global bladder function during filling and voiding (minimally invasive procedure that involves placement of catheters in the urethra and rectum and electrodes on the perineum or thigh). These components collectively make up a urodynamics study. Cystourethroscopy is direct visualization of the urethra, prostate, and bladder. It may further aid in evaluating prostate size, diagnose urethral stricture disease, or identify other causes for urinary tract symptoms such as a bladder mass or stones.

OVERACTIVE BLADDER

The following section will review the diagnosis and treatment of patients with idiopathic OAB and neurogenic OAB.

Idiopathic overactive bladder as described in the overview is a symptom complex of urinary frequency, urgency, and nocturia. Incontinence may exist with urgency when no other cause is identified such as an obvious UTI, bladder cancer, or stones.

Management of Idiopathic OAB

The first line treatment of patients with OAB are conservative measures like lifestyle modifications. Patients should always be counseled regarding their fluid intake with particular attention paid to caffeine intake. Smoking cessation and regular exercise to aid in weight loss are important points of counseling as well. The bladder diary is a critical tool. It helps the patient and clinician potentially identify the cause of one's voiding symptom. Furthermore, with the aid of questionnaires, it will provide a means for tracking progress during the treatment phase. When the physical examination reveals either increased or decreased pelvic floor muscle tone, pelvic floor muscle therapy should be offered. Although physical therapy is widely accepted as a useful adjunct in the treatment of OAB in females, there is a relative dearth of research of its use in males and specific recommendations cannot be made at this time (Dmochowski & Gomelsky, 2009).

Second-line treatment for OAB is pharmacological. AUA and SUFU have well-established guidelines on various medications consisting of antimuscarinic and beta-3 adrenergic agents. Acetylcholine stimulates M3 muscarinic receptors via parasympathetic pathways and antimuscarinics antagonize these receptors, decreasing the strength and frequency of detrusor contraction. Alternatively, mirabegron, the only beta-3 receptor agonist available, stimulates beta-3 receptors. These receptors are normally active during bladder filling (thus aiding in bladder relaxation) by way of the sympathetic nervous system (Chai, 2016).

Owing to the concern for polypharmacy and potential interactions, all of the patient's medications should be checked for interactions prior to beginning therapy. Table 32.1 lists the available medications for use in the United States, and all the listed medications have been shown to have similar efficacy in the treatment of OAB. It is important to keep in mind that the side effect profiles do differ among the drugs, and the costs of the medication (and insurance restrictions) frequently preclude clinician's choice of which medication to start.

Antimuscarinic medications have a side effect profile that at times are more bothersome to patients than the actual OAB symptoms. These side effects include dry eyes, dry mouth, constipation, and cognitive effects. Extreme caution is advised in starting these medications on patients with any degree of cognitive impairment, constipation, or any other confounding illnesses or medications that exacerbate anticholinergic effects. Treatment with these medications in patients with untreated narrow-angle glaucoma is contraindicated. Antimuscarinic use in patients who have gastroparesis or gastric outlet obstruction should be used cautiously as well. Extended release or transdermal oxybutynin is a better choice than the oral route because of its more favorable side effect profile. Often the medications work well for patients; however, the side effects can be overwhelming. An attempt at side effect management is warranted in these cases before abandoning treatment.

Mirabegron is the only medication of its class and may be used as monotherapy or in conjunction with antimuscarinics (Gormley et al., 2014). Mirabegron has similar efficacy in males with OAB as other anticholinergics and is better tolerated as its side effect profile is minimal (Chung et al., 2016; Tubaro et al., 2017). Mirabegron should be used cautiously in patients with hypertension as it has been shown to exacerbate high blood pressure through its adrenergic properties.

TABLE 32.1 Medications for Overactive Bladder

Generic	Trade Name	Dosages	Mechanism of Action	Other Notes
Oxybutynin chloride	Ditropan Ditropan XL Oxytrol (Patch)	5 mg BID to TID 5 mg to 15 mg QD 3.9 mg/d	Antimuscarinic	Transdermal or oral
Tolterodine tartrate	Detrol Detrol LA	2 mg BID 4 mg QD	Antimuscarinic	
Fesoterodine fumarate	Toviaz	4 mg to 8 mg QD	Antimuscarinic	
Solifenacin succinate	Vesicare	5 mg to 10 mg QD	Antimuscarinic	M3 selective
Darifenacin hydrobromide	Enablex	7.5 mg to 15 mg QD	Antimuscarinic	Most M3 selective
Trospium chloride	Sanctura Sanctura XR	20 mg BID 60 mg Q AM	Antimuscarinic	Quaternary amine structure decreases chance of crossing blood-brain barrier
Mirabegron	Myrbetriq	25 mg to 50 mg QD	Beta Adrenergic	No dry mouth, constipation, cognitive side effects

AM, morning; BID, twice a day; Q, every; QD, every day; TID, three times a day.

If patients fail to control their symptoms with conservative behavioral management and pharmacological treatment, third-line treatments can be offered. The AUA/SUFU OAB guidelines place intravesical botulinum toxin, peripheral tibial nerve stimulation (PTNS), and sacral neuromodulation (SNS) as third-line treatments for idiopathic OAB. These three procedures are performed by a urologist typically. Intravesical botulinum toxin or onabotulinum toxinA (Botox) is directly injected into the detrusor muscle with cystoscopy and is performed by a urologist during a procedure can be performed in the office or the operating room. Botulinum toxin acts at the parasympathetic nerve terminal where it inhibits neurotransmitter release. Through this action, detrusor contraction is inhibited. As such, acute urinary retention is of paramount concern. The studies show that the retention rate is less than 10% in nondiabetic patients and 10% to 20% in diabetics. Patients with a PVR greater than 150 mL are also at risk for urinary retention (Rahnama'i, Marcelissen, Brierley, Schurch, & de Vries, 2017).

S3 is the dominant nerve innervating the detrusor muscle. Through S3 neuromodulation it is possible to ameliorate OAB symptoms. There are two methods of achieving this. PTNS targets the posterior tibial nerve, which originates at S3. PTNS can be performed in the clinic without the need for systemic anesthesia. Qualified midlevel providers and physicians are authorized to deliver the weekly treatments for 12 weeks. Each session lasts 30 minutes. Some patients may benefit from further maintenance therapy. Sacral neuromodulation directly modulates the S3 nerve root via placement of the leads into the S3 sacral foramen through a two-step process. The initial step is performed with local anesthesia. Leads are percutaneously implanted with fluoroscopic guidance, and an external pulse generator is left. If patient response is satisfactory after a trial period, an implantable pulse generator is surgically placed under sedation. Patients are taught how to adjust settings with a patient-controlled programmer (Vasavada & Rackley, 2016).

The last line of treatment is augmentation cystoplasty or cystectomy and urinary diversion. These are dramatic measures and rarely used (Gormley et al., 2014). It is very important to note that indwelling catheters or suprapubic catheters are not recommended for the treatment of OAB or incontinence due to high complication rates.

Neurogenic OAB is a broad term inclusive of any bladder dysfunction rooted in a neurological cause, such as spinal cord injuries, strokes, and multiple sclerosis. Spinal cord injury patients, depending on the level, may lose coordinated control of voiding leading to detrusor-sphincter dysynergia (DSD). This can be dangerous as it can lead to high detrusor pressures, which in turn can lead to upper urinary tract damage. Symptomatically, these patients will present with incontinence and small functional bladder volumes. Because these patients are at risk of developing upper urinary tract damage, they should undergo periodic upper tract imaging and monitoring of their renal function. They should also be referred to a urologist as they may need urodynamics testing, anticholinergic/antimuscarinic pharmacotherapy to reduce bladder pressures, and bladder drainage management. This may include intermittent catheterization, indwelling suprapubic catheter, urinary diversion, a continent catheterizable channel, or, least preferably, an indwelling Foley catheter. In contrast, stroke victims will never develop DSD. Instead, they are at risk of losing the guarding reflex, which can lead to urinary frequency and urgency urinary incontinence (Wieder, 2014).

Men with longstanding *bladder outlet obstruction (BOO)* may develop OAB. BOO occurs in men with BPH or urethral stricture disease. Chronic BOO may lead to bladder remodeling, which may cause irritative symptoms, such as frequency, urgency, and nocturia. Incontinence is less likely unless overflow is present. Irritative lower urinary tract symptoms are expected to resolve in approximately 70% of men after treatment of their obstruction (Wieder, 2014). Patients with OAB and BOO may benefit from combined alpha blocker and anticholinergic therapy with a low risk of urinary retention if urinary flow is not severely impaired (Lee et al., 2004).

Detrusor overactivity with impaired contractility (DOIC) is diagnosed with urodynamics studies. These patients present with the same symptoms as an OAB patient but will also have an elevated PVR urine test. Diabetes and bladder outlet obstruction lead to DOIC. These patients are treated with surgery, intermittent catheterization, and/or medications (Liu, Chan, & Tse, 2014).

URINARY INCONTINENCE

As discussed previously, there are many different types of incontinence. Although urge urinary incontinence will be the more commonly encountered type of incontinence, it is important to keep in mind the other types that exist and may need further evaluation by a specialist.

Urge urinary incontinence (UUI) is defined as the strong desire to void followed by involuntary loss of urine. Up to 90% of men with UUI will have associated OAB (Abrams et al., 2002; Hashim & Abrams, 2016). This is treated in the same algorithm as described above for OAB. Other causes of urgency with or without incontinence can be due to inflammation within the urinary tract such as UTIs, bladder cancer, or stones that will cause irritative voiding symptoms.

Stress urinary incontinence (SUI) is defined as the involuntary loss of urine with physical activity or exertion. History is the primary means of diagnosis. The typical patient will admit to loss of urine with laughing, coughing, sneezing, or lifting heavy objects. SUI in the male is often seen after radical prostatectomy for prostate cancer due to damage or weakness of the external urinary sphincter and absence of the internal sphincter. Patients with certain levels of spinal cord injury may also develop SUI. For example, sacral spinal cord disease can lead to an atonic external urinary sphincter, resulting in SUI.

Conservative and surgical options vary depending on the severity of SUI. Conservative measures include penile clamps. Surgical treatment includes urethral bulking agents, artificial urinary sphincters, and suburethral slings (Maleb, 2016).

Urethral bulking agents such as Durasphere, Deflux, and Macroplastique are used in patients with a mild degree of SUI only. This treatment has not been shown to be as effective in patients with moderate to severe SUI.

Artificial urinary sphincters are typically a three-piece implantable device that includes a cuff that fits around the urethra, a pump that will fit into the scrotum that the patient can use for deactivation of the sphincter, and a reservoir that is placed ectopically through the inguinal canal. This option is the gold standard for treatment of SUI in male patients. The cuff, which is the artificial sphincter component, is constantly in an activated state to coapt the urethra and prevent incontinence. When the patient desires to void, he will squeeze the pump within the scrotum to deflate the sphincter. The sphincter will reinflate after several minutes. Implantable devices are always at risk for becoming infected; therefore, a patient with recurrent UTIs will be ineligible. The healthcare provider should assess patients for sufficient manual dexterity and cognitive function when considering implantation. Two types of slings exist for the treatment of male SUI. *Transobturator slings, AdVance*, can be offered to men with mild to moderate symptoms. A recent study, TOMS, showed a 50% improvement in symptoms measured in the number of pads used per day (Yiou et al., 2016). The second available sling is *Virtue*, a quadratic sling, which traverses the obturator foramen and has prepubic arms. Although the details of such slings are beyond the scope of this chapter, it is important to know that various treatment options do exist and that appropriate referral to a urologist is necessary for further therapy.

Mixed urinary incontinence (MUI) encompasses patients who have symptoms of stress incontinence and urgency incontinence. This is seen in men who have had a prostatectomy and should be managed on an individual basis on bother symptoms (Hashim & Abrams, 2016). Although it is rare, spinal cord injury patients may have MUI. Management strategies include a combination of anticholinergic and alpha blocker medication plus a catheterization regimen. Many of these patients need referral to a urologist for management and urodynamic studies.

Overflow incontinence occurs with urinary retention. As the bladder becomes overdistended, urine will "overflow" the bladder and leak through the urethra. Causes of urinary retention can be due to an obstructive process from urethral strictures or an enlarged prostate. Other times, neurogenic causes (acute strokes, spinal cord injuries, abdominal perineal resection, Parkinson's disease, multiple sclerosis, etc.) lead to an atonic or flaccid bladder causing urinary retention. Treatment of the underlying condition and managing the urinary retention will treat the incontinence. These patients should be referred to a urologist for further management.

Nocturnal enuresis is usually seen in children, but 2% to 3% of patients can experience it into their adult years and some may even have adult onset (Vande Walle et al., 2012). This is different from nocturia as nocturnal enuresis is urinary incontinence during sleep. These patients may have upper urinary tract damage which can be seen as hydronephrosis and/or impaired renal function. This is due to dysfunctional, high-pressure voiding or even longstanding urinary retention. Nocturnal enuresis onset as an adult can be due to multiple factors including sedative medication usage, underlying neurogenic bladder, baseline OAB, obstructive sleep apnea, or voiding dysfunction (Hashim & Abrams, 2016; van Kerrebroeck et al., 2002; Vande Walle et al., 2012). A distinction should be made between nocturnal enuresis and nocturnal polyuria.

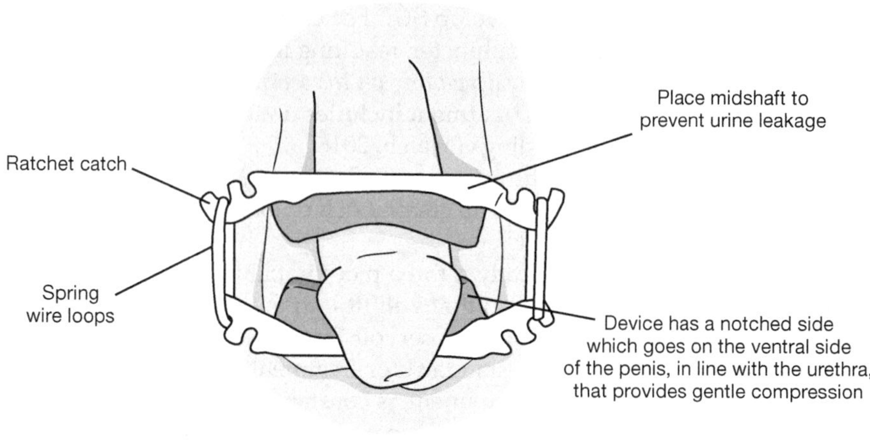

FIGURE 32.3 Cunningham penile clamp, AUS diagram.

Nocturnal polyuria occurs when one voids more than 30% of his total voided volume during sleeping hours. This is seen in patients with other comorbid conditions such as obstructive sleep apnea or congestive heart failure. These patients are often very bothered by their symptoms. Elimination of offending agents and/or treatment of the underlying medical condition is the treatment modality of choice (Lee, Dillon, & Lemack, 2017).

Continuous incontinence is defined and the constant loss of urine without voluntary control. Continuous incontinence is suggests the presence of a fistula (Toozs-Hobson et al., 2012). Although it is rare, urethrocutaneous or rectovesical fistulas should be on the clinician's radar if the patient has a history of cancer, radiation, prior surgery, or inflammatory bowel disease. If a fistula is suspected the patient should be referred to a urologist and/or general surgeon. Many patients may describe severe urgency and have a history of recurrent UTIs.

Insensible incontinence occurs when the patient tells you he cannot tell when he is experiencing incontinence. This could be due to neurological conditions (stroke, spinal cord injury, altered mental status) causing impaired sensation or functional incontinence, overflow from urinary retention, or a fistula causing continuous incontinence (Toozs-Hobson et al., 2012). Nonambulatory patients may require assistance to the toilet, absorbent pads, and/or timed voiding reminders during the day to promote dryness.

Many patients may mistake incontinence for postvoid dribbling. Postvoid dribble is defined as a small amount of urine remaining in the urethra after avoid. The urine will dribble out after a void and can be seen in patients with BPH or previous urethral surgery. It is important to quantify the amount of urine leakage they are experiencing (Abrams et al., 2002) The patient should be reminded that this may be a normal phenomenon and the urine can be eliminated by milking the urethra after voiding.

Constipation

The gastrointestinal and the genitourinary system are closely related and dysfunction with one system may lead to dysfunction in the other. Bowel and bladder dysfunction is seen in young children as a symptom complex of voiding dysfunction and most commonly constipation. As patients become older this once again becomes a functional problem. It is not uncommon to see patients with constipation who have difficulty with voiding. When the rectum is overstretched with stool, it may compress the bladder and affect common nerves and pelvic floor muscles, leading to incomplete bladder emptying, overactivity, UTIs, and even incontinence. Urinary incontinence and constipation are both problems encountered with the aging population; therefore, constipation should be addressed during workup and treated aggressively (Fusgen & Wiedemann, 2016).

CONCLUSION

History and physical examination form the cornerstone in the diagnosis of the OAB and incontinence. Common conditions that share the differential diagnosis of OAB, such as UTI and urinary retention, must be ruled out before arriving at the diagnosis of OAB. Indeed, OAB is a diagnosis of exclusion. Urinalysis is mandatory. Urine culture and PVR urine should be assessed as indicated. It is important to recognize that OAB is not a disease. It is a complex of symptoms that can be managed but not necessarily cured. Proper patient education is paramount. Expectations should be managed and goals should be set early. Only then should treatment be initiated, progressing in a step-wise fashion beginning with first-line therapy. Nonurologists can certainly provide treatment up to the second-line; however, patients who require further treatment should be referred to a specialist. One should always remember that indwelling catheters are not recommended in the treatment of OAB owing to an unacceptably low benefit-to-risk ratio.

CLINICAL PEARLS

- Urge urinary incontinence will be the more commonly encountered type of incontinence in outpatient clinics.
- OAB can be socially isolating, preventing men from engaging in activities for fear of inability to find a bathroom.
- A bladder diary is an important adjunct to the diagnosis of OAB.
- If treatment of BPH symptoms in men is not successful (especially frequency/urgency), consider trial of a medication for OAB.
- Men should be educated about normal lower urinary tract function, risks and benefits of treatment, and that satisfactory symptom control may require trials of multiple medication.
- Treatments must be given adequate time to determine success; combination therapy should be considered only after a reasonable trial of single therapy is unsatisfactory.

RESOURCES

Questionnaires are a useful tool in assessing the bother scores and degree of incontinence. Several questionnaires are available. Listed are just a few that you can use in your practice as a screening tool. All of these questionnaires are available with a simple online search.

1. American Urological Association Symptom Score (AUASS): www.asui.org/client_files/file/AUA-Symptom-Score.pdf
2. International Consultation on Incontinence Modular Questionnaire (ICIQ): www.iciq.net/ICIQ-UIshortform.html
3. International Prostate Symptom Score (IPSS): www.urospec.com/uro/Forms/ipss.pdf

CLINICIAN AND PATIENT EDUCATION

A comprehensive review of the diagnosis and management of overactive bladder guidelines can be found online. Diagnosis and Treatment of Non-Neurogenic Overactive Bladder (OAB) in Adults: AUA/SUFU Guideline: www.auanet.org/guidelines/overactive-bladder-(oab)-(aua/sufu-guideline-2012-amended-2014)

The National Institute on Aging also offers easy to read information on urinary incontinence in aging patients. Information can be found at: www.nia.nih.gov/health/urinary-incontinence-older-adults

Urology Care Foundation through the AUA has several educational resources for patients and healthcare providers on several men's health topics including OAB and incontinence. These references are in a easy-to-read, downloadable format: www.urologyhealth.org

REFERENCES

Abrams, P., Cardozo, L., Fall, M., Griffiths, D., Rosier, P., Ulmsten, U., … Wein, A. (2002). The standardisation of terminology of lower urinary tract function: Report from the Standardisation Sub-committee of the International Continence Society. *Neurourology and Urodynamics, 21*(2), 167–178. doi:10.1002/nau.10052

Buckley, B. S., & Lapitan, M. C.; Epidemiology Committee of the Fourth International Consultation on Incontinence. (2010). Prevalence of urinary incontinence in men, women, and children—Current evidence: Findings of the Fourth International Consultation on Incontinence. *Urology, 76*(2), 265–270. doi:10.1016/j.urology.2009.11.078

Carter, H. B., Albertsen, P. C., Barry, M. J., Etzioni, R., Freedland, S. J., Greene, K. L., … Zietman, A. L. (2013). Early detection of prostate cancer: AUA guideline. *The Journal of Urology, 190*(2), 419–426. doi:10.1016/j.juro.2013.04.119

Chai, T. (2016). Physiology and pharmacology of the bladder and urethra. In A. Wein, L. R. Kavoussi, A. W. Partin, & C. A. Peters (Eds.), *Campbell-Walsh urology* (11th ed., Vol. 3, pp. 1631–1684). Philadelphia, PA: Elsevier.

Chung, A., Noguchi, N., Chan, L., & Tse, V. (2016). Voiding dysfunction in older men. *Current Opinion in Urology, 26*(2), 177–183. doi:10.1097/MOU.0000000000000265

Clemens, Q. (2016). Urinary incontinence in men. *Up To Date, Topic 14611 V 35.0*. Retrieved from https://www.uptodate.com/contents/urinary-incontinence-in-men

Dmochowski, R. R., & Gomelsky, A. (2009). Overactive bladder in males. *Therapeutic Advances in Urology, 1*(4), 209–221. doi:10.1177/1756287209350383

Drake, M. J. (2007). The integrative physiology of the bladder. *The Annals of the Royal College of Surgeons of England, 89*(6), 580–585. doi:10.1308/003588407X205585

Drake, M. J. (2016). Overactive bladder. In A. Wein, L. R. Kavoussi, A. W. Partin, & C. A. Peters (Eds.), *Campbell-Walsh urology* (11th ed., Vol. 3, pp. 1796–1806). Philadelphia, PA: Elsevier.

Drake, M. J., Mills, I. W., & Gillespie, J. I. (2001). Model of peripheral autonomous modules and a myovesical plexus in normal and overactive bladder function. *The Lancet, 358*(9279), 401–403. doi:10.1016/S0140-6736(01)05549-0

Fusgen, I., & Wiedemann, A. (2016). Chronic constipation: A geriatric syndrome with urological implications. *Aktuelle Urologie, 47*(1), 51–53. doi:10.1055/s-0041-106175

Gerber, G., & Brendler, C. (2016). Evaluation of the urologic patient: History, physical examination, and urinalysis. In A. Wein, L. R. Kavoussi, A. W. Partin, & C. A. Peters (Eds.), *Campbell-Walsh urology* (11th ed., Vol. 1, pp. 1–25). Philadelphia, PA: Elsevier.

Gorina, Y., Schappert, S., Bercovitz, A., Elgaddal, N., & Kramarow, E. (2014). Prevalence of incontinence among older americans. *Vital and Health Statistics, 3*(36), 1–33.

Gormley, A., Lightner, D., Burgio, K., Chai, T., Clemens, Q., Culkin, D., … Vasavada, S. (2014). Diagnosis and Treatment of Overactive Bladder (Non-Neurogenic) in Adults: AUA/SUFU Guideline. American Urological Association. Retrieved from http://university.auanet.org/common/pdf/education/clinical-guidance/Overactive-Bladder.pdf

Hashim, H., & Abrams, P. (2016). Evaluation and management of men with urinary incontinence. In A. Wein, L. R. Kavoussi, A. W. Partin, & C. A. Peters (Eds.), *Campbell-Walsh urology* (11th ed., Vol. 3, pp. 1701–1717). Philadelphia, PA: Elsevier.

Juszczak, K., Ziomber, A., Wyczolkowski, M., & Thor, P. J. (2009). Urodynamic effects of the bladder C-fiber afferent activity modulation in chronic model of overactive bladder in rats. *Journal of Physiology and Pharmacology, 60*(4), 85–91.

Kavoussi, P. (2016). Surgical, radiographic, and endoscopic anatomy of the male reproductive system. In A. Wein, L. R. Kavoussi, A. W. Partin, & C. A. Peters (Eds.), *Campbell-Walsh urology* (11th ed., Vol. 1, pp. 498–515). Philadelphia, PA: Elsevier.

Lee, D., Dillon, B. E., & Lemack, G. E. (2017). Adult onset nocturnal enuresis: Identifying causes, cofactors and impact on quality of life. *Lower Urinary Tract Symptoms*. doi:10.1111/luts.12183

Lee, J. Y., Kim, H. W., Lee, S. J., Koh, J. S., Suh, H. J., & Chancellor, M. B. (2004). Comparison of doxazosin with or without tolterodine in men with symptomatic bladder outlet obstruction and an overactive bladder. *BJU International, 94*(6), 817–820. doi:10.1111/j.1464-410X.2004.05039.x

Liu, S., Chan, L., & Tse, V. (2014). Clinical outcome in male patients with detrusor overactivity with impaired contractility. *International Neurourology Journal, 18*(3), 133–137. doi:10.5213/inj.2014.18.3.133

Malaeb, B. (2016). Surgery for male SUI. Retrieved from https://university.auanet.org/core_topic.cfm?coreid=137

Mangera, A., & Chapple, C. R. (2014). Application of guidelines to the evaluation of the male patient with urgency and/or incontinence. *Current Opinion in Urology, 24*(6), 547–552. doi:10.1097/MOU.0000000000000110

Palleschi, G., Pastore, A. L., Maggioni, C., Fuschi, A., Pacini, L., Petrozza, V., & Carbone, A. (2014). Overactive bladder in diabetes mellitus patients: A questionnaire-based observational investigation. *World Journal of Urology, 32*(4), 1021–1025. doi:10.1007/s00345-013-1175-3

Rahnama'i, M. S., Marcelissen, T. A., Brierley, B., Schurch, B., & de Vries, P. (2017). Long-term compliance and results of intravesical botulinum toxin A injections in male patients. *Neurourology and Urodynamics, 36*(7), 1855–1859. doi:10.1002/nau.23196

Shamliyan, T. A., Wyman, J. F., Ping, R., Wilt, T. J., & Kane, R. L. (2009). Male urinary incontinence: Prevalence, risk factors, and preventive interventions. *Reviews in Urology, 11*(3), 145–165.

Solmaz, V., Albayrak, S., Tekatas, A., Aksoy, D., Gencten, Y., Inanir, S., & Erdemir, F. (2017). Evaluation of overactive bladder in male antidepressant users: A prospective study. *International Neurourology Journal, 21*(1), 62–67. doi:10.5213/inj.1732652.326

Stothers, L., Thom, D., & Calhoun, E. (2005). Urologic diseases in America project: Urinary incontinence in males—Demographics and economic burden. *The Journal of Urology, 173*(4), 1302–1308. doi:10.1097/01.ju.0000155503.12545.4e

Toozs-Hobson, P., Freeman, R., Barber, M., Maher, C., Haylen, B., Athanasiou, S., ... Swift, S. (2012). An International Urogynecological Association (IUGA)/International Continence Society (ICS) joint report on the terminology for reporting outcomes of surgical procedures for pelvic organ prolapse. *Neurourology and Urodynamics, 31*(4), 415–421. doi:10.1002/nau.22238

Tubaro, A., Batista, J. E., Nitti, V. W., Herschorn, S., Chapple, C. R., Blauwet, M. B., ... Oelke, M. (2017). Efficacy and safety of daily mirabegron 50 mg in male patients with overactive bladder: A critical analysis of five phase III studies. *Therapeutic Advances in Urology, 9*(6), 137–154. doi:10.1177/1756287217702797

van Kerrebroeck, P., Abrams, P., Chaikin, D., Donovan, J., Fonda, D., Jackson, S., ... Weiss, J. (2002). The standardisation of terminology in nocturia: Report from the Standardisation Sub-committee of the International Continence Society. *Neurourology and Urodynamics, 21*(2), 179–183. doi:10.1002/nau.10053

Vande Walle, J., Rittig, S., Bauer, S., Eggert, P., Marschall-Kehrel, D., & Tekgul, S.; American Academy of Pediatrics; European Society for Paediatric Urology; European Society for Paediatric Nephrology; International Children's Continence Society. (2012). Practical consensus guidelines for the management of enuresis. *European Journal of Pediatrics, 171*(6), 971–983. doi:10.1007/s00431-012-1687-7

Vasavada, S., & Rackley, R. R. (2016). Electrical Stimulation and Neuromodulation in Storage and Emptying. In A. Wein, L. R. Kavoussi, A. W. Partin, & C. A. Peters (Eds.), *Campbell-Walsh urology* (11th ed., Vol. 3, pp. 1899–1917). Philadelphia, PA: Elsevier.

Wein, A. (2016). Pathophysiology and Classification of Lower Urinary Tract Dysfunction: Overview. In A. Wein, L. R. Kavoussi, A. W. Partin, & C. A. Peters (Eds.), *Campbell-Walsh Urology* (11th ed., Vol. 3, pp. 1685–1696). Philadelphia, PA: Elsevier.

Wieder, J. (2014). *Pocket Guide to Urology* (5th ed.). Oakland, CA: J. Wieder Medical.

Wu, N., Marshall, T. S., Boulanger, L., Bui, C. N., Lamothe, K., Janning, S., & Haas, G. P. (2014). Antimuscarinic use among individuals with urinary incontinence who reside in long-term care facilities. *International Urology and Nephrology, 46*(1), 285–296. doi:10.1007/s11255-013-0507-y

Yehoshua, A., Chancellor, M., Vasavada, S., Malone, D. C., Armstrong, E. P., Joshi, M., … Pulicharam, R. (2016). Health resource utilization and cost for patients with incontinent overactive bladder treated with anticholinergics. *Journal of Managed Care and Specialty Pharmacy, 22*(4), 406–413. doi:10.18553/jmcp.2016.22.4.406

Yiou, R., Butow, Z., Parisot, J., Lingombet, O., Augustin, D., de la Taille, A., … Audureau, E. (2016). Update on 2-year outcomes of the TOMS transobturator male sling for the treatment of male stress urinary incontinence. *Neurourology and Urodynamics, 35*(1), 44–47. doi:10.1002/nau.22668

CHAPTER 33

Cardiovascular Prevention: Hypertension and Dyslipidemia

Joanne Thanavaro

HYPERTENSION: INTRODUCTION AND INCIDENCE

Hypertension is a significant modifiable risk factor for cardiovascular disease, stroke, renal disease, and death. Despite many years of public health education, awareness and control of hypertension remain a significant healthcare problem. About 75 million American adults (32%) have high blood pressure and one in three adults have prehypertension; prevalence is highest in older populations, and almost 20% of young adults are hypertensive (Go et al., 2013). High blood pressure was the primary or contributing cause of death for more than 410,000 Americans in 2014, and costs the nation $48.6 billion each year including cost for healthcare services, medications, and missed days of work (Centers for Disease Control and Prevention [CDC], 2011; Everett & Zajacova, 2015; Kochanek, Xu, Murphy, Minino, & Kung, 2011).

Men younger than age 45 have higher levels of hypertension compared to women of the same age group; this difference is most pronounced in early adulthood. From ages 45 to 64, the percentage of men and women with hypertension is similar; after 64 years of age a much higher percentage of women than men have high blood pressure (Go et al., 2013). Observed gender differences are due to biological factors (sex hormones, chromosomal differences, and biological sex differences that are protective against hypertension in women) as well as behavioral risk factors including high body mass index, smoking, and low physical activity (Everett & Zajacova, 2015; Go et al., 2013).

As with many chronic diseases, disparities exist between gender, race, and ethnicity. Among adult men 20 years and older in the United States, the following have high blood pressure:

- Among non-Hispanic whites: 33.4% of men and 30.7% of women
- Among non-Hispanic blacks: 42.6% of men and 47% of women
- Among Mexican Americans: 30.1% of men and 28.8% of women (Eckel et al., 2013)

By 2030, it is projected that the prevalence of hypertension will increase 7.2% from 2013 estimates (Go et al., 2013). For adults over 45 without hypertension at present, there is a 40-year risk for developing hypertension of 93% for African-Americans, 92% for people of Hispanic descent, 86% risk for Caucasians, and an 84% chance of developing hypertension for Chinese adults (Whelton et al., 2017).

PATHOPHYSIOLOGY

The pathogenesis of hypertension is complex and involves the interaction of multiple organ systems; hypertension is a polygenic disorder with multiple contributing causes. Arterial blood pressure is a product of cardiac output and peripheral vascular resistance. Cardiac output is the product of stroke volume and heart rate; stroke volume is influenced by sodium intake, renal function, and mineralocorticoids. The inotropic effects occur by increases in heart rate and contractility as well as extracellular fluid volume augmentation. Peripheral vascular resistance is dependent on the sympathetic nervous system, humoral factors, and local autoregulation.

Hypertension contributes to cerebrovascular, ocular, cardiovascular, renal, and metabolic diseases. Chronic hypertension increases arterial stiffness and widens pulse pressures, resulting in decreased coronary perfusion and an increase in myocardial oxygen consumption. Additionally, longstanding hypertension results in cardiac structural changes including left atrial enlargement, aortic root dilatation, and development of left ventricular hypertrophy (LVH). Long term, the presence of LVH impairs diastolic function, resulting in arrhythmias, heart failure, and ischemic heart disease. As a result, LVH is associated with an increased risk of premature death and morbidity.

Cerebrovascular changes related to hypertension alter cerebral blood flow and result in alterations in intracranial pressure and frequently cerebral edema. Patients with chronic hypertension tolerate higher mean arterial pressures initially, but ultimately have disruption of their autoregulatory system and an increase in cerebrovascular resistance and are more prone to cerebral ischemia when flow decreases.

Renovascular hypertension is the clinical consequence of renin-angiotension-aldosterone system (RAAS) activation. Renal artery occlusion creates ischemia and the release of renin and secondary elevation in blood pressure (BP). Hyperreninemia promotes the conversion of angiotension I to angiotension II causing severe vasoconstriction and aldosterone release. The reduction in renal blood flow, accompanied by increased afferent glomerular resistance, further impairs renal function. Despite widespread treatment of hypertension, the incidence of end-stage renal disease continues to rise.

The pathophysiological effects of hypertensive ocular changes include acute changes related to malignant hypertension and chronic changes from long-term hypertension. Malignant hypertension may lead to acute retinal lesions including focal intraretinal periarteriolar transudates, inner retinal ischemic spots, microaneurysms, and collateral and shunt vessels. Chronic retinal changes include arteriosclerosis (narrowing of vessels), retinal hemorrhages, increased vascular tortuosity, and remodeling changes due to capillary nonperfusion.

Hypertension is one of many widely recognized metabolic risk factors along with dyslipidemia and hyperglycemia. The combination of these risk factors results in prothrombotic and proinflammatory changes that elevates the risk for atherosclerotic cardiovascular disease (Hamrahian & Batuman, 2017).

Risk Factors for Hypertension

According to the American College of Cardiology/American Heart Association (ACC/AHA) Task Force on Clinical Practice Guidelines, healthcare providers should access for all risk factors associated with cardiovascular disease (CVD) (Whelton et al., 2017). Risk factors are divided into modifiable and nonmodifiable risk factors; the goal being to promote lifestyle strategies to reduce those risk factors that are modifiable. Modifiable risk factors include obesity, dyslipidemia, diabetes mellitus, cigarette smoking, and physical inactivity. Healthy lifestyle is widely recommended for all individuals. Recommendations for lifestyle modification to manage hypertension is summarized in Table 33.1. For overall cardiovascular risk reduction smoking cessation and good control of diabetes are recommended. Nonmodifiable risk factors for CVD include age (older than 55 for men) and a family history of premature CVD (men under age 55).

■ HISTORY

Hypertension is likely to be due to several synergistic factors that must be evaluated during the initial patient assessment. These factors include age, obesity, family history,

TABLE 33.1 Lifestyle Modifications to Manage Hypertension

Lifestyle Modification	Recommendation	Approximate SBP Reduction
Weight reduction	Maintain normal body weight (body mass index 18.5–24.9 kg/m^2	5–20 mmHg/10 kg of weight loss
DASH (dietary approaches to stop hypertension) eating plan	Consume a diet rich in fruits, vegetables, and low-fat dairy products with a reduced content of saturated total fat	8–14 mmHg
Dietary sodium reduction	Reduce dietary sodium intake to no more than 100 mmol per day (2–4 g of sodium or 6 g of sodium chloride)	2–8 mmHg
Physical activity	Engage in regular aerobic physical activity at least 30 min daily on most days of the week	4–9 mmHg
Moderation of alcohol	Limit consumption to no more than two drinks per day (1 ounce or 30 mL ethanol; 24 ounces of beer, 10 ounces of wine or 3 ounces of 80-proof whiskey) in most men. Women and lower weight persons should limit alcohol to one drink daily.	2–4 mmHg

SBP, systolic blood pressure.

race, reduced number of nephrons in the kidney, high-sodium diet, excessive alcohol consumption, and physical inactivity. Men should be asked about their history of obstructive sleep apnea, endocrine issues such as pheochromocytoma or aldosteronism, Cushing's syndrome, thyroid conditions, chronic kidney disease, and coarctation of the aorta (although this is less common in adults). The initial history should also include assessment for the presence or absence of target organ damage including damage to the heart, brain, or kidneys; peripheral artery disease; and retinopathy. The evaluation of men with documented hypertension should include an exploration of lifestyle behaviors and concomitant disorders that may affect prognosis and guide the treatment of elevated BP. This includes investigation of modifiable risk factors (see Table 33.1) and unmodifiable risk factors, including age and family history.

Other pieces of the history that are important in the assessment of hypertension in men are use of nonsteroidal anti-inflammatory agents (particularly chronic use), use of corticosteroids, use of antidepressants, use of decongestants, and use of weight loss medication or sodium-containing antacids. Other medication use to consider includes erythropoietin, cyclosporine or tacrolimus, methylphenidate or amphetamines, atypical antipsychotics, (e.g., clozapine, olanzapine), angiogenesis inhibitors, and tyrosine kinase inhibitors.

The review of systems should focus on symptoms including chest pain, palpitations, shortness of breath (SOB), dyspnea on exertion (DOE), fatigue, orthopnea, and paroxysmal nocturnal dyspnea (National Heart, Lung and Blood Institute, 2004). Men may also present as "otherwise healthy" with little previous contact with the healthcare system but have developed issues with their erectile or sexual function; many men may have no symptoms of coronary artery disease until their first cardiac event. Additionally it is possible to have an event even after normal diagnostic evaluation.

Overall cardiovascular risk can be calculated by utilizing the atherosclerotic cardiovascular disease (ASCVD) risk factor calculator to determine the 10-year risk of developing heart disease. This score is helpful in motivating patients to undertake healthy lifestyle choices and guides therapy for dyslipidemia, an important risk factor for hypertension (American College of Cardiology, 2017).

PHYSICAL EXAMINATION

All adult men with normal BP should nevertheless have a reassessment of their BP every year; if risk factors for hypertension are present, their BP should be evaluated every 6 months. The physical examination should include vital signs and the ausculatory method of BP measurement with a properly calibrated and validated instrument should be used. Patients should be seated for at least 5 minutes in a chair (not on an exam table) with their feet on their floor and the arm supported at heart level. An appropriate-size cuff (cuff bladder should encircle at least 80% of the arm) should be used and at least two measurements should be taken. Ideally there should be an average of at least two readings on two separate occasions to indicate the individual's true BP. Clinicians should provide patients their BP numbers and goals both verbally and in writing. Recommended goals for BP according to ACC/AHA Task Force (American College of Cardiology, 2017) guidelines state (Whelton et al., 2017):

- Normal BP is less than 120/80 mmHg
- Elevated BP is 120 to 129/<80 mmHg
- Stage I hypertension is 130 to 139/80 to 89 mmHg
- Stage II hypertension is ≥140/≥90 mmHg

The physical examination for the male with hypertension should also include (Alexander, 2018):

- Examination of optic fundus
  - Flame hemorrhages due to extreme elevation of BP
  - Preretinal hemorrhages characterized by a rounded inferior margin
  - Microaneurysms due to dilation of retinal arteries
  - Cotton-wool exudates or areas of "fluffy" ischemia associated with hypertensive retinopathy
  - Hard exudates: yellow to white lesions in a discrete circular pattern associated with hypertensive retinopathy
- Palpation of the thyroid gland
  - Nodules that may indicate malignancy
  - Enlargement that may indicate hypothyroidism
- Auscultation for carotid, abdominal, and femoral bruits
- Thorough examination of the heart and lungs
  - Evidence of fluid collection in the lungs
  - Evidence of regurgitation or murmurs
- Examination of the abdomen for enlarged kidneys, masses, and abdominal aortic pulsations
- Palpation of the lower extremities for edema and pulses
- Neurological assessment for potential sequelae related to perfusion or ischemic issues
- Calculation of body mass index

DIAGNOSTIC TESTS

Routine laboratory tests that are recommended before initiating antihypertensive therapy include (Whelton et al., 2017):

- Liver function tests (LFTs) including alanine transaminase (ALT) and aspartate aminotransferase (AST)
- Electrolytes
- Urinalysis

- Thyroid-stimulating hormone (TSH)
- Fasting blood sugar (FBS)
- Blood urea nitrogen/creatinine (BUN/Cr)
- Electrocardiogram (ECG)
- Carotid duplex (only if there is evidence of carotid artery disease) if a carotid bruit is found

This initial evaluation should also include calculation of the 10-year ASCVD event risk for the individual.

MEDICAL MANAGEMENT

According to ACC/AHA 2017 Guidelines (Whelton et al., 2017) all adults aged ≥18 years of age with hypertension should implement lifestyle modifications. BP goals should be set in accordance with guidelines, and initiation of BP-lowering medications should be instituted if BP goals cannot be attained with lifestyle changes. The 2017 guidelines from ACC/AHA 2017 (Whelton et al., 2017) recommend a BP goal of 130/80 mmHg for adults with hypertension and known CVD or a 10-year ASCVD event risk of 10% or higher. These guidelines also suggest that in adults with hypertension and no additional risk factors a goal of 130/80 mmHg remains reasonable as well.

Three strategies for initiation of antihypertensive medications have been suggested: (a) start with one drug, titrate to maximum dose, and then add a second drug, (b) start one drug, then add a second drug before achieving maximum dose first, or (c) begin with two drugs at the same time, either as separate or combination pills. Initial combination therapy is recommended if the BP is greater than 20/10 mmHg above goal.

Home BP measurement is recommended as a method to create a more complete picture of an individual's BP and offer a better prediction of cardiovascular morbidity and mortality risks than office measurements. However, the existing literature is inconclusive regarding the accuracy of BP measurements taken at home; one of the key recommendations is that the BP device used by the patient has been validated with an internationally accepted protocol (O'Brien & Stergiou, 2017). Home BP guidelines have been endorsed by the American Heart Association and the American Society of Hypertension. These recommendations should be shared with men as they begin and continue management of hypertension:

- Use a validated device.
- Take a measurement before your office visit.
- Take 2 morning and 2 evening readings every day for 1 week.
- Discard reading from day 1.
- Come to an office visit with a total of 12 BP readings over 1 week to help your provider make a sound clinical decision regarding your BP and possible need for medication (Pickering et al., 2008).

Compelling Indications for Hypertension Management

Providers should be aware of which medications are particularly useful for preexisting CVD and choose these agents as appropriate (Whelton et al., 2017). For example:

1. Heart failure: angiotensin-converting enzyme inhibitor (ACEI)/angiotensin receptor blocker (ARB) + beta blocker (BB) + diuretic + spironolactone
2. Following myocardial infarction (MI) or clinical coronary artery disease (CAD): ACEI/ARB and BB
3. CAD: ACEI, BB, diuretic, calcium channel blocker (CCB)

4. Diabetes: ACEI/ARB, CCB, diuretic
5. Chronic kidney disease: ACEI/ARB
6. Recurrent stroke prevention: ACEI, diuretic

There is no preferential drug efficacy according to race: when treating African Americans, select a thiazide or CCB alone or in combination. When treating Non–African Americans, consider thiazides, ACEI, ARB, or CCB, alone or in combination to a target BP of <130/80 mmHg.

For the management of hypertension, a "rule of 10" and a "rule of 5" have been helpful in predicting the drug effects of lowering BP. With a standard dose of any one of the five major classes of antihypertensive agents, one can anticipate approximately a 10-mmHg decrease in systolic BP and a 5-mmHg decrease in diastolic BP. When doses of the same drug are doubled, there is only a 2-mmHg incremental decrease in systolic BP and a 1-mmHg incremental decrease in diastolic BP. Preferably, when two drugs with different mechanisms are taken together, the decrease in BP is the sum of the decrease of the individual agents (approximately 20 mmHg in systolic BP and 10 mmHg in diastolic BP). Early combination therapy, especially single-pill combination (SPC), is recommended (Chiang et al., 2015).

It is important that clinicians are aware of the causes of resistant hypertension so that men are not prescribed unnecessary or inappropriate medications. Some causes of resistant hypertension include (Yaxley & Thambar, 2015):

- Incorrect technique in measuring BP
- Pseudohypertension
- Lack of adherence to lifestyle interventions
- High-sodium food and over-the-counter medications
- Suboptimal therapies
- Lack of patient adherence to antihypertensive medications
- Sleep apnea
- Paroxysmal hypertension
- Hypertension related to secondary causes

Initial Drugs of Choice for Hypertension

ACC/AHA guidelines recommend the following four agents for initial treatment of hypertension: ACEIs, ARBs, thiazide diuretics, and CCBs (Whelton et al., 2017).

BBs are no longer considered first-line treatment for hypertension because of lack of evidence in randomized controlled trials demonstrating decreases in mortality or morbidity risks with these drugs (Whelton et al., 2017). However, a BB may be indicated based on compelling indications. Should BBs be used, the following beta-1 selective medications are possibly safer in patients with chronic obstructive pulmonary disease (COPD), asthma, diabetes, and peripheral vascular disease: metoprolol, bisoprolol, betaxolol, and acebutolol.

A full discussion of the variations in recommended medical treatment for hypertension and recommendations for special groups (such as patients with valvular heart disease and preoperative management) is beyond the scope of this chapter, and the reader is referred to the published ACC/AHA 2017 guidelines for full details.

Nonpharmacological Management

Nonpharmacological management of contributing issues to hypertension is an important adjunct, and for men who have an elevated BP and minimal risk factors nonpharmacological management may be sufficient to reduce their BP reading. Nonpharmacological management is also an option at any point, and in combination with medications. For example, weight reduction has the potential to reduce BP by as much as 5 to 20 mmHg per 10 kg of weight loss. Weight loss should be a slow process with a goal of 1 to 2 lb weekly. The most effective approach involves both diet and physical activity.

Two dietary patterns are recommended according to the most recent AHA/ACC Guideline on Lifestyle Management including a DASH (dietary approaches to stop hypertension) pattern and a macronutrient pattern (Eckel et al., 2014). The DASH pattern is high in vegetables, fruits, low-fat dairy products, whole grains, poultry, and fish and low in sweets, sugar-sweetened beverages, and red meats. When all foods were supplied to adults with a BP range of 120-159/80-95 mmHg, and body weight was held stable, the DASH pattern of eating lowered BP in men and women, African Americans and whites, older and younger adults, and patients with and without hypertension. In addition to eating a DASH diet, patients should aim for restricting total sodium intake to no more than 2,400 mg daily.

There is no accepted uniform definition of the macronutrient pattern of eating. However, these diets are higher in fruits and vegetables (particularly fresh fruits and root and green varieties of vegetables); whole grains including cereals, breads, rice, and pasta; and fatty fish that are rich in omega-3 fatty acids and are lower in red meat. Recommendations also include substituting lower-fat or fat-free dairy products in lieu of higher-fat dairy foods and use of oils (olive or canola), nuts (walnuts, almonds, or hazelnuts), and margarines blended with rapeseed or flaxseed instead of butter and other fats. The macronutrient patterns tended to be moderate in total fat (32% to 35% of total calories), low in saturated fats (9%–10% of total calories), and high in fiber and polyunsaturated fats in the studies reviewed for this guideline. Counseling to eat a macronutrient pattern, compared to minimal advice to eat a low-fat diet, in free-living middle-age and older adults (with type 2 diabetes or at least three CVD risk factors) reduced BP by 6–7/2–3 mmHg.

One approach to patients who are motivated by tracking their progress is to suggest the free app, *MyFitnessPal*, which allows the patient to chart calories, carbohydrates, fats, proteins, and other nutrient details and is helpful for assessing both dietary patterns recommended for BP reduction.

Higher levels of physical activity contribute to lower rates of chronic disease, including CVD. Mechanisms offered to explain the relationship between physical activity and CVD rates include beneficial effects on both BP and lipid levels. Aerobic and resistance exercise training, and a combination of both, have demonstrated beneficial effects on BP if the exercise was continued for at least 12 weeks, including 3 to 4 sessions a week with a session lasting 40 minutes and involving moderate-to-vigorous intensity.

Men of all ages should be encouraged to choose an exercise program that they find appealing and that fits into their overall work and family responsibilities. Scheduling exercise times on personal calendars helps to keep the commitment to physical activity. Setting reasonable goals for activity is paramount and starting a program one to two times weekly, with the intent to gradually increase exercise, is a good way to start (Eckel et al., 2014).

Smoking Cessation

Providers can follow the 5As and 5Rs for assessing and implementing strategies for smoking cessation. The 5As approach is a goal-directed way to help assess for readiness to make a quit attempt (Larzelere & Williams, 2012):

- Ask about tobacco use at every visit.
- Assess the patient's current readiness to quit tobacco.
- Advise the tobacco user to quit smoking.
- Assist with smoking cessation readiness by listening, discussing barriers to cessation and providing information on support groups. Offer medications as needed.

- Arrange for follow-up contact. This can be accomplished via telephone or additional office visits. Follow-up is particularly helpful when patients are in the first few weeks of smoking cessation.

Motivational interviewing is helpful for patients who are not ready to make a quit attempt, following the 5Rs approach:

- Relevance: encourage the patient to indicate why quitting is personally relevant.
- Risks: help the patient identify potential negative effects of continued smoking.
- Rewards: ask the patient to explore potential consequences of smoking cessation. This may include financial savings, better health, or responding to requests to stop smoking from family members.
- Roadblocks: help the patient identify potential barriers to quitting. Discuss strategies to lessen barriers.
- Repetition: repeat the 5Rs with every follow-up visit.

DYSLIPIDEMIA: OVERVIEW AND INCIDENCE

Elevated blood cholesterol is a major risk factor for CVD. According to the Centers for Disease Control and Prevention nearly 31 million adults in the United States have a total serum cholesterol (TC) level above 240 mg/dL. The percentage of adults age 20 years and older with high TC levels was 12.1% between 2011 and 2014. Seventy-four million adults (31.7%) also have high low-density lipoprotein (LDL) values (CDC, 2017).

The National Cholesterol Treatment Guidelines outline the importance of using cholesterol-lowering medications for the prevention of coronary heart disease (CHD) (Third Report of the National Cholesterol Education Program, 2017). During 2003 to 2012, the percentage of adults aged 40 and over using a cholesterol-lowering medication in the past 30 days increased from 20% to 28%. Ninety-three percent of adults using a cholesterol-lower medication used a statin agent. Approximately 71% of adults with CVD and 54% of adults with hypocholesteremia used a cholesterol-lowering medication. Medication use increased with age including 17% of adults aged 40 to 59 and 48% of adults aged 75 or older (CDC, 2017). Despite these trends, less than half of patients with a high LDL value are getting treatment and fewer than 1 out of 3 adults with high LDLs are controlled. Adults with health insurance were more likely than those without health insurance to use a cholesterol-lowering medication.

High cholesterol levels vary by race and ethnicity. Although 31% of men and 32% of women have LDL levels greater than 130 mg/dL, Mexican American males have higher LDL levels compared to Mexican American females. LDL levels in females are higher than men in non-Hispanic black and white populations (CDC, 2017).

PATHOPHYSIOLOGY

Atherosclerosis results from chronic inflammation associated with interactions between modified lipoproteins, macrophages, immunity responses, and normal arterial cellular structures. Elevated cholesterol levels are central to the initiation and progression of vascular atherosclerosis evidenced by the clinical consequences of MI, stroke, peripheral vascular disease, and heart failure. Atherosclerotic clinical events are uncommon in people with lifelong low plasma cholesterol levels. The plasma lipids—cholesterols, triglycerides, phospholipids, and free fatty acids—are derived from exogenous dietary courses and endogenous lipid synthesis. Hyperlipidemia can be primary or secondary to another underlying condition, such as hypothyroidism or poorly controlled diabetes. Triglycerides and cholesterol are essential to cellular structure and metabolism. They are not water soluble and require apolipoproteins for lipid transport in the form of various lipoproteins. There are six classes of apolipoproteins (A to H) and several subclasses (designated by arabic numbers or roman numerals) that are important in lipid transport and interaction between lipoprotein and tissue receptors, enzymes, and coenzymes. Apolipoproteins A (apo A) and B (apo B) are two major components of lipid transport.

Lipoproteins comprise apolipoproteins, phospholipids, triglycerides, and cholesterol. The classification of lipoproteins depends on the relative contents of major apolipoproteins and lipid components. There are four major lipoprotein classes based on their density and sizes: ultralow density lipoprotein (ULDL—chylomicrons), very low density lipoprotein (VLDL), low-density lipoprotein (LDL), and high-density lipoprotein (HDL). The density and size of lipoproteins are inversely related; the less dense lipoproteins, the larger the size of the particles, and vice versa. There are also spectrums of particle sizes in each lipoprotein category. The number and size of LDLs as measured by nuclear magnetic resonance (NMR) are a better indicator of atherogenesis than the LDL cholesterol level; the small dense LDL particles appear to be more atherogenic.

The chylomicrons and VLDLs are richest in triglyceride, and LDLs and HDLs contain the largest proportion of cholesterol. Triglycerides during lipid absorption after a meal predominantly reside in chylomicrons, whereas fasting plasma triglycerides are found mostly in VLDLs. VLDLs are produced by the liver and are responsible for supplying free fatty acids to tissues: they are also the major carriers of circulating triglycerides. LDLs are by-products of VLDL metabolism and are primary carriers of plasma cholesterol. Chylomicrons, VLDLs, and LDLs all carry apo B and other apolipoproteins, and HDLs carry apo AI and apo AII. HDL particles are produced by the liver and intestine and as they mature become enriched with other apolipoproteins and lipids by exchanges with chylomicrons and VLDLs.

The clinical application of NMR measurement of LDL is limited by its lack of availability and expense. Distinguishing patterns of lipoprotein elevation facilitates medical management and coronary disease risk predictions. A total cholesterol elevation may reflect an increase in LDL or HDL, but only LDL elevation is associated with increased coronary disease risk; HDL elevations actually decreases risk of CVD. A pattern of increased elevation of VLDL, increased small LDL particles, and low HDL cholesterol is prominent in atherogenic dyslipidemia. These abnormalities usually occur together and have a common metabolic basis. The term atherogenic dyslipidemia is used because this pattern frequently occurs in patients with premature CHD and diabetes (Brunzell et al., 2008).

It is unclear whether lipoprotein parameters other than LDL or non-HDL cholesterol provide clinically significant additional prognostic information regarding CVD risk, yield additional information about the effectiveness of therapy, or indicate more appropriate treatment. The newest national guidelines for the treatment of dyslipidemia encourage all providers to determine risk of CAD as a guide to help determine and manage dyslipidemia (Jellinger et al., 2017).

Risk Factors for Dyslipidemia

Increased probability for dyslipidemia includes the presence of any one of the risk factors listed below. The greatest risk of CHD is conferred by a combination of multiple factors:

- Diabetes
- Personal history of CHD or noncoronary atherosclerosis (abdominal aortic aneurysm, peripheral artery disease, carotid artery stenosis)

- Family history of CVD before 50 years of age in male relatives or 60 years of age in female relatives
- Tobacco use
- Hypertension
- Obesity (body mass index of 30 kg/m^2 or greater)

HISTORY

The evaluation of patients with dyslipidemia should focus on risk factors. In addition to the risk factors above, the American Association of Clinical Endocrinologists includes the following as major risk factors for dyslipidemia and atherosclerosis (American Association of Clinical Endocrinologists and American College of Endocrinology, 2017):

- Elevated serum total cholesterol levels
- Elevated levels of non-HDL levels
- Elevated LDL levels

Hypertriglyceridemia is usually asymptomatic until triglycerides are greater than 1,000 to 2,000 mg/dL. Patients may report midepigastric pain due to acute pancreatitis. Severe hypertriglyceridemia may also cause skin lesions called xanthomas.

Clinicians should evaluate for possible secondary causes of elevated lipids. Secondary causes for elevated total cholesterol and LDL cholesterol (LDL-C) include hypothyroidism, nephrosis, dysgammaglobulinemia, systemic lupus erythematosus and multiple myeloma, progestin or anabolic steroid treatment, cholestatic diseases of the liver (as seen in primary biliary cirrhosis), and protease inhibitors used in the treatment of HIV infections (Vodnala, Rubenfire, & Brook, 2012). Elevations in triglycerides and VLDL may be secondary to chronic renal failure, diabetes mellitus type 2, obesity, excessive alcohol ingestion, hypothyroidism, antihypertension medications (especially thiazides and beta-adrenergic blockers), corticosteroid use, orally administered estrogens, oral contraceptives agents, pregnancy, and protease inhibitors in the treatment of HIV (Egan, Li, Qanungo, & Wolfman, 2013).

In this context, much like with hypertension, men may present as "otherwise healthy" and a history of little previous contact with the healthcare system but have developed issues with their erectile or sexual function that have driven them to seek evaluation.

PHYSICAL EXAMINATION

Hyperlipidemia may present with a myriad of clinical signs. Recognition of these signs enables the identification of the underlying lipid disorder and facilitates the most appropriate therapies to reduce the likelihood of potential sequelae. In addition to a complete cardiovascular examination, the provider should evaluate for dermatological and ophthalmological signs of high cholesterol levels. There are five types of xanthomas (Nezafati, 2017):

- Xanthoma striata palmaris: Orange-yellow discolorations of the palmar creases that may be raised and are considered pathognomonic for dysbetalipoproteinemia.
- Tuberoeruptive xanthomas: Nonpainful, raised, erythematous, nodular lesions approximately 0.5 cm in diameter that are usually found on the elbows and knees.
- Tuberous xanthomas: Larger, coalesced tuberoeruptive xanthomas that are raised, moderately firm nontender lesions found predominately on the elbows and knees.

- Tendon xanthomas: More common in familial hypercholesterolemia. They are usually slow growing and may present as a firm-to-hard subcutaneous nodule with normal overlying skin. Common sites include the Achilles tendons and extensor tendons of the digits. Small tendon xanthomas are usually asymptomatic but massive tendon xanthomas can develop in two rare disorders (cerebrotendinous xanthomatosis and beta-sitosterolemia) from accumulation of unusual sterols transported by LDL
- Eruptive xanthomas: Small nodular papules seen over the trunk, buttocks and thighs and associated with the cylomicronemia syndrome (CS). This syndrome affects patients with triglycerides levels usually greater than 2,000 mg/dL and includes recurrent episodes of abdominal pain that may be accompanied by nausea, vomiting, or dyspnea. Pancreatitis is not necessarily present with CS. If pancreatitis or CS is present, upper right or left quadrants of the abdomen may be tender to palpation, and hepatomegaly and splenomegaly may be appreciated.

Ophthalmological signs may include the presence of corneal arcus which is a grayish white opacification at the periphery of the cornea and/or xanthelasmas, which are pale yellow raised lesions around the eyelids (Miller, 2008).

DIAGNOSTIC TESTS

A lipid profile is required for the diagnosis of dyslipidemia, and should be obtained after a 9- to 12-hour fast. Recommended optimal goals in patients without ASCVD or diabetes mellitus (DM) include (Third Report of the National Cholesterol Education Program [NCEP] Expert Panel):

- Total cholesterol
  - Desirable <200 mg/dL
  - Borderline high 200 to 239 mg/dL
  - High ≥240 mg/dL
- LDL cholesterol
  - Optimal <100 mg/dL
  - Near optimal/above optimal 100–129 mg/dL
  - Borderline high 130–159 mg/dL
  - High 160–189 mg/dL
  - Very high ≥190 mg/dL
- HDL cholesterol
  - Low <40 mg/dL
  - High ≥60 mg/dL
- Triglycerides
  - Desirable ≤150 mg/dL

According to the ACC/AHA Guideline on the Treatment of Blood Cholesterol to Reduce Atherosclerotic Cardiovascular Risk in adults, dyslipidemia treatment should be recommended based on ASCVD risk reduction. The ASCVD risk algorithm is a standardized guideline to predict 10-year risk for a first ASCVD event and provides recommendations for statin drug use. ASCVD risk is calculated using the variables of gender, age, race, total cholesterol, HDL, systolic BP, receiving hypertension treatment, diabetes, and smoking history. These factors are entered into a pooled cohort equation that determines 10-year risk. The free app to calculate ASCVD risk is available for mobile devices in digital media stores and can be accessed at my.americanheart.org/cvriskcalculator (American College of Cardiology, 2017).

The ASCVD risk estimator is intended for use in patients without known ASCVD or DM and with LDL cholesterol levels <190 mg/dL. Risk should be calculated every 4 to 6 years in adults between the ages of 45 and 75 who are not taking medication to reduce cholesterol levels. Although the ASCVD risk score was developed and validated in large populations, several studies have suggested that the risk calculator substantially overestimates 10-year risk but other studies suggest that its risk estimates are accurate.

Other risk assessment tools are available including the Framingham Risk Assessment Tool, the Multi-Ethic Study of Atherosclerosis (MESA) 10-year ASCVD Risk with Coronary Artery Calcification Calculator, the Reynolds Risk Score and the United Kingdom Prospective Diabetes Study (UKPDS) risk engine, all of which are recommended by the American Association of Clinical Endocrinologists (AACE).

MEDICAL MANAGEMENT

Nonpharmacological management takes many forms. Lifestyle is the foundation of ASCVD risk reduction efforts; lifestyle modification including adhering to a heart healthy diet, regular exercise habits, avoidance of tobacco, and maintenance of a healthy weight remain crucial to health promotion and ASCVD risk reduction. Clinicians should regularly monitor adherence to lifestyle and manage other risk factors for CVD. In individuals who are not receiving cholesterol-lowering medications, it is recommended that a 10-year ASCVD risk score be calculated every 4 to 6 years in persons aged 40 to 75 years without clinical ASCVD or diabetes, and with LDL-C levels between 70 to 189 mg/dL.

The 2013 ACC/AHA Blood Cholesterol Guidelines (17) have updated several key treatment parameters including a focus on ASCVD risk reduction with four identified statin benefit groups, a new perspective on LDL-C and/or non-HDL cholesterol treatment goals and safety recommendations.

The four major statin benefit groups in whom ASCVD risk reduction outweigh the risk of adverse events include:

- Individuals with clinical ASCVD
- Primary elevations of LDL-C ≥190 mg/dL
- Diabetics aged 40 to 75 with LDL-C 70-189 mg/dL and without clinical ASCVD
- Individuals without clinical ASCVD or diabetes with LDL-C 70 to 189 mg/dL and an estimated 10-year ASCVD risk ≥7.5%

Clinical ASCVD is defined as acute coronary syndromes, a history of MI, stable or unstable angina, coronary or other arterial revascularization, stroke, transient ischemic attack (TIA), or peripheral artery disease presumed to be of atherosclerotic origin. For the primary prevention of ASCVD in individuals without clinical ASCVD and LDL-C 70 to 189 mg/dL, the estimated absolute 10-year risk of ASCVD should be used to guide the initiation of statin therapy. The 10-year ASCVD risk should be estimated using the Pooled Cohort Equations For Estimating Atherosclerotic Cardiovascular Disease Risk.

For individuals with diabetes (diabetes mellitus type 1 and type 2) and ASCVD, an estimated 10-year ASCVD risk can also be used to guide the intensity of statin therapy. For those with clinical ASCVD or with LDL-C ≥190 mg/dL who are already in a statin benefit group, it is not appropriate to estimate 10-year ASCVD risk.

Prior to the release of the ATP IV treatment guidelines, it was recommended that statin therapy should be titrated to achieve a specific LDL goal. Because the Expert Panel found no randomized controlled trials (RCTs) to support this type of titration, the new recommendation is to select the appropriate intensity of statin agent that can be expected to reduce ASCVD risk. The RCTs reviewed in the most recent guideline either compared fixed doses with placebo or untreated control subjects, or compared fixed doses of higher intensity with moderate intensity statins. The intensity of statin therapy should be considered for both primary and secondary prevention of dyslipidemia. The Expert Panel defined the intensity of a statin agent based on the average expected LDL response to a specific drug.

High-intensity statin therapy should lower LDL-C on average by ≥50%. High-intensity agents include atorvastatin 40 to 80 mg and rosuvastatin 20 to 40 mg. High-intensity statin drugs are recommended as follows:

- Secondary prevention in adults 75 years of age and younger
- Primary prevention in adults with LDL 190 mg/dL (5 mmol/L) or higher
- Primary prevention in adults 40 to 75 years of age with LDL 70 to 189 mg/dL (1.8 to 4.9 mmol/L) and an estimated 10-year risk of ASCVD of 7.5% or higher (moderate-dose also an option)
- Primary prevention in diabetes patients 40 to 75 years of age with LDL 70 to 189 mg/dL (1.8 to 4.9 mmol/L) and an estimated 10-year risk of ASCVD

A moderate-intensity statin should, on average, lower LDL-C on average by approximately 30% to 50% (Miller, 2008). Agents in this category include lower doses of atorvastatin and rosuvastatin, as well as simvastatin, pravastatin, and lovastatin. Moderate-intensity statin therapy should be considered in patients who:

- Require secondary prevention and are older than 75 years of age.
- Cannot tolerate a high-dose statin.
- Require primary prevention, are 40 to 75 years of age with LDLs between 70 and 189 mg/dL (1.8 to 4.9 mmol/L) and have an estimated 10-year risk of ASCVD of 7.5% or higher. A higher dose for these patients is also a recommended option.
- Require primary prevention and are diabetics between the ages of 45 to 75 years of age with LDL levels between 70 and 189 mg/dL (1.8 to 4.9 mmol/L) and an estimated 10-year risk of ASCVD of less than 7.5% (Miller, 2008).

A daily dose of a low-intensity statin can be expected to lower LDL levels, on average, by less than 30% and include lower doses of medium-intensity drugs. They are indicated primarily for patients who cannot tolerate a high- or moderate-dose statin.

The ACC/AHA 2017 guidelines also make recommendations for considering a statin for those patients who are not in the four statin benefit groups. For example, primary prevention with a statin could be an option for patients with an LDL of 160 mg/dL or higher or who have other evidence of genetic hyperlipidemia. Known CVD onset in a first-degree male relative before the age of 55 may be another reason for starting a lipid-lowering agent. Patients with these issues may opt for starting a statin because they believe that being proactive may help decrease their genetic predisposition for dyslipidemia. It is particularly important to have a discussion of risk and benefits of taking a statin drug when starting medication is requested by the patient. Additional reasons for considering a statin for patients who fall outside the four statin benefit groups include a high sensitivity C-reactive protein of 2 mg/dL or higher, an ankle-brachial index less than 0.9, and a coronary artery calcium (CAC) score of 300 Agatston units or higher, or in the 75th percentile or higher for age, gender, and/or ethnicity.

Clinician-patient discussion is crucial prior to starting therapy. Discussion topics recommended include:

- The potential for ASCVD risk-reduction benefits
- The potential for adverse effects and drug-drug interactions
- The importance of a heart healthy lifestyle even if medications are used
- The management of other risk factors

CONCLUSION

All men with hypertension should have a detailed, clear, and evidence-based plan of care to manage their current hypertension symptoms and prevent future comorbid symptoms due to dyslipidemia. Management often requires a multidisciplinary approach that includes recommendations for behavioral and motivational changes, as well as overall lifestyle changes to promote greater levels of activity and decreased use of tobacco and alcohol. Furthermore, men older than age 40 without preexisting CVD or diabetes should be screened for risk factors every 4 to 6 years; this interval changes if risk factors develop, especially as risk for CVD increases directly with age.

CLINICAL PEARLS

- A "rule of 10" and a "rule of 5" have been helpful in predicting the drug effects of lowering BP when treating hypertension.
- Although some patients may be intolerant to statins, data from RCTs suggest that more than 90% of patients with an adverse event from a statin can tolerate it when it is reintroduced after a drug holiday.
- Nonstatin drugs, such as niacin and fenofibrate, have shown no benefits in lowering cardiovascular effects.
- Fish oil is a low-risk intervention with uncertain benefits.
- The rule of 20: The degree of LDL reduction, and not the absolute LDL value, is the heart of the new lipid guideline. Lowering LDL by 20, 40, and 60 mg/dL translates into a corresponding ischemic heart disease reduction by approximately 20%, 30%, and 50%.
- If you still want to achieve an LDL level of ≤70 mg/dL in a given patient, ezetimibe adds more benefit in high-risk patients who are statin intolerant or who are already on a maximum statin dose.
- When lifestyle modification is not possible, "statins are king."
- Atorvastatin provides "the most bang for your buck" regarding the efficacy and pricing of all statins.
- Up to half of hypertensive patients are not adequately controlled.

CLINICIAN RESOURCES

- 2017 Guideline for High Blood Pressure in Adults. American College of Cardiology.
- The Seventh Report of the Joint National Committee on Prevention, Detection, Evaluation, and Treatment of High Blood Pressure (JNC 7). National Heart, Lung, and Blood Institute (2003).
- 2014 Evidence-Based Guidelines for the Management of High Blood Pressure in Adults: Report from the Panel Members Appointed to the Eighth Joint National Committee (JNC 8).
- 2013 AHA/ACC Guidelines on Lifestyle Management to Reduce Cardiovascular Risk. A Report of the American College of Cardiology/American Heart Association Task Force on Practice Guidelines.
- Treatment of Hypertension in Adults Over Age 60 to Higher vs. Lower Targets. American College of Physicians and the American Academy of Family Physicians (2017).
- 2013 ACC/AHA Guideline on the Treatment of Blood Cholesterol to Reduce Atherosclerotic Cardiovascular Risks in Adults.
- American Association of Clinical Endocrinologist and American College of Endocrinology Guidelines for Management of Dyslipidemia and Prevention of Cardiovascular Disease (2017).

PATIENT RESOURCES

AHA Diet and Lifestyle Recommendations: AHA Diet and Lifestyle Recommendation Article: www.heart.org/HEARTORG/HealthyLiving/Diet-and-Lifestyle-Recommendations_UCM_305855_Article.jsp#.WYHwA4WcFPY

DASH Eating: Your Guide to Lowering Your Blood Pressure with DASH. Dietary Approaches to Stop Hypertension:www.nhlbi.nih.gov/files/docs/public/heart/hbp_low.pdf

Framingham Risk Assessment Tool: www.framinghamheartstudy.org/risk-functions/coronary-heart-disease/hard-10-year-risk.php

Reynolds Risk Score, designed to predict the risk of having a future heart attack, stroke, or other major heart disease in the next 10 years: www.reynoldsriskscore.org

The Multi-Ethnic Study of Atherosclerosis (MESA) Calculator: www.mesa-nhlbi.org/MESACHDRisk/MesaRiskScore/RiskScore.aspx

The UK Prospective Diabetes Study (UKPDS): Clinical and therapeutic implications for type 2 diabetes:www.thecalculator.co/health/UKPDS-Cardiac-Risk-Calculator-945.html

Your Guide to Lowering Your Blood Pressure with DASH brochure: h/www.nhlbi.nih.gov/files/docs/public/heart/dash_brief.pdf

REFERENCES

Alexander, M. R. Hypertension clinical presentation. Retrieved from https://emedicine.medscape.com/article/241381-clinical

American College of Cardiology. (2017). ASCVD risk estimator plus. Retrieved from http://tools.acc.org/ASCVD-Risk-Estimator-Plus/#!/calculate/estimate

Brunzell, J. D., Davidson, M., Furberg, C. D., Goldberg, R. B., Howard, B. V., Stein, J. H., & Witztum, J. L. (2008). Lipoprotein management in patients with cardiometabolic risk. Consensus conference report from the American Diabetes Association and the American College of Cardiology Foundation. *Journal of the American College of Cardiology, 51*, 1512–1524. doi:10.1016/j.jacc.2008.02.034

Centers for Disease Control and Prevention. (2011). Vital signs: prevalence, treatment, and control of hypertension. United States, 1999–2002 and 2005–2008. *MMWR. Morbidity and Mortality Weekly Report, 60*, 103–108.

Centers for Disease Control and Prevention. (2017). High cholesterol facts. Retrieved from https://www.cdc.gov/cholesterol/facts.htm

Chiang, C. E., Wang, T. D., Ueng, K. C., Lin, T. H., Yeh, H. I., Chen, C. Y., … Lin, S. J. (2015). 2015 guidelines of the Taiwan Society of Cardiology and the Taiwan Hypertension Society for the management of hypertension. *Journal of the Chinese Medical Association, 78*, 1–47. doi:10.1016/j.jcma.2014.11.005

Durkin, M. (2016). Pearls for lowering lipids. Retrieved from https://acpinternist.org/archives/2016/07/lipids.htm

Eckel, R. H., Jakicic, J. M., Ard, J. D., Hubbard, V. S., de Jesus, J. M., & Lee, I. M. (2013). 2013/AHA/ACC Guideline on lifestyle management to reduce cardiovascular risk. *Circulation, 129*(25 suppl 2), S76–S99. doi:10.1161/01.cir.0000437740.48606.d1

Egan, B. M., Li, J., Qanungo, S., & Wolfman, T. E. (2013). Blood pressure and cholesterol control in hypertensive hypercholesterolemic patients: National health and nutrition examination surveys 1988–2010. *Circulation, 128*, 29–41. doi:10.1161/CIRCULATIONAHA.112.000500

Everett, B., & Zajacova, A. (2015). Gender differences in hypertension and hypertension awareness among young adults. *Biodemography and Social Biology, 61*, 1–17. doi:10.1080/19485565.2014.929488

Go, A. S., Mozaffarian, D., Roger, V. L., Benjamin, E. J., Berry, J. D., Borden, W. B.. … Turner, M. B.; on behalf of the American Heart Association Statistics Committee and Stroke Statistics Subcommittee. (2013). Heart disease and stroke statistics—2013 update: A report from the American Heart Association. *Circulation, 127*, e6–e245. doi:10.1161/CIR.0b013e31828124ad

Hamrahian, S. M., & Batuman, V. (2017). Pathophysiology of hypertension. Retrieved from http://emedicine.medscape.com/article/1937383-overview#a4

Jellinger, P. S., Handelsman, Y., Rosenblit, P. D., Bloomgarden, Z. T., Fonseca, V. A., Garber, A. J., ... Davidson, M. (2017). American Association of Clinical Endocrinologist and American College of Endocrinology guidelines for management of dyslipidemia and prevention of cardiovascular disease. *Endocrine Practice, 23*(Suppl 2), 1–87. doi:10.4158/EP171764.APPGL

Kochanek, K. D., Xu, J. Q., Murphy, S. L., Minino, A. M., & Kung, H. C. (2011). Deaths: Final data for 2009. *National Vital Statistics Reports, 60*(3), 1–116.

Larzelere, M. M., & Williams, D. E. (2012). Promoting smoking cessation. *American Family Physician, 85*, 591–598.

Miller, M. (2008). Signs and symptoms of dyslipidemia. Retrieved from http://www.medscape.org/viewarticle/585045_4

National Heart, Lung and Blood Institute. (2004). The seventh report of the Joint National Committee on prevention, detection, evaluation and treatment of high blood pressure. Retrieved from https://www.nhlbi.nih.gov/health-pro/guidelines/current/hypertension-jnc-7

Nezafati, K. A. (2017). Tendon Xanthoma. *Clinical Advisor*. Retrieved from http://www.clinicaladvisor.com/dermatology/xanthoma-tendon/article/592290

O'Brien, E., & Stergiou, G. S. (2017). The pursuit of accurate blood pressure measurement: A 35-year travail. *The Journal of Clinical Hypertension, 19*, 746–752. doi:10.1111/jch.13005

Pickering, T. G., Miller, N. H., Ogedegbe, G., Krakoff, L. R., Artinian, N. T., & Geoff, D. (2008). Call to action on use and reimbursement for home blood pressure monitoring: A joint statement from the American Heart Association, the American Society of Hypertension, and Preventive Cardiovascular Nurses Association. *Hypertension, 52*, 1–9. doi:10.1161/HYPERTENSIONAHA.107.189011

Third Report of the National Cholesterol Education Program (NCEP) Expert Panel on detection, evaluation and treatment of high blood cholesterol in adults (Adult Treatment Panel III) Final Report. (2017). Retrieved from https://www.nhlbi.nih.gov/files/docs/resources/heart/atp-3-cholesterol-full-report.pdf

Vodnala, D., Rubenfire, M., & Brook, R. D. (2012). Secondary causes of dyslipidemia. *American Journal of Cardiology, 110*, 823–825. doi:10.1016/j.amjcard.2012.04.062

Whelton, P. K., Carey, R. M., Aronow, W. S., Casey, D. E., Collins, K. R., Himmelfarb, C. D., ... Wright J. T. Jr. (2017). 2017 ACC/AHA/AAPA/ABC/ACPM, AGS, APHA, ASH/ASPC/NMA/PCNA guideline for the prevention, detection, evaluation, and management of high blood pressure in adults. *Journal of the American College of Cardiology, 71*(19), e127–e248. doi:10.1016/j.jacc.2017.11.006

Yaxley, J. P., & Thambar, S. V. (2015). Resistant hypertension: an approach to management in primary care. *Journal of Family Medicine and Primary Care, 4*, 193–199. doi:10.4103/2249-4863.154630

CHAPTER 34

Evaluation and Management of Stroke in Men

Adriana R. Messina

INTRODUCTION

Cerebral vascular accident (CVA) or stroke is defined as a compromise in cerebral blood flow that can temporarily or permanently cause alterations in motor, sensory, or cognitive function. A stroke occurs once every 4 minutes in the United States with rates expected to rise (Wilson, 2013). CVAs are the fifth leading cause of death and have a total incidence (male and female) of 700,000 cases per year (Prabhakaran, Ruff, & Bernstein, 2015). The effects of stroke can be debilitating to patients' quality of life, and the fastest care ensures the best outcomes. Strokes cause devastating effects making it one of the top reasons people are unable to return to work (National Stroke Association, 2017). New protocols to ensure rapid care within the first 90 minutes of onset have been established in the emergency room setting and by paramedic personnel to reduce the chance of permanent disability in those discovered to have stroke symptoms. Outcomes for patients improve when treatment is established in less than 3 hours of symptom onset (Mayo Clinic, 2017). All patients who may be experiencing a stroke will be prioritized by emergency responders and taken to designated stroke centers for optimal care.

There are multiple causes of a stroke, and some can be altered and others cannot. Nonmodifiable risk factors include age, sex, ethnicity, and family history. Health-related risk factors or modifiable risk factors include diet, body mass index, physical activity, chronic illness, acute illness, heart disease, diabetes, hypertension, hypercholesterolemia, smoking, and alcohol and drug use. Ischemic strokes are four and a half times more common than hemorrhagic strokes, which include intracranial hemorrhage (ICH) and subarachnoid hemorrhage (SAH) (Wetmore et al., 2014). Ischemic CVAs represent dying brain tissue with varying levels of infarction and ischemia. Ischemia is active loss or compromise of tissue due to blockage of blood flow. Infarction occurs from lack of blood perfusion and results in death of brain tissue and loss of function. The center of the lesion is referred to as the ischemic core or area of irreversible effects and the ischemic penumbra is the area surrounding the infarct that could be restored with timely reperfusion (Prabhakaran et al., 2015). It takes only 3 minutes without adequate oxygen therapy to cause irreversible tissue loss.

A hemorrhagic CVA is bleeding from uncontrolled hypertension, causing blood to leak from weakened vessels, ruptured aneurysms, or arteriovenous malformations. Time is crucial during a period of occluded blood flow or uncontrolled bleeding to the cerebral tissues. For every minute that passes after the onset of a stroke, 2 million neurons die which can equivocate to years of aging without rapid treatment (Prabhakaran et al., 2015).

Transient ischemic attacks (TIAs), or ministrokes, reflect a focused area of ischemia without complete infarction that usually resolves quickly within 24 hours of symptom onset. TIA occurrence can increase the risk of a subsequent CVA, recurrent TIAs, and death. A precluding TIA or stroke can increase the risk of stroke to 3% to 4% in the days to weeks following the first event (Kernan et al., 2014).

The ABCD2 scoring system is a tool that can assist in determining a patient's risk for stroke following a TIA. It takes five factors into consideration to calculate a score:

- Patient's age is greater than or equal to 60 years
- Duration of symptoms ranging from a couple of minutes to greater than or equal to 60 minutes
- History of diabetes
- Blood pressure >140 mmHg systolic and >90 mmHg diastolic
- If symptoms at presentation include unilateral weakness or speech complications

The added score ranges from 0 to 7, low risk to high risk, revealing a percentage of likely stroke occurrence at 2, 7, and 90 days (Kernan et al., 2014). Low-risk scores range from 0 to 3, moderate risk is 4 to 5, and high risk is 6 to 7.

INCIDENCE

Populations that are increasingly predisposed to a CVA include African Americans, Hispanics, and those older than 50 years of age (National Institutes of Health & National Institute of Neurological Disorders and Stroke, 2017). Men have a higher incidence of CVA than women at different ages of the life span: child, adolescent, and the older adult. Women have the protective properties of estrogen until menopause when their incidence and severity of stroke worsens. Oral contraceptives can also increase their risk for a CVA as young adults and increases as they age with continued use. Preliminary research reveals that Caucasian men studied from age 70 to 85 with decreased plasma levels of testosterone and dihydrotestosterone were at a greater risk for stroke (Yeap et al., 2014). Those that experience a TIA have an increased risk of a CVA during their lifetime. The incidence of TIA is known to increase with age and is more prevalent among men.

Factors such as diabetes mellitus and myocardial infarction increase the risk of stroke and subsequent death from stroke over time in men. Undiagnosed cardiac disorders, uncontrolled hypertension, or hyperlipidemia can also cause detrimental effects for increased stroke rates for men. Stroke risk for African Americans increases threefold higher than for Caucasians for every 10 mmHg increase in systolic blood pressure (Mozaffarian et al., 2016). Fifteen percent of Mexican Americans who suffered a TIA will subsequently endure a stroke (Mozaffarian et al., 2016). However, African American men were slightly less likely to have a stroke, 3.9%, than African American females at 4.0% (Mozaffarian et al., 2016). Men are more at risk for uncontrolled and undiagnosed health concerns because they are more likely to delay or avoid seeking medical care than women. It is noted that perception of self-worth, embarrassment, unwillingness to express emotions about health, anxiety, fear, and overall poor communication with healthcare providers inhibit men from seeking care (Yousef, Grunfeld, & Hunter, 2015). Incidence of stroke in men exponentially rises for those of African American and Hispanic descent. This reality composes of a multitude of factors such as social situations, economic disparities, lack of resources, and genetic precursors.

ANATOMY AND PHYSIOLOGY

CVAs can occur at multiple areas within the brain tissue, which directly correlates to the type of deficit the patient is experiencing. It is crucial to determine which areas of the central or peripheral nervous system are affected. The lesion could be in the brain, brainstem, or spinal cord if located in the central nervous system, or it can affect the peripheral nervous system, which consists of the 12 cranial nerves and peripheral nerves. Examining the patient for deficits with a full neurological assessment will obtain important clues for diagnosis.

The brain is composed of four sections—the cerebrum, cerebellum, brainstem, and diencephalon—and brain tissue is separated into gray and white matter. Four lobes make up each cerebral hemisphere: the frontal, temporal, occipital, and the brainstem. Additional gray matter areas include the basal ganglia, which direct movement. The thalamus and hypothalamus lie in the diencephalon and are responsible for sensory communicative functions and regulating temperature, heart rate, and blood pressure, respectively. The white matter from cerebral cortex, deemed the internal capsule, leads to brainstem in three parts, namely, the midbrain, pons, and medulla. The cerebellum is responsible for body movement and coordination. The spinal cord is composed of cervical spine (C1-C7), thoracic spine (T1-T12), lumbar spine (L1-L5), sacral spine (S1-S5), and the coccygeal spine.

The peripheral nervous system is made up of cranial nerves and peripheral nerves that connect to bodily organs, skin, heart, and extremities. It controls the somatic nervous system, which monitors the pain center and muscle movements and the reactions to sensation and touch.

The autonomic nervous system, also controlled by the peripheral nervous system, innervates internal organs and formulates reflex responses to stimuli. The sympathetic and parasympathetic nervous system are included in the autonomic nervous system and respond either in times of stress (sympathetic) or to maintain expected normal functioning of tissues for periods of rest and for homeostasis (parasympathetic).

There are 12 cranial nerves; some are sensory, motor, or both or consist of a unique function. The peripheral nerves include 31 pairs along the spinal cord, 8 cervical, 12 thoracic, 5 lumbar, 5 sacral, and 1 coccygeal, that transmit sensory or motor messages. Many of the peripheral nerves have both sensory and motor fibers. Each is responsible for a specific set of functions. Motor communication includes messages that are transmitted from the cerebral cortex and brainstem centers and extend down to the periphery via motor pathways. The corticospinal tract communicates to start or stop voluntary muscle movements that are intricate and specialized and is responsible for muscle tone. These fibers converge to form the shape of a pyramid at the medulla and then cross to the other side of the body below. The basal ganglia system controls gross body movements and muscle tone traveling from cerebral cortex, basal ganglia, brainstem, and spinal cord. The cerebellar system regulates coordination with movement and maintains posture and balance, receiving both sensory and motor signals.

When there is a compromise of the corticospinal tract, it directly correlates with the area of deficit. An upper motor lesion above the pyramid will cause a contralateral deficit exhibited in body functioning, whereas a lower lesion below the pyramid will result in an ipsilateral impairment. The range of weakness varies depending upon the damage to the neurons. Finer detailed movements are greatly impaired or absent especially with damage to the descending pathways of motor neurons that control arms and legs. Deep tendon reflexes and muscle tone will reflect hypertonicity when the lesion exists in the upper tract; contrarily, reflexes and tone are greatly diminished or absent with the presence of a lower neuron lesion (Trompetto et al., 2014). Basal ganglia and cerebellar defects do not cause detrimental paralysis but can change patient function. Cerebellar effects can lead to gait, coordination, and balance impairment, and basal ganglia changes can cause hypersensitive muscle tone and compromised involuntary movement response (Trompetto et al., 2014).

Sensory pathways travel from receptors in skin, muscle, and mucous membranes through the spinal cord and up to the brain. There are two ways the sensory messages travel to the brain: the spinothalamic tract, which includes smaller cells, and the posterior column, which is made up of thicker, larger cells. Spinothalamic neurons transmit touch, pain, and temperature sensations, whereas the posterior columns send messages of pressure, fine touch, vibration, and proprioception. These communicative transmissions reach the thalamus, where they are briefly recognized, then travel to the sensory cortex for complete perception of the signals. Knowing these fundamental pathways can help to identify lesions along the spinal cord when relating to deficits found on physical examination. Each spinal nerve connects to a specific area of skin identified as a dermatome. Recognizing impairment involving specific dermatomes can give clues to the affected sensory nerve.

Deep tendon reflexes (DTRs) can consist of as few as two neurons, one sensory and one motor, to multiple neurons. A sensory message travels to the spinal cord across the neuromuscular pathway and down to the corresponding muscle that triggers the involuntary response. Loss or reduced tone can be assessed by performing DTRs immediately following a brain injury (Trompetto et al., 2014).

HISTORY

Common presentation of CVAs can include one or several symptoms, namely, sudden onset of speech impairment, facial droop on one side, loss of motor function, syncope, drooling, weakness, or confusion. Further signs of a CVA include seizures, tremors, or involuntary movements. Changes that transpire quickly, in comparison with gradual onset, indicate TIA or CVA, and some patients state that they had "the worst headache of their life," which may specify a subarachnoid hemorrhage (Becske, 2017). Other signs may present as weakness, ranging from fine to gross motor skills, such as grasping or dropping items, to being unable to move a limb/leg/arm or one side of the body. The provider needs to know whether the deficits are symmetrical, proximal, or distal, or include loss of sensation or consciousness, which can represent the extent of impairment. Investigating the timing and start of the weakness is crucial: was it sudden, gradual, or noticeable, or did it greatly or negligibly affect daily activities?

The most common symptoms in altered neurological presentation are headache and dizziness. It is crucial to determine associated symptoms and characteristics such as severity, onset, location, and duration to rule out differential diagnoses. Define if the patient has experienced an aura, sneezing, coughing, fever, stiff neck, or altered vision, which may represent a different disease process than a CVA. When patients report dizziness, it is crucial to determine if coexisting symptoms such as weakness, lightheadedness, fainting, head-spinning, or balance issues are present. Identify triggers and the timing of the symptoms to effectively triage potential stroke patients (Kerber & Newman-Toker, 2015).

Various symptoms or effects of a stroke can include altered mood, sudden outbursts of emotions, fatigue, loss of bowel or bladder control, and lack of awareness. Some signs may be subtle and require careful observation of a patient by a family member or friend to recognize a change.

RISK FACTORS

The risk factors for a CVA range from a multitude of health concerns as well as social and financial challenges. The most common risk factor for hemorrhagic stroke is uncontrolled hypertension and aneurysms greater than 7 mm (Backes et al., 2014). Smoking, alcohol use, and history of a first-degree relative are important risk factors for ruptured aneurysms occurring most frequently in the middle cerebral artery within the circle of Willis (Backes et al., 2014). Health-related risk factors include diet, body mass index, physical activity, chronic illness, acute illness, heart disease, diabetes, personal history of hypertension, hypercholesterolemia, alcohol use, and drug use. It is likely that prevention could be more difficult to achieve if a patient is surrounded by others with the same risk factors and medical conditions.

It is optimal to have a young adult with unknown risk factors begin screening at age 30, but yearly visits could begin sooner depending on family history. Lower socioeconomic status can expose a patient to increased risk factors due to decreased income; predisposed social situation; access to healthcare, education, and transportation; and lack of public resources. Interestingly, occupational psychological stress was not found to have any effect on the incidence of stroke but did increase the likelihood of coronary heart disease in smokers and blue collar workers (Torén et al., 2014). It is unlikely that stress would be considered a directly modifiable risk factor for stroke. However, it is interesting that stress can affect the onset of heart disease and hypertension, which would eventually increase the risk of stroke if not managed properly.

A research study completed in Western Australia showed that Caucasian men older than 65 years with ongoing diabetes are at increasingly higher risk of stroke-related deaths as they age and recurrent stroke rates rise in the 10 to 20 years after the first CVA (Yeap et al., 2015). The decade in which the patients were initially diagnosed with diabetes was taken into account, with surprising ratios of subjects with an early recognition of the disease within their 30s and 40s (Yeap et al., 2015). These authors validated that diabetes is predictive of overall health and progressive disease.

POTENTIAL CULTURAL CONSIDERATIONS

There are numerous health disparities to consider when evaluating vulnerable populations that are at risk for cerebral vascular compromise. Individuals who have less access to education, less family or community support, and decreased or no access to health-related services tend to be exposed to increased risk factors. African Americans have an increase of 40% in mortality rate for heart disease than whites (Moore et al., 2016). Additional social factors that may interfere with improved outcomes of compromised populations can include medical mistrust, poor health literacy, and segregation from family, transportation, and house services (Moore et al., 2016).

These clues tell healthcare providers of all disciplines that the male population needs focused attention when addressing these risk factors during a healthcare visit. Some details can be missed if the assessment questions do not directly focus on their concerns. Yousef et al. (2015) has discussed recurring barriers to help seeking among men in a study conducted from age 15 to 80 and recognized embarrassment, anxiety, fear, miscommunication with healthcare providers, and unwillingness to share concerns about health. It is important to target men to eliminate these obstacles allowing them to feel more comfortable seeking care. Providers that approach their male patients with statements of concern could be more effective at encouraging clients who return for follow-up visits.

Lower education and smoking are more prevalent in men who have experienced ischemic stroke. Smoking overall directly correlates to low education but not necessarily to hypertension (Nordahl et al., 2014). Similarly, hypertension in combination with low education and smoking revealed an increase of ischemic stroke among men as well (Nordahl et al., 2014). Smoking and hypertension increases risk for ischemic and hemorrhagic CVAs but did not prove to be gender specific.

Literature has shown that incidence of ischemic strokes have reduced in the white population compared to blacks. The rate of hemorrhagic strokes, however, has not changed for both populations and remains stable. Interestingly, rates of intracerebral hemorrhage (ICH) and subarachnoid hemorrhage (SAH) are higher among Mexican American communities than among Caucasians (Mozaffarian et al., 2016).

PHYSICAL EXAMINATION

Upon hospital admission, the provider will be performing a comprehensive physical examination to assess the male patient's condition and triage for the appropriate testing and treatment. This process begins with an overall assessment of consciousness, first establishing orientation by having patient recall person, place, and time. The Glasgow Coma Scale (GCS) can also be used for patients who have an altered level of consciousness (LOC), calculating a score for a patient's behavior, response to eye opening, and verbal and motor replies. The National Institutes of Health Stroke Scale (NIHSS) will likely be completed by a neurologist and/or provider in charge of the patient's care. It comprises a numerical value for several tested areas including motor, sensory, visual, and language functions; a higher score corresponds to severe neurological alterations.

The best way to continue, after assessing LOC, is with a complete neurological examination from head to toe. Ensure that tests are done bilaterally and check for symmetrical versus asymmetrical function. The cranial nerves are the hallmark testing points (Table 34.1) to determine deficits and their severity. The olfactory nerve can be tested by using oils or a mild scent to have patient sense smell. This nerve test is not completed often for a stroke diagnosis, but it requires that the patient has the eyes closed and check that each nostril is patent after occluding each one. Cranial nerve II controls visual perception and is tested by using the ophthalmoscope and finding the optic disks. It is essential to ensure that the edges are not blurry, discolored, or enlarged and to assess the patient for partial loss or peripheral loss of vision as well as visual fields by confrontation (Suter & Harvey, 2016).

Optic and oculomotor nerves (cranial nerves II and III) control the motor function of the pupil by using light to inhibit the reaction. The response to movement close and far away tests the near response, convergence, and accommodation of the lens and pupils. Observe for ptosis on one side, and note if the pupils are different in size and become larger or smaller with reaction to light. To evaluate oculomotor, trochlear, and abducens nerves (cranial nerves III, IV, and VI, respectively), check six directions of extraocular movements and observe for loss

TABLE 34.1 Cranial Nerve Reference Guide

Cranial Nerves	Name	Classification	Function
I	Olfactory	Sensory	Sense of smell
II	Optic	Sensory	Vision
III	Oculomotor	Motor	Movement of eyes
IV	Trochlear	Motor	Movement of eyes
V	Trigeminal	Sensory, motor	Facial perception Jaw muscle strength
VI	Abducens	Motor	Lateral movement of eyes
VII	Facial	Motor, sensory	Motor movement of face Taste sensation
VIII	Acoustic	Sensory	Hearing
IX	Glossopharyngeal	Motor, sensory	Swallowing, movement of tongue Voice
X	Vagus	Motor, sensory	Gag reflex, uvula/soft palate rise
XI	Spinal accessory	Motor	Strength of trapezius muscles
XII	Hypoglossal	Motor	Tongue movement, side to side

of coordination. It is essential to rule out diplopia, double vision, in one or both eyes. Ruling out nystagmus, the quick or repetitive movement of the eyes in one direction, is important for determining cerebellar disease. Test the motor function of the trigeminal nerve V by having the patient clench the jaw and move it side to side while placing hands on masseter and temporal muscles to evaluate strength. The sensory portion of the examination tests the sensation of a sharp and dull object bilaterally on the face. Specific areas to test include the forehead, cheeks, and jaw while the patient's eyes are closed. The corneal reflex is blinking when a cotton swab or object is used to touch the corneas of the patient from their periphery (Bickley, 2014).

Assessing the facial nerve (cranial nerve VII) requires that the patient smile, frown, raise eyebrows, puff out cheeks, and hold eyes closed against the pressure of opening them from the provider. To assess the acoustic nerve (cranial nerve VIII) test the patient's hearing by initially performing a whisper test on both ears. The provider stands about 2 feet behind the patient and whispers softly toward each ear while having the patient repeat what is said immediately following. It is recommended to change the word or phrase used for each ear. If the patient is found to have hearing loss in one or both ears, assess whether it is conductive or sensorineural by using a tuning fork with the Rinne and Weber tests. Cranial nerve IX involves listening to the patient's voice for alterations in phonation. To test cranial nerve X, which controls swallowing, have the patient open the mouth, stick out the tongue, and say "Ah" while watching for the characteristic uvula rise. The gag reflex is also a part of the vagus nerve and is assessed by targeting touch to the back of the throat, eliciting the response.

Testing the spinal accessory nerve (XI) involves having the patient move against force of the provider's hands placed on the patient's shoulders while he performs a shrug. Have the patient continue by applying slight pressure to both sides of the face while patient is applying muscular force. It is necessary to assess for strength, symmetry, and abnormal movements. Testing the last twelfth cranial nerve, hypoglossal, proceeds with having the patient move the tongue from cheek to cheek while checking masseter muscle strength and assessing symmetry. Pay close attention to the patient's speech and assess the tongue inside the mouth for abnormal movements (Bickley, 2014).

The cranial nerve assessment most likely will give clues to the patient's motor and sensory status, and here it is important to continue with a thorough examination. The motor assessment deciphers differences by applying mild force to the limbs and observing the patient's positioning and response to movements. Observe for involuntary actions, tics, fasciculations, tone, bulk of muscle mass, and strength. Compare patient's movements symmetrically and take notice of any deviations from normal. Hold the limbs in your arms while flexing the joints of the hands and wrists, elbows, and knees while applying energy, stimulating the patient to elicit resistance. Observe if the movement is controlled and how strong it is and evaluate the tone. Strength evaluation includes having the patient flex and extend at specific joints to test the function of the spinal nerves.

The cervical spine is tested while flexing and extending at the elbows and wrists in addition to finger abduction, opposition of the thumb with resistance, and grip strength. The lumbar spine nerves are stimulated with the flexion and extension of the hip, knee, and ankles in addition to the abduction and adduction of the hips. Grading motor strength ranges from 0, which is no movement against gravity, to 5, which represents full movement and strength against gravity.

The cerebellar examination includes checking for nystagmus, coordinating movements from finger of examiner to nose of patient, rapid alternating movements with hands on lap, sliding heel on opposite leg from knee to shin, walking heel to toe, ruling out wide or staggering gait or leaning to side of lesion. The movements coordinated by the cerebellar system are crucial to evaluate synchronized and purposeful function while ensuring gait is not compromised. Some additional tests include small knee bends, hopping in place, and the Romberg test, which is performed by standing in place with both eyes closed for 30 to

60 seconds and feet together without loss of balance. The pronator drift test is performed by having the patient hold the arms straight out, pronated, with eyes closed, while either sitting or standing. The provider applies quick downward pressure to arms and releases, observing for patient's arms to quickly return to the original position (Bickley, 2014).

Deep tendon reflexes represent the joining tissue strength of the muscle as it responds to the elicited stimulus on the connective tissue. A reflex hammer is used at several different locations testing corresponding nerves: biceps (C5 and C6), brachioradialis (C6), triceps (C7), patellar (L4), Achilles tendon (S1). The provider holds the limb to eliminate the effect of gravity and directs the patient to relieve all muscle tone and resistance, thereby making the limb flaccid. With a swift and steady motion the provider applies mild pressure to tap the tendon area and grades the reflex from 0, representing no reflex, to +4, which is hyperreflexive. Grade +2 represents a normal response to the stimuli.

The sensory assessment includes testing pain, temperature, light touch, vibration, and position or proprioception. For pain, a dull pointed object can be used to elicit a response while quizzing the patient where it is felt while eyes are closed. A cotton ball is ideal for light touch sensation while asking where the patient feels it. Vibration is tested with the use of a 128-Hz tuning fork applied to joints for the patient to sense with eyes closed. Ask the patient when the vibration stops. The joints that can be used are interphalangeal joints of the patient's finger, the joint of the big toe, patella, medial malleolus, and other prominent bony areas. Proprioception testing includes keeping the patient's eyes closed and moving the position of the big toe up and down. Temperature could be tested using hot and cold water but is not needed if pain perception is not compromised. It is important to remember to remind the patient to keep the eyes closed and compare that the proximal and distal assessment of each sensory exam are equal. Additional sensation tests include stereognosis, or identifying an object by touch; two-point discrimination, or having the patient identify two areas touched at the same time and telling how far apart they are; number identification or graphesthesia; point localization having the patient identify where they were touched while eyes were closed. Extinction is tested by touching the patient on both sides of the body in the same area while his eyes are closed and having the patient identify both spots (Bickley, 2014).

ABNORMAL FINDINGS

Alterations in sensory, motor, or behavioral changes are determined by the area of injury and reflect the functional compromise of the correlating tissue. Middle cerebral artery infarctions, which are the most common type of ischemic CVAs, cause sensory decline and aphasia, whereas the right middle cerebral artery causes neglect to one entire side of the body.

Each brain lobe is representative of a specific function and can be compromised if an infarct occurs within this area. The frontal lobe controls impulsive behavior, memory, emotions, creativity, and social interactions. Personality changes are commonly seen in those affected in the frontal lobes and can fluctuate dramatically. Temporal lobe infarctions can cause aphasia or inability to express thoughts or interpret communication. The temporal lobe is responsible for hearing, enjoying music, recognition of written and verbal communication, and memory. Occipital lobe infarcts can commonly cause changes in vision or perception. Compromise of the cerebellum can affect balance, coordination, muscle tone, and distance perception. The brainstem can affect breathing, changes in heart rate, blood pressure, taste, smell, and appetite.

The absence of muscle tone with application of mild force is regarded as flaccidity; the patient's limb will completely flop down with gravity. Contrary to flaccidity is increased tone, which manifests as spasticity and repetitive shaking that can become more prominent with movement. Rigidity can occur with increased tone and resistance with tense muscles compromising flexibility and movement. Table 34.2 can guide the provider in interpreting abnormal

TABLE 34.2 Neurological Deficit Terms and Descriptions

Term for Neurological Deficit	Definition/Description
Aphasia	May be expressive or receptive; difficulty in saying what the brain is commanding, or difficulty in processing what is being said, inability to understand, inability to communicate through speech
Agnosia	Inability to recognize/comprehend sights, sounds, words, sensory information
Amnesia	Partial/total, permanent/transient loss of memory
Ataxia	Difficulty walking/gait, defective muscular coordination with voluntary movements
Apraxia	Inability to perform purposeful acts
Alexia	Inability to comprehend written words
Akinesia	Complete/partial loss of muscle movement
Agraphia	Loss of ability to write
Dyskinesia	Defect affecting voluntary movement, disorder characterized by uncontrolled or involuntary movements
Dysphonia	Difficulty with phonation, loss of voice
Dysphagia	Difficulty swallowing
Dysphasia	Impairment of speech resulting from brain lesion/neurodevelopmental disorder
Dyslexia	Difficulty using/interpreting written forms of communication by an individual whose vision and general intelligence are unimpaired
Hemiparesis	Loss of function on one side of the body
Hemiplegia	Weakness on one side of the body
Homonymous hemianopia	Blindness in one half of visual field
Ptosis	Drooping of upper eyelid
Dysarthria	Difficulty with speech and forming words
Diplopia	Double vision
Bradykinesia	Slowness of movement/gait

findings in CVA patients by using these descriptions for assessment purposes and aids in communication among providers concerning the extent of deficits found on examination.

DIAGNOSTICS

Initial diagnostic tools utilized will depend on the setting in which the stroke patient is found. Those who are in the community or in their homes will be assessed first by emergency responders, who will perform a concise neurological examination. They will likely give aspirin and transport the patient to the designated stroke center in the area unless the CVA is likely to be hemorrhagic. Once the patient reaches a hospital setting, the most important test to be done is a noncontrast CT scan or MRI of the brain to establish whether the CVA is ischemic or hemorrhagic. The patient will also have an immediate echocardiogram to rule out the chance of a cardiac event such as a ST-segment elevated myocardial infarction or occlusion. Laboratory testing will include a basic metabolic panel, complete blood count, and PT/INR/PTT (prothrombin time/international normalized ratio/partial thromboplastin time) initially. A lipid panel and glycosylated hemoglobin can be added as well or could wait until the patient is stable. A neurologist and nurse will be performing a neurological examination and the NIHSS to comprehensively assess for all possible deficits.

Additional diagnostic studies may include angiography of collateral circulation to assess for a blockage or thrombus. A carotid artery MRI can be completed to rule out occlusion and determine if an immediate intervention is needed. It is recommended that the patients with a presumed TIA have brain imaging done within 24 hours of symptom onset in addition to vessel imaging to rule out and prevent an acute infarct (Nanda, 2017).

MANAGEMENT

Recommendations for health promotion are essential in management of stroke, both for men who have already experienced a CVA and those who have not. It is essential to spread awareness among young men to be proactive in their well-being from an early age. Prevention of cardiac disease, high cholesterol, high blood pressure, and diabetes can ensure patients years of an optimal quality of life. Patients who already have acquired these diseases can learn to improve in managing their symptoms and decrease the chance of a detrimental health event. Educational programs including heart healthy diet counseling, weight loss goals, and exercise plans tailored to each patient's lifestyle can inspire them to follow through. Furthermore, teaching patients what each disease process means and what could happen in the future can offer insight to prevention and care as necessary. It is imperative to teach patients the warning signs of a stroke so that they can recognize when to call for help. The American Heart Association uses the acronym FAST to quickly identify stroke symptoms and prompts patients to seek help immediately: Face drooping, Arm weakness, Speech difficulty, and Time to call 911 (FAST), with or without these additional symptoms, "sudden numbness or weakness of face, arm or leg, sudden confusion, trouble speaking or understanding, sudden trouble seeing in one or both eyes, sudden trouble walking, dizziness, loss of balance and coordination, sudden severe headache." Use this guidance to educate patients and families to pursue prompt medical attention (American Heart Association, 2017b).

Different cultures may present challenges in management of prevention of stroke, acute stroke, and those with permanent disabilities following stroke. A survey showed that African Americans prefer to learn about health through their physicians first and then at barbershops and churches (Moore et al., 2016). Patients for whom English is a second language may find more comfort in trusting information given to them through their familiar cultural community.

MEDICAL MANAGEMENT

After ruling out alternative diagnoses and stroke has been confirmed, it is important to determine what the patient's plan will be going forward. Identifying the individual's risk factors for stroke will provide a preliminary guideline for management of the patient. Those with known diabetes mellitus (DM) or with subclinical disease can start with nutrition counseling and lifestyle modifications, which prove to be most beneficial over medications (Kernan et al., 2014). Medications may also be necessary in order for the patient to maintain glycemic control. Blood pressure (BP) stabilization and monitoring of those with a systolic BP greater than 140 mmHg and a diastolic BP greater than 90 mmHg is imperative. Introduction of statin therapy for those with hyperlipidemia, with low-density lipoprotein (LDL) greater than 100 mg/dL, or those with DM diagnosis with or without evidence of LDL elevation has also been shown to reduce cardiovascular events. Current smokers must be provided with tobacco cessation education and counseling. It must be stressed that continued use of tobacco can greatly affect the recurrence of subsequent detrimental health concerns. It can take at least 5 to 15 years for a smoker who has stopped smoking to reach a decreased risk of stroke as a nonsmoker (World Health Organization, 2018). Smoking can at least double the risk of an ischemic stroke and can triple the risk of hemorrhage stroke (The Internet Stroke Center, 2017). Nonsmokers who have exposure to second-hand smoke have an increased risk of stroke between 20% and 30% (Centers for Disease Control and Prevention, 2017). Continued smoking and exposure to smoke can greatly increase patient mortality risk, and ongoing education is crucial to improve quality of life for individuals.

Patients who drink alcohol in moderate to excessive amounts should stop drinking entirely or reduce frequency to occasional use. Weight loss can also assist in reduction of health events, especially in those who are overweight, obese, and with known risk factors. Obesity is not clearly linked to increased risk of stroke; however, the sequelae that accompany it can provoke a cardiovascular event (Kernan et al., 2014). Physical activity, in contrast, can prevent and may reduce recurrence of CVAs. Anticoagulation can also play a role for some patients. Aspirin may be recommended for antiplatelet aggregation therapy for those with DM or more aggressive anticoagulation like warfarin may be indicated for patients with coagulopathies.

Physical, occupational, and speech therapy may also be indicated for patients with weakness, hemiplegia, aphasia, and gait disturbances. Most, if not all, CVA diagnosed patients will receive a consult for physical therapy to ensure that any deficits are examined. This is usually done within days of diagnosis in order to prevent stagnation and persistence of complications. The severity of the deficit will determine how long their course of therapy will be and if they can be discharged home or to a rehabilitation facility until their strength is restored. They will receive inpatient and outpatient therapy as well as exercises to perform on their own that can last for several weeks to months. Occupational therapy aids in the everyday functioning activities such as getting dressed, eating, cooking, and bathing. Speech therapy is especially crucial for those CVA patients suffering with speech impairments and cognitive changes related to communication.

CRITERIA FOR REFERRALS

Patients presenting with any neurological change in the hospital or clinic setting, from alteration of mental status to loss of function, can prompt a consult for neurology. However, it is crucial to determine how acute the change is and the best course of action. Neurological deficits, especially when acute, are time sensitive in regard to regaining function and maintain a patient's quality of life. It is important to make sound medical judgments especially with understanding of the patient's baseline. The patient's medical history is also a clue for whom to involve in a patient's care, especially relating to the acute presentation. A cardiologist is crucial for patients with cardiac disease and to rule out myocardial infarction. Factors that may prompt a cardiac consult include elevated troponin levels, abnormal heart sounds on physical examination that are not characteristic of patient's current history, and any patient report of chest pain, shortness of breath, indigestion, or fatigue.

OVERVIEW OF POTENTIAL INVASIVE PROCEDURES/SURGERY

Reperfusion therapy is the most essential piece of treatment in order to regain as much function as possible at the area of the lesion. Tissue plasminogen activator (tPA) is considered the gold standard of treatment for an ischemic stroke, and is the only drug currently approved by the Food and Drug Administration (FDA) for this indication. If the stroke was determined to be ischemic by CT scan, tPA can be administered, with the goal of clot eradication, attempting to promote recovery of as much ischemic brain tissue as possible. This is essential to administer within the first 3 hours of symptom onset (American Heart Association, 2017a), but a second source outlines that tPA can be beneficial in patients who are within a 4.5-hour window of when symptoms began (Prabhakaranet al., 2015). If tPA fails, then the clot needs to be removed surgically by a physician. In addition, if a patient seeking medical treatment passed the recommended time frame, the procedure approach is preferred and intravenous thrombolysis is contraindicated (Prabhakaranet al., 2015). A wired cage-like device is inserted through the femoral artery to travel to the area of ischemia to retrieve the clot. This procedure is called a thrombectomy, uses coil retrievers, and needs to be completed within 6 hours of symptom onset (American Heart Association, 2017a). Another management method uses a stent retriever, which occludes the clot at the site and restores blood flow immediately upon removal. Suction could also be applied to help in removing the clot by aspirating through a guide catheter (Prabhakaranet al., 2015).

Hemorrhagic CVAs are treated with a procedure to stop the source of the bleed. Physicians perform vascular surgery, placing a coil to occlude the outlet of bleeding in ruptured blood vessels (American Heart Association, 2017a).

PREVENTION AND CONCLUSIONS

The Healthy People 2020 initiative, created by the American Heart Association, encompasses guidelines for prevention of stroke and cardiovascular disease in primary care. Providers can teach their patients how to control these risk factors: hypertension, smoking, dyslipidemia, diabetes, excess weight, lack of exercise, and alcohol use. Controlling diseases such as atrial fibrillation and carotid artery disease can greatly reduce the risk of ischemic strokes (American Heart Association, 2017a). It is crucial to target lower socioeconomic groups to educate in the community for many reasons. They have reduced access to resources as well as being targeted as consumers of unhealthy habits such as smoking and fast food and should be educated about the harmful effects of smoking and potential complications related to smoking (Nordahl et al., 2014).

Increased physical activity, specifically walking, can significantly reduce the risk of stroke in men. Certain factors need to be determined, such as the number of hours per week spent walking, pace of walking, and distance (Jefferis, Whincup, Papacosta, & Wannamethee, 2014). Men who walk more than 22 hours per week can reduce the probability of stroke by half, and walking for intervals greater than 3 hours can make a significant difference (Jefferis et al., 2014). The risk was further reduced in those with more vigorous activity. Heart rate and forced expiratory volume over 1 minute (FEV_1) are related to physical activity and can also be predictive factors of cardiovascular health and a reduced risk for stroke.

CLINICAL PEARLS

- Rapid stroke treatment is crucial for tissue preservation and restoration of motor and sensory function.
- Men with a suspected CVA must be evaluated at a designated stroke center, have an extensive neurological examination, have a head CT scan as soon as possible, with an electrocardiogram to rule out a myocardial infarction, embolus, or occlusions.
- Ensure the time when the symptoms first occurred to determine if tPA is indicated in an ischemic stroke.
- Rapid reperfusion is the goal to restore compromised brain function and improve outcomes for patients with ischemic stroke.
- Consult with neurology as soon as possible.
- Initiate the proper medical management and establish a plan of care quickly.
- Lifestyle teaching for prevention of CVA recurrence is the key to health promotion and reduction of stroke incidence.

RESOURCES FOR THE PROVIDERS

ABCD2 scoring system for TIA and stroke occurrence: www.stroke.org/sites/default/files/resources/tia-abcd2-tool.pdf?docID
Healthy People 2020: www.healthypeople.gov
NIHSS—National Institutes of Health Stroke Scale: www.stroke.nih.gov/resources/scale.htm

RESOURCES FOR THE PATIENTS

Healthy People 2020: www.healthypeople.gov
Know Stroke. Know the signs. Act in time: www.stroke.nih.gov
Recognizing Symptoms of Stroke: www.stroke.nih.gov/privacy.htm
Returning to work after a stroke: www.stroke.org/we-can-help/survivors/living-stroke/lifestyle/returning-work-after-stroke
Tips from Former Smokers: Smoking, Heart Disease and Stroke: www.cdc.gov/tobacco/campaign/tips/diseases/heart-disease-stroke.html

REFERENCES

American Heart Association. (2017a). About stroke, treatment. Retrieved from http://www.strokeassociation.org/STROKEORG/AboutStroke/Treatment/Stroke-Treatment_UCM_492017_SubHomePage.jsp

American Heart Association. (2017b). Warning signs. Retrieved from http://www.strokeassociation.org/STROKEORG/WarningSigns/Stroke-Warning-Signs-and-Symptoms_UCM_308528_SubHomePage.jsp#

Backes, D., Vergouwen, M. D. I., Velthuis, B. K., van der Schaaf, I. C., Bor, A. S. E., Algra, A., & Rinkel, G. J. E. (2014). Difference in aneurysm characteristics between ruptured and unruptured aneurysms in patients with multiple intracranial aneurysms. *Stroke, 45*(5), 1299–1303. doi:10.1161/strokeaha.113.004421

Becske, T. (2017). Subarachnoid hemorrhage clinical presentation. *Medscape*. Retrieved from https://emedicine.medscape.com/article/1164341-clinical

Bickley, L. (2014). *Bates' guide to physical examination and history taking* (11th ed., 681–740). Philadelphia, PA: Lippincott, Williams & Wilkins.

Centers for Disease Control and Prevention. (2017). Tips from former smokers: Smoking, heart disease and stroke. Retrieved from https://www.cdc.gov/tobacco/campaign/tips/diseases/heart-disease-stroke.html

Jefferis, B. J., Whincup, P. H., Papacosta, O., & Wannamethee, S. G. (2014). Protective effect of time spent walking on risk of stroke in older men. *Stroke, 45*(1), 194–199. doi:10.1161/STROKEAHA.113.002246

Kerber, K., & Newman-Toker, D. (2015). Misdiagnosing dizzy patients, common pitfalls in clinical practice. *Neurology Clinics, 33*, 565–575. doi:10.1016/j.ncl.2015.04.009

Kernan, W. N., Ovbiagele, B., Black, H. R., Bravata, D. M., Chimowitz, M. I., … Wilson, J. A.; On behalf of the American Heart Association Stroke Council, Council on Cardiovascular and Stroke Nursing, Council on Clinical Cardiology, and Council on Peripheral Vascular Disease. (2014). Guidelines for the prevention of stroke in patients with stroke and transient ischemic attack: A guideline for healthcare professionals from the American Heart Association/American Stroke Association. *Stroke, 45*(7), 216–236. doi:10.1161/STR.0000000000000024

Mayo Clinic. (2017). Stroke, treatment outcomes. Retrieved from https://www.mayoclinic.org/diseases-conditions/stroke/diagnosis-treatment/treatment-outcomes/txc-20135630

Moore, N., Wright, M., Gipson, J., Jordan, G., Harsh, M., Reed, D., … Murphy, A. (2016). A survey of African American Men in Chicago barbershops: Implications for the effectiveness of the barbershop model in the health promotion of African American Men. *Journal of Community Health, 41*(4), 772–779. doi:10.1007/s10900-016-0152-3

Mozaffarian, D., Benjamin, E. J., Go, A. S., Arnett, D. K., Blaha, M. J., Cushman, M., … Howard, V. J. (2016). Heart disease and stroke statistics—2016 update: A report from the American Heart Association. *Circulation, 133*(4), e38–e360. doi:10.1161/CIR.0000000000000485

Nanda, A. (2017). Transient ischemic attack workup. *Medscape.* Retrieved from https://emedicine.medscape.com/article/1910519-workup

National Institute of Health, & National Institute of Neurological Disorders and Stroke. (2017). Know Stroke. Know the signs. Act in time. Retrieved from https://stroke.nih.gov

National Stroke Association. (2017). Returning to work after stroke. Retrieved from http://www.stroke.org/we-can-help/survivors/living-stroke/lifestyle/returning-work-after-stroke

Nordahl, H., Osler, M., Frederiksen, B. L., Andersen, I., Prescott, E., Overvad, K., Diderichsen, F., & Naja Hulvej Rod, N. H. (2014). Combined effects of socioeconomic position, smoking, and hypertension on risk of ischemic and hemorrhagic stroke. *Stroke, 45*, 2582–2587. doi:10.1161/STROKEAHA.114.005252

Prabhakaran, S., Ruff, I., & Bernstein, R. A. (2015). Acute stroke intervention. A systematic review. *JAMA, 313*(14), 145–162. doi:10.1001/jama/2015.3058

Suter, P. S., & Harvey, L. H. (2016). *Vision rehabilitation: Multidisciplinary care of the patient following brain injury*. Boca Raton, FL: CRC Press.

The Internet Stroke Center. (2017). Stroke statistics. Retrieved from http://www.strokecenter.org/patients/about-stroke/stroke-statistics

Torén, K., Schiöler, L., Giang, W. K., Novak, M., Söderberg, M., & Rosengren, A. (2014). A longitudinal general population-based study of job strain and risk for coronary heart disease and stroke in Swedish men. *BMJ Open, 4*(3), e004355. doi:10.1136/bmjopen-2013-004355

Trompetto, C., Marinelli, L., Mori, L., Pelosin, E., Currà, A., Molfetta, L., & Abbruzzese, G. (2014). Pathophysiology of spasticity: Implications for neurorehabilitation. *BioMed Research International, 2014*, 354906. doi:10.1155/2014/354906

Wetmore, J. B., Phadnis, M. A., Mahnken, J. D., Ellerbeck, E. F., Rigler, S. K., Zhou, X., & Shireman, T. I. (2014). Race, ethnicity, and state-by-state geographic variation in hemorrhagic stroke in dialysis patients. *Clinical Journal of the American Society of Nephrology, 9*(4), 756–763. doi:10.2215/cjn.06980713

Wilson, M. E. (2013). Stroke: Understanding the differences between males and females. *Pflügers Archive—European Journal of Physiology, 465*(5), 595–600. doi:10.1007/s00424-013-1260-x

World Health Organization. (2018). Fact Sheet about health benefits of smoking cessation. Tobacco free initiati*ve.* Retrieved from http://www.who.int/tobacco/quitting/benefits/en

Yeap, B. B., Alfonso, H., Chubb, S. A. P., Hankey, G. J., Handelsman, D. J., Golledge, J., … Norman, P. E. (2014). In older men, higher plasma testosterone or dihydrotestosterone is an independent predictor for reduced incidence of stroke but not myocardial infarction. *The Journal of Clinical Endocrinology & Metabolism, 99*(12), 4565–4573. doi:10.1210/jc.2014-2664

Yeap, B. B., McCaul, K. A., Flicker, L., Hankey, G. J., Almeida, O. P., Golledge, J., & Norman, P. E. (2015). Diabetes, myocardial infarction and stroke are distinct and duration-dependent predictors of subsequent cardiovascular events and all-cause mortality in older men. *The Journal of Clinical Endocrinology & Metabolism, 100*(3), 1038–1047. doi:10.1210/jc.2014-3339

Yousef, O., Grunfeld, E., & Hunter, M. (2015). A systematic review of the factors associated with delays in medical and psychological help-seeking among men. *Health Psychology Review, 9*(2), 264–276. doi:10.1080/17437199.2013.840954

CHAPTER 35

Men and Heart Health

Kathleen Fasing

INTRODUCTION

This chapter will provide highlights of the recent data and overall current care of the gentleman with heart disease. Within this chapter, the intent is to promote excitement for the changes within this cardiology realm which help the patient direct his own care and his own daily activities and gain insight into methods that may improve his quality of life. Cardiology has transformed from a division of care focused upon diagnosing the sick and performing procedures to fix or temporize the condition to a different philosophy. This emergent philosophy is to mingle the needed procedures and diagnosis with an ongoing diligence of self-care. This self-care includes daily improvements in diet, exercise, mindfulness, and psychological wellness that promote and maintain healthy cardiac function. The chapter is meant as a review and guide to both the clinician and the patient for whom it may benefit.

MEN AND HEART HEALTH: BACKGROUND

This is a very exciting time within cardiology and many changes have occurred over the years, from the early 1980s to 2018 and beyond. There has been progression within the cardiology department from a focus on diagnosing an acute myocardial infarction (MI) and performing immediate angioplasty to providing angiolytics to open blocked arteries to the current wellness focus. This wellness framework promotes such activities as yoga, a plant-based diet, mindfulness, and stress reduction activities (Kahn, 2016). Just as these changes have been very progressive and have instituted a proactive and patient ownership framework for heart health, this chapter will highlight a few of the new findings, studies, recommendations, and progressive care models first and then review conventional workups and treatment recommendations. This style of tipping the information on its head is much like the "flipping the classroom" technique, which is used within educational departments across this nation (Brame, 2013). The intent of giving the reader initial assignments, articles, and data and letting the reader digest that information, prior to moving deeper within the subject, has been wildly successful within the teaching business (Brame, 2013).

The adoption of this framework is utilized to gain enthusiasm and interest in a few of the philosophical changes within cardiology and mingle these changes with progressing data of the conventional thinking. Conventional knowledge determines the diagnosis and treatment criteria utilized daily within cardiology. The separation of men's and women's heart health is sometimes a difficult process and often notes distinct differences and not so distinct differences. The aim in this chapter is to relate both findings to highlight the differences in presentation and treatment and how this difference can affect men's health and how we have learned to treat men's cardiac health (Box 35.1).

BOX 35.1 MEN'S HEALTH SUBJECT AREAS

- The young man and development of coronary artery disease (CAD) from teenage years
- Statistics on men's acute myocardial infarctions (AMIs), CAD, heart attacks, and overall cardiac events
- Country of origin and ethnic differences
- The aging man and increased risks of MI
- Encompassing full body interaction within cardiac illness and wellness
- Metabolic syndrome
- Controlling one's diet, physical activity, sleep, mindfulness, fear and anger management
- Risk factors for CAD or coronary heart disease (CHD)
- Diagnosing MI, ischemia, injury, and infarct
- Diagnostic and laboratory testing
- Clot formation, endothial changes, and lipid management
- MI versus cardiac arrest
- Interventions for CAD
- Long-term management of CAD; where wellness tactics meet pharmacological care and men's reaction to cardiac medications
- Psychological impact of cardiac diagnosis and decreased functional status
- The young man and steroid use
- Atrial fibrillation
- Valvular heart disease and previous treatment versus current updates
- Angioplasty, stents, medications, coronary artery bypass grafts (CABG) and semi-invasive procedures
- Congestive heart failure (CHF) and new medications
- Genetic factors and implications; inflammation and immune responses

HALLMARK STUDIES: CHANGING THE MINDSET AND LIFESTYLE MODIFICATIONS

In previous years modifiable risk factors and nonmodifiable risk factors for coronary artery disease (CAD) have been identified, with nonmodifiable risk factors including genetics and family history of CAD, age, and gender (American Heart Association [AHA], 2017). Modifiable risk factors for CAD include hypertension (HTN), insulin resistance and diabetes, diet, and physical activity (AHA, 2015).

Studies on Prevention of CAD

Within the last 5 to 7 years there have been dramatic changes in our understanding of these risk factors for CAD and recommendations for prevention of CAD. Kolata (2016) sites four recent studies that utilize diet modification and increased physical activity to decrease one's genetic risk of CAD. The first study involves Dr. Khera and colleagues at Massachusetts General Hospital (MGH) in which they utilized large data sets to determine the effects of genes and lifestyle in the development of heart disease. They cited the statistic of about 365,000 individuals who die annually within the United States of heart disease and 17.3 million who die of heart disease worldwide. In their study, they note that certain genes can double the risk of heart disease, while a good lifestyle may cut this risk in half. They also site that the opposite may be true for those with terrible lifestyle habits; those with poor lifestyles may erase nearly half of the benefits of having good genetics (Khera et al., 2016).

This observation was gained by evaluating four large prospective cohort studies involving 55,685 participants. Genetics and lifestyle factors were independently associated with a susceptibility to CAD. The study points to those adopting a favorable lifestyle associated with a nearly 50% lower relative risk for CAD (Khera et al., 2016). Dr. Michael Lauer, a cardiologist with the National Institutes of Health (NIH), who was not involved with the study, evaluated the data and noted the consensus was impressive and the subjects utilized four large studies, yet the results were convincing and consistent. The analysis from the studies involved lifestyle changes: not smoking, exercising moderately, and eating a healthy diet heavy in fruits, vegetables and grains, fish and dairy products, less processed meats, less sugar-sweetened beverages, and less trans fats and sodium (Carroll, 2016; Kolata, 2016). The four studies started in 1987 and ended in 2008, involving 50 different genetic variations of single-nucleotide polymorphisms (SNP), which researchers utilized to create a risk score. Lifestyle factors were associated with outcomes and included nonobesity (body mass index [BMI] of less than 30), performing physical activity at least once weekly, and having a healthful diet pattern.

Very similar recommendations are derived and urged in the 2013 American Heart Association (AHA) and American College of Cardiology (ACC) Guideline on Lifestyle Management to Reduce Cardiovascular Risk (Eckel et al., 2013). These guidelines give specific recommendations for lifestyle changes and grade the science and knowledge leading into the recommendations as either strong or moderate and in other cases, less than convincing evidence. The data was derived starting in 2008 and involved rigorous systematic evidence reviews for each topic. The aim of the guidelines involved the decrease risk of CAD, the leading cause of morbidity and death worldwide (Eckel et al., 2013). This AHA/ACC review noted that with physical activity, substantial epidemiological evidence links higher levels of aerobic physical activity to lower rates of cardiovascular disease (CVD) and other chronic disease such as diabetes mellitus (DM) type 2. They also noted a dose-dependent inverse relationship between levels of physical activity and rates of CVD (Eckel et al., 2013). Recommendations included a diet of whole grains, low-fat dairy, poultry, fish, and legumes, vegetables, fruits, and nuts; decreasing caloric intake; and lowering sodium intake, which are named as strong recommendations and correlates in lowering blood pressure. They cited large bodies of data associated with higher levels of physical activity, lower rates of chronic diseases such as CVD, and enhanced longevity. The beneficial effects of exercise are related to a decreased lipid profile and decreased blood pressure (Eckel et al., 2013). They recommend aerobic exercise for a 40-minute duration three to four times per week to gain the benefit of decreased blood pressure and decreased low-density lipoproteins (LDLs) and triglycerides. The gestalt of their recommendations in gaining these healthier lifestyles is an effort to decrease the contributing disease products that lead to a higher risk of CVD. The control of HTN, control of BMI and resultant DM type 2, weight loss and improved diet profile, and increased activity and exercise level are all rated as strong and moderate levels of evidence for decreasing one's risk of CVD.

In a related fashion, the evidence and recommendations for decreased caloric intake and reduction in BMI have also proved true within the world of electrophysiology and the management of atrial fibrillation. Atrial fibrillation is associated with hospital readmissions, increased rates of congestive heart failure (CHF), decreased tolerance of daily activities, and several morbidity indicators. In 2005, about 3 million Americans had atrial fibrillation and it is projected that in 2050, 8 million Americans will have atrial fibrillation. About 70% of the people with atrial fibrillation are between ages of 65 and 85 and there is a higher incidence of atrial fibrillation in women. In the United States 2.3% of people over 40 years of age have atrial fibrillation. The associated disease states with atrial fibrillation are CAD, HTN, rheumatic heart disease and pericarditis, hyperthyroidism, obesity, DM or metabolic syndrome, lung and kidney disease, sleep apnea, and family history of atrial fibrillation (Pietrangelo,

2014). Those with atrial fibrillation on the average are five times more likely to have a stroke. Symptoms associated with atrial fibrillation are lethargy and fatigue, palpitations, activity intolerance, sleep disturbances, and emotional and psychological sequelae (Pietrangelo, 2014). Atrial fibrillation is treated with rate control, rhythm control, and ablative treatment options, but it often returns and is difficult to manage (Shukla et al., 2015).

The Long-Term Effect of Goal-Directed Weight Management in an Atrial Fibrillation Cohort: The LEGACY Trial

A hallmark 2014 study was presented at the ACC meeting in March 2015, which astonished observants and had an immense impact. Rather than the typical presentation of a new heart angioplasty technique, stent, or invasive device, this presentation concerned the LEGACY trial, which involved the long-term effect of goal-directed weight loss in the reduction of atrial fibrillation symptoms (Pathak et al., 2015). The conclusion of this trial involved the study of numerous independent variables of atrial fibrillation. The initial aim of the study was to determine which lifestyle changes and what variables had the most statistically significant risk reduction for atrial fibrillation (Pathak et al., 2015). The most significant independent variable in relation to recurrence of atrial fibrillation was weight reduction and the extent of weight reduction. The most important information involved lifestyle modification and a concentrated effort to change diet and activity, which resulted in a 10% reduction in BMI. A single variable, the 10% reduction in BMI, was noted as effective as a second ablation in minimizing the recurrence of atrial fibrillation and noted as statistically significant. The next group of a 3% to 7% reduction in BMI was also noted as statistically significant in reducing the recurrence rate of atrial fibrillation, and less than a 3% reduction in BMI had no effect upon the recurrence rate of atrial fibrillation (Pathak et al., 2015). The LEGACY study was then further discussed and analyzed and additional authors question another significant group, focusing on those patients with decreased atrial fibrillation symptoms resulting from a hypothesized increase in aerobic exercise (measured by metabolic equivalents [METS] noted with treadmill exercise). It was postulated that those with less recurrence of atrial fibrillation are those who had >2 METs fitness gained via aerobic exercise in comparison with no benefit gained and no decreased atrial fibrillation symptoms within the category of those with <2 METs improvement in fitness, measured with treadmill testing. Their interpretation of the LEGACY trial is that not only did significant weight reduction as measured with a decrease in BMI of 10% or greater have a profound effect upon atrial fibrillation occurrence, but that increased exercise also had a significant impact. They indicate that further study is needed, but they advise increased exercise, as a significant lifestyle change, in decreasing atrial fibrillation and atrial fibrillation symptoms (Atreya & Guigliano, 2015).

SHIFT IN MANAGEMENT OF CAD TO PREVENTION OF CAD

The overall emerging consensus among experts who manage CAD and atrial fibrillation involves a shift in the treatment paradigm to a more preventive risk reduction paradigm. Within clinics and care centers the importance of dietary changes, exercise protocols, referrals to nutritionists who are experts in cardiac health and cardiac rehabilitation, and prescriptions for a healthy lifestyle are becoming the mainstream in recommendations for both patient populations (AHA, 2017). The adherence to such healthy lifestyle changes including reduction in BMI, avoidance of high sugar content foods, the utilization of aerobic exercises for at least 30 to 40 minutes four times weekly, nonsmoking, and the utilization of a diet high in fruits, vegetables, and grains is recommended for improvement in cardiac health and overall risk reduction for of chronic diseases such as HTN, CAD, DM, and metabolic syndrome (AHA, 2015). There is an obvious move to a more progressive disease avoidance framework and one that involves diet and exercise maximization leading to CAD, HTN, stroke, and atrial fibrillation disease prevention (Kahn, 2016).

CORONARY HEART DISEASE INCIDENCE

As of 2017, the AHA announced the fact that CHD, HTN, and stroke remain top causes of death in the United States. CHD accounts for 1 in every 7 deaths in the United States each year, killing more than 360,000 individuals yearly. There are about 790,000 heart attacks per year in the United States, with 114,000 of them resulting in death. Of these 790,000 heart attacks each year, 580,000 are new heart attacks and 210,000 are recurrent heart attacks (AHA, 2017). The average age for a heart attack is 65.3 years in men and 71.8 years in women (AHA, 2017).

The AHA compiles data on CHD (also known as CAD) in combination with HTN and stroke data and present it as an overall risk for death. The combination of the three disease states accounts for 801,000 deaths per year and 1 out of every 3 deaths within our country (AHA, 2017). Additionally, 2,200 Americans die of CVD each day, averaging 1 cardiac death every 40 seconds (AHA, 2017). In the U.S. population, the incidence of men having deadly MIs per year in 2013 was 321,000, and MI was noted as the leading cause of death for men. This equated with 1 in every 4 men dying of a lethal MI in 2013 (Centers for Disease Control and Prevention [CDC], 2013).

The sudden cardiac death is often the only symptom of CAD, and in the United States, in 2013, between 70% and 89% of those reported with sudden cardiac death were men (CDC, 2013). Heart disease was noted as the leading cause of death for men in racial and ethnic groups in the United States, and these groups comprise African Americans, American Indians or Alaskan Natives, Hispanics, and Caucasian Americans. For American men who are of Asian descent and Pacific Islanders, heart disease as a cause of death is rated as number 2 behind cancer as the leading cause of death (CDC, 2013).

HISTORY: PRESENTING SYMPTOMS

Classic presenting symptoms for the man who is having a heart attack include jaw pain, crushing substernal chest pain, left arm pain or bilateral arm pain, pain across the back, nausea, and fatigue. Less commonly reported, but nevertheless suspicious, complaints include fatigue that may be rather sudden in onset, unexplained sudden depression, or erratic behavior combined with tooth pain or jaw pain. A good rule of thumb may be if the story sounds a bit suspicious and is not explained by some other diagnosis, consider an MI. It is better to err on the side of being too cautious in making this diagnosis, rather than missing an MI. The patient should be directed to the nearest emergency room, and if his condition is compromised, he should be transported via ambulance.

The matching of physical signs with the history and an accurate interview of the patient's symptoms is key in the diagnosis. As above, some symptoms are classic for ischemia or heart attack, while others are deceiving. The patient with DM will often have no symptoms or a silent MI and presents with a family member noting they are exhausted, not acting right, or simply speculating if the patient is coming down with something. Other patients present with extra heart sounds as an S_3 or an S_4, which can correlate with leaky valves, as caused by a flail mitral valve and chordae tendineae rupture associated with an acute MI (Davies, 2001). The S_3 will coordinate with the leaky valve, while S_4 is more often associated with left ventricular dysfunction and left ventricular failure (Sato et al., 2017). With wide open mitral regurgitation there will be a very prominent S_3, grade III or greater. With the presence of S_4 and overall pump failure, there is often very prominent jugular venous distention (Sato et al., 2017). Twenty percent of the presenting MIs are associated with ventricular arrhythmias and most often ventricular tachycardia (Davies, 2001). There are frequently associated atrioventricular node delays and pauses seen with those having ischemia or infarctions of the right coronary artery and at times the circumflex artery (Davies, 2001). With the presenting arrhythmias, it is key to verify if there is suspected cardiomyopathies as source of the arrhythmia versus an ischemic origin of the arrhythmia (Davies, 2001). Additional symptoms often associated with MIs include dyspnea, wheezing, dizziness and/or syncope, cough, nausea and vomiting, and diaphoresis (Zafari & Yang, 2017).

RISK FACTORS

Areas of interest in the evaluation of each male patient presenting for care include risk factors for CAD, presenting symptoms and signs of angina, family history, age group and challenges and risks associated with age ranges, and the workup and evaluation of CAD. Risk factors associated with CAD include HTN, elevated LDL cholesterol, and smoking (CDC, 2013). Associated medical conditions that relate directly to these components of CAD include DM, overweight and obesity status, poor diets, physical inactivity, and excessive alcohol use, drug use, and use of steroids (CDC, 2013; Kolata, 2016).

As an overview and examination of cardiac topics and men, it seems only logical to touch upon HTN, lipid management, sugar and glucose control, congenital defects, arrhythmia disturbances, valvular heart disease, social stressors, and risk factors. Other pressing issues for men and cardiology include medication effects, such as beta blockers, calcium channel blocker, or angiotensin-converting enzyme (ACE), and their potential overall effects on one's life. Many men are concerned that if these effects could limit energy or virility, "why would I (the patient) take such a medication?"

Providers often simply recommend a treatment without fully understanding the patient's obvious question. Men may be cautious about asking questions that relate to the rationale for such medications and the need to follow a provider's orders and recommendations. Often the man will agree to the prescription from the provider, but avoid taking the medication for reasons that can include cost and perceived sexual function effects. This avoidance may be due to denial, or lack of education regarding medications or the disease state.

Early-Onset CAD and Ethnic Distribution of CAD in Men

It makes sense to first cover the subject of angina, ischemia, and CAD and the risks they may impose upon the patient. The development of CAD is felt to have started early in life and can be noted as early as 17 and 18 years of age, when warning signs of premature heart disease can appear (Arts, Fernandez, & Lofgren, 2014). CAD has been noted in deceased 18-year-old men, at the time of their autopsy (AHA, 2017). An estimated 23.4 million American adults have DM, and 8.0% of them are white men, 14.1% are African American men, 12.6% are Hispanic men, and 11.8% are Asian men (AHA, 2017).

Determining the presence of ischemia avoids missing the diagnosis and losing critical time to provide treatment for CAD. If the diagnosis is missed and the patient continues to have chest pain (angina) or chest pain–related symptoms; these problems may progress to occlusions of coronary vessels with a significant blockage of over 90%, with or without clot disruption and an acute MI (Zafari & Yang, 2017).

Risk Factors for Heart Disease and Metabolic Syndrome

Previously discussed risk factors for heart disease and stroke include family history of heart disease, DM, HTN, age, and gender (Grundy, 2016). Additionally, there has been an

BOX 35.2 DIAGNOSIS OF METABOLIC SYNDROME = THREE OF FIVE FEATURES

Abdominal obesity with a waist circumference of 102 cm (40 inches) or more in men and 88 cm (35 inches) or more in women
Serum triglycerides of 150 mg/dL or above
High-density lipoprotein cholesterol of 40 mg/dL or more in men and 50 mg/dL or more in women
Blood pressure of 130/85 mmHg or higher
Fasting glucose of 100 mg/dL or above

identified grouping of risk factors, which when coexisting, formulate a cluster of features that greatly increase the risk of CAD. This group of risk factors (Box 35.2) is designated metabolic syndrome, which represents a predisposition to developing CAD (Grundy, 2016).

With three of these five features, one may be diagnosed with metabolic syndrome. Approximately 32% of the U.S. population has metabolic syndrome and about 85% of those with DM type 2 have metabolic syndrome (Grundy, 2016). The outlook or prediction in this metabolic syndrome is noted because of the rise in obesity rates among young adults, and it is predicted that metabolic syndrome (also known as syndrome X) will overtake smoking as the leading risk factor for heart disease (Grundy, 2016).

ASSESSMENT OF THE MAN WITH POSSIBLE CAD

Each presenting male patient—young, middle aged, or elderly—must first be asked about any presenting symptoms, risk factors, likelihood of discovering actual disease, and consequences for missing a diagnosis of CAD. Despite age, two of the most important questions to be asked are regarding the family history for CAD, angina, or MI and the age at which relatives were diagnosed with CAD or actually suffered an MI. If the answer is a first-degree relative such as mother, father, sister, or brother who had a procedure for CAD, heart attack, or death related to heart attack, prior to age 50 to 60 years, the provider must move forward with suggest a stress test to assess for CAD (Laurance, 2012). If the answer is 30 to 35 years of age when an MI or death occurred, the stress test should be scheduled urgently, ideally within a day to a week at the most.

Of equal magnitude is the discussion regarding a history of DM and questioning the patient if he is being treated for DM or prediabetes, and the last blood glucose or hemoglobin A_{1c} (glycosylated hemoglobin) test. Regardless of any symptoms or complaints, or even no symptoms or complaints, the criterion for a stress test is immediately met with a history of DM. Patients with DM are considered to have CAD until they are proved to have no CAD; quite often there are absolutely no symptoms present but there is silent ischemia, which would otherwise be undetected (Al-Nozha, Ismail, & Al Nozha, 2016). Stated in other terms, if DM is present, this primary risk category requires moving directly to an ischemic workup with an exercise stress test (Al-Nozha et al., 2016). For years, it has been accepted that DM is treated as a CAD equivalent in risk stratification and requires ordering of diagnostic testing to evaluate for CAD (Wannamethee, Shaper, & Lennon, 2004).

Once past these two key questions, other questions can include family history of other cardiac abnormalities, cholesterol level, typical exercise patterns, weight gain over time, and questions regarding areas of retained weight such as increased midsection or abdominal girth. Increased abdominal girth measurements over time are a direct risk factor for CAD (Grundy, 2016). Much of what is seen and managed within cardiology (as is true of many other areas of medicine) is the less urgent or acute findings, complaints, and details, which entail the remainder of the care of the man with heart disease. The term heart disease clearly entails the blockage within the coronary artery, or CAD. The other entities of diagnosis include congenital disorders, cardiomyopathies, arrhythmias, and valvular heart disease. These diagnoses can involve mild disease states with only minor limitations in functional capacity versus advanced disease states and very limiting or debilitating symptoms.

There is subtlety within the diagnosis and decisions on how to medically treat partial blockages or partially occluded coronary arteries. These partial findings and variable level of the disease progression is where medical treatment and lifestyle modifications are applicable. This is the window of time in which the provider can maximize medical therapy and the patient may optimize his own healthcare activities. There has been a larger transformation of providing patient explanations of the disease process and discussing diet, exercise, increased activity, smoking cessation, mindfulness, and stress reduction techniques. The current gestalt is the overall interplay which all these issues have in determining the health of the man's heart.

Physical Examination

The physical examination may be very benign in nature, assessing subtle clues for possible coronary disease, versus advanced or worrisome findings. The examination should be approached utilizing the same head to toe focus of systems and review of any abnormal findings. The examination of the head and neurologic system may give clues of delayed answering, poor reasoning or memory, and subtle changes in cognition (especially if there are previous established exams for comparison) which can be early or subtle signs of ischemia. A specific ear marking, known as the earlobe crease or Frank's sign, is noted as being associated with CAD (Agouridis, Elisaf, Nair, & Mikhailidis, 2015). This sign must be correlated with age and other risk factors for CAD, and studies have shown variable association with CAD, with some believing it is associated with CAD and others not. Additional signs of vascular disease are carotid bruits and the indication of vascular disease in the carotid vessels. Additional findings include superficial veins on the chest wall, suggesting revascularization and collateral circulation within other vessels and vasculature (Davies, 2001). Other examination findings include the presence of S_3 heart sounds, indicating volume or regurgitation toward the atrium, and S_4 heart sound, which is indicative of a stiff and noncompliant left ventricle (Sato et al., 2018). Additional assessment of bruits at the femoral or radial artery may be telling of other vascular issues, and the overall visual inspection of skin, capillary refill, and signs of chronic venous stasis are also keys to the overall physical examination. Systolic and diastolic murmurs are helpful in identifying valvular issues. The identification of a loud versus soft systolic murmur is associated with aortic stenosis or mitral regurgitation, and diastolic murmurs are associated with mitral stenosis and aortic insufficiency (Shipton & Haney, 2001).

■ DIAGNOSTIC TESTS

The initial evaluation within an acute setting is the standard by which acute myocardial injury and infarct is determined and evaluated, and patients are triaged to the best available modality to allow opening of a blocked artery and flow to the myocardium, avoiding any long-term damage to the myocardium. These evaluation and treatment issues within the acute setting must be dealt with quickly, effectively, and with the proper tests ordered that will bring the most direct and effective treatment. This review of the acute process is one which at times must be answered and dealt with directly by the advanced practice provider, either the nurse practitioner (NP), physician assistant (PA), or the physician. This timely and astute evaluation of an urgent or emergent set of patient symptoms and data must be diagnosed, managed, and treated immediately.

ECG Evaluation

Regardless of the acuity of the presenting rhythm and the acuity of ECG changes, one must always evaluate the presenting rhythm, changes in rhythm, and changes in QRS complex, QT interval, and ST segment to determine an initial diagnosis. The standard in ECG interpretation was developed by Dubin and exists today. The initial review of the ECG involves five questions (Box 35.3). The importance of ECG comparison to an earlier or the last ECG cannot be overstated. In the acute setting, changes in ECG morphology become quite obvious. However, much more subtle changes, which indicate changes in the patient's health status, may be determined by the comparison of a previous ECG or the last ECG to the current ECG tracing (Palsenon, 2016).

The ECG is likely to show rhythm abnormalities, changes in the ECG pattern with ST-segment changes, which may indicate ischemia (lack of oxygen), injury (prolonged lack of oxygen), or infarct (death of tissue/myocardium; Paulsenon, 2016). The ECG is often coupled in the acute setting with cardiac enzymes, such as troponins, which are obtained to determine if an active infarct is present (Butala & Yeh, 2015).

One of the greatest challenges in ECG interpretations is diagnosing an MI in the setting of a left bundle branch block. Both QRS complex morphologies can be wide, include ST-segment depression and at times ST-segment elevation. In this setting, ECG alone will not make the diagnosis (Palsenon, 2016). It will be coupled with the patient's complaints, history, presenting symptoms, physical examination findings, and laboratory markers.

BOX 35.3 BASICS OF ECG INTERPRETATION

What is the heart rhythm and what is the heart rate?

Is there a P wave for each QRS complex? No distinct P waves indicate atrial fibrillation or atrial flutter or junctional rhythm.

Is the QRS complex narrow, wide, irregular? Irregular, fast, and erratic may be ventricular tachycardia or ventricular fibrillation.

What is the ST segment activity? Is there ST depression (indicating ischemia), ST elevation (injury pattern), or ST elevation which is pronounced in two to three of the correlating leads (infarct pattern).

Is there a definitive connection between the atrial signal and the ventricular signal, or is there an AV (atrioventricular) delay? With an AV delay, is it a first-degree AV delay, second-degree AV delay, or complete heart block?

Additional questions: Is there a bundle branch block or widened QRS complex? Is this a new or old finding?

Laboratory Evaluation

In addition to the ECG, laboratory tests will be obtained and include the standard complete blood count (CBC) with differential and platelets, a comprehensive metabolic panel, cardiac troponins, CK-MB (creatine kinase-muscle/brain; older and less used cardiac marker), and any other testing that is applicable to the patient's current history. The troponin lab test must be drawn as a set with the first marker drawn immediately and a follow-up marker drawn in 6 hours. The patient will often want to check out of the emergency department (ED) prior to the second blood draw. It is always a wise discussion to let the patient know that the evaluation within the ED involves the two lab markers and an exercise stress test. This test, when there are equivocal findings with laboratory tests and patient data, will determine the presence of ischemia and injury and determine the likelihood of a cardiac event (Mattu et al., 2015). The troponins must be obtained as a set—initial troponins 2 hours apart and a final troponin 6 hours later—and must show a combined consensus of whether an MI is occurring. These tests are performed within an acute setting and once it is determined that the patient is having an MI, the providers must then decide how to open the occluded vessel and make the choice to use thrombolytics (as in the late 1980s) or perform acute coronary intervention (ACI) utilizing angioplasty and stenting versus coronary artery bypass grafting (CABG; Van de Werf, 2014).

Stress Test Modalities

The ED-ordered and directed stress test has become the norm for evaluation of angina throughout the United States. The stress test is done to determine the risk profile for a "hard" cardiac event, such as an MI. If the man is having a MI, the stress test is not performed in this acute setting. In the face of an MI, the patient will then undergo either transfer to the cardiac catheterization laboratory for a heart catheterization, angioplasty, and cardiac stent placement, as deemed appropriate (Kapur, 2015).

Once these questions are answered the provider must determine which type of stress test, echocardiogram, and further investigation or workup will be required. The workup for a stress test includes a general question: can the patient achieve a desired elevated heart rate and can the patient run or walk on a treadmill to gain this exercise state? Exercise stress tests include walking on the treadmill and combining an echocardiogram with this treadmill stress test.

Alternatively, the target heart rate may be achieved with a medication such as dobutamine, which is used to raise the patient's heart rate to an exercise state equivalent and then an echocardiogram can be obtained. This from of stress test includes a medication to increase the rate and bring about an exercise state, in the setting in which any comorbid conditions limit the man's ability to exercise or run on the treadmill. Contraindications to such a test can include a history of paroxysmal or persistent atrial fibrillation (relative contraindication depending on test modality), history of ventricular arrhythmia which may be prompted by the dobutamine, or known allergy to the medications.

A nuclear medicine stress test with technetium may be ordered as an alternative. This stress test is definitive in assessing for existing CAD. An MRI and PET scan may also be ordered and show previous MI scar tissue and "hibernating myocardium" (Bhola & Lin, 2015). The term *hibernating myocardium* refers to myocardial tissue that may have been involved in an ischemic event or partial thickness damage to the myocardium. This may include a subendocardial MI with some retained functional myocardium, and may also include areas that were previously thought to entail a full thickness MI, but in fact contain some degree of intact or resting or hibernating myocardium (Bhola & Lin, 2015). The significance of the test is in determining if there is some remaining and hibernating myocardium, which in the setting of an angioplasty or stent placement could begin to behave in a viable action. With improvement in function and perfusion it can then become involved in a recovery process and improved overall pump and ejection fraction function (Bhola & Lin, 2015).

Unfortunately, health insurance carriers have recently begun to require preapprovals for stress tests and have set up barriers to ordering such tests. Often a stress echocardiogram is rejected by the insurance company, which requests a separate baseline echocardiogram and a treadmill stress test. These can be ordered and may be mildly or moderately positive. But the provider should note that when performed separately, neither test fully assesses CAD and does not provide risk stratification for further treatment. Once these separate tests are completed, the patient comes back to the facility for the combined stress echocardiogram. Similar issues exist with the nuclear medicine stress test, and often the provider must provide information of the patient's early family history, DM, or combined risk factor details, which will encourage approval of the correct stress test.

STRESS TEST INTERPRETATION

What does this mean and what do the tests indicate? Echocardiograms show valvular disorders and Doppler flow displaying normal or abnormal flow patterns; wall motion abnormalities; measurements of chambers, valves, and muscular tissues; and septal measurements. The echocardiogram is an excellent noninvasive test that uses sound waves to gain motion implications via ultrasound technology. It is often used with the initial workup and uncovers global versus segmental akinesis, or dyskinesis of particular areas of the heart (such as the anterior, medial, or inferior walls or segments of the heart). If there appears to be damage to these segments and an existing cardiomyopathy (decreased muscle contraction function), then one may move on to further assess this with a stress test, if causes are thought to be ischemic, or another test if the cardiomyopathy is thought to be related to other causes (Armstrong & Ryan, 2009). The echocardiogram often will give the initial insight of the overall pump function and other structural abnormalities (Armstrong & Ryan, 2009).

Diagnostic Procedures

Once the presence of an acute MI is recognized, the decision of the next best step is needed. The window of moving to intervention in the cardiac catheterization laboratory is generally a 4-hour window in which intervention is deemed appropriate. The previous treatment paradigm during the 1980s and 1990s was often having the patient undergo an acute angioplasty. Stents were not readily available, and the standard of care was not immediate stent placement, as it is currently. At that time, there were often failed angioplasties and frequently dissected coronary arteries. The patient was often treated within the cardiac catheterization lab, only to be sent emergently down the hall to the operating room suite for an emergent CABG surgery. The previous dosing on heparin, lytic therapies, and antiplatelet therapies were stacked upon each other, and included a significant risk of bleeding with the surgery being performed on an acute basis.

Over time the period from presentation within the ED to accomplishment of balloon inflation was increasingly shortened. The national goal became door to balloon time in less than 1 hour. The EDs across the nation had moved to a less than 1 hour time frame, from calling the on-call cardiac catheterization team to time of the start of the angioplasty procedure. This became known as "door to balloon" time (Kapur, 2015). Currently, there are drug-eluting stents, which are designed to remain patent, avoid accumulation of platelets, avoid interstitial accumulation of sludge and plague, and prevent plaque rupture and further clot formation. These stents have become rather specialized and are designed with specific drug coatings to the intraluminal surface and specific designs and shapes. There are also stents specifically designed for bifurcations.

Additional technology includes Doppler flow wires, which are designed to evaluate intracoronary flow. These devices, known as fractionated flow wires, can assess the degree of blockage down a coronary artery. This assessment of the degree of blockage helps the cardiologist judge the need for angioplasty or stenting versus treating a partial dissection with medical management. Typically, a blockage within a coronary artery is not treated with angioplasty or stenting unless the vessel is 70% to 100% occluded. At less than a 70% occlusion the cardiologist will not intervene because the lower grade lesions are not flow limiting, as are the higher degree blockages. The coronary artery needs to be at least 70% occluded prior to performing angioplasty versus stenting procedures. The less occluded vessels will be treated with maximizing beta-blocking agents, taking a long-acting nitrate such as isosorbide mononitrate or isosorbide dinitrate, and considering the use of a calcium channel blocker. Antiplatelet aggregation medications such as clopidigrel is considered and often utilized.

Additional treatment modalities can be based upon the cardiac catheterization and can include utilizing the left internal mammary artery for grafting the left anterior descending coronary artery. Modalities may also include CABG, which may be performed as a lateral access minimally invasive CABG procedure (Weigang et al., 2004). This procedure requires an MRI to image the epicardial fat pad.

Many of the invasive procedures performed in the workup are very technically advanced and highly mechanized evaluations and involve the latest in technology, patient care, balloon catheterization, and stent interventions. These "diagnose and fix" modalities are currently utilized within all cardiology departments in this country and are at the core of what we do in cardiology.

With these technological breakthroughs and advanced treatments, one must not forget to utilize traditional diagnostic techniques: to listen to what the patient is saying and to utilize the history and physical examination to the fullest. By maximizing the approach to history taking and the physical examination, one gains numerous clues to the source of the diagnosis and possible treatment options. This workup involves then prescribing a treatment plan, which often swings back to the focus of increased self-care and insight discussed at the start of the chapter.

MANAGEMENT PRINCIPLES

When focusing on the man with heart disease and risk of heart disease, one must focus upon the continued care and progression of disease. With a historical approach the cardiologist and care team may have allowed the patient to recover from the heart attack and simply rest or "take it easy." The new framework is that of maximizing rehabilitation and even in advanced heart disease, investigating treatments that help keep the patient active and promote the best case scenario for the patient to continue to be active as possible in performing activities of daily living.

Introduction to Heart Failure and Ventricular Remodeling

This framework concerns utilizing medical management in concert with patient exercise improvement techniques and progressively improving and increasing exercise modalities (Van Craenenbroeck, 2017). The advent of care involving medications to treat heart failure with drugs such as ACE inhibitors, beta blockers, spironolactone, and furosemide (Lasix) have improved afterload reduction and have aided in ventricular remodeling. The process of taking a very accurate history often leads to the diagnosis of a cardiomyopathy or the

BOX 35.4 EVALUATION AND TESTING OPTIONS FOR MEN WITH KNOWN OR SUSPECTED CARDIAC DISEASE

Holter Monitors: Utilized to determine rhythm irregularities; will detect percentages or overall burdens of premature ventricular contractions (PVCs) and other trends. Most frequently used to evaluate arrhythmias. Are often ordered as a 24- or 48-hour study and may utilize 3 leads or 12 leads; 12-lead monitors are ordered specifically to determine morphology and sites of PVCs and to determine if PVCs are unifocal or multifocal and where they originate.

Event Monitor: Gives the percentage of atrial fibrillation or burden of atrial fibrillation. Will also give information on atrial flutter, premature atrial contractions (PACs), and PVCs and their occurrence rates.

12-Lead ECG: Determines heart rate and heart rhythm, shows normal P wave or atrial contraction, QRS ventricular contraction, and T wave and ST segments, which correspond to ventricular relaxation. Will display ischemia (ST-segment inversion), injury (ST-segment elevation), and infarct (ST-segment elevation in the acute setting and Q wave in the chronic setting). Will also show atrioventricular (AV) blocks and bundle branch blocks. Gives an electrical picture of all that is happening in the heart, based upon 12 separate leads.

CT of heart: Shows anatomical relationship of structures and valves and can give an image of the heart structures, which can then be manipulated with additional software to create a road map for electrophysiological studies.

Heart MRI: Utilized in PVC ablations and can show scar of delayed enhancement or scar tissue, which helps locate sites of PVCs. Utilized in the workup of cardiomyopathies, and delayed enhancement may indicate sites of possible amyloid infiltration (Gheorghiade et al., 2016).

Echocardiogram: Used in assessment of the heart with baseline studies, studies in the setting of ischemia, studies with the workup of valvular disorders, and the workup of cardiomyopathies.

Transesophageal Echocardiogram (TEE): TEEs are used to pass an esophageal probe down the throat, while the patient is sedated, to visualize the back of the heart and the left atrium. The left atrium is not visualized in the standard transthoracic echocardiogram. The TEE will determine if there is clot present within the left atrium.

CT Angiography/Calcium Score: CT angiography (CTA) and calcium scoring is a relatively new noninvasive procedure that predicts the likelihood of a coronary blockage and major cardiac event and notes the level of calcium within the coronary arteries. In one large study of 5,007 patients, 8.2% of the patients, 363 persons, in follow-up were noted to have a major cardiac event (MACE), including death, myocardial infarction, or cardiac intervention such as angioplasty, following CTA and calcium scoring, which was deemed statistically significant. These tests allow a noninvasive insight into the patient's coronary anatomy, calcium deposits within the coronary arteries, and likelihood of having a blocked coronary artery. The calcium score is the overall collection or deposit of calcium that exists throughout the coronary tree or bed of vessels rather than any individual site within a specific coronary artery (Boyar, 2016). The advantage is early identification of risk factors and early treatment such as stringent lipid management prior to a cardiac event (Hou et al., 2012).

(continued)

BOX 35.4 EVALUATION AND TESTING OPTIONS FOR MEN WITH KNOWN OR SUSPECTED CARDIAC DISEASE (*continued*)

Catheterization: The cardiac catheterization is an invasive test performed in a radiography suite utilizing computerized imaging equipment which takes angiograms gained via arterial access, typically from the groin area and femoral artery with a catheter that is directed to the coronary ostia or opening of the coronary artery with contrast agent injected into the artery to produce the image. These direct images of the coronary arteries will show blockages and irregularities in the arteries. These suites and departments also intervene during myocardial infarctions and at nonurgent times to deliver stents to these arteries and opening blockages within the arteries (Mayo Clinic Newsletter, 2017).

These testing modalities allow the provider to give a full assessment of the heart's function, limitations, and areas that will require intervention. These are simply examples of the most common tools that may be used in the assessment and workup of patients with suspected coronary or electrical malfunction of the heart.

diagnosis of heart failure. The workup includes a thorough history-taking process and delineation of when and how decreasing energy levels took place, surrounding events and symptoms, worsening symptoms and activities that may improve symptoms, and the prior workup, which may have been accomplished at the primary care office or local hospital. With this very precise history, one can then utilize the correct echocardiogram, CT, MRI, Holter monitor, event monitor, or other diagnostic tools to help diagnose the condition that is leading to the symptoms of fatigue, dyspnea (shortness of breath), postural nocturnal dyspnea (PND), orthopnea (shortness of breath while lying down), peripheral edema, palpitations, agitation, depression, and anxiety (Box 35.4).

These symptoms are hallmarks of a constellation of features known as heart failure, or traditionally as congestive heart failure. The renaming of the condition to heart failure is prompted as not all forms of heart failure include a degree of congestion. The term is delineated from the overall decreased pump function of the heart and decreased left ejection fraction (EF), which leads to less blood being pumped out per heartbeat (stroke volume as the milliliters of blood per second and EF as the amount of blood in liters per minute ejected from the heart). This blood is ejected from the heart during systole, but depends upon the degree of filling of the heart in diastole and the smooth muscle contraction, condition, and performance of this muscle to expand and fill in the diastole and snap back and eject blood in systole.

The Importance of the Ejection Fraction

The EF is the fraction derived by the equation *End-diastolic volume (EDV) −End-systolic volume (ESV)/End-diastolic volume.* The classic good or maximum EF is = 70% in the very healthy heart and may be represented by (Gheorghiade et al., 2016):

$$\text{EDV of 100 mL} - \text{ESV of 30 mL/EDV of 100 mL} = 70/100\text{ mL} = 70\%$$

This concept of the stretch of the myocardium exhibited with passive filling or diastole, followed by the rebound and force of contraction with systole is known as the Frank-Starling curve, which is named after the two cardiologists who first studied this phenomenon (Fukuta & Little, 2008). This pump ability of the left ventricle gives a very good idea of the condition of the muscle of the ventricle and its ability to both relax (diastole) and passively fill and maximize the amount of blood in which it holds and then actively contract (systole) and eject this blood to the aorta, head, rest of the body, and ultimately to vital organs and tissues. This ejection of blood is dependent upon the passively filling cycle and the process works in concert together and is dependent upon the time of filling (two thirds of the cardiac cycle) and the time of ejection (one third of the cardiac cycle) (Fukuta & Little, 2008). This timing of the filling and contracting phases of the mechanical reaction follows the electrical reaction of the ECG's P wave for atrial filling, QRS complex for ejection of blood, and QT interval for ventricular relaxation or passive filling.

The electrical activity precedes the mechanical action of the heart by 0.4 millisecond (ms) to 0.8 ms. This process of systole and diastole is prompted by the electrical action of the heart, and then the ensuing mechanical action of the heart is repeated with each heartbeat. This ability of the heart to pump can be influenced by the condition of its muscle tissue or myocardium, damage to the myocardium, electrical abnormalities of the heart, physiological tachycardia (normally elevated heart rates in response to illness or stress), infection, disease states involving the myocardium, and other illness (Fukuta & Little, 2008). The comprehension of the normal cycle of the heart and the normal systolic and diastolic function is key in understanding the abnormal conditions of the myocardium, which are grouped into the category of cardiomyopathies or conditions which alter the muscle health of the heart and result in a lowered EF of the heart (Fukuta & Little, 2008).

Cardiomyopathy

Cardiomyopathy can be defined as a decreased EF of 40% or less and is classified within the categories of ischemic cardiomyopathy (ICM) and nonischemic cardiomyopathies (NICMs). The NICMs have been used as equivalents to dilated cardiomyopathies (Bozkurt et al., 2016). Cardiomyopathies can be further subdivided into those resulting from pressure overloads or hypertrophy, such as the hypertrophic obstructive cardiomyopathy, versus those resulting from fluid or volume overload, such as the alcoholic cardiomyopathy (Bozkurt et al., 2016). The AHA published a scientific statement regarding dilated cardiomyopathies in 2016 (Bozkurt et al., 2016) and delineated the most severe cardiomyopathies from the treatable cardiomyopathies, which may improve via medications such as beta blockers and antiarrhythmics, increased physical activity on an ongoing basis, and the use of permanent pacemakers (PPMs), intracardiac defibrillators (ICDs also described as AICDs, automatic implantable cardioverter defibrillators), and cardiac resynchronization therapy (CRT) with ICDs. Resynchronization therapy aims at timing the pacing and contraction of the right ventricle and the left ventricle in a more physiological and synergistic fashion (Mayo Clinic, 2018).

Dilated cardiomyopathies: Overall grouping involving the following (previously described as heart muscle disease) dilated cardiomyopathies (DCMs): hypertrophic, restrictive, arrhythmogenic right ventricular (ARVC), or nonclassified cardiomyopathies in the 1980s.

Inflammatory and viral cardiomyopathies: The World Health Organization and International Society and Federation of Cardiology classification system added inflammatory and viral cardiomyopathies in 1996 (Bozkurt et al., 2016).

Genetic, nongenetic, and acquired cardiomyopathies: The AHA then further subdivided cardiomyopathies into two groups based upon predominant organ involvement. They were divided into primary cardiomyopathies (genetic, nongenetic, and acquired) and secondary cardiomyopathies with generalized systemic (multiorgan) disorders including amyloidosis, hemochromatosis, autoimmune and collagen disorders, vascular diseases, toxins, cancer therapy, and endocrine disorders such as DM (Bozkurt et al., 2016).

European Society of Cardiology classification of cardiomyopathies: The European Society of Cardiology (ESC) took a different approach and classified cardiomyopathies into specific morphological and functional phenotypes, which include hypertrophic cardiomyopathies, DCM, ARVC, restrictive cardiomyopathies, and unclassified cardiomyopathies (Bozkurt et al., 2016).

The term dilated cardiomyopathy is defined as a heterogeneous myocardial disorder that is characterized by ventricular dilation and depressed myocardial performance in the absence of HTN and valvular, congenital, or ischemic heart disease. The degree of the myocardial depression and treatment of the patient's functional status are highly variable. The approach to these patients includes medications, devices, and exercise modalities that minimize damage to the myocardial tissue, increase EF and functional status, and bring about myocardial remodeling.

Myocardial remodeling is defined as alteration in the structure, mass, shape, and dimensions of the heart. This remodeling is in response to hemodynamic load and/or cardiac injury in association with neurohormonal activation. Remodeling may be described as pathological or physiological and is referred to as adaptive and maladaptive or remodeling and reverse remodeling (Cohn, 2017). The extent of damage caused by this remodeling process in the setting of a cardiac infarct is determined by the overall size of the MI (Abouzaki & Abbate, 2016).

Like many other features of cardiology in men and women, there is a distinct difference in how this remodeling process takes place. With MIs, there is an initial increase in the end-diastolic volume of the left ventricle within the early stages of the infarct, which is a reaction to the larger preload at the time of the infarct and an effort to compensate for decreased heart muscle contractility (Abouzaki & Abbate, 2016). With the increase in volume, there is an increase in wall stress on the ventricle and a resultant increase in overall left ventricle (LV) chamber volumes. The stretch of the LV results in adverse ventricular remodeling. In men, LV dilation prevails over the hypertrophy or pressure overload LV remodeling that often occurs with women and cardiac infarcts. The process with men includes LV dilatation, resulting in an eccentric phenotype and leading to further wall motion stress, neurohormonal activation, a progressive dilation, and systolic dysfunction with worse long-term heart failure outcomes than the hypertrophic pattern of remodeling that is common with women and MIs (Abouzaki & Abbate, 2016).

Recommendations for initial treatment and prompt diagnosis of the heart attack and expedited intervention with angioplasty and stent placements, prior to further stress upon the myocardium and promoting immediate reperfusion, is the recommended treatment within the population of men who are actively having the MI (Abouzaki & Abbate, 2016). In the setting of the acute MI many factors can highlight a man's response to symptoms. The recommendations are prompt identification of the MI, determination of extent of MI with ECG interpretation, and immediate care within the cardiac catheterization laboratory for reperfusion of the blocked coronary artery (Covino, Stern, & Stern, 2011). There is often a problem with the man responding to signals of chest pain, jaw pain, perfuse sweating or diaphoresis, or fatigue or acute changes in energy levels (Covino et al., 2011). The existence of increased stress in the man's job or home life, anxiety, denial, need to appear as a strong man who can handle pain (stoic behavior), and depression and fear are all key issues that often keep men from seeking medical attention and waiting for several days to investigate causes of chest pain (Mayor, 2015). This hesitancy of denial of the problem at hand is often a male trait, in light of symptoms of an MI. This is not a universal male response to an MI, but it is often witnessed and may be based upon years of societal expectations that men should adapt and cope with pain (Mayor, 2015).

STRESS COMPONENTS OF MYOCARDIAL INFARCTION, ATRIAL FIBRILLATION, AND MALE COPING

Additional variables such as stress, depression, and anger are partial determinates in men's heart health. The emotional impact upon heart disease may become the classic chicken or egg question; it may be difficult to determine if the heart attack or the stress, depression, and anger management issue was the initial symptom. Steptoe (2016) notes that individuals with heart disease and previous heart attacks are depressed in 15% of the large-scale studies within the United States and additional studies in other countries. This average of 15% of those suffering post-MI depression is a repeated finding in these studies. Another 25% of those who have experienced a heart attack suffer milder levels of depressive symptoms and anxiety symptoms. Steptoe (Steptoe, 2016) moves on to note the ways in which men and women utilized social support in coping with these variables. He describes women as utilizing friends' and family's opinion, support, and backing. On the other hand, the man who has a heart attack, and especially the older male within the family, is expected to cope on his own and to keep a strong exterior and rely only on himself during this time of stress. He describes the delicate balance of expected social norms and the increased sense of one's frailty and one's own possible death (Steptoe, 2016). Additional areas of study are posttraumatic stress disorder after heart attack, depression after heart attack, and well-being after heart attack.

The AHA (2017), on its website, approaches stress and heart disease from the angle of those who smoke and drink to cope with daily stress, who then develop HTN or worsen preexisting HTN, with the use of these coping strategies (AHA, 2017). They cite drinking and smoking in excess and its effects upon damaging the walls of arteries throughout the body. Schiffrin (Schiffrin, 2014) recommends stress reduction tactics of exercising, maintaining a positive attitude, eating a healthy diet, reducing caffeine, and maintaining a healthy weight. His research notes that medications are helpful for other features of heart disease, but not in lowering stress.

In addition to the stress response associated with heart attacks, there has been identification of anger and anger-related diagnosis. The anger response and emotion of anger have been associated with atrial fibrillation. There is a direct correlation between increased anger and a higher risk of atrial fibrillation (Patterson, 2015). This correlation exists for men with anger and atrial fibrillation, but does not correlate with women who have anger issues (Patterson, 2015). Anger in men has been tied to higher C reactive protein and homocysteine levels and higher cortisol levels (Patterson, 2015). Recommendations include stress reduction techniques, practicing anger management, and reducing factors in one's life that are known to stimulate the anger response (Patterson, 2015).

Atrial fibrillation alters one's sense of wellness in life and may cause feelings of uneasiness, stress, anxiety, fear, worry, confusion, frustration, depression, and anger. Ryan (2017) has several suggestions for coping with the stress associated with atrial fibrillation, and recommends keeping an anxiety log, which allows the man to review previous stressors and anxiety and to acknowledge the stress. He also suggests planning a 20-minute period for stress each day and then clearing one's brain of the stressful thoughts thereafter. He recommends such techniques as yoga, relaxation, meditation, and walking. He also recommends natural remedies such as lavender oil, chamomile, and aromatherapy (Ryan, 2017). There are many peer-reviewed studies and journals on atrial fibrillation, but in the most recent years several of the well-known cardiology centers across the country are integrating wellness tactics and "whatever works" in helping male patients reach a better state of coping and wellness with atrial fibrillation. Ryan has worked on coping tactics and strategies to assist in quality of life changes that can benefit the patient since 2002. This focus on wellness and changes in daily tactics is an area of further study that will be needed in the future.

FURTHER DISCUSSION OF STRESS TEST CHOICES

In determining the type of stress test utilized, providers must chose the most suitable test based on the patient history and which type of stress test is most appropriate. The first question one should ask is if the patient is capable or walking fast or running on a treadmill, and if the patient (given his comorbid conditions) can tolerate an increased heart rate, sweating, and exercising for 8 to 12 minutes on the incline of the treadmill. Additionally, the issue of preexisting medical conditions that would limit a particular type of stress test must be addressed.

An example of a poor choice of stress test would include a dobutamine stress test to determine CAD in the setting of atrial fibrillation with rapid ventricular response. In this test, the dobutamine is utilized in its ability to increase the heart rate and bring about a hyperemic (increased blood flow and heart rate) exercise state for the individual who may have difficulty walking upon a treadmill. In this setting, the increased heart rate will trigger atrial fibrillation, rather than simply bringing about an exercise state. The preferred alternative would be a nuclear medicine stress test. In this type of test, the patient with atrial fibrillation would have a scanned nuclear study. With a nuclear stress test, the nuclear agent is delivered and provides the imaging medium, which lights up areas of decreased coronary perfusion, but will not bring about or trigger the atrial fibrillation.

This example highlights the importance of knowing the stress test and matching the test with the patient's known symptoms and history. Other questions to be answered are simple questions regarding the patient's medications and results of a stress test. A patient who is on large doses of beta blockers will be unable to reach a peak cardiac exercise state via studies aimed chiefly at reaching an exercise state via heart rate increasing measures. This patient will hold the beta blocker in the morning of the test, but will still be unable to reach a maximum exercise status due to the large dosing of beta blockers over time. In this setting a pharmacological study which mimics a hyperemic or exercise state is recommended. Additionally, it is important to remember exercise stress tests should never be simply ordered as a screening tool and ordered due to some symptom, event, or prompting occurrence, which gives the provider the direct clue that there is a likelihood for CAD or chronotropic incompetence (Askew, Chareonthaitawee, & Arruda-Olson, 2017).

Types of stress tests and medications utilized in these stress tests include the following:

1. *Treadmill ECG stress test*: Test in which the patient exercises upon the treadmill with increasing speed and inclines and based upon the Bruce Protocol Stress Test in which the energy derived is quantified in metabolic equivalents (METS). No medication is given to accelerate the heart rate or exercise response.
2. *Treadmill/echocardiogram stress test*: Test in which one is exercised as above, but baseline echocardiogram images are assessed prior to exercising upon the treadmill and post-treadmill maximum exercise level is met. The echocardiogram will show any valvular disorders potentiated with exercise, wall motion abnormalities, and heart rate responses that may have effects upon the myocardium.
3. *Stress tests that utilize agents to speed the heart rate or mimic an exercise state:*
    A. *Adenosine*—A naturally occurring substance found throughout the body in various tissues, which functions to regulate blood flow in many vascular beds, such as in the myocardium. There are specific pathways which produce adenosine including the *S*-adenosyl homocysteine and the adenosine triphosphate pathway (which plays a role during ischemia); 80% of those receiving adenosine reach a maximal exercise state.
    B. *Regadenoson (Lexiscan)*—Produces a hyperemic or exercise state very quickly and maintains it for an optimal duration. Coronary vasodilation and an increase in coronary blood flow result from the activation of the A2A adenosine receptor by regadenoson.

C. *Dobutamine*—A cardiac inotrope and chronotrope. Stimulates beta-1 and beta-2 receptors. Increases regional myocardial blood flow.
D. *Dipyridamole (Persatine)*—An indirect coronary vasodilator that works by increasing intravascular adenosine levels; 66% of those receiving dipyridamole reach a maximum exercise state (Akinpelu & Yang, 2016).

Typically, several of the agents which patients with preexisting angina or cardiac disease are taking are stopped prior to stress testing. Such medications should be stopped 24 hours prior to the test or on the morning of the test and include beta blockers (such as metoprolol tartrate, metoprolol succinate, and propranolol) and isosorbide mononitrates and dinitrates. A few patients will be taking dipyridamole, which should be stopped 48 hours prior to the stress test (Schwartz, 2017).

Two New Medications for the Management of Heart Failure

As noted previously, heart failure is the condition in which the heart has a decreased ejection described as an EF of 35% to 40% in which there becomes growing concern of the likelihood of arrhythmias, which may be associated with such a poor pump function. These are discussed previously and may entail the placement of an ICD. The patient with decreased pump function is unable to pump enough blood through the heart to provide sufficient blood to the rest of the body and meet the metabolic demands of the organs and tissues (Tse, 2015).

It was discovered that ventricular remodeling could be altered by a process of reverse ventricular remodeling utilizing the drugs in the class of angiotensin-converting enzymes, ACEs, angiotensin receptor blockers (ARBs), diuretics, digoxin, and beta blockers (Tse, 2015). This discovery of utilizing both medications was a hallmark breakthrough in the management of those with heart failure. In the same light and significance, there have been two recent breakthrough discoveries and medications in the management of heart failure (HF) as of recent times, which include ivabradine (Corlanor) and the combination sacubitril/valsartan (Entresto) (AHA, 2017). These two drugs entail great breakthroughs in the management of HF. Ivabradine controls heart rate without any negative inotropic effect (forward pump function of the heart). It is the first selective I_f channel inhibitor (Tse, 2015). Entresto is a combination medication which includes an ARB (valsartan) and a neprilysin inhibitor, which is showing great improvement in treating those with New York Heart Association class II to IV symptoms and systolic heart dysfunction (Fala, 2015). These medications must be monitored closely and are not applicable in every situation. There are many interactions with additional medications and a dedicated HF team is necessary for ongoing treatment with these medications. These discoveries are encouraging in treating a disease that is a major clinical concern and affects 5 million people within the United States, is the leading cause for hospitalization for those over 65 years of age, and for which an excess of 500,000 new cases are diagnosed each year (Tse, 2015).

Historically we referred to HF in terms of diastolic and systolic dysfunction and we discussed previous MIs, viral infiltration of the heart, and many other disorders (Rodriguez & Ruel, 2016). HF has adopted new terms known as HFpEF, pronounced *hefpef,* which refers to heart failure with a preserved EF. Another term, HFrEF, pronounced *hefref,* refers to a stiff ventricle that is noncompliant (Rodriguez & Ruel, 2016). When one does not work within these clinics, the terms may become confusing. HFpEF is noted as increasing in frequency, owing to our aging population and rising incidence rates of diabetes and obesity. Also noted is the fact that we have made headway in reducing mortality rate with HFrEF, but we haven't done much with HFpEF (Rodriguez & Ruel, 2016). As clinicians, our focus must be on reducing mortality risk, but at times as important and often more important is reducing morbidity and assisting the patient in reducing overall symptoms.

WHEN TO REFER

The question often becomes evident when one service within patient care wants an opinion of another service; when do we ask for a consultation and when do we refer to cardiology? The answer to this question is straightforward and easy, if there is a thought that further expertise is needed, just refer or call. Cardiology services across the country will easily inform the primary service if the matter should be handled by cardiology. Thus, if the primary service questions if a referral is needed, then refer. If the cardiology issue is very simplistic, the cardiology service will walk the primary through a direct care approach. There are specific times to refer, such as in the setting of ischemia, injury or an MI, second or third degree AV block requiring pacing, or an EF of 35% or less for consideration of an ICD.

New Surgical Procedures for the Treatment of Coronary Artery Disease and Valve Disorders

This exciting time within cardiology is not limited to new medications for HF. There are several changes within interventional cardiology and surgical cardiology, with a growing synergy among those in interventional, surgical, and electrophysiology cardiology departments. One of the most exciting changes involves procedures that utilize minimally invasive surgery, which is done in conjunction with interventional cardiology and placements of stents within adjoining vessels (Rodriguez & Ruel, 2016). Hybrid operating room suites allow these complementary groups to achieve the least invasive, best directed, and most effective combination of skills in order to treat specific areas of the heart by utilizing all available skills. This combination treatment approach can also utilize an electrophysiology ablation in a setting of minimally invasive surgery (Rodriguez & Ruel, 2016).

Other advances in the cardiac catheterization laboratory include the use of transcatheterization aortic valve replacement surgery for those who have severe aortic stenosis and are not a candidate for an open surgical valve replacement (Nissen, 2015). Generally, this technique is used more frequently with the female population with aortic stenosis, due to the small caliber of their aortic valves and overall smaller vessel size (Nissen, 2015). This procedure is also used to a lesser degree in the male population, especially with those patients who have no other treatment option for their aortic stenosis, which is often causing a great decline in functional status (Nissen, 2015). The final advancement in the surgical cardiology forum is that of minimally invasive CABG procedures involving a lateral approach, a minimally invasive approach, which often does not involve a full bypass procedure. Such surgeries are named minimally invasive coronary surgery (MICS) and minimally invasive direct coronary artery bypass (CAB). MICS involves a small thoracotomy and CAB involves a small thoracotomy and use of endoscopic revascularization techniques (Nissen, 2015). The term HCR refers to hybrid coronary revascularization with a combined CABG grafting with percutaneous coronary interventions, a state-of-the-art group of revascularization techniques that result in less blood loss, decreased hospital stays, decreased pain level, and combined modalities that ultimately can be more patient specific than previous surgeries (Nissen, 2015).

CONCLUSION

There are specific differences between the management of cardiac diagnoses with men and women. There is a general idea among many caregivers that most of the previous research has been done on the male patient and that there are few new ideas or concepts to grasp regarding men and the heart. The emerging body of knowledge views cardiac diagnosis as a multi-system phenomenon and one which has interlinking causation. This chapter has been aimed at showing the interlinking nature of risk factors, coexisting cardiac diagnosis, and learned and instinctual coping strategies. The emerging belief entails connecting the medical treatments and the supportive nursing interventions aimed at self-care with the great impact of sequential exercise and diet improvement. This focus upon self-care and determining ways in which the man can become imbedded in his own treatment has been supported with studies showing CAD can be reversible and atrial fibrillation can be greatly controlled via weight loss.

This exciting time in cardiology involves gaining an accurate diagnosis, developing a medical and nursing treatment plan, and combining these plans with a patient-focused care plan of improved diet, exercise, and overall self-care.

CLINICAL PEARLS

- If the history story sounds a bit suspicious and is not explained by another diagnosis, consider an MI.
- DM is the equivalent to a known MI; those with DM often do not have symptoms but it is accepted to assume an individual with DM has CAD, until proven otherwise.
- Cardiomyopathies may be tachycardia mediated and once the rate is controlled, the cardiomyopathy can often be reversed.
- Myocardial infarctions can have classic presentations and atypical presentations. Atypical presentations can include acute onset depression, fatigue and lethargy and a feeling of uneasiness, and a feeling that something is just not right. If the provider has a mild suspicion, it is smarter to evaluate than ignore this suspicion. Follow one's instinct.
- Like any other practice area, know the criteria for pacing, ICD placement, and cardiac rehabilitation. These criteria are standards checked by insurance companies to determine if they are met, when reviewing patient care charts.
- Become familiarized with cardiomyopathies and know to refer sarcoid and amyloid and other infiltrative processes, as these may be more aggressive than other cardiomyopathies.
- Anticoagulate in the presence of atrial fibrillation and become familiar with risk factors for stroke.
- Men who respond to stress with anger are three times more likely to be diagnosed with heart disease and five times more likely to have a heart attack before turning 55.

RESOURCES FOR THE CLINICIAN

American Heart Association: www.heart.org
Healthy People 2020: www.healthypeople.gov
Men's Health Network: www.menshealthresourcecenter.com

RESOURCES FOR THE PATIENT

Academy of Nutrition and Dietetics, Heart Health Tips for Men: www.eatright.org/resource/health/wellness/heart-and-cardiovascular-health/heart-health-for-men
American Heart Association: www.heart.org

Harvard Men's Health Watch: www.health.harvard.edu/mens-health/the-essentials-to-keep-a-mans-heart-healthy
Healthy People 2020: www.healthypeople.gov
Men's Health Network: www.menshealthresourcecenter.com

REFERENCES

Abouzaki, N., & Abbate, A. (2016). Causes and prevention of ventricular Remodeling after MI. *American College of Cardiology*. Retrieved from http://www.acc.org/latest-in-cardiology/articles/2016/07/21/07/28/causes-and-prevention-of-ventricular-remodeling-after-mi

Agouridis, A. P., Elisaf, M. S., Nair, D. R., & Mikhailidis, D. P. (2015). Ear lobe crease: A marker of coronary artery disease? *Archives of medical science: AMS, 11*(6), 1145–1155. doi:10.5114/aoms.2015.56340

Akinpelu, D., & Yang, K. H. (2016). Pharmacologic stress testing: Background, indications, contraindications. *Medscape*. Retrieved from http://emedicine.medscape.com

Al-Nozha, M. M., Ismail, H. M., & Al Nozha, O. M. (2016). Coronary artery disease and diabetes mellitus. *Journal of Taibah University Medical Sciences, 11*(4), 330–338. doi:10.1016/j.jtumed.2016.03.005

American Heart Association. (2015). Heart Disease and Stroke Statistics-2015 update. *Circulation, 131*(4), e29–e322. doi:10.1161/CIR.0000000000000152

American Heart Association. (2017). Heart disease and stroke statistics 2017, at a glance. *Circulation, 135*(10), e146–e603. doi:10.1161/CIR.0000000000000485

Armstrong, W., & Ryan, T. (2009). *Feigenbaum's echocardiography*. Philadelphia, PA: Lippincott, Williams and Wilkins.

Arts, J., Fernandez, M. L., & Lofgren, I. E. (2014). Coronary heart disease risk factors in college students. *Advances in Nutrition (Bethesda, MD), 5*(2), 177–187. doi:10.3945/an.113.005447

Askew, J., Chareonthaitawee, P., & Arruda-Olson, A. (2017). Selecting the optimal cardiac stress test. Retrieved from https://www.uptodate.com/contents/selecting-the-optimal-cardiac-stress-test

Atreya, A. R., & Guigliano, G. R. (2015), The heavy LEGACY: Should weight Management be part of every atrial fibrillation clinic? *Global Cardiology Science & Practice, 2015*(4), 57. doi:10.5339/gcsp.2015.57

Bhola, R., & Lin, E. C. (2015). Hibernating and stunned myocardium imaging. *Medscape*. Retrieved from http://emedicine.medscape.com/article/352588-overview

Boyar, A. (2016). EBT Coronary calcium scoring guide; Advanced body scan of Newport. Retrieved from http://www.newportbodyscan.com/ebt-coronary-calcium-scoring-guide

Bozkurt, B., Colvin, M., Cook, J., Cooper, L. T., Deswal, A., Fonarow, G. C., … Yancy, C. (2016). Current diagnostic and treatment strategies for specific dilated cardiomyopathies: A scientific statement from the American heart association. *Circulation, 134*, e579–e646. doi:10.1161/CIR.0000000000000455

Brame, C. J. (2013). Flipping the classroom. Vanderbilt center for teaching. Retrieved from http://cft.vanderbilt.edu/guides-sub-pages/flipping-the-classroom

Butala, N., & Yeh, R. (2015). Is door-to-balloon time a misleading metric? American College of Cardiology. Retrieved from http://www.acc.org/latest-in-cardiology/articles/2015/06/03/13/23/is-door-to-balloon-time-a-misleading-metric

Carroll, A. E. (2016). The power of simple life changes to prevent heart disease. *The New York Times*. Retrieved from https://www.nytimes.com/2016/12/12/upshot/the-power-of-simple-life-changes-to-prevent-heart-disease.html

Centers for Disease Control and Prevention. (2013). Men and heart disease fact sheet. Retrieved from https://www.cdc.gov/dhdsp/data_statistics/fact_sheets/fs_men_heart.htm

Cohn, J. N. (2017). Cardiac remodeling: Basic aspects. Up to Date. Retrieved from https://www.uptodate.com/contents/cardiac-remodeling-basics-aspects

Covino, J., Stern, T., & Stern, J. (2011). Denial of cardiac illness: Consequences and management. *The Primary Care Companion to CNS Disorders, 13*(5), PCC.11f01166. doi:10.4088/PCC.11f01166

Davies, S. (2001). Clinical presentation and diagnosis of coronary artery disease: Stable angina. *British Medical Journal, 59*, 17–27. doi:10.1093/bmb/59.1.17

Eckel, R, Jakicic, J., Ard, J., Hubbard, V., de Jesus, J., Lee, I., … Yanovski, S. (2013). AHA/ACC Guideline on lifestyle management to reduce cardiovascular risk: A report of the American college of cardiology and American heart association task force on practice guidelines. *Circulation, 63*(25 pt B), 2960–2984. doi:10.1161/01.cir.0000437740.48606.d1

Fala, L. (2015). Entresto (Sacubitril/Valsartan): First in class angiotensin receptor neprilysin inhibitor FDA approved for patients with heart failure. *Engage Healthcare Communications, 8*(6), 330–334.

Fukuta, H., & Little, W. C. (2008). The cardiac cycle and the physiological basis of left ventricular contraction, ejection, relaxation, and filling. *Heart Failure Clinic, 4*(1), 1–11. doi:10.1016/j.hfc.2007.10.004

Gheorghiade, M., Larson, C., Shah, S., Greene, S., Cleland, J., Colucci, W., … Butler, J. (2016). Developing new treatments for heart failure, focus on heart, *Circulation: Heart failure, 9*(5), e002727. doi:10.1161/Circheartfailure.115.002727

Grundy, S. (2016). Metabolic syndrome update. *Trends in Cardiovascular Medicine, 26*(4), 364-373. doi:10.1016/j.tcm.2015.10.004

Hou, Z., Lu, B., Gao, Y., Jiang, S., Wang, Y., Li, W., & Budoff, M. J. (2012). Prognostic value of coronary CT angiography and calcium score for major adverse cardiac events in outpatients. *JACC: Cardiovascular Imaging, 5*(10), 990–999. doi:10.1016/j.jcmg.2012.06.006

Kahn, J. (2016). 4 foods shown to reverse artery disease. *Huffington Post.* Retrieved from https://Huffingtonpost.com

Kapur, N. K. (2015). From door-to-balloon to door-to-unload time, an emerging View on the management of STEMI complicated by cardiogenic shock. Retrieved from https://citoday.com/2015/04/from-door-to-balloon-to-door-to-unload-time

Khera, A., Connor, A., Phil, D., Drake, I, Natarajan, P., Bick, A., … Kathiresan, S., (2016). Genetic risk adherence to a healthy lifestyle & coronary Disease. *New England Journal of Medicine, 375*, 2349–2358. doi:10.1056/NEJMoa1605086

Kolata, G. (2016). Genetic heart disease risk eased by healthy habits, study finds. *The New York Times.* Retrieved from https://nyti.ms/2ev50ek

Laurance, J. (2012). Male gene increases risk of hereditary heart disease for one in five. Retrieved from https://www.independent.co.uk

Mattu, A., Chanmugum, A., Swardon, S., Woodridge, D., Winters, M., & Marcucci, L., (2015). *Avoiding common errors in the emergency department.* Philadelphia, PA: Lippincott.

Mayo Clinic Staff. (2017). Cardiac stents. Retrieved from https://www.mayoclinic.org/tests-procedures/coronary-angioplasty/about/pac-20384761

Mayo Clinic Staff. (2018). Cardiac resynchronization therapy. Retrieved from https://www.mayoclinic.org/tests-procedures/cardiac-resynchronization-therapy/pyc-20385014

Mayor, E. (2015). Gender roles and traits in stress and health. *Frontiers in Psychology, 6*, 779. doi:10.3389/fpsyg.2015.00779

Newport-site. (2013). Advanced body scan of Newport. Retrieved from https://www.newportbodyscan.com

Nissen, S. (2015). Answers for heart disease. *Healthy Living.* Retrieved from http://everydayhealth.com

Palsenon, S. (2016). *Rapid interpretation of EKGs. Dale Dubin's text* (6th ed.). Tampa, FL: Cover Publishing.

Pathak, R., Middeldorp, M., Meredith, M., Mehta, A., Majajan, R., Wong, C., … Sanders, P. (2015). Long-term effect of goal-directed weight management in an atrial fibrillation cohort: A long-term follow-up study (LEGACY). *Journal of the American College of Cardiology, 65*(20), 2159–2169. doi:10.1016/j.jacc.2015.03.002

Patterson, E. (2015). Dealing with AFib and anger. New life outlook. Retrieved from https://afib.newlifeoutlook.com/afib-and-anger

Pietrangelo, A. (2014). Atrial fibrillation by the numbers: Facts, statistics, and you. Healthline Media. Retrieved from https://www.healthline.com/health/living-with-atrial-fibrillation/facts-statistics-infographic

Rodriguez, M., & Ruel, M. (2016), Minimally invasive multivessel coronary Surgery and hybrid coronary revascularization: Can we routinely achieve less invasive coronary surgery? *Methodist Debakey Cardiovascular Journal, 12*(1), 14–19. doi:10.14797/mdcj-12-1-14

Ryan, S. S. (2017). Coping with the fear and anxiety of atrial fibrillation. Retrieved from https://a-fib.com/seven-ways-to-cope-with-fear-and-anxiety-a-fib

Sato, Y., Kawasaki, T., Honda, S., Harimoto, K., Miki, S., Kamitani, T., … Matoba, S., (2017). Third and fourth heart sounds and myocardial fibrosis in hypertrophic cardiomyopathy. *Circulation Journal, 82*(2), 509–516. doi:10.1253/circj.CJ-17-0650

Schiffrin, E. L. (2014). Stress and heart health, AHA/ASA 2015-2016 annual report. Retrieved from http://www.heart.org/HEARTORG/HealthyLiving/StressManagementHowDoesStressAffectYou/Stress-and-Heart-Health_UCM_437370_Article.jsp#.Ww5C2tSFOM8

Schwartz, R. (2017). Nuclear cardiology tests frequently asked questions. Department of cardiology. Retrieved from https://urmc.rochester.edu/cardiology

Shipton, B., & Haney, W. (2001). Valvular heart disease: Review and update. American Family Physician. Retrieved from http://www.aafp.org/afp/2001/0601/p2201.html

Shukla, A., Aizer, A., Holems, D., Fowler, S., Park, D. S., Bernstein, S., … Chinitz, L. (2015). Effects of obstructive sleep apnea treatment on atrial Fibrillation recurrence. *JACC: Clinical Electrophysiology, 1*(1–2), 41–51. doi:10.1016/j.jacep.2015.02.014

Steptoe, A. (2016). Could stress increase your risk of a heart attack. British Heart Foundation. Retrieved from https://blog.bhf.org.uk/could-stress-increase-your-risk-of-a-heart-attack-4ac39d11d65b

Tse, S. (2015). Ivabradine (Corlanor) for heart failure: The first selective and specific I-f inhibitor. *Daily PT News Updates, 40*(12), 810–814.

Van Craenenbroeck, E. M. (2017). Exercise training as therapy for chronic heart failure. *European Society of Cardiology, 14*, 43.

Van de Werf, F. (2014). The history of coronary reperfusion. *European Heart Journal, 35*, 2510–2515. doi:10.1093/eurheartj/ehu268

Wannamethee, S. G., Shaper, A. G., & Lennon, L. (2004). Cardiovascular disease incidence and mortality in older men with diabetes and in men with coronary heart disease. *Heart, 90*(12), 1398–1403. doi:10.1136/hrt.2003.026104

Weigang, E., Royl, J., Dencker, A., Schoelhorn, J., Van de Loo, A., & Beyersdorf, F. (2004). Results after MIDCAB and OPCAB surgeries: Problems and Consequences of incomplete angiographic follow up in the mid-term course. *Interactive Cardiovascular and Thoracic Surgery, 3*(2), 302–308. doi:10.1016/j.icvts.2004.01.003

Zafari, A. M., & Yang, E. H. (2017). Myocardial infarction: Practice essentials, background, definitions. *Medscape*. Retrieved from http://emedicine.medscape.com/article/155919-overview

Index